Infectious Diseases of the Nervous System

Commissioning editor: Melanie Tait
Editorial assistant: Myriam Brearley
Production controller: Chris Jarvis
Desk editor: Claire Hutchins
Cover designer: Alan Studholme

Infectious Diseases of the Nervous System

Edited by

Larry E. Davis MD FACP
Chief, Neurology Service, New Mexico VA Health Care System
and Professor of Neurology, Neuroscience and Microbiology,
University of New Mexico School of Medicine,
Albuquerque, New Mexico, USA

Peter G. E. Kennedy MD PhD DSc FRCP FRSE FMedSci
Burton Professor of Neurology, Glasgow University
Department of Neurology, Institute of Neurological Sciences,
Glasgow, Scotland, UK

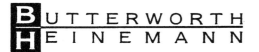

OXFORD   AUCKLAND   BOSTON   JOHANNESBURG   MELBOURNE   NEW DELHI

Butterworth-Heinemann
Linacre House, Jordan Hill, Oxford OX2 8DP
225 Wildwood Avenue, Woburn, MA 01801-2041
A division of Reed Educational and Professional Publishing Ltd
First published 2000

Ⓡ A member of the Reed Elsevier plc group

Every effort has been made to ensure that the drug dosage schedules within
this text are accurate and conform to standards accepted at time of publication.
However, as treatment recommendations vary in the light of continuing research
and clinical experience, the reader is advised to verify drug dosage schedules herein
with information found on product information sheets. This is especially true in
cases of new or infrequently used drugs.

British Library Cataloguing in Publication Data
A catalogue record for this book is available from the British Library

Library of Congress Cataloguing in Publication Data
A catalogue record for this book is available from the Library of Congress

ISBN 0 7506 4213 0   100 1930734

Printed and Bound in Great Britain
Data manipulation by David Gregson Associates, Beccles, Suffolk

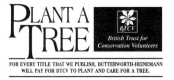

Contents

About the editors

Larry E. Davis graduated in medicine from Stanford University and completed a medical residency at Stanford. He then worked for the Centers for Disease Control and Prevention, USPHS, as an epidemiologist and virologist. After finishing a residency in neurology at Johns Hopkins Hospital, he undertook a fellowship in neurovirology at Johns Hopkins Hospital under Richard T. Johnson, MD. He has conducted clinical and basic research in the pathogenesis of infections of the nervous system for over 30 years, particularly in the fields of Reye's syndrome, inner ear infections, tuberculous meningitis and neuromuscular manifestations of influenza.

Peter G. E. Kennedy received his medical training at University College London, and his postgraduate training in neurology at the National Hospital, Queen Square, London. His scientific training started in neuroimmunology with Martin Raff at University College, and continued with research at the Institute of Virology, Glasgow, the Institute of Neurology, London and Johns Hopkins University School of Medicine. He has held the Burton Chair of Neurology at Glasgow University since 1987. For 20 years he has carried out clinical and basic research into the pathogenesis of viral infections of the CNS, particularly herpes simplex and varicella-zoster viruses, and more recently of human African trypanosomiasis.

Contributors

J. Richard Baringer MD
Professor of Neurology and Pathology, HA and Edna Benning Professor and Chair, Department of Neurology, University of Utah School of Medicine, Salt Lake City, UT, USA

James E. Childs ScD
Chief, Viral and Rickettsial Zoonoses Branch, National Center for Infectious Diseases, Centers for Disease Control and Prevention, Atlanta, GA, USA

Randall J. Cohrs PhD
Associate Professor, Department of Neurology, University of Colorado Health Sciences Center, Denver, CO, USA

Patricia K. Coyle MD
Professor of Neurology, School of Medicine, State University of New York, Stony Brook, NY, USA

Nicholas Day MA BM BCh MRCP
Honorary Consultant Physician in Infectious Diseases and Tropical Medicine, Centre for Tropical Medicine, Nuffield Department of Clinical Medicine, The John Radcliffe Hospital, Oxford, UK

Jorge L. M. de Atouguia MD
Infectious Diseases Specialist, Tropical Medicine Specialist, Institute of Hygiene and Tropical Medicine, University of Lisbon, Portugal

Rajith de Silva MD MRCP(UK)
Consultant Neurologist, Essex Centre for Neurological Sciences, Oldchurch Hospital, Romford, UK

Roberta L. DeBiasi MD
Assistant Professor of Pediatrics and Neurology, University of Colorado Health Sciences Center, Denver, CO, USA and Associate Investigator, Denver Veterans Affairs Medical Center, Denver, CO, USA

Anita Desai MSc PhD (Neurovirology)
Senior Scientific Officer, Department of Neurovirology, National Institute of Mental Health and Neurosciences, Bangalore, India

Donald H. Gilden MD
Professor and Chairman, Departments of Neurology and Microbiology, University of Colorado Health Sciences Center, Denver, CO, USA

M. Gourie-Devi MBBS MD (General Medicine), DM (Neurology)
Director – Vice Chancellor and Professor of Neurology, National Institute of Mental Health and Neuro Sciences, Bangalore, India

Thiravat Hemachudha MD
Professor of Neurology, Department of Medicine, Neurology Division, Chulalongkorn University Hospital, Bangkok, Thailand

J. Simon Kroll MA FRCPCH FRCP
Professor of Paediatrics and Molecular Infectious Diseases, Imperial College School of Medicine, St Mary's Hospital, London, UK

James J. LaGuardia MD
Department of Neurology, University of Colorado Health Sciences Center, Denver, CO, USA

Ehud Lavi MD
Associate Professor, Division of Neuropathology, Department of Pathology and Laboratory Medicine, University of Pennsylvania School of Medicine, Philadelphia, PA, USA

Jennifer M. MacLennan MA BM BCh MRCP
Research Fellow, Oxford Vaccine Group, Department of Paediatrics, The John Radcliffe Hospital, Oxford, UK

Ravi Mahalingam PhD
Associate Professor, Department of Neurology, University of Colorado Health Sciences Center, Denver, CO, USA

Christina M. Marra MD
Associate Professor, Neurology and Medicine (Infectious Diseases), University of Washington, Seattle, WA, USA

Justin C. McArthur MB BS MPH
Professor of Neurology and Epidemiology, Deputy Director, Department of Neurology, Johns Hopkins University, Baltimore, MD, USA

Erawady Mitrabhakdi MD
Assistant Professor of Neurology, Department of Medicine, Neurology Division, Chulalongkorn University Hospital, Bangkok, Thailand

Christopher D. Paddock MD
Medical Officer, Viral and Rickettsial Zoonoses Branch, National Center for Infectious Diseases, Centers for Disease Control and Prevention, Atlanta, GA, USA

V. Ravi MD MAMS
Associate Professor and Head, Department of Neurovirology, National Institute of Mental Health and Neuro Sciences, Bangalore, India

S. K. Shankar MD FAMS
Professor and Head, Department of Neuropathology, National Institute of Mental Health and Neuro Sciences, Bangalore, India

Alex Tselis MD PhD
Assistant Professor, Department of Neurology, Wayne State University, Detroit, MI, USA

Gareth Turner MA BM BCh DPhil
Wellcome Trust Career Development Fellow in Clinical Tropical Medicine, The Nuffield Department of Clinical Laboratory Sciences, The John Radcliffe Hospital, Oxford, UK

Kenneth L. Tyler MD
Vice-Chair and Professor of Neurology, Medicine, Microbiology and Immunology, University of Colorado Health Sciences Center, Denver, CO, USA and Chief, Neurology Service, Denver Veterans Affairs Medical Center, Denver, CO, USA

Tiffany M. White BS
Department of Neurology, University of Colorado Health Sciences Center, Denver, CO, USA

Robert G. Will FRCP FRCP(Ed) MD MB BChir
Professor of Clinical Neurology, Director of CJD Surveillance Unit, Western General Hospital, Edinburgh, UK

Foreword

Neurological infections continue to be major causes of mortality and morbidity worldwide. Nevertheless, when I completed my residency in neurology almost 40 years ago, I was discouraged from pursuing my prior training and interest in virology and infectious diseases, since 'no one in neurology would be interested'. Even in internal medicine the subspecialty of infectious diseases was fading in perceived importance and interest. The discovery of antibiotics, the public health control of tuberculosis and rabies, and the successful prevention of paralytic poliomyelitis by vaccines all portended the demise of infections as important challenges in industrialized countries.

Three factors were not foreseen in these predictions. First, agents would be related to chronic diseases not previously regarded as infectious. This occurred first in neurology between 1966 and 1971 with the transmissions of kuru and Creutzfeldt-Jakob disease and the recovery of viruses from subacute sclerosing panencephalitis and progressive multifocal leucoencephalopathy. Since then studies of the possible role of infectious agents in multiple sclerosis, rheumatoid arthritis, atherosclerosis, schizophrenia, and many other chronic diseases have flourished.

Second, the biological adaptability of infectious agents was underestimated. Mutations, shifts in hosts, and altered modes of transmission have presented new challenges at an astonishing rate. The development of antibiotic resistance has led to a new importance of nosocomial infections, and drug resistant strains of tuberculosis now pose a new worldwide threat. For example, the incidence of tuberculosis in Russia has tripled in recent years. The shift of a simian lentivirus into humans led to the appalling AIDS epidemic, and the resultant immunodeficiency has given new importance to progressive multifocal leucoencephalopathy and new clinical neurological presentations related to toxoplasma, cytomegalovirus, and herpes zoster virus. Last year Nipah virus abruptly appeared in Southeast Asia; the new virus may have spread from fuit-bats, to pigs, to humans. Its origin is still uncertain, but several hundred people developed a unique multifocal encephalitis and some survivors have relapsed with progressive disease – a new virus causing a new disease.

Third, the changing global ecology of infectious agents has accelerated the emergence of new agents and their spread. The swelling world population increases the opportunities for mutations, encounters with zoonotic agents, and the likelihood of sustaining the new agent in human populations. At the same time, the shrinking world secondary to rapid travel provides more contacts and the spread of agents; now, thanks to jet travel, formerly exotic agents of other continents can be in any village in North America or Europe within one incubation period. In recent years I have seen numerous patients with neuro-cystocercosis, several patients with cerebral malaria and a patient with Japanese encephalitis in Baltimore among visitors and travellers. The potential for exotic infectious agents to establish natural cycles in new sites was exemplified last summer with the sudden appearance of African West Nile virus in New York City and the resultant seven human deaths from enceph-alitis. Similar events can be anticipated in the future.

Selected infections that involve the nervous system are updated in this volume. These include a newly recognized neurological disease (Ehrlichiosis), several infections that are spreading geographically (Lyme disease, Japanese encephalitis and neurotuberculosis), several infections that have become more prevalent or modified in presentation because of the AIDS epidemic (herpes-viruses), and a number that can be prevented with new vaccines (bacterial meninigitis and rabies). They represent an interesting potpourri of changing infections in a changing world.

Richard T. Johnson MD
Baltimore and Singapore

Preface

Research in the last decade has allowed major advances in the understanding of nervous system infections. This book is for clinicians who now have the opportunity to use this new information to treat previously devastating diseases. As such, the chapters in this book are written for practising neurologists and internists to help synthesize selected diseases into a clinically useful format. This book does not cover every infectious agent that harms the nervous system. Instead, we chose topics that represent important infections of the nervous system and in which there have been recent improvements in diagnosis, pathogenesis and management. We asked internationally recognized experts to summarize the large body of information in their field into a comprehensive and understandable chapter.

In 1987 Butterworth-Heinemann published a book, *Infections of the Nervous System*, edited by Peter G. E. Kennedy and Richard T. Johnson that was well received by the neurology and infectious disease communities. It has been 13 years since that publication and we felt it was timely to produce a similar book as there have been many advances in the understanding and treatment of nervous system infections. The use of polymerase chain reaction assays to detect the aetiologic agent is now faster and often more sensitive than the time-honoured method of culturing the infectious agent. Magnetic resonance imaging has improved our ability to localize and characterize the infectious lesion within the central nervous system. Moreover, we now have a wider spectrum of antimicrobial agents to treat nervous system infections.

The chapters address prions, viruses, bacteria, and parasites. Selected viruses (herpes simplex, varicella zoster, cytomegalovirus, Japanese B, human immunodeficiency and rabies), bacteria (*Borrelia burgdorferi*, *Treponema pallidum*, *Mycobacterium tuberculosis* and common bacteria causing acute meningitis), and parasites (*Trypanosoma* species, *Plasmodium falciparum* and *Ehrlichia* species) were chosen because of their increasing clinical importance.

In viruses, Baringer discusses the changing spectrum of clinical presentations of herpes simplex encephalitis, the usefulness of polymerase chain reaction assays to rapidly establish the diagnosis and recently recommended changes in the treatment with acyclovir. Gilden, LaGuardia, Mahalingam, White and Cohrs discuss the newly recognized spectrum of herpes zoster encephalomyelitis and new antiviral drugs that are available. Tselis and Lavi analyse an emerging spectrum of brain and spinal cord cytomegalovirus infections that develop in immunocompromised patients and discuss new antiviral treatments. DeBiasi and Tyler discuss the most complete differential diagnosis of recurrent aseptic meningitis available with attention to the diagnosis, treatment and prophylaxis of recurrent herpes simplex virus type 2, the most common cause. Ravi, Desai, Shankar and Gourie-Devi cover comprehensively the diagnosis and management of Japanese B encephalitis, a frequently fatal encephalitis in Asia. Hemachudha and Mitrabhadki describe the changing picture of rabies that continues to cause fatal encephalitis in many parts of the world and the new recommendations for post-exposure prophylaxis. Coyle discusses the clinical picture, neuroimaging and treatment of post-infectious encephalomyelitis, an increasingly recognized encephalitis that follows systemic viral infections and vaccinations.

Two important infectious causes of dementia are covered. De Silva and Will cover the exciting history of prion diseases, the many clinical pictures it can produce and biochemical details of this fascinating infectious protein. McArthur discusses the diagnosis and treatment of AIDS dementia likely due to human immunodeficiency virus and the exciting impact that new antiretroviral treatments have made in preventing and treating the dementia.

In bacteria, Coyle highlights the spectrum of clinical signs and symptoms that occur in CNS Lyme disease from *Borrelia burgdorferi* and the difficulty in the diagnosis and treatment of the chronic CNS infection. Marra discusses the evolving clinical picture of neurosyphilis due to *Treponema pallidum* and recent changes in the recommendation for treatment. Kroll and MacLennan discuss new bacterial vaccines that have or will soon reduce the incidence of acute bacterial meningitis and demonstrate that bacterial vaccines may be the major way bacterial meningitis is prevented. Davis discusses the clinical presentations of tuberculous meningitis that occur in the United States, new methods of diagnosis, and the recent changes in antibiotic treatment regimens.

Parasites continue to cause important CNS infections worldwide. Day and Turner discuss new concepts in the pathogenesis and treatment of cerebral malaria. Atouguia and Kennedy discuss the diagnosis, pathogenesis and new treatments of African trypanosomiasis. Davis *et al.* present information on the clinical features, diagnosis and treatment of CNS ehrlichiosis, a new emerging group of rickettsial infections in the United States.

Clinicians now have opportunities as never before to improve outcomes for many patients with infections of the nervous system. It is our hope that this book will enhance the ability of clinicians to care for these patients.

Larry E. Davis MD FACP
Peter G. E. Kennedy MD PhD DSc FRCP FRSE FMedSci

Acknowledgements

We thank everyone who helped in the preparation of this book. In particular, we are indebted to all the authors for their outstanding contributions. We thank Melanie Tait, Myriam Brearley, Chris Jarvis and Claire Hutchins, staff at Butterworth-Heinemann for their immense help in editing and assembling the book. Finally, we thank our wives, Ruth and Catherine, and our children, Meredith, Colin and Charles, and Luke and Vanessa for their encouragement, support and patience during the many hours required to bring this book to publication.

1

Cerebral malaria

Nicholas Day and Gareth Turner

Introduction

Malaria is caused by the protozoan parasite *Plasmodium*, which is transmitted by the bite of infected anopheline mosquitoes in tropical and semi-tropical countries. Four species infect man, including *P. falciparum*, *P. vivax*, *P. malariae* and *P. ovale*. Of these only *P. falciparum* commonly causes severe disease. Falciparum malaria is the most important parasitic infection of man, with between 300 and 500 million cases per year causing an estimated 800 000 deaths in sub-Saharan Africa alone (World Health Organization, 1992). The vast majority of fatal cases occur in African children, and although high quality epidemiological data are difficult to obtain, many of these succumb to the severe 'cerebral' form of the disease, which has a mortality of 15–20%. Thus falciparum malaria is the commonest and potentially the most serious parasitic infection of the human central nervous system.

Although of great importance and of particular interest to neurologists, coma is only one of a wide spectrum of clinical manifestations of malaria infection. These range from asymptomatic parasitaemia to acute multisystem failure with coma, jaundice, renal failure, severe acidosis and haemodynamic shock. The factors responsible for this variation are not fully understood, though it is clear that intensity of transmission and consequent immunity to infection play important roles.

Because of its geographical distribution severe malaria occurs predominantly outside the experience of Western physicians. When rare cases of cerebral malaria are seen in returning tourists, this lack of familiarity can lead to critical delays in diagnosis and treatment of an illness which can evolve into a life-threatening condition with surprising rapidity. Because visitors to endemic areas have no acquired immunity they are particularly susceptible to the multisystem form of the disease. For this reason this review will discuss aspects of the clinical diagnosis and treatment of severe malaria in general, and will not be confined to the cerebral aspects of the disease. Treatment options have improved over the past two decades with the introduction of new powerful antimalarial drugs, but these advances have been tempered by the continuing march of drug-resistance and the failure of a number of promising ancillary therapies.

In this review we will also discuss recent advances in our understanding of the pathophysiology of malaria. Pathological and molecular techniques have provided many putative mechanisms by which parasite–host interaction might produce neurological dysfunction and damage to other organs, though despite these insights the exact mechanism of coma in cerebral malaria remains unknown and controversial.

The parasite life cycle

Asexual cycle

Pre-erythrocytic hepatic phase

P. falciparum infection develops following injection of sporozoites by an infected anopheline mosquito. The sporozoites initially invade hepatocytes via specific receptor-mediated binding between the host cell surface and the parasite's circumsporozoite protein (Cerami *et al.*, 1992). This is one of several cell receptor-ligand interactions central to the successful completion of the parasite's complex life cycle. Once in the hepatocytes the parasite multiplies, and after a median of around 6 days the 'hepatic schizont' ruptures, releasing tens of thousands of merozoites into the bloodstream.

Erythrocytic phase

The motile merozoites rapidly attach to and invade erythrocytes, probably via sialic acid residues on blood group glycoproteins (Hadley, 1986). Once within the erythrocyte the young ring form (which in the case of *P. falciparum* often looks like a pair of ear-muffs, with darkly staining dumbbell-shaped nuclear chromatin material and a thin ring of cytoplasm) begins eating the contents of the red cell, which is mainly haemoglobin. A by-product of haemoglobin proteolysis is pigment, or haemozoin, which consists of a polymer of haem groups linked by iron-carboxylate bonds (Slater *et al.*, 1991). The appearance of visible dirty brown-black crystals of pigment within the digestive vacuole of the developing parasite marks the transition to the trophozoite stage of the erythrocytic cycle. About midway through this 48-hour cycle the parasitized erythrocytes develop increased adhesiveness, mediated by parasite-derived ligands localized at protein-dense 'knobs' on the erythrocyte cell surface (Figure 1.1). This causes binding to endothelial cells (sequestration within blood vessels), other uninfected red cells (rosetting), and other parasitized erythrocytes (autoagglutination). The parasite undergoes further development and nuclear division, and at schizogony (merogony) the mature sequestered parasite bursts releasing a new generation of daughter merozoites into the bloodstream to reinvade new erythrocytes. Each schizont can release up to 32 merozoites, of which in a non-immune patient 10–20 successfully reinvade. This logarithmic increase in the parasitaemia continues through several 2-day cycles before the parasites are detectable in the blood (usually around 11 days post-infection at a parasitaemia of about 50/μl). Fever usually occurs on about day 13, which represents the median clinical incubation period of the disease.

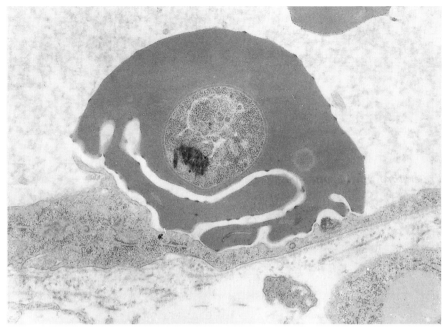

Figure 1.1 Transmission electron micrograph showing a *Plasmodium falciparum*-infected erythrocyte adherent to an endothelial cell. The points of contact between the red cell and endothelial cell are made by electron dense knob proteins which are derived from the parasite and inserted into the red cell membrane.

This may be up to 5 days shorter or considerably longer depending on the size of sporozoite innoculation and the degree of host immunity.

Sexual cycle

Host phase

After several asexual erythrocytic cycles some of the parasites differentiate into sexual gametes (gametocytogony), which can live for weeks in the bloodstream waiting to be taken up by a female anopheline mosquito taking a blood feed.

Mosquito phase

Within the mosquito the male gametes divide, develop flagella, and seek the activated female macrogamete. Fusion and meiosis take place, forming a zygote which then becomes motile (the ookinete) and encysts in the midgut. Here the oocyst (as it is now termed) rapidly enlarges as thousands of sporozoites develop. The oocyst ruptures and the sporozoites make their way to the salivary glands, from where they are injected into the next human host when the mosquito feeds. This whole process is termed sporogony and takes at least 8 days, the exact time depending on the ambient temperature and the species of mosquito.

Epidemiology

Malaria transmission

Transmission of malaria occurs throughout much of the tropics, and depends on a number of factors. Human host and vector must be present in sufficient densities, and conditions must allow not only for survival of the mosquitoes, but also for successful sporogony to be possible within the life-time of individual insects. Hence transmission does not occur at altitudes over 2000 m or if the temperature is too hot or too cold. Occasionally malaria can be transmitted via blood transfusion or infected needles. This mosquito-less route lacks a hepatic phase and depending on the inoculum, the incubation period can be quite short.

Rates of transmission of malaria vary widely from area to area, ranging in entomological terms from less than one to several hundred infected bites per year. In clinical epidemiology malaria endemicity has traditionally been measured in terms of parasite rates or 'spleen rates', though these measures give only a rough yes/no guide to infection and say nothing of the severity or burden of disease. This was reasonable in the days of the malaria eradication programme of the 1950s and 1960s, when the aim was to eliminate all transmission. Now it has been generally accepted that the battle to eradicate malaria is lost, and interventions can only reduce the level of transmission. In this setting insight into the relationship between transmission level and malaria-attributable morbidity and mortality is essential. Over the past 10–15 years considerable research effort has been directed at this question, often with surprising results.

Malaria-attributable mortality

Most malaria-attributable deaths world-wide occur in areas where there is no system of death certification, and often patients die without reaching any form of health care. Estimation of malaria-attributable mortality is fraught with difficulties. Attempts using 'verbal autopsies' (detailed post-mortem questioning of relatives) in the Gambia indicated that malaria was responsible for 25% of all deaths in children aged 1–4 years (Greenwood et al., 1987) though this technique has since been shown to have serious limitations (Snow et al., 1992). Indeed 25% may be a gross underestimate; an intervention study of insecticide-impregnated bednets aimed at reducing malaria transmission found a 50% fall in all cause mortality in the intervention arm (Alonso et al., 1991).

Clinical epidemiology

The clinical manifestations of malaria vary with age and geographical area. In parts of tropical Africa where malaria is holoendemic (spleen or parasite rates in children > 75%), people may receive as many as one to two infected bites per day. In this setting the main clinical manifestation of malaria is severe anaemia in children aged 1–3 years, and cerebral malaria is rare. In other areas of Africa where transmission is less intense the predominant severe disease syndrome is cerebral malaria occurring in slightly older children (Brewster and Greenwood, 1993; Snow *et al.*, 1994). One recent study of severe malaria in five different areas found an inverse relationship between transmission intensity and incidence of severe disease (Snow *et al.*, 1997). Severe malaria never occurs in African adults living in holoendemic or hyperendemic (spleen or parasite rates in children 50–75%) areas, but does occur in areas where transmission is sporadic (Endeshaw and Assefa, 1990). In contrast in south-east Asia, where falciparum malaria transmission is unstable, severe malaria in adults is relatively common (Hien *et al.*, 1996). The above observations are consistent with the acquisition of immunity playing a major role in the clinical epidemiology of malaria. In areas of high transmission, children have frequent infections and their burden of disease is high. However, once (and if) they reach around 10 years of age they have acquired sufficient immunity (premunition) to prevent development of the severe manifestations of disease, though not to prevent infection and (often completely asymptomatic) parasitaemia. In areas of low, sporadic, transmission all ages are susceptible to severe disease, though this is mainly manifest in young adults who are more likely to be working in the forest or migrants seeking employment in an endemic area. Tourists and other overseas travellers from temperate climes also fall into this category.

Malaria and HIV infection coexist in many parts of the world, and much interest and concern has focused on the possibility of an interaction between the two (Chandramohan and Greenwood, 1998). There are theoretical grounds for suspecting that malaria could hasten HIV progression and that HIV infection could worsen the severity of any malaria infection. So far no convincing evidence for such an interaction exists, though adequately powered studies in severe malaria have not yet been carried out.

Clinical features

Uncomplicated malaria

The symptoms of uncomplicated falciparum malaria are qualitatively similar to those caused by the three benign human malarias, and may even be less severe initially than in *P. vivax*. Fever is often preceded by 24–48 h of headaches, myalgias and a general feeling of lethargy and dysphoria. It is usually accompanied by shivering and chills, and occasionally by violent rigors. Headache and muscle pains worsen, and anorexia is the rule. The classical tertian (alternate day) fever is rarely seen in naturally occurring falciparum infections, the fever chart more commonly showing a continuous, gently fluctuating pyrexia with occasional peaks of $>39°C$. Respiratory symptoms such as cough and tachypnoea can occur, though respiratory examination is usually unremarkable. Splenomegaly and hepatosplenomegaly, and mild abdominal discomfort are all common, and nausea and vomiting, diarrhoea, or constipation may also feature. The symptom complex associated with malaria infection is very non-specific and diagnostically unhelpful; any patient returning from or living in an endemic area who presents with fever alone must be assumed to have malaria until proven otherwise.

The proportion of acute malaria infections which progress to severe disease varies between areas and populations, and is greatly influenced by the availability of antimalarial treatment. It has been estimated that around one in 100 acute infections in Gambian children develop complications (Greenwood *et al.*, 1991), and in adult malaria in Thailand the mortality was found to be about one per 1000 (Meek, 1988; Luxemburger *et al.*, 1997).

Comparison between adults and children

Severe malaria has been studied mainly in two groups of patients, African children and non-immune south-east Asian adults. The clinical syndromes vary markedly between these two groups (Table 1.1). African children present with either severe anaemia, the newly-recognized syndrome of malaria with severe respiratory distress, or with cerebral malaria (Marsh *et al.*, 1995). In non-immune adult patients coma is much more likely to occur as part of a multisystem disorder; cerebral malaria may coexist with one or more of jaundice, acute renal failure, blackwater fever, severe metabolic acidosis, and haemodynamic shock ('algid' malaria) (Hien, *et al.*, 1996). As noted above, African adults from high transmission areas do not get severe malaria. Severe malaria in Asian children has not been studied to the same extent, though there is some evidence that as relatively young non-immune individuals they develop a syndrome midway between those seen in African children and Asian adults (Cao *et al.*, 1997). As an example, dialysis-requiring renal failure occurs at an

Table 1.1 Severe malaria: differences between African children and South-east Asian adults.

Feature	African children	South-east Asian adults
Sex	Males = females	Male predominance, probably as exposure is related to work pattern (often economic migrants)
Symptom duration before onset of complications	Typically 1–2 days	Often 4–5 days
Convulsions	Common; may occur without cerebral malaria	Uncommon. Usually a feature of cerebral malaria
Renal failure	Very rare	Common (∼30%)
Jaundice	Rare	Very common (∼50%)
Hypoglycaemia	∼40%, usually disease-related	∼20%, often quinine-related
Coma duration in cerebral malaria following treatment	Usually 1–2 days	Usually 2–5 days
Neurological sequelae post cerebral malaria	∼10%	∼1–2%
Overall mortality	20–30%	20–30%

incidence of around 5%, compared with 0% in African children and 11% in non-immune adults (Waller *et al.*, 1995; Hien *et al.*, 1996; D. Bethell, personal communication).

Cerebral malaria

The causes of impairment of consciousness in severe malaria include cerebral malaria *per se*, ictal activity, hypoglycaemia, severe acidosis and systemic hypotension (shock). Although the 'non-cerebral' causes of coma complicate any strict definition of cerebral malaria, in practice any patient with proven *P. falciparum* infection and impairment of consciousness or other signs of cerebral dysfunction is severely ill, and requires parenteral antimalarial therapy and intensive care monitoring.

Cerebral malaria in adults

This usually presents as a diffuse symmetrical encephalopathy, which may develop over several hours or start abruptly following a generalized seizure. A strict definition of cerebral malaria requires the presence of asexual forms of *P. falciparum* on the peripheral blood film, unrousable coma which persists for at least 30 minutes following a seizure, and exclusion of any other cause of encephalopathy (including bacterial meningitis and viral encephalopathies, common in much of the tropics) (World Health Organization, 1990). Hypoglycaemia should also be excluded. 'Unrousable coma' requires a best motor response on the Glasgow Coma Scale (GCS) of ≤ 3 (i.e. non-localizing) and best verbal response of ≤ 2 (at best incomprehensible sounds) (Warrell *et al.*, 1982). The eye opening part of the GCS is of limited value, as in cerebral malaria the eyes may remain open despite deep coma. In general, focal neurological signs are unusual. The marked meningism characteristic of bacterial meningitis with photophobia and board-like neck rigidity is not seen, though mild neck stiffness can occur. Pupillary reflexes are usually intact, as are the corneal reflexes. Disorders of conjugate gaze are very common, though oculocephalic and oculovestibular reflexes are normal. Primitive reflexes such as the pout reflex may be present, and the jaw jerk is often brisk. There may be generalized hypertonia with symmetrical brisk tendon reflexes and easily elicitable ankle clonus, though less frequently hypotonia is also seen. In true cerebral malaria abdominal reflexes are invariably absent. In severe cases, abnormal posturing (Plum and Posner, 1980) including decerebrate (abnormal arm flexion with extension of legs) and decorticate (abnormal extensor response in arms and legs) rigidity may occur either spontaneously, in the presence of hypoglycaemia, or in response to a noxious stimulus.

In non-immune adults convulsions are much less common than in children, occurring in around 20% of cases of cerebral malaria (Hien *et al.*, 1996). Convulsions occur rarely in the absence of impairment of consciousness, and are not associated with episodes of hypoglycaemia (Hien *et al.*, 1996; Waruiru *et al.*, 1996).

In adults, coma usually resolves after 1–5 days (median ∼2 days), but may occasionally continue for up to 2 weeks (Hien *et al.*, 1996). The vast majority of adults who survive cerebral malaria emerge from coma with no discernible residual neurological abnormalities.

Cerebral malaria in children

A strict definition of cerebral malaria in African children includes an inability to localize painful stimuli, which is difficult to assess in the very young. The Blantyre coma scale is commonly used, with a cut-off score for defining cerebral malaria of ≤2/5, though this is subject to a number of intrinsic inaccuracies (Molyneux *et al.*, 1989; Newton *et al.*, 1997a). Older children can be assessed as adults using the GCS. For all children other causes of impaired consciousness must be considered, such as convulsions (which may have a longer post-ictal period than the average febrile convulsion), hypoglycaemia (which should respond to intravenous glucose in the early stages), and the administration of sedative drugs. Although for research purposes accurately defining cerebral malaria is important, in practice it has been suggested that any 'prostrated' child with malaria (with or without impairment of consciousness) should be treated as severe malaria (Marsh *et al.*, 1995). Prostration is defined as the inability to sit unassisted in a child normally able to do so. In children not able to sit it is defined as an inability to feed. In a clinical setting prostration is easily defined prospectively and indicates a need for urgent treatment.

In cerebral malaria the time from the onset of febrile symptoms to onset of coma in African children is typically around 48 h, considerably shorter than commonly seen in non-immune adults (Molyneux *et al.*, 1989; Mabeza *et al.*, 1995). They also regain consciousness more quickly, usually within 2–3 days (Molyneux *et al.*, 1989; Waller *et al.*, 1995). In profound coma conjugate gaze abnormalities, hypotonia, hypertonia, decorticate and decerebrate posturing, and opisthotonus may all occur. Death may be preceded by brainstem signs consistent with (but not necessarily caused by) brainstem herniation (Newton *et al.*, 1991, 1996).

Convulsions are the commonest neurological manifestations of malaria in African children, and can occur either as part of cerebral malaria or as an independent entity. Over 70% of children with cerebral malaria have convulsions, and in one study 25% of those with seizures following admission had electroencephalographic evidence of covert status epilepticus (Crawley *et al.*, 1996). In these children the clinical manifestations of seizure activity between overt fits was minimal and easily overlooked. They included irregular breathing patterns, nystagmus and minor twitching movements of a finger or corner of the mouth. The overall clinical condition of these children often improved dramatically with administration of anticonvulsants. In children infected with falciparum malaria without background impairment of consciousness seizures are also common, particularly in the under 3-year-old age group. Although some of these may represent childhood febrile convulsions, in a study of

Kenyan children presenting to hospital with convulsions and malaria 54% had rectal temperatures less than 38°C (Waruiru *et al.*, 1996).

Neurological sequelae

A proportion of African children who survive cerebral malaria develop long-term neurological complications. These include ataxia, cortical blindness and hemiparesis, and represent a massive human and social burden. Sequelae have been clinically associated with protracted and deep coma, repeated convulsions, and hypoglycaemia (Brewster *et al.*, 1990; Bondi, 1992; Bajiya and Kochar, 1996; van Hensbroek *et al.*, 1997). The incidence of these complications has been underestimated but is probably over 20%, though this falls to <5% 6 months post-illness (van Hensbroek *et al.*, 1997). There is conflicting evidence regarding the presence of persistent minor neuropsychiatric sequelae (Muntendam *et al.*, 1996; Varney *et al.*, 1997), and it is unknown whether there is any long term effect of cerebral malaria on the psychosocial and intellectual development of children.

Other neurological manifestations

Coma, seizures and neurological sequelae are not the only neurological manifestations of falciparum malaria. In Vietnamese adults a self-limiting 'post-malaria neurological syndrome' has been described (Nguyen *et al.*, 1996). Patients present with an acute confusional state, psychosis, seizures, or tremor. In the 22 patients studied the median (range) time from parasite clearance to onset of neurological symptoms was 96 hours (6 h to 60 days). It occurred in 0.12% of all falciparum malaria patients, but was 300 times more common following severe rather than uncomplicated malaria. In addition in a randomized trial, it was significantly more likely to occur in patients given mefloquine rather than the combination of quinine and sulfadoxine/pyrimethamine to complete antimalarial treatment.

A syndrome of delayed cerebellar ataxia has been described following falciparum malaria in Sri Lanka and more recently in the Sudan (Senanayake and de Silva *et al.*, 1994; Abdulla *et al.*, 1997). There is no impairment of consciousness, and symptoms resolve spontaneously a median (range) of 10 weeks (3–16) after their onset.

The pathophysiology of these post-infectious neurological conditions is unknown, though from Sri Lanka there is some evidence of an immunological mechanism; compared with appropriate controls patients with ataxia had significantly raised tumour necrosis factor and interleukin-6 in both serum and cerebrospinal fluid (de Silva *et al.*, 1992).

Hypoglycaemia

Hypoglycaemia is associated with severe malaria in both adults and children, and carries a poor prognosis (White *et al.*, 1983b, 1987). It can be a consequence of severe malaria *per se* (Looareesuwan *et al.*, 1985; Taylor and

Molyneux, 1988; White *et al.*, 1983b 1987), or a side-effect of treatment with quinine or quinidine (White *et al.*, 1983b). Hypoglycaemia of both aetiologies is particularly common and refractory to treatment in pregnant women. Often the classical signs of hypoglycaemia are either inconstant or mistaken for clinical features of severe malaria itself (sweating, anxiety, confusion, and coma). If there is doubt and blood glucose measurement is not instantly available, a therapeutic trial of 50% glucose should be administered; if hypoglycaemia is present this will often lead to a dramatic improvement in symptoms.

Acidosis

The pathophysiological and prognostic importance of metabolic acidosis in both adult and childhood severe malaria is only now becoming apparent. The clinical syndrome of respiratory distress in African children, previously either unrecognized or incorrectly attributed to heart failure secondary to severe anaemia, is now thought to be mainly caused by acidosis (Marsh *et al.*, 1995; English *et al.*, 1996, 1997). Metabolic acidosis is strongly associated with fatal outcome in both adults and children (Taylor *et al.*, 1993; Krishna *et al.*, 1994b; Hien *et al.*, 1996), and appears to be caused by a combination of lactic acidosis and poor renal handling of bicarbonate. The latter is particularly true in non-immune adults in whom renal failure is common, but is also true in African children, where severe renal impairment never occurs (English *et al.*, 1997). Hypovolaemia and anaemia are associated with lactic acidosis in the same population. Metabolic acidosis can occur with or without cerebral involvement, though in one study of adults with cerebral malaria cerebrospinal fluid lactate was a powerful predictor of death (White *et al.*, 1985).

Severe anaemia

Malaria is a parasitic infection of red cells, and anaemia is a common and inevitable consequence of severe malaria. When marked, it is itself a criterion for severe malaria (World Health Organization, 1990). Severe anaemia (Hb < 5 g/dl) was present in 29% of 2433 children admitted to a Kenyan hospital with malaria, and was associated with a mortality of 18% compared with an 8% overall mortality (Marsh *et al.*, 1995). It is particularly severe if associated with respiratory distress. In Vietnamese adults severe anaemia (haematocrit < 21%) was present in 16% of patients admitted with severe malaria, though in 90% of these it was accompanied by at least one other manifestation of severe malaria and was not in itself a useful predictor of poor outcome (Hien *et al.*, 1996; Day, unpublished observations).

Renal failure

Renal involvement in malaria may take a number of forms, the most important of which is an 'acute tubular necrosis'-like syndrome similar to that seen in sepsis. This particularly affects non-immune patients, and is not uncommon in the context of imported severe malaria. Blackwater fever, once the scourge of colonial administrations, still occurs occasionally. The nephrotic syndrome-causing glomerulonephritis associated with *P. malariae* is a chronic manifestation of malaria and will not be discussed here.

Acute renal failure

Acute renal failure (ARF) accounts for a significant proportion of the morbidity and mortality associated with severe malaria in non-immune individuals. In Vietnam 158 of 560 cases (28%) of severe adult malaria had renal failure (plasma creatinine >288 µmol/l (3 mg/dl)) on admission, and a total of 41% had renal failure at some stage during their illness (Hien *et al.*, 1996). Overall, 14% required dialysis. Renal failure on admission (oliguric or non-oliguric) was associated with a marked increase in the risk of death (29% in those with renal failure, 9.2% in those without). This is in marked contrast to severe malaria in African children, where any renal dysfunction is usually subclinical and the need for dialysis vanishingly rare (Waller *et al.*, 1995).

ARF in severe malaria may present either acutely as part of a fulminant multisystem disorder, or develop over several days in patients recovering from the initial acute phase of severe disease. Patients developing renal failure acutely tend to be oliguric or anuric, frequently have jaundice and coexisting lactic acidosis, and usually require immediate or early dialysis. When renal failure develops after the acute phase of the disease patients are more likely to have non-oliguric renal failure, and are less likely to require dialysis. If dialysis is required in this group the indication is more likely to be uraemic symptomatology or (non-lactic) acidosis than hyperkalaemia or fluid overload.

The clinical features of malaria-associated ARF are very similar to those of the 'acute tubular necrosis' (ATN) syndrome seen in patients with bacterial sepsis or hypovolaemia, suggesting that the pathological processes may be similar. In support of this the few renal biopsies taken in malaria-associated ARF have tended to show pathological changes in the tubules consistent with ATN (Sitprija *et al.*, 1967; Stone *et al.*, 1972), and reports of glomerulonephritis are rare.

Blackwater fever

Blackwater fever is an enigmatic condition characterized by fever, massive intravascular haemolysis and haemoglobinuria, which, in severe cases, can lead to acute renal failure. Its exact aetiology is unclear, though it occurs only in areas of the tropics endemic for malaria, and is associated with malaria infection, quinine ingestion, and glucose-6-phosphate dehydrogenase deficiency. How the presence of one or more of these factors leads to haemolysis is not known, though it is clear that no single factor can explain all cases of blackwater fever. Once a major cause of renal failure and malaria-associated mortality, it is now relatively uncommon and rarely leads to severe ARF. In a recent descriptive study of 50 cases of blackwater fever, just three patients required dialysis and only a single patient died (Tran *et al.*, 1996).

Jaundice

Jaundice is even more common than ARF in non-immune adults (60% in one series (Hien *et al.*, 1996)), and like ARF is very unusual in children. It is associated with renal failure, cerebral malaria, and hyperparasitaemia, and is caused by a combination of haemolysis and mild hepatic dysfunction (the serum bilirubin is often a mixture of conjugated and unconjugated forms). Serious hepatic dysfunction with asterixis and hepatic encephalopathy never occurs. However, serum transaminases may be elevated, and low hepatic blood flow is associated with raised plasma lactate concentrations, suggesting that reduced hepatic function may contribute to lactic acidosis (Pukrittayakamee *et al.*, 1992).

Pulmonary oedema

This serious complication of severe malaria is particularly common in pregnant women, and is usually fatal if facilities for mechanical ventilation are not on hand (which they usually are not). Clinically it resembles the adult respiratory distress syndrome (Fein *et al.*, 1978; Martell *et al.*, 1979), and though it can be precipitated by fluid overload, it is usually associated with normal central venous and pulmonary artery occlusion pressures (Blanbeil *et al.*, 1980; James, 1985).

Haemodynamic shock (Algid malaria)

Severe hypotension as a consequence of severe malaria is haemodynamically similar to bacterial septic shock, characterized by a very low systemic vascular resistance and normal or raised cardiac output (Day, unpublished observations). Shock usually occurs on the background of other severe complications of malaria, and is associated with raised plasma lactate levels and metabolic acidosis. The prognosis is poor despite inotropic support. Bacterial septicaemia is occasionally implicated, though blood cultures are usually sterile (Bygbjerg and Lanng, 1982).

Abnormalities of haemostasis

Patients with severe malaria have an increased risk of bleeding, particularly if they have multisystem dysfunction. Epistaxis, bleeding gums, and, more seriously, upper gastrointestinal bleeds can occur, though life-threatening haemorrhage is rare. Thrombocytopenia is usual in malaria, though counts below 25 000/µl are rare except with very severe disease. Laboratory tests for disseminated intravascular coagulation are usually normal.

Factors associated with poor prognosis

Respiratory distress or impaired consciousness predicted 84% of deaths among Kenyan children admitted to hospital with malaria (Marsh *et al.*, 1995). Other

Table 1.2 Laboratory features of severe malaria.

	Associated with poor prognosis if:
Haematology	
Normochromic normocytic anaemia	Haematocrit < 15% or Hb < 5 g/dl
Thrombocytopenia	
Hypofibrinogenaemia (rare)	
Pigment-containing leucocytes	> 4% of circulating neutrophils
Haemoglobinaemia	
Parasitaemia	> 10% or 500 000/dl; mature parasites seen in peripheral blood
Decreased red cell deformability	Deformability reduced
Biochemistry	
Hyponatraemia	
Hypochloraemia	
Hypophosphataemia	
Hypoglycaemia	Present
Metabolic acidosis	Standard base deficit > 3.3 mmol/l; pH < 7.300
Lactic acidosis	> 4 mmol/l
Raised CSF lactate	Raised
Hyperbilirubinaemia*	
Azotaemia*	Raised. In adults renal failure associated with threefold increase in mortality
Moderately raised hepatic transaminases	
Raised creatine kinase and myoglobin	

* Rare in African children

features particularly associated with fatal outcome are hypoglycaemia, increased plasma lactate or acidosis, and increased cerebrospinal fluid lactate concentration (Table 1.2). The presence on the peripheral blood film of mature parasites (> 20% with visible pigment) is also associated with a poor prognosis (Waller *et al.*, 1995).

In adults depth of coma, agitation, oliguria, jaundice and shock are important clinical predictors of poor outcome. Prognostically useful laboratory markers include several measures of acidosis (raised plasma or cerebrospinal fluid lactate, or low pH), the presence of leucocyte pigment and/or mature parasites on the peripheral blood film, and hypoglycaemia. Peripheral parasite count is also positively associated with the occurrence of complications or death; non-immune patients with a parasitaemia of > 4% should probably be treated as having severe malaria (Luxemburger *et al.*, 1995).

Overall the mortality from cerebral malaria is 20–30% in both adults and children. However in non-immune adults the mortality depends on the number of coexisting complications. In one series of 560 cases patients with cerebral malaria alone had a case fatality of around 6% (ND, unpublished observations). This rose to 15% if another complication was present (one of shock, jaundice, renal failure, hypoglycaemia, severe anaemia and hyperparasitaemia), 25% with two complications, and > 40% if three or more complications were present. There are no large series of severe malaria patients treated in

ITUs in the developed world, though what evidence there is suggests that mortality rates are very similar to those cited above.

The Pathological Features of Cerebral Malaria

The study of the pathology of cerebral malaria (CM) began with the pioneering work of Marchiafava and his group in Italy in the late 19th century (Bignami and Bastianelli, 1889; Marchiafava and Bignami, 1894). Numerous other studies have been published since, although they vary in size and in the degree and nature of the correlation between clinical details and pathological findings (Ewing, 1902; Dudgeon and Clarke, 1917; Durck, 1925; Gaskell and Miller, 1920; Kean and Smith, 1944; Rigdon, 1944; Spitz, 1946; Clark and Tomlinson, 1949; Lemercier *et al.*, 1966; Edington, 1967; Macpherson *et al.*, 1985; Oo *et al.*, 1987; (Aikawa *et al.*, 1990; Polder *et al.*, 1991; Pongponratn *et al.*, 1991; Walker *et al.*, 1992; Patnaik *et al.*, 1994; Lucas *et al.*, 1996). A major hindrance to the identification of specific pathological features of CM in these studies has been the confusing heterogeneity within and between these studies. However, some common features have been recognized, though their significance and pathogenesis remain open to much debate. The introduction of WHO clinical diagnostic criteria and the new experimental methods of electron microscopy (EM), immunohistochemistry and molecular biology have led to a number of recent clinicopathological studies addressing specific questions concerning the pathogenesis of cerebral malaria (Turner, 1997; Newton and Krishna, 1998).

1 Sequestration of parasitized erythrocytes

Marchiafava's group were the first to document the process of sequestration; 'Those of them (the erythrocytes) which have been invaded by the parasite offer greater resistance to the circulation than the normal ones, whence it happens that they accumulate towards the circumference of the larger vessels, and their circulation is either stopped or retarded in certain portions of the capillaries . . .' (Bignami and Bastianelli, 1889).

Histological and EM examinations of post-mortem brain tissue from CM show cerebral microvessels distended by numerous parasitized erythrocytes, which are attached to cerebral endothelial cells via electron dense 'knob proteins' on their surface. The key to this appearance is the selective disappearance from the general circulation of erythrocytes infected with the late trophozoite and schizont stages of the parasite, and their preferential sequestration within the microvascular beds of vital organs. This process is the clinical correlate of the *in vitro* phenomenon of cytoadherence, which is characterized by receptor-mediated adhesion of PRBC to endothelial cells (Berendt *et al.*, 1994a).

Attempts to link the process of sequestration in the brain to the incidence of coma have shown a significant quantitative association between the presence of coma in severe malaria and the level of cerebral microvascular sequestration

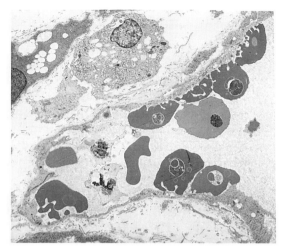

Figure 1.2   Transmission electron micrograph showing ruptured 'ghosted' erythrocyte membranes adherent to endothelial cells. These are left behind following the rupture of the mature, multi-segmented schizont, but can adhere to the endothelial cell due to the retention of knob proteins on the surface of the ruptured red cell membrane.

(MacPherson *et al.*, 1985; Pongponratn *et al.*, 1991). Other studies cite cases where coma was not associated with any significant histological evidence of sequestration (Patnaik *et al.*, 1994), though these have not allowed for factors which may influence the histological observation of sequestration, such as the duration of treatment before death.

2 Pigment deposition and phagocytosis

When sequestered parasites undergo schizogony, erythrocyte membrane ghosts are left adherent to cerebral endothelial cells (Figure 1.2). These ghosts contain unneeded parasite remnants, including malaria pigment, the breakdown products of haemoglobin digestion by the developing parasite. Pigment deposition can be seen lining cerebral vessels after erythrocytes newly infected with immature ring form parasites have re-entered the circulation. Circulating monocytes phagocytose ghost erythrocyte membranes and the pigment, which is known to have toxic and stimulatory effects on monocytes *in vitro* (including stimulation of TNFα release (Taverne *et al.*, 1990) and decrease in motility). Pigment left behind after PRBC rupture may also have a direct pathophysiological effect on cerebral endothelial cells (Taramelli *et al.*, 1998).

3 Haemorrhages

Multiple small petechial haemorrhages, often within the immediate subcortical rim of white matter, are frequently seen on macroscopic examination of the fresh brain from a case of cerebral malaria. Histological examination reveals three separate types of haemorrhage. The first is the simple petechial haemorrhage, which can also be seen in other conditions such as carbon monoxide poisoning and barotrauma (Spitz, 1946). There are also ring haemorrhages, characterized by a central necrotic vessel, surrounding ring of uninfected red cells and outer ring of PRBC and leucocytes (Rigdon, 1944). The third type of haemorrhage is the eponymous Dürck's granuloma, with a rim of reactive microglial cells and astrogliosis surrounding a central vessel (Dürck, 1925). Interpretation of the nature, frequency, distribution and importance of these lesions varies, but the consensus from multiple studies is that haemorrhages are a common pathological feature in the post mortem brain in CM.

4 Cerebral oedema and brain swelling

Evidence from radiological (Looareesuwan *et al.*, 1995) and intracranial pressure monitoring (Newton *et al.*, 1991; 1997b) supports a role for brain swelling in some cases of severe malaria. However, pathological evidence of cerebral oedema, including perivascular, parenchymal and intracellular oedema, is much harder to find. Post-mortem examination of adult Vietnamese patients shows little evidence for widespread cerebral oedema, brainstem herniation or increased brain weight (Mai *et al* unpublished data). Some data from African children also show no significant pathological evidence of cerebral oedema (Lucas *et al.*, 1996). Ongoing studies of Malawian children do however show brain oedema, so there is clearly some disparity between patient groups. The apparent increased susceptibility of children to brain swelling may reflect differences in vascular autoregulation or maintenance of the blood–brain barrier in younger patients. A key question is whether brain swelling and raised intracranial pressure necessarily always mean cerebral oedema. Massive intravascular sequestration may be sufficient to increase brain volume in the intravascular component due to the burden of sequestered PRBC. However, there remains no doubt that cerebral oedema can be seen in brains of individual fatal CM cases.

5 Leucocyte and astroglial inflammatory responses

Observations of leucocytes within the cerebral vasculature in cerebral malaria vary. Some studies report the presence of leucocytes to be a common feature (Patnaik *et al.*, 1994), and several authors have proposed that they underlie the pathophysiological mechanisms of endothelial cell damage (Toro and Roman, 1978; Polder *et al.*, 1991). There is evidence for intravascular sequestration of host leucocytes from the murine model of cerebral malaria. The consequent pro-inflammatory cytokine production (Grau *et al.*, 1986) may play a major role in the pathology of malaria in this model. Leucocyte migration into the brain itself is not a feature of human CM, apart from extravasation around areas of haemorrhage.

Production of pro-inflammatory cytokines by circulating leucocytes or astroglial cells is felt to contribute significantly to the pathology of murine malaria (Medana *et al.*, 1997a), which has been likened to an encephalitis (Jennings *et al.*, 1997). There is evidence in Vietnamese CM patients for activation of cerebral endothelial cells (Turner *et al.*, 1994), and local disruption of blood–brain barrier junctional proteins, with associated activation of perivascular macrophages (Brown *et al.*, 1999). Perivascular macrophage activation may reflect dysfunction of the blood–brain barrier (Maegraith, 1948), which is known to occur in the murine model (Chan-Ling *et al.*, 1992). However, murine malaria shows important differences from the human disease, most notably the lack of infected erythrocyte sequestration in the brain. The murine model presents an interesting opportunity to study pathophysiological mechanisms, but remains a model which is unlikely to accurately reflect human disease.

6 Neuronal toxicity and degeneration

Little evidence for neurodegeneration has been reported in cerebral malaria, although given the degree of PRBC sequestration it is perhaps surprising that widespread ischaemic neuronal or endothelial cell damage is not commonly seen. Marchiafava and Bignami reported chromatolysis in brain cells and related this to several cases where bulbar (brainstem) symptoms were prominent clinically (Marchiafava and Bignami, 1894). Rigdon reported depletion of the Purkinje cells of the cerebellum and focal degeneration of brain tissue (Rigdon, 1944). There is also evidence from *in vitro* studies that circulating antibodies in human cerebral malaria patients can inhibit Purkinje cell growth *in vitro* (Calvet *et al.*, 1993). There has been recent interest in the potential role of excitotoxic neurotransmitters from the Kyneurinine pathway in mediating coma in the murine CM model (Sanni *et al.*, 1998). The role of neurotoxicity in the pathogenesis of human CM should become clearer with the results of current investigations into neuronal cell death through reperfusion injury, excitotoxic neurotransmitter release and apoptosis.

Pathophysiological mechanisms in cerebral malaria

As an infection of the central nervous system cerebral malaria has a number of interesting features. First, the mechanism of coma is completely unknown. The pathological hallmark of cerebral malaria is cytoadherence of parasitized erythrocytes to endothelial cells in the deep microvasculature of the brain, but how this leads to coma is deeply controversial. Secondly, if the patient survives, the coma is usually completely reversible; this is particularly true in non-immune adults with cerebral malaria, in whom the rate of neurological sequelae is about 1%.

Parasite cytoadherence and host sequestration receptors

Cultured parasitized erythrocytes infected with *P. falciparum* bind to endothelial cells. They also display other cytoadherent phenotypes such as binding to uninfected red cells (rosetting), leucocytes and platelets as well as autoagglutination with other infected cells. Studies *in vitro* have demonstrated that cytoadherence is a specific receptor-mediated process (Berendt *et al.*, 1994a), and a number of different host molecules have been shown to support PRBC binding, both as recombinant proteins and expressed on endothelial cell monolayers. These include thrombospondin (TSP), CD36, ICAM-1, VCAM-1 and E-selectin, CD31, chondroitin sulphate A and the integrin $\alpha3\beta v$. Immunohistochemical studies of the distribution of these sequestration receptors has confirmed that they are expressed in the brain during cerebral malaria, and that some are up-regulated (Turner et al., 1994). However, the pattern of receptor expression does not account for specific cerebral sequestration, as the same receptors are expressed in numerous other vascular beds in the body. Up-regulation of sequestration receptor expression appears to be due to a systemic endothelial activation, not specific for malaria, which can be seen in other vascular beds during malaria and other systemic infections (Turner et al., 1998).

There is controversy as to whether parasite sequestration can be directly linked to the causation of coma in CM (Berendt et al., 1994b; Clark and Rockett, 1994). Studies of 50 Vietnamese adults with severe malaria with and without coma confirmed that, allowing for time to death and thus the duration of treatment, all patients with CM showed evidence of cerebral sequestration, although some patients with sequestered parasitized red blood cells (PRBC) in the brain had not developed coma by the time of death (Turner G, unpublished observations). Sequestration is thus necessary but not wholly sufficient to cause coma in CM. Other authors propose that sequestration is merely an epiphenomenon, and that all the symptoms of CM may be mediated by soluble circulating factors such as cytokines or nitric oxide (Clark et al., 1991, 1992). It is more likely that following sequestration of PRBC, a chain of events is initiated, probably involving release of soluble mediators from PRBC or host cells in the brain, which leads indirectly to coma.

Parasite adhesion ligands

Much less is known about the parasite ligand responsible for binding to host sequestration receptors on endothelial cells. In vitro experiments using micromanipulation to develop clonal lines of parasites showed that binding to ICAM-1 and CD36 were separate and could vary independently (Roberts et al., 1992). Antigenic phenotype was co-modulated with changes in cytoadherence, suggesting that the same molecule was responsible for both phenotypes. The cytoadherence properties of laboratory isolates have been investigated using biochemical techniques (Chaiyaroj et al., 1994; Gardner et al., 1996) and suggest a role for the Plasmodium falciparum erythrocyte membrane protein-1 (PfEMP-1) molecule. Long-term attempts to clone PfEMP-1 have recently come to fruition with the identification of a large family of genes in the falciparum genome termed the var genes (Baruch et al., 1995; Smith et al., 1995; Su et al., 1995). These are a multigene family randomly dispersed throughout the P. falciparum genome but favouring telomeric expression sites. They have several domains including a Duffy binding like (DBL) domain similar to binding sequences for the Duffy blood group antigen. Studies of the ligand binding sequences should help to elucidate the mechanisms underlying differences in cytoadherence phenotype between parasite strains, and their interaction with host receptors.

Events at the blood–brain barrier: endothelial activation

Evidence from both human disease and animal models indicates that PRBC sequestration in the cerebral microvasculature is associated with endothelial cell activation (Chan-Ling *et al.*, 1992; Turner *et al.*, 1994). Immunophenotypic changes have been demonstrated and electron microscopy shows blebbing of endothelial cell membranes and formation of pseudopodia. Cultured brain endothelial cells derived from Saimiri monkeys show marked morphological changes including phagocytosis of some parasitized erythrocytes, although this has not been observed in human cases (Robert *et al.*, 1996). It is plausible that binding of PRBC to cerebral endothelial cells may cause receptor-mediated cell signalling via molecules like ICAM- 1 and CD31, which could lead to alterations in the structural or functional integrity of the blood–brain barrier. PRBC binding to cerebral endothelial cells may thus have significance not just because of physical obstruction to blood flow but functional disturbance of the blood–brain barrier. Leakage of the blood–brain barrier associated with perivascular astrocyte activation and TNFα secretion has been shown in the murine model of CM (Medana *et al.*, 1997a, b).

Soluble neuroactive mediators

The rapidly reversible nature of malaria coma has led some authors to propose that soluble rapidly diffusible mediators might mediate the symptoms of CM. These could represent parasite toxins, host cytokine release induced by infection, or local release of neuroactive mediators within the CNS which could have an 'anaesthetic'-like action (Clark and Rockett, 1994).

TNFα

By analogy with severe sepsis, TNFα and other pro-inflammatory cytokines are strong candidates for the putative mediators responsible for the multisystem organ failure and hypotension seen in cases of severe malaria. Raised levels of plasma TNFα in malaria have been associated with disease severity in African children (Grau *et al.*, 1989; Kwiatkowski *et al.*, 1990). However, many other diseases, including *Plasmodium vivax* infection, are associated with high circulating TNFα levels, most of which do not have coma as a clinical feature; so raised systemic TNFα alone is unlikely to be the sole mediator of cerebral symptoms.

Nitric oxide

Release of nitric oxide (NO) within the brain parenchyma has also been proposed as a mechanism that might explain the coma of cerebral malaria.

Studies of serum and cerebrospinal fluid (CSF) NO metabolites (reactive nitrogen intermediates, or RNI) have provided conflicting results. Some studies have found a positive correlation between plasma RNI and severity of disease (Cot et al., 1994; Nussler et al., 1994; Kremsner et al., 1996; al-Yaman et al., 1997), whereas others have shown either no association (Agbenyega et al., 1997; Taylor et al., 1998) or even an inverse association (Anstey et al., 1996). CSF levels have also been uninformative (Agbenyega et al., 1997; Dondorp et al., 1997). It is likely that if NO plays a role in the pathogenesis of cerebral malaria it does so at a local level. Measurement of relative plasma or CSF levels of NO metabolites may be too blunt a tool.

Intracranial pressure, cerebral blood flow and cerebral oedema

Measurement of intracranial pressure (ICP) in malaria can be estimated from the CSF opening pressure of lumbar puncture, or by intracranial pressure monitoring. CSF opening pressures are not raised in South-East Asian adult patients with CM (White, 1991), but raised ICP levels have been associated with fatal outcome in African children (Waller et al., 1991a; Newton et al., 1997b). Raised intracranial pressure may also contribute to decreased cerebral perfusion pressure and consequent cytotoxic oedema, and in African children can be associated with a neurological syndrome consistent with brainstem herniation (Newton et al., 1991). However, the frequency of herniation in post-mortem series from Vietnam was very low, and radiological imaging of adult South-East Asian patients does not indicate that cerebral oedema is present in the majority of cases (Looareesuwan et al., 1995). Thus there may be differences in the contribution of ICP to CM in different patient groups.

Host genetic polymorphisms in susceptibility and resistance factors to cerebral malaria

A variety of host genetic polymorphisms have now been associated with resistance or susceptibility to cerebral malaria. The best known and first described of these are the inherited red cell disorders. The genes coding for these mutations are maintained at high levels in populations exposed to endemic malaria, because although they are associated with a potentially deleterious phenotype in the homozygous state, heterozygotes have an advantage under the selection pressure exerted by malaria infection. These conditions include red cell disorders such as sickle cell anaemia, hereditary ovalocytosis, and the alpha- and beta-thalassaemias. The protection they confer on the host is thought to be mediated by the decreased ability of the parasite to invade or survive in the erythrocyte (Weatherall et al., 1988). Some HLA alleles, notably HLA-B53 in Gambian children, have also been linked to protection against severe malaria (Hill et al., 1991). These associations are not constant between populations, and their full pathophysiological significance remains unclear. A further disease-associated polymorphism has recently been discovered in the promoter region of the TNFα gene (McGuire et al., 1994); this could theoretically influence disease by varying individual cytokine responses to infection.

In addition a polymorphism in domain 1 of the sequestration receptor ICAM-1 has been identified which is associated with increased levels of cerebral malaria in Kenyan children (Fernandez-Reyes *et al.*, 1997). The field of genetic host susceptibility is in its infancy but shows great promise; it looks certain to contribute greatly to our understanding of the pathophysiology of severe malaria over the coming decades.

Management

Cerebral malaria is a medical emergency, and priority should be given to rapid assessment of the patient's condition including a search for complications, prompt institution of antimalarial therapy and any other necessary supportive treatment, and careful monitoring by experienced nursing staff in the best-equipped location available.

Diagnosis

Cerebral malaria should be suspected in any patient with impaired consciousness or seizures who has been in an endemic area in the previous year, whether or not they were taking antimalarial prophylaxis. Malaria can be transmitted by modes other than mosquito bites; failure to consider the possibility of transmission by blood transfusion, contaminated needles or organ transplantation may lead to a dangerous delay in diagnosis. If malaria is strongly suspected in a severely ill patient with a first negative smear, it is reasonable to start antimalarial treatment empirically.

The blood smear

The most sensitive and specific test remains the peripheral blood film. This is a microscopic count of infected erythrocytes in a peripheral blood smear stained using either a modified Giemsa method or reversed Field stain. If the film is fixed with alcohol before staining the parasites can be seen within intact erythrocytes (a thin film), and the count expressed as a percentage of erythrocytes parasitized. Alternatively a thicker blood film can be stained directly, allowing the erythrocytes to lyse leaving the parasites visible alongside leucocyte nuclei (a thick film). Counts are then expressed per 200 or 400 leucocytes. The thin film is easier to read, the thick vastly more sensitive; a skilled microscopist should be able to detect parasitaemias of 20–50 parasites per µl on a thick film (Day *et al.*, 1996a). Thick films are not routinely done in Western laboratories, and in the era of automated cell counters even manual microscopic examination of a thin film has to be explicitly requested; if malaria is suspected this should be specifically stated and manual examination of both a thick and thin film requested. With experience the parasite species can be determined on morphological grounds from the blood film. If there is any doubt the film should be sent to a reference centre, and for the purposes of initial treatment falciparum malaria assumed.

Patients who have lived their lives in endemic areas may have low levels of parasitaemia in association with fever caused by an unrelated illness, which might easily be overlooked. Conversely peripheral blood films can be initially 'negative' if the parasitaemia is low due to sequestration in a synchronous infection or prior treatment with antimalarials; the film should be repeated if clinical suspicion remains. In non-immune patients with signs and symptoms associated with severe malaria the presence on light microscopy of lumps of malaria pigment in the cytoplasm of circulating leucocytes is a strong indicator that severe falciparum malaria is the true diagnosis (Phu *et al.*, 1995; Day *et al.*, 1996a).

PCR

The use of polymerase chain reaction (PCR)-based techniques has also been investigated, and shows higher specificity and similar sensitivity compared to thick blood film diagnosis. At present the technology is too complex for use in the field, but its potential as a research technique is high; PCR-based nucleic acid techniques can be used to speciate, to detect strain variation (useful for epidemiological and immunological research, and to distinguish recrudescence from reinfection in clinical studies), and to detect parasite developmental stage (analysis of mRNA). They can even be applied to stored Giemsa-stained blood films (Li *et al.*, 1997).

Rapid diagnostic tests

A number of methods for the rapid diagnosis of malaria infection have been developed recently. The first of these was based on an acridine orange fluorescence technique, and improved and developed commercially as the quantitative buffy coat (QBC) method. More recent dipstick tests are based around detection in blood of either falciparum-derived histidine rich protein 2 (HRP2) or of parasite lactate dehydrogenase (Pieroni *et al.*, 1998; Piper *et al.*, 1999). The latter is able to detect malaria and speciate, whereas the former is specific to *Plasmodium falciparum*. Neither are quite as sensitive as a thick film in experienced hands, but undoubtedly have a role in laboratories in the developed world where malaria is an uncommon diagnosis.

Initial assessment

After checking the airway and weighing the patient (if possible), an appropriate dose of antimalarial can be started if the diagnosis is known or clinical suspicion high. A rapid clinical assessment should follow including assessment of conscious level (including formal decomposed coma score), state of hydration, and haemodynamic and respiratory status. Blood should be taken for bedside glucose testing, peripheral blood smear, full blood count (or haematocrit), arterial blood gases (if available) and biochemistry. Hypo-glycaemia should be treated if present or not excluded. Oxygen should be given if there is respiratory distress or hypoxia. Start intravenous rehydration if indicated. If initial assessment confirms the presence of severe malaria or suspected severe malaria the patient should be transferred to the highest dependency unit available (preferably an intensive care unit).

The role of lumbar puncture in cerebral malaria

Because of the possible pathophysiological role of raised intracranial pressure in patients (particularly children) with cerebral malaria, the role of lumbar puncture (LP) in initial management of the comatose malaria patient is controversial. For while it is vital to exclude bacterial meningitis in any patient with impairment of consciousness (or seizures in the under 1 age group) (Wright et al., 1993), there is a concern that lumbar puncture in a child with a swollen brain may precipitate coning. This is a theoretical (if very reasonable) worry which remains unproven. Whereas imaging studies have shown that the majority of children or adults with cerebral malaria have no evidence of cerebral oedema (Newton et al., 1994; Looareesuwan et al., 1995), opening pressures at LP are raised in about 80% of children (Newton et al., 1991; Waller et al., 1991b; White, 1991). Opinion is divided as to whether an admission LP is safe in children with severe malaria (Newton et al., 1991), though we consider the case for delay unproven. If lumbar puncture is delayed appropriate antimeningitis cover must be given. An LP can then be performed either after a CT scan has excluded significant brain swelling or after 48 h following neurological improvement. If early LP is undertaken, considerations concerning desirability of pre-LP CT (if available) are the same as those for the investigation of suspected meningitis in any other circumstances. In adults there is little evidence for a major role for raised intracranial pressure, and LP is generally considered a safe manoeuvre. In all cases it is important that antimalarial therapy should not be delayed by the LP.

Treatment of malaria

A working party working under the auspices of WHO recently drew up recommendations for the antimalarial chemotherapy of severe malaria (Table 1.3 – taken from Transactions Supplement (in press)), which vary according to the level of health care available. Their guidelines for 'facilities with maximal possible health care' are given in Table 1.3.

Quinine

The cinchona alkaloids first came to medical attention in the 1630s, when bark from the cinchona tree was used successfully for the treatment of agues. Quinine remained the mainstay of antimalarial therapy until the 1950s, when it was supplanted by chloroquine and other synthetic antimalarials. However, with the inexorable spread of chloroquine resistance, quinine has once again come into widespread use, and is currently the most widely used antimalarial in the treatment of severe malaria. It is usually given by slow intravenous infusion via an infusion pump, though careful monitoring is

Table 1.3 Treatment of severe malaria.

Chloroquine-resistant or sensitivity unknown	Chloroquine-sensitive
1 Quinine 20 mg dihydrochloride salt/kg (loading dose)[a] diluted in 10 ml/kg isotonic fluid by intravenous infusion over 4 h, followed 8 h after the start of the loading dose by 10 mg/kg[b] over 4 h, 8-hourly until patient can swallow. Then quinine tablets 10 mg quinine salt/kg (maximum 600 mg) 8–12 hourly to complete 7 days treatment.[c] Alternatively the oral component can be replaced by a single dose of 25 mg/kg sulfadoxine and 1.25 mg/kg pyrimethamine (maximum 1500 mg sulfadoxine/75 mg pyrimethamine)	**1 Chloroquine** 10 mg base/kg in isotonic fluid by constant rate intravenous infusion over 8 h, followed by 15 mg/kg over 24 h
or	or
2 Artesunate 2.4 mg/kg intravenously on the first day followed by 1.2 mg/kg daily for a minimum of 3 days until the patient can take oral therapy of another effective antimalarial	**2 Chloroquine** 5 mg base/kg in isotonic fluid by constant rate intravenous infusion over 6 h, every 6 h, to a total dose of 25 mg/kg over 30 h
or	or
3 Artemether 3.2 mg/kg intramuscularly on the first day followed by 1.6 mg/kg daily for a minimum of 3 days until the patient can take oral therapy of another effective antimalarial	**3 Quinine, artesunate, artemether or quinidine** (see left hand column)
or	
4 Quinidine 15 mg base/kg (loading dose) by intravenous infusion over 4 h, followed 8 h after the start of the loading dose by 7.5 mg base/kg[b] over 4 h, 8-hourly until the patient can take oral medication, then quinine tablets or sulfadoxine/pyrimethamine as in *1* above.	

[a] Loading dose should not be given if patient has received quinine, quinidine or mefloquine within the preceding 12 h.

[b] In patients needing more than 48 h parenteral therapy, reduce the maintenance dose to 5–7 mg quinine dihydrochloride/kg or to 3.75–5 mg quinidine base/kg, 8-hourly.

[c] In areas where a 7-day course of quinine is not curative (e.g. Thailand and Vietnam) add a course of oral tetracycline 4 mg/kg four times daily or doxycycline 3 mg/kg once daily (except for children under 8 years and pregnant women), or clindamycin 10 mg/kg twice a day, for 7 days.

Reproduced with permission from *Severe and Complicated Malaria*, third edition by the World Health Organization, supplement to Transactions of the Royal Society of Tropical Medicine and Hygiene, 2000.

necessary due to the risk of cardiotoxicity (prolongation of the QTc interval on the ECG). In settings where close monitoring are unavailable adequate drug levels can be rapidly achieved using intramuscular injection (Waller *et al.*, 1990). Severe malaria can rapidly progress to death, so it is important that therapeutic blood levels of drug are attained as quickly as possible. For this reason it is recommended that all patients who have not been adequately treated previously with quinine should receive an initial loading dose (White *et al.*, 1983a; White, 1996). In areas where there is no quinine resistance, quinine can be given 12 hourly after the loading dose, but in quinine resistant areas the dosing interval should be shortened to 8 h. Oral therapy can be commenced once the patient is well enough to tolerate it, though a minimum of three doses of parenteral quinine is prudent. Alternatives to oral quinine include sulfa-doxine/pyrimethamine (in some areas) and mefloquine, though in this context this was associated with a 5% incidence of serious neuropsychiatric reactions in Vietnamese adults (Nguyen *et al.*, 1996).

Quinine commonly causes a complex of minor side-effects collectively known as cinchonism (tinnitus, high frequency hearing loss, and nausea), which although reversible is responsible for much of the poor compliance with oral courses. More seriously quinine can cause hyperinsulinaemic hypogly-caemia, which is difficult to detect in the unconscious patient and particularly common in pregnant women (White *et al.*, 1983b). Intramuscular quinine may cause sterile abscesses, and in Vietnam tetanus following intramuscular quinine administration is almost invariably fatal (Yen *et al.*, 1994). Quinine use is epidemiologically associated with blackwater fever, though the pathophysio-logical basis for this is not understood (Tran *et al.*, 1996).

Quinidine

Quinidine is a diastereomer of quinine, and although it is intrinsically more active as an antimalarial than quinine it is also more cardiotoxic (Phillips *et al.*, 1985). Consequently, when it is infused parenterally, cardiac monitoring is mandatory. It is most often used for the treatment of severe malaria when quinine or artemisinin derivatives are unavailable, usually in a first world setting.

Chloroquine

Chloroquine, a 4-aminoquinoline, is a synthetic antimalarial first used extensively in the 1950s (though first synthesized by German chemists in the 1930s). It is more rapidly acting than quinine and has a better side-effect profile, but because of the spread of chloroquine resistance its use in cerebral and other forms of severe malaria is limited to a few restricted geographical areas (parts of central America, Argentina, North Africa and the Middle East). Although with truly chloroquine-sensitive parasites there is a sugges-tion that chloroquine is more effective than quinine, when there is any doubt about sensitivity quinine or an artemisinin derivative should be used. Like quinine, chloroquine should be given by slow controlled intravenous infusion to avoid cardiotoxicity. It can also be given effectively by the intramuscular and subcutaneous routes, though as absorption remains very rapid care should still be taken.

Sulfadoxine/pyrimethamine

This combination of a long-acting sulphonamide and a dihydrofolate reductase inhibitor is used as an alternative to quinine or an artemisinin derivative for the treatment of chloroquine-resistant (or presumed chloroquine-resistant) falciparum malaria. It is given as a single dose intramuscularly, and can be used in the treatment of cerebral malaria when alternatives are unavailable. However, the likelihood of increasing clinical resistance and questions over absorption in critically ill patients make it a second line treatment in severe malaria.

Artemisinin derivatives

Artemisinin (Qinghaosu) is a sesquiterpene lactone peroxide extracted from the leaves of the plant *Artemisia annua* (sweet wormwood). Artemisinin and its derivatives artemether and artesunate are the most rapidly acting antimalarial drugs in terms of clearance of parasitaemia. The medicinal use of *Artemisia annua* as a remedy for fever (Qinghao) was mentioned in the Chinese medical literature almost 2000 years ago (Hong, AD 340). The active ingredient (Qinghaosu) was extracted by Chinese scientists in the 1970s, and shown to have powerful antimalarial activity. Clinical studies in China followed (Qinghaosu Antimalarial Coordinating Group, 1979), and since the late 1980s and early 1990s artemisinin and its derivatives have been used extensively in South-East Asia and increasingly in Africa. Animal toxicity studies have raised concerns about possible nerve cell damage with high doses of these drugs, but so far no neurotoxicity has been reported in man. In fact the Qinghaosu drugs appear very well tolerated, with no significant side-effects reported despite their use in several million patients with uncomplicated malaria. They have also been widely and successfully used for the treatment of cerebral and other forms of severe malaria. Early studies with artemether suggested that it might both shorten the duration of coma in cerebral malaria and substantially decrease mortality. Unfortunately these findings have not been confirmed by two large randomized controlled trials in severe malaria, one in Gambian children ($n = 576$) and the other in Vietnamese adults ($n = 560$). These showed no difference in mortality between artemether and quinine. Artemisinin and artesunate in suppository form have been successfully used for the treatment of severe malaria including cerebral malaria, leading to the exciting prospect of early and safe treatment of cerebral malaria in remote rural areas where parenteral administration is unavailable.

Supportive therapy and the treatment and prevention of complications

Nursing care

The importance of good nursing care in the management of severe malaria cannot be overemphasized. Essential areas include monitoring and nursing of the unconscious patient, accurate fluid balance, maintenance of the airway in the unconscious or fitting patient, and vigilance with respect to hypoglycaemia and the onset of other complications.

Hypoglycaemia

This dangerous complication of both severe malaria and quinine treatment should be actively excluded in all patients with severe malaria, especially those with impaired consciousness. If bedside blood glucose testing is not available, unconscious patients should be given 50 ml of 50% dextrose solution intravenously over 5–10 minutes as a therapeutic trial. Hypoglycaemia can recur repeatedly, and in the case of quinine-induced hypoglycaemia may occur several days after the initiation of therapy; constant vigilance is required. Failure to treat adequately severe or protracted hypoglycaemia may lead directly to death or permanent brain damage.

Convulsions

Convulsions should be treated promptly with either diazepam (rectally or intravenously) or intramuscular paraldehyde. Often convulsions are single and easily terminated with diazepam. Second line drugs used for refractory or repeated seizures include parenteral phenytoin and phenobarbitone. Prophylaxis of seizures with a single dose of phenobarbitone (3.5 mg/kg) significantly reduced fit frequency in a small study of non-immune children and adults in Thailand (White *et al.*, 1988), though a higher dose (10 mg/kg) failed to have an effect on fit frequency in Kenyan children (Winstanley *et al.*, 1992). A subsequent randomized double-blind trial of a single 20 mg/kg dose of phenobarbitone in Kenyan children with cerebral malaria demonstrated a significant reduction in seizures in the phenobarbitone group, but with a significantly higher overall mortality (Crawley *et al.*, 2000).

Hyperpyrexia

Paracetamol is the usual antipyretic treatment given in malaria, and can be given down a nasogastric tube or as a suppository. However, a recent study has suggested that paracetamol may prolong parasite clearance (Brandts *et al.*, 1997). Non-steroidal anti-inflammatories are probably as effective but are associated with an increased risk of gastrointestinal bleeding.

Fluid and electrolyte balance

Patients with severe malaria are usually somewhat dehydrated on presentation, but volume repletion should be undertaken cautiously as in malaria pulmonary oedema can develop at relatively low or even normal filling pressures (James, 1985). Isotonic saline should normally be used, though severely anaemic patients may require blood. In the presence of shock or ARF or any doubt about fluid status either the central venous pressure (CVP) or the pulmonary artery occlusion pressure (PAOP) should be monitored, keeping the CVP at

$\sim 5\,\mathrm{cmH_2O}$, and the PAOP between 8 and 12 mmHg. Despite these words of caution rehydration is essential in the dehydrated patient, and may lead to a dramatic improvement in any hypovolaemia-related metabolic acidosis.

Renal failure

In general, the management of malaria-associated ARF is similar to that of 'ATN' of any cause, though particular care should be taken not to fluid overload the patient, especially if facilities for mechanical ventilation are not on hand. In a retrospective study the mortality of malaria-associated ARF in the absence of dialysis facilities was found to be 70%; this was halved to 35% after the introduction of peritoneal dialysis (Trang et al., 1992). Although this and other studies demonstrate that acute peritoneal dialysis is generally effective in malaria-associated ARF (Canfield et al., 1968), a comparison with pumped veno-venous haemofiltration suggests that haemofiltration is more effective in terms of clearance of acidosis, creatinine and potassium and leads to a shorter period of dialysis dependence and a significant reduction in mortality (Day, unpublished data). Intermittent haemodialysis may also be used (Jackson and Woodruff, 1962), though a continuous form of renal replacement therapy is preferable in haemodynamically unstable patients. The standard indications for dialysis apply (metabolic acidosis, hyperkalaemia, fluid overload and signs or symptoms of the uraemic syndrome), though in rapid onset disease the threshold for dialysis should be low. Hyperkalaemic patients ($K^+ > 7\,\mathrm{mmol/l}$) should be given intravenous calcium followed by a glucose and insulin infusion while awaiting dialysis. There is no convincing evidence to support the use of 'renal dose' dopamine or high-dose frusemide in either incipient or established renal failure. Patients with very fulminant severe malaria are hypercatabolic and often develop a severe metabolic acidosis before the serum creatinine or potassium have a chance to rise; such patients may benefit from early dialysis.

The presence or development of blackwater fever should not be an indication for stopping quinine, unless a qinghaosu drug can be substituted (none is presently licensed in the UK). In general the presence of blackwater fever should not alter the principles of management described above.

Haemodynamic shock

Shock should be treated with oxygen and volume expansion (monitoring of central venous or pulmonary arterial pressures is mandatory). Massive haemorrhage (from GI tract or rarely a ruptured spleen) should be sought and excluded. A septic screen including blood cultures should be carried out, and appropriate broad spectrum antibiotics started to cover the possibility of bacterial sepsis. When necessary a dopamine infusion for inotropic support should be started (Day et al., 1996b; Bruneel et al., 1997). Dobutamine or noradrenaline may also be used, though there is little experience with their use in malaria. Adrenaline should be avoided as it induces serious lactic acidosis (Day et al., 1996b).

Treatment of malaria in pregnancy

Non-immune pregnant women with falciparum malaria are at increased risk of developing severe complications, particularly hypoglycaemia, pulmonary oedema, heart failure and post-partum haemorrhage. The fetus is also prone to hypoglycaemia, fetal distress and, like the mother, is at high risk of dying.

Pregnant women should if possible be nursed on an intensive care unit and contractions and fetal heart rate monitored. Blood glucose should be checked regularly. Quinine may worsen hypoglycaemia and theoretically may increase uterine contractions, but it is the drug most often used in this setting (Looareesuwan *et al.*, 1985). Artemether and artesunate appear so far to be safe in pregnancy, and can be given when available.

Adjuvant therapies

Over the years a wide range of adjuvant therapies have been proposed for the treatment of cerebral and other forms of severe malaria. Most have been suggested on theoretical grounds, often on the basis of unproven pathophysiological hypotheses. Some have fallen by the wayside after larger trials failed to confirm benefits claimed following preliminary studies. Others, though promising, remain largely untested but have failed to find a place in standard practice. A problem faced by those sorting through the large number of candidate adjuvant therapies is the relative lack of available study sites and resources to conduct large clinical studies in cerebral malaria; hence not every theoretically promising compound can be tested. At the time of writing no properly powered randomized drug trial of a study drug (antimalarial or otherwise) in severe malaria has ever shown a significant improvement in mortality over existing standard treatment.

Exchange blood transfusion

There exists a weak but significant positive correlation between peripheral parasite count and severity of malaria, and on this basis it has been suggested that patients with hyperparasitaemia might benefit from physical removal of parasitized erythrocytes (and any associated humoral toxins) by exchange blood transfusion. This has the added theoretical advantage of correcting any anaemia and replacing damaged unparasitized erythrocytes with fresh healthy ones. However, transfusion is not a risk-free practice, particularly in the developing world. The blood has to be properly cross-matched and adequately screened for blood-borne pathogens such as hepatitis B and HIV, and medical and nursing care of a standard sufficient to minimize the risks of over or under-transfusion is necessary. Exchange transfusion is still recommended by some, particularly in non-immune patients with very high parasitaemias (> 30%). No adequately powered randomized controlled trial has yet been conducted, and as such this rather dramatic treatment cannot be routinely recommended.

Corticosteroids

Because of their strong anti-inflammatory action and efficacy in treating vasogenic cerebral oedema, glucocorticoids such as dexamethasone have in the past been recommended for the treatment of cerebral malaria. This was based on the assumption that an increase in microvascular permeability and consequent cerebral oedema played a critical role in the pathophysiology of the condition (the 'permeability hypothesis') (Maegraith and Fletcher, 1972). There is evidence for a mild increase in systemic microvascular permeability in severe malaria (Davis *et al.*, 1992), but imaging studies show that most patients with cerebral malaria do not have marked cerebral oedema (Looareesuwan *et al.*, 1995; Cordoliani *et al.*, 1998). In a double-blind study of 100 Thai adults with strictly defined cerebral malaria, 2 mg/kg of dexamethasone over 48 h had no effect on mortality and increased coma duration (Warrell *et al.*, 1982). A smaller study with a higher dose of dexamethasone in Irian Jaya also failed to demonstrate any benefit (Hoffman *et al.*, 1988). However, neither of these studies was large enough to show a mortality difference, and there has not been any trial of corticosteroids in the patient group who on theoretical pathophysiological grounds might be expected to benefit most, African children with cerebral malaria.

Osmotic anticerebral oedema agents

The rationale for the use of mannitol and urea in invert sugar in cerebral malaria is similar for that offered for glucocorticoids. In a small study of Kenyan children with cerebral malaria and raised intracranial pressures (as measured by intracranial monitors) mannitol was successful in reducing intracranial pressure for short periods (Newton *et al.*, 1997b). However, no convincing clinical evidence exists to support the routine use of osmotic agents, and the danger of causing fluid and electrolyte derangements is real.

Iron chelators (desferrioxamine B)

By interfering with iron-dependent parts of the malaria parasite metabolism desferrioxamine, an iron chelator, is a weak antimalarial. Although a double-blind randomized trial in 83 Zambian children with cerebral malaria demonstrated a relatively reduced coma recovery time (Gordeuk *et al.*, 1992), a much larger study ($n = 352$) has recently failed to repeat this finding and demonstrated a slightly increased mortality in the desferrioxamine group (Thuma *et al.*, 1998).

Anti-TNF antibodies

The use of anti-TNF antibodies in the treatment of cerebral malaria was suggested following discovery of an association between high plasma TNFα levels and poor outcome in cerebral malaria (Grau *et al.*, 1989; Kwiatkowski *et al.*, 1990). However, a recent study of cytokine profiles in non-immune adults with severe falciparum malaria demonstrated that compared with other forms of severe malaria (such as hypoglycaemia and jaundice) cerebral malaria was associated with significantly lower pro-inflammatory cytokine levels, including TNFα (Day *et al.*, 1999). In a randomized double-blind placebo-controlled trial of anti-TNF antibodies in 302 Gambian children there was no influence on survival, and an increased number of neurological sequelae in the treatment group (van Heusbroek *et al.*, 1996).

Dichloroacetate

Lactic acidosis is a serious complication of severe malaria which often accompanies cerebral malaria, both in African children and in non-immune adult patients. By activating the pyruvate dehydrogenase complex, dichloracetate has been shown to lower plasma lactate concentrations in a number of conditions including severe falciparum malaria (Krishna *et al.*, 1994a). No survival effect has yet been shown for any disease. A large clinical trial in African children is now underway.

Conclusion

Cerebral malaria is a common and important CNS infection, which escapes the attention of many Western physicians. However, it is a major cause of mortality and neurological morbidity in developing countries, and increasingly affects travellers returning to developed countries from the tropics. Early clinical recognition of the disease is vital, as is early institution of effective treatment. The pathophysiology of the disease remains controversial, although modern studies using agreed clinical guidelines are having some success in addressing the roles of different mechanisms in malaria pathogenesis. These have led to a vastly improved understanding of the mechanisms underlying parasitized-erythrocyte sequestration, the roles of cytokines and neuroactive mediator release in cerebral malaria, and the importance of systemic acidosis in the pathogenesis of severe malaria in general in both adults and children. Several new adjuvant treatments are being evaluated in an attempt to exploit this new information.

Acknowledgements

Both authors are supported by the Wellcome Trust of Great Britain, as Career Development Fellows. We would like to thank the other members of the Oxford Tropical Network for discussions which have contributed to the ideas and research reported in this article, especially Professor Nick White, Professor Kevin Marsh and Professor Chris Newbold. We would like to acknowledge Dr David Ferguson (Electron Microscopy Unit, Department of Cellular Pathology, The John Radcliffe Hospital, Oxford) for permission to use the electron micrographs. All photomicrographs are from samples collected by the staff of the Wellcome Trust Clinical Research Unit, Centre for Tropical Diseases, Ho Chi Minh City, Vietnam.

References

Abdulla, M. N., Sokrab, T. E., Zaidan, Z. A., Siddig, H. E. and Ali, M. E. (1997). Post-malarial cerebellar ataxia in adult Sudanese patients. *East Afr. Med. J.*, **74**, 570–572.

Agbenyega, T., Angus, B., Beddu-Addo, G. *et al.* (1997). Plasma nitrogen oxides and blood lactate concentrations in Ghanaian children with malaria. *Trans. R. Soc. Trop. Med. Hyg.*, **91**(3), 298–302.

Aikawa, M., Iseki, M., Barnwell, J., Taylor, D., Oo, M. and Howard, R. (1990). The pathology of human cerebral malaria. *Am. J. Trop. Med. Hyg.*, **43**, 30–37.

al-Yaman, F., Awburn, M. M. and Clark, I. A. (1997). Serum creatinine levels and reactive nitrogen intermediates in children with cerebral malaria in Papua New Guinea. *Trans. R. Soc. Trop. Med. Hyg.*, **91**, 303–305.

Alonso, P. L., Lindsay, S. W., Armstrong, J. R. *et al.* (1991). The effect of insecticide-treated bed nets on mortality of Gambian children [see comments]. *Lancet*, **337**, 1499–1502.

Anstey, N. M., Weinberg, J. B., Hassanali, M. Y. *et al.* (1996). Nitric oxide in Tanzanian children with malaria: inverse relationship between malaria severity and nitric oxide production/nitric oxide synthase type 2 expression. *J. Exp. Med.*, **184**, 557–567.

Bajiya, H. N., and Kochar, D. K. (1996). Incidence and outcome of neurological sequelae in survivors of cerebral malaria. *J. Assoc. Physicians India*, **44**, 679–681.

Baruch, D., Pasloske, B., Singh, H. *et al.* (1995). Cloning the *P. falciparum* gene encoding PfEMP-1, a malaria variant antigen and adherence receptor on the surface of parasitized human erythocytes. *Cell*, **82**, 77–87.

Berendt, A., Ferguson, D., Gardner, J. *et al.* (1994a). Molecular mechanisms of sequestration in malaria. *Parasitology*, **108**, 19–28.

Berendt, A., Turner, G. and Newbold, C. (1994b). Cerebral malaria: the sequestration hypothesis. *Parasitol. Today*, **10**, 414–416.

Bignami, A. and Bastianelli, A. (1889). Observations of estivo-autumnal fever. *Riforma Med.*, **6**, 1334–1335.

Blanloeil, Y., Baron, D., de Lajartre, A. Y. and Nicolas, F. (1980). [Acute respiratory distress syndrome (ARDS) in cerebral malaria (author's transl.)]. *Sem. Hop.*, **56**, 1088–1090.

Bondi, F. S. (1992). The incidence and outcome of neurological abnormalities in childhood cerebral malaria: a long-term follow-up of 62 survivors. *Trans. R. Soc. Trop. Med. Hyg.*, **86**, 17–19.

Brandts, C. H., Ndjave, M., Graninger, W. and Kremsner, P. G. (1997). Effect of paracetamol on parasite clearance time in *Plasmodium falciparum* malaria [see comments]. *Lancet*, **350**, 704–709.

Brewster, D. R. and Greenwood, B. M. (1993). Seasonal variation of paediatric diseases in The Gambia, west Africa. *Ann. Trop. Paediatr.*, **13**, 133–146.

Brewster, D. R., Kwiatkowski, D. and White, N. J. (1990). Neurological sequelae of cerebral malaria in children. *Lancet*, **336**, 1039–1043.

Brown, H., Hien, T. T., Day, N. P. J., Mai, N. T., Chuong, L. V., Chau, T. T., Loc, P. P., Phu, N. H., Bethell, D., Farrar, J., Gatter, K., White, N. and Turner, G. (1999). Evidence of blood–brain barrier dysfunction in human cerebral malaria. *Neuropathol. Appl. Neurobiol.*, **25**, 331–340.

Bruneel, F., Gachot, B., Timsit, J. F. *et al.* (1997). Shock complicating severe falciparum malaria in European adults. *Intensive Care Med.*, **23**, 698–701.

Bygbjerg, I. and Lanng, C. (1982). Septicaemia as a complication of falciparum malaria (letter). *Trans. R. Soc. Trop. Med. Hyg.*, **76**, 705.

Calvet, M. C., Druilhe, P., Camacho-Garcia, R. and Calvet, J. (1993). Culture model for the study of cerebral malaria: antibodies from *Plasmodium falciparum*-infected comatose patients inhibit the dendritic development of Purkinje cells. *J. Neurosci. Res.*, **36**, 235–240.

Canfield, C. J., Miller, L. H., Bartelloni, P. J., Eichler, P. and Barry, K. (1968). Acute renal failure in *Plasmodium falciparum* malaria. Treatment by peritoneal dialysis. *Arch. Int. Med.*, **122**, 199–203.

Cao, X. T., Bethell, D. B., Pham, T. P. *et al.* (1997). Comparison of artemisinin suppositories, intramuscular artesunate and intravenous quinine for the treatment of severe childhood malaria. *Trans. R. Soc. Trop. Med. Hyg.*, **91**, 335–342.

Cerami, C., Frevert, U., Sinnis, P. *et al.* (1992). The basolateral domain of the hepatocyte plasma membrane bears receptors for the circumsporozoite protein of *Plasmodium falciparum* sporozoites. *Cell*, **70**, 1021–1033.

Chaiyaroj, S. C., Coppel, R. L., Magowan, C. and Brown, G. V. (1994). A *Plasmodium falciparum* isolate with a chromosome 9 deletion expresses a trypsin-resistant cytoadherence molecule. *Mol. Biochem. Parasitol.*, **66**, 21–30.

Chan-Ling, T., Neill, A. and Hunt, N. (1992). Early microvascular changes in murine cerebral malaria detected in retinal wholemounts. *Am. J. Pathol.*, **140**, 1121–1130.

Chandramohan, D. and Greenwood, B. M. (1998). Is there an interaction between human immunodeficiency virus and *Plasmodium falciparum*? *Int. J. Epidemiol.*, **27**, 296–301.

Clark, H. and Tomlinson, W. (1949). The pathological anatomy of malaria. In: *Malariology* Vol. 2, (M. F. Boyd, ed.). Philadelphia: WB Saunders. pp. 845–903.

Clark, I and Rockett, K. (1994). The cytokine theory of human cerebral malaria. *Parasitol. Today*, **10**, 410–412.

Clark, I., Rockett, K. and Cowden, W. (1992). Possible central role of nitric oxide in conditions clinically similar to cerebral malaria. *Lancet*, **340**, 894–896.

Clark, I. A., Rockett, K. A. and Cowden, W. B. (1991). Role of TNF in cerebral malaria [letter; comment]. *Lancet*, **337**, 302–303.

Cordoliani, Y. S., Sarrazin, J. L., Felten, D., Caumes, E., Leveque, C. and Fisch, A. (1998). MR of cerebral malaria. *Am. J. Neuroradiol.*, **19**, 871–874.

Cot, S., Ringwald, P., Mulder, B. *et al.* (1994). Nitric oxide in cerebral malaria [letter] [see comments]. *J. Infect. Dis.*, **169**, 1417–1418.

Crawley, J., Smith, S., Kirkham, F., Muthinji, P., Waruiru, C. and Marsh, K. (1996). Seizures and status epilepticus in childhood cerebral malaria [see comments]. *Q. J. Med.*, **89**, 591–597.

Crawley, J., Waruiru, C., Mithwani, S., Mwangi, I., Watkins, W., Ouma, D., Winstanley, P., Peto, T. and Marsh, K. (2000). Effect of phenobarbital on seizure frequency and mortality in childhood cerebral malaria: a randomised, controlled intervention study. *Lancet*, **355**(9205), 701–6.

Davis, T. M., Suputtamongkol, Y., Spencer, J. L. *et al.* (1992). Measures of capillary permeability in acute falciparum malaria: relation to severity of infection and treatment. *Clin. Infect. Dis.*, **15**, 256–266.

Day, N. P., Pham, T. D., Phan, T. L. *et al.* (1996a). Clearance kinetics of parasites and pigment-containing leukocytes in severe malaria. *Blood*, **88**, 4694–4700.

Day, N. P., Phu, N. H., Bethell, D. P. *et al.* (1996b). The effects of dopamine and adrenaline infusions on acid-base balance and systemic haemodynamics in severe infaction [see comments] [published erratum appears in *Lancet* 1996 Sep 28; 348(9031): 902]. *Lancet*, **348**, 219–223.

Day, N. P. J., Hien, T. T., Schollaardt, T., Loc, P. P., Chuong, L. V., Chau, T. T. H., Mai, N. T. H., Phu, N. H., Sinh, D. X., White, N. J. and Ho, M. (1999). The prognostic and pathophysiological role of pro- and anti-inflammatory cytokines in severe malaria. *J. Infect. Dis.*, **180**, 1288–1297.

de Silva, H. J., Hoang, P., Dalton, H., de Silva, N. R., Jewell, D. P. and Peiris, J. B. (1992). Immune activation during cerebellar dysfunction following *Plasmodium falciparum* malaria. *Trans. R. Soc. Trop. Med. Hyg.*, **86**, 129–131.

Dondorp, A., Angus, B., Hardeman, M. *et al.* (1997). Prognostic significance of reduced red cell deformability in severe falciparum malaria. *Am. J. Trop. Med. Hyg.*, **57**, 507–511.

Dudgeon, L., and Clarke, C. (1917). A contribution to the microscopical histology of malaria. *Lancet,* **ii**, 153–156.

Dürck, H. (1925). Uber die mit herdformingen Glialproduktionen einhergehenden Ekrankungen des Zentralnervensystems. *Arch. Schiffs- u. Tropen-Hyg.*, **29**, 43–76.

Edington, G. M. (1967). Pathology of malaria in West Africa. *Br. Med. J.*, **1**, 715–718.

Endeshaw, Y. and Assefa, D. (1990). Factors affecting outcome of treatment in a suboptimal clinical setting. *J. Trop. Med. Hyg.*, **93**, 44–47.

English, M., Sauerwein, R., Waruiru, C. *et al.* (1997). Acidosis in severe childhood malaria [see comments]. *Q. J. Med.*, **90**, 263–270.

English, M., Waruiru, C. and Marsh, K. (1996). Transfusion for respiratory distress in life-threatening childhood malaria. *Am. J. Trop. Med. Hyg.*, **55**, 525–530.

Ewing, J. (1902). Contribution to the pathological anatomy of malaria fever. *J. Exp. Med.*, **6**, 119–180.

Fein, I. A., Rackow, E. and Shapiro, L. (1978). Acute pulmonary edema in *Plasmodium falciparum* malaria. *Am. Rev. Resp. Dis.*, **118**, 425–429.

Fernandez-Reyes, D., Craig, A. G., Kyes, S. A. *et al.* (1997). A high frequency African coding polymorphism in the N-terminal domain of ICAM-1 predisposing to cerebral malaria in Kenya. *Hum. Mol. Genet.*, **6**, 1357–1360.

Gardner, J. P., Pinches, R. A., Roberts, D. J. and Newbold, C. I. (1996). Variant antigens and endothelial receptor adhesion in *Plasmodium falciparum*. *Proc. Natl. Acad. Sci. USA*, **93**, 3503–3508.

Gaskell, J. Miller, W. (1920). Studies on malignant malaria in Macedonia. *Q. J. Med.*, **13**, 381–426.

Gordeuk, V., Thuma, P., Brittenham, G. *et al.* (1992). Effect of iron chelation therapy on recovery from deep coma in children with cerebral malaria [see comments]. *N. Engl. J. Med.*, **327**, 1473–1477.

Grau, G. E., Piguet, P. F., Engers, H. D., Louis, J. A., Vassalli, P. and Lambert, P. H. (1986). L3T4+ T lymphocytes play a major role in the pathogenesis of murine cerebral malaria. *J. Immunol.*, **137**, 2348–2354.

Grau, G. E., Taylor, T. E., Molyneux, M. E. *et al.* (1989). Tumor necrosis factor and disease severity in children with falciparum malaria. *N. Engl. J. Med.*, **320**, 1586–1591.

Greenwood, B., Bradley, A., Greenwood, A. *et al.* (1987). Mortality and morbidity from malaria among children in a rural area of the Gambia, West Africa. *Trans. R. Soc. Trop. Med. Hyg.*, **81**, 478–486.

Greenwood, B., Marsh, K. and Snow, R. (1991). Why do some African children develop severe malaria? *Parasitol. Today*, 7, 277–281.

Hadley, T. J. (1986). Invasion of erythrocytes by malaria parasites: a cellular and molecular overview. *Ann. Rev. Microbiol.*, **40**, 451–477.

Hien, T. T., Day, N. P. J., Phu, N. H. *et al.* (1996). A controlled trial of artemether or quinine in Vietnamese adults with severe falciparum malaria. *N. Engl. J. Med.*, **355**, 76–83.

Hill, A., Allsop, C., Kwaiatkowski, D. *et al.* (1991). Common West African HLA antigens are associated with protection from severe malaria. *Nature*, **352**, 595–600.

Hoffman, S. L., Rustama, D., Punjabi, N. H. *et al.* (1988). High-dose dexamethasone in quinine-treated patients with cerebral malaria: a double-blind, placebo-controlled trial. *J. Infect. Dis.*, **158**, 325–331.

Hong, G. (AD 340). *Handbook of Emergency Treatments*.

Jackson, R. and Woodruff, A. (1962). The artificial kidney in malaria and blackwater fever. *Br. Med. J.*, **i**, 1367–1372.

James, M. (1985). Pulmonary damage associated with falciparum malaria: a report of ten patients. *Ann. Trop. Med. Parasitol.*, **79**, 123–138.

Jennings, V. M., Actor, J. K., Lal, A. A. and Hunter, R. L. (1997). Cytokine profile suggesting that murine cerebral malaria is an encephalitis. *Infect. Immun.*, **65**, 4883–4887.

Kean, B. and Smith, J. (1944). Death due to estivo-autumnal malaria. *Am. J. Trop. Med.*, **24**, 317–322.

Kremsner, P., Winkler. S., Wilding, E. *et al.* (1996). High plasma levels of nitrogen oxides are associated with severe disease and correlate with rapid parasitological and clinical cure in *Plasmodium falciparum* malaria. *Trans. R. Soc. Trop. Med. Hyg.*, **90**, 44–47.

Krishna, S., Supanaranond, W., Pukritayakamee, S. *et al.* (1994a). Dichloroacetate for lactic acidosis in severe malaria: a pharmacokinetic and pharmacodynamic assessment. *Metabolism*, **43**, 974–981.

Krishna, S., Waller, D. W., ter Kuile, F. *et al.* (1994b). Lactic acidosis and hypo-glycaemia in children with severe malaria: pathophysiological and prognostic significance. *Trans. R. Soc. Trop. Med. Hyg.*, **88**, 67–73.

Kwiatkowski, D., Hill, A. V., Sambou, I. *et al.* (1990). TNF concentration in fatal cerebral, non-fatal cerebral, and uncomplicated *Plasmodium falciparum* malaria. *Lancet*, **336**, 1201–1204.

Lemercier, G., Rey, M. and Collomb, H. (1966). [Cerebral lesions of malaria in children]. *Bull Soc. Pathol. Exot. Filiales*, **59**, 533–548.

Li, J., Wirtz, R. A. and McCutchan, T. F. (1997). Analysis of malaria parasite RNA from decade-old Giemsa-stained blood smears and dried mosquitoes. *Am. J. Trop. Med. Hyg.*, **57**, 727–731.

Looareesuwan, S., White, N., Karbwang, J. *et al.* (1985). Quinine and severe falciparum malaria in late pregnancy. *Lancet*, **ii**, 4–8.

Looareesuwan, S., Wilairatana, P., Krishna, S. *et al.* (1995). Magnetic resonance imaging of the brain in patients with cerebral malaria. *Clin. Infect. Dis.*, **21**, 300–309.

Lucas, S., Hounnou, A., Bell, J. *et al.* (1996). Severe cerebral swelling is not observed in children dying with malaria. *Q. J. Med.*, **89**, 351–353.

Luxemburger, C., Nosten, F., Raimond, S. D., Chongsuphajaisiddhi, T. and White, N. J. (1995). Oral artesunate in the treatment of uncomplicated hyperparasitemic falciparum malaria. *Am. J. Trop. Med. Hyg.*, **53**, 522–525.

Luxemburger, C., Ricci, F., Nosten, F., Raimond, D., Bathet, S., and White, N. J. (1997). The epidemiology of severe malaria in an area of low transmission in Thailand. *Trans. R. Soc. Trop. Med. Hyg.*, **91**, 256–262.

Mabeza, G. F., Moyo, V. M., Thuma, P. E. *et al.* (1995). Predictors of severity of illness on presentation in children with cerebral malaria. *Ann. Trop. Med. Parasitol.*, **89**, 221–228.

MacPherson, G. G., Warrell, M. J., White, N. J., Looareesuwan, S. and Warrell, D. A. (1985). Human cerebral malaria. A quantitative ultrastructural analysis of parasitized erythrocyte sequestration. *Am. J. Pathol.*, **119**, 385–401.

Maegraith, B. (1948). Synthesis: the pathogenesis of malaria. In: *Pathological Processes In Malaria and Blackwater Fever*, Oxford: Blackwell Scientific Publications, pp. 378–379.

Maegraith, B. and Fletcher, A. (1972). The pathogenesis of mammalian malaria. *Adv. Parasitol.*, **10**, 49–75.

Marchiafava, E., and Bignami, A. (1894). On summer–autumnal malarial fevers. In: *Malaria and the Parasites of Malaria Fevers*, vol. 150, London: The New Sydenham Society, pp. 1–234.

Marsh, K., Forster, D., Waruiru, C. *et al.* (1995). Indicators of life-threatening malaria in African children [see comments]. *N. Engl. J. Med.*, **332**, 1399–1404.

Martell, R., Kallenbach, J. and Zwi, S. (1979). Pulmonary oedema in falciparum malaria. *Br. Med. J.*, **i**, 1763–1764.

McGuire, W., Hill, A. V., Allsopp, C. E., Greenwood, B. M. and Kwiatkowski, D. (1994). Variation in the TNF-alpha promoter region associated with susceptibility to cerebral malaria. *Nature*, **371**, 508–510.

Medana, I. M., Hunt, N. H. and Chan-Ling, T. (1997a). Early activation of microglia in the pathogenesis of fatal murine cerebral malaria. *Glia*, **19**, 91–103.

Medana, I. M., Hunt, N. H., and Chaudhri, G. (1997b). Tumor necrosis factor-alpha expression in the brain during fatal murine cerebral malaria: evidence for production by microglia and astrocytes. *Am. J. Pathol.*, **150**, 1473–1486.

Meek, S. R. (1988). Epidemiology of malaria in displaced Khmers on the Thai–Kampuchean border. *Southeast Asian J. Trop. Med. Publ. Hlth*, **19**, 243–252.

Molyneux, M. E., Taylor, T. E., Wirima, J. J. and Borgstein, A. (1989). Clinical features and prognostic indicators in paediatric cerebral malaria: a study of 131 comatose Malawian children [see comments]. *Q. J. Med.*, **71**, 441–459.

Mutendam, A. H., Jaffar, S., Bleichrodt, N. and van Hensbroek, M. B. (1996). Absence of neuropsychological sequelae following cerebral malaria in Gambian children. *Trans. R. Soc. Trop. Med. Hyg.*, **90**, 391–394.

Newton, C. R., Chokwe, T., Schellenberg, J. A. *et al.* (1997a). Coma scales for children with severe falciparum malaria. *Trans. R. Soc. Trop. Med. Hyg.*, **91**, 161–165.

Newton, C. R., Crawley, J., Sowumni, A. *et al.* (1997b). Intracranial hypertension in Africans with cerebral malaria. *Arch. Dis. Child.*, **76**, 219–226.

Newton, C. R., Kirkham, F. J., Winstanley, P. A. *et al.* (1991). Intracranial pressure in African children with cerebral malaria [see comments]. *Lancet*, **337**, 573–576.

Newton, C. R. and Krishna, S. (1998). Severe falciparum malaria in children: current understanding of pathophysiology and supportive treatment. *Pharmacol. Ther.*, **79**, 1–53.

Newton, C. R., Marsh, K., Peshu, N. and Kirkham, F. J. (1996). Perturbations of cerebral hemodynamics in Kenyans with cerebral malaria. *Pediatr. Neurol.*, **15**, 41–49.

Newton, C. R., Peshu, N., Kendall, B. *et al.* (1994). Brain swelling and ischaemia in Kenyans with cerebral malaria. *Arch. Dis. Child.*, **70**, 281–287.

Nguyen, T. H., Day, N. P., Ly, V. C. *et al.* (1996). Post-malaria neurological syndrome [see comments]. *Lancet*, **348**, 917–921.

Nussler, A., Eling, W. and Kremsner, P. (1994). Patients with *Plasmodium falciparum* malaria and *Plasmodium vivax* malaria show increased nitrite and nitrate plasma levels. *J. Infect. Dis.*, **169**, 1418–1419.

Oo, M. M., Aikawa, M., Than, T. *et al.* (1987). Human cerebral malaria: a pathological study. *J. Neuropathol. Exp. Neurol.*, **46**, 223–231.

Patnaik, J. K., Das, B. S., Mishra, S. K., Mohanty, S., Satpathy, S. K. and Mohanty, D. (1994). Vascular clogging, mononuclear cell margination, and enhanced vascular permeability in the pathogenesis of human cerebral malaria. *Am. J. Trop. Med. Hyg.*, **51**, 642–647.

Phillips, R. E., Warrell, D. A., White, N. J., Looareesuwan, S. and Karbwang, J. (1985). Intravenous quinidine for the treatment of severe falciparum malaria. Clinical and pharmacokinetic studies. *N. Engl. J. Med.*, **312**, 1273–1278.

Phu, N., Day, N., Diep, T., Fergusson, D. and White, N. (1995). Intraleukocytic malaria pigment and prognosis in severe malaria. *Trans. R. Soc. Trop. Med. Hyg.*, **89**, 200–204.

Pieroni, P., Mills, C. D., Ohrt, C., Harrington, M. A. and Kain, K. C. (1998). Comparison of the ParaSight-F test and the ICT Malaria Pf test with the polymerase chain reaction for the diagnosis of *Plasmodium falciparum* malaria in travellers. *Trans. R. Soc. Trop. Med. Hyg.*, **92**, 166–169.

Piper, R., Lebras, J., Wentworth, L. (1999). Immunocapture diagnostic assays for malaria using Plasmodium lactate dehydrogenase (pLDH). *Am. J. Trop. Med. Hyg.*, **60**, 109–118.

Plum, F. and Posner, J. (1980). *The Diagnosis of Stupor and Coma*. Philadelphia: FA Davis Company.

Polder, T. W., Jerusalem, C. R. and Eling, W. M. (1991). Morphological characteristics of intracerebral arterioles in clinial (*Plasmodium falciparum*) and experimental (*Plasmodium berghei*) cerebral malaria. *J. Neurol. Sci.*, **101**, 35–46.

Pongponratn, E., Riganti, M., Punpoowong, B. and Aikawa, M. (1991). Microvascular sequestration of paratisized erythrocytes in human falciparum malaria: a pathological study. *Am. J. Trop. Med. Hyg.*, **44**, 168–75.

Pukrittayakamee, S., White, N. J., Davis, T. M. *et al.* (1992). Hepatic blood flow and metabolism in severe falciparum malaria: clearance of intravenously administered galactose. *Clin. Sci. (Colch)*, **82**, 63–70.

Qinghaosu Antimalarial Coordinating Group. (1979). Antimalarial studies on qinghaosu. *Chinese Med. J.*, **98**, 811–816.

Rigdon, R. (1944). The pathological lesions in the brain in malaria. *Southern Med. J.*, **37**, 687–694.

Robert, C., Peyrol, S., Pouvelle, B., Gay-Andrieu, F. and Gysin, J. (1996). Ultrastructural aspects of *Plasmodium falciparum*-infected erythrocyte adherence to endothelial cells of Saimiri brain microvasculature. *Am. J. Trop. Med. Hyg.*, **54**, 169–177.

Roberts, D., Craig, A., Berendt, A. *et al.* (1992). Rapid switching to multiple antigenic and adhesive phenotyps in malaria. *Nature*, **357**, 689–692.

Sanni, L. A., Thomas, S. R., Tattam, B. N. *et al.* (1998). Dramatic changes in oxidative tryptophan metabolism along the kynurenine pathway in experimental cerebral and noncerebral malaria. *Am. J. Pathol.*, **152**, 611–619.

Senanayake, N. and de Silva, H. J. (1994). Delayed cerebellar ataxia complicating falciparum malaria: a clinical study of 74 patients. *J. Neurol.*, **241**, 456–459.

Sitprija, V., Indraprasit, S., Pochanugool, C., Benyajati, C. and Piyaratn, P. (1967). Renal failure in malaria. *Lancet*, **i**, 186–188.

Slater, A. F., Swiggard, W. J., Orton, B. R. *et al.* (1991). An iron-carboxylate bond links the heme units of malaria pigment. *Proc. Natl. Acad. Sci. USA*, **88**, 325–329.

Smith, J., Chitnis, C., Craig, A. *et al.* (1995). Switches in expression of *Plasmodium falciparum var* genes correlate with changes in antigenic and cytoadherent phenotypes of infected erythrocytes. *Cell*, **82**, 101–110.

Snow, R. W., Armstrong, J. R., Forster, D. *et al.* (1992). Childhood deaths in Africa: uses and limitations of verbal autopsies. *Lancet*, **340**, 351–355.

Snow, R. W., Bastos de Azevedo, I., Lowe, B. S. *et al.* (1994). Severe childhood malaria in two areas of markedly different falciparum transmission in east Africa. *Acta Trop*, **57**, 289–300.

Snow, R. W., Omumbo, J. A., Lowe, B. *et al.* (1997). Relation between severe malaria morbidity in children and level of *Plasmodium falciparum* transmission in Africa [see comments]. *Lancet*, **349**, 1650–1654.

Spitz, S. (1946). The pathology of acute falciparum malaria. *Mil. Surg.*, **99**, 555–572.

Stone, W., Hanchett, J. and Knepshield, J. (1972). Acute renal insufficiency due to falciparum malaria. Review of 42 cases. *Arch. Int. Med.*, **129**, 620–628.

Su, X.-z., Heatwole, V., Wertheimer, S. *et al.* (1995). The large diverse gene family *var* encodes proteins involved in cytoadherence and antigenic variation of *Plasmodium falciparum*-infected erythrocytes. *Cell*, **82**, 89–100.

Taramelli, D., Basilico, N., De Palma, A. M. *et al.* (1998). The effect of synthetic malaria pigment (beta-haematin) on adhesion molecule expression and interleukin-6 production by human endothelial cells. *Trans. R. Soc. Trop. Med. Hyg.*, **92**, 57–62.

Taverne, J., Bate, C. A., Kwiatkowski, D., Jakobsen, P. H. and Playfair, J. H. (1990). Two soluble antigens of *Plasmodium falciparum* induce tumor necrosis factor release from macrophages. *Infect. Immun.*, **58**, 2923–2928.

Taylor, A. M., Day, N. P., Sinh, D. X. *et al.* (1998). Reactive nitrogen intermediates and outcome in severe adult malaria. *Trans. R. Soc. Trop. Med. Hyg.*, **92**, 170–175.

Taylor, T. E., Borgstein, A. and Molyneux, M. E. (1993). Acid-base status in paediatric *Plasmodium falciparum* malaria [see comments]. *Q. J. Med.*, **86**, 99–109.

Taylor, T. E. and Molyneux, M. E. (1988). Blood glucose levels in Malawian children before and during administration of intravenous quinine for severe malaria. *N. Engl. J. Med.*, **319**, 1040–1047.

Thuma, P. E., Mabeza, G. F., Biemba, G. *et al.* (1998). Effect of iron chelation therapy on mortality in Zambian children with cerebral malaria [In Process Citation]. *Trans. R. Soc. Trop. Med. Hyg.*, **92**, 214–218.

Toro, G. and Roman, G. (1978). Cerebral malaria. A disseminated vasculomyelinopathy. *Arch. Neurol.*, **35**, 271–275.

Tran, T. H., Day, N. P., Ly, V. C. *et al.* (1996). Blackwater fever in southern Vietnam: a prospective descriptive study of 50 cases. *Clin. Infect. Dis*, **23**, 1274–81.

Trang, T. T., Phu, N. H., Vinh, H. *et al.* (1992). Acute renal failure in patients with severe falciparum malaria. *Clin. Infect. Dis.*, **15**, 874–880.

Turner, G. (1997). Cerebral malaria. *Brain Pathol.*, **7**, 569–582.

Turner, G. D., Ly, V. C., Nguyen, T. H. *et al.* (1998). Systemic endothelial activation occurs in both mild and severe malaria. Correlating dermal microvascular endothelial cell phenotype and soluble cell adhesion molecules with disease severity. *Am. J. Pathol.*, **152**, 1477–1487.

Turner, G. D., Morrison, H., Jones, M. *et al.* (1994). An immunohistochemical study of the pathology of fatal malaria. Evidence for widespread endothelial activation and a potential role for intercellular adhesion molecule-1 in cerebral sequestration. *Am. J. Pathol.*, **145**, 1057–1069.

van Hensbroek, M. B., Palmer, A., Jaffar, S., Schneider, G. and Kwiatkowski, D. (1997). Residual neurologic sequelae after childhood cerebral malaria. *J. Pediatr.*, **131**, 125–129.

van Hensbroek, M. B., Palmer, A., Onyiorah, E., Schneider, G., Jaffar, S., Dolan, G., Memming, H., Frenkel, J., Enwere, G., Bennett, S., Kwiatkowski, D., Greenwood, B. (1996). The effect of a monoclonal antibody to tumor necrosis factor on survival from childhood cerebral malaria. *J. Infect. Dis.*, **174**(5), 1091–7.

Varney, N. R., Roberts, R. J., Springer, J. A., Connell, S. K, and Wood, P. S. (1997). Neuropsychiatric sequelae of cerebral malaria in Vietnam veterans. *J. Nerv. Ment. Dis.*, **185**, 695–703.

Walker, O., Salako, L., Thomas, J., Sodeine, O. and Bondi, F. (1992). Prognostic risk factors and post mortem findings in cerebral malaria in children. *Trans. R. Soc. Trop. Med. Hyg.*, **86**, 491–493.

Waller, D., Crawley, J., Nosten, F. *et al.* (1991a). Intracranial pressure in childhood cerebral malaria. *Trans. R. Soc. Trop. Med. Hyg.*, **85**, 362–364.

Waller, D., Crawley, J., Nosten, F. *et al.* (1991b). Intracranial pressure in childhood cerebral malaria. *Trans. R. Soc. Trop. Med. Hyg.*, **85**, 362–364.

Waller, D., Krishna, S., Craddock, C. *et al.* (1990). The pharmacokinetic properties of intramuscular quinine in Gambian children with severe falciparum malaria. *Trans. Roy. Soc. Trop. Med. Hyg.*, **84**, 488–491.

Waller, D., Krishna, S., Crawley, J. *et al.* (1995). Clinical features and outcome of severe malaria in Gambian children. *Clin. Infect. Dis.*, **21**, 577–587.

Warrell, D., Looareesuwan, S., Warrell, M. *et al.* (1982). Dexamethasone proves deleterious in cerebral malaria: a double-blind trial in 100 comatose patients. *N. Engl. J. Med.*, **306**, 313–319.

Waruiru, C. M., Newton, C. R., Forster, D. *et al.* (1996). Epileptic seizures and malaria in Kenyan children. *Trans. R. Soc. Trop. Med. Hyg.*, **90**, 152–155.

Weatherall, D., Bell, J., Clegg, J. *et al.* (1988). Genetic factors as determinants of infectious disease transmission in human communities. *Philos. Trans. R. Soc. Lond. Biol.*, **321**, 327–348.

White, N. (1996). The treatment of malaria. *N. Engl. J. Med.*, **335**, 800–806.

White, N. J. (1991). Lumbar puncture in cerebral malaria [letter]. *Lancet*, **338**, 640–641.

White, N. J., Looareesuwan, S., Phillips, R. E., Chanthavanich, P. and Warrell, D. A. (1988). Single dose phenobarbitone prevents convulsions in cerebral malaria. *Lancet*, **2**, 64–66.

White, N. J., Looareesuwan, S., Warrell, D. A. *et al.* (1983a). Quinine loading dose in cerebral malaria. *Am. J. Trop. Med. Hyg.*, **32**, 1–5.

White, N. J., Marsh, K., Turner, R. C. *et al.* (1987). Hypoglycaemia in African children with severe malaria. *Lancet*, **1**, 708–711.

White, N. J., Warrell, D. A., Chanthavanich, P. *et al.* (1983b). Severe hypoglycemia and hyperinsulinemia in falciparum malaria. *N. Engl. J. Med.*, **309**, 61–66.

White, N. J., Warrell, D. A., Looareesuwan, S., Chanthavanich, P., Phillips, R. E. and Pongpaew, P. (1985). Pathophysiological and prognostic significance of cerebrospinal-fluid lactate in cerebral malaria. *Lancet*, **1**, 776–778.

Winstanley, P. A., Newton, C. R., Pasvol, G. *et al.* (1992). Prophylactic phenobarbitone in young children with severe falciparum malaria: pharmacokinetics and clinical effects. *Br. J. Clin. Pharmacol.*, **33**, 149–154.

World Health Organization. (1990). Severe and complicated malaria. *Trans. Roy. Soc. Trop. Med. Hyg.*, **84**, 1–65.

World Health Organization. (1992). World malaria situation 1990. Division of Control of Tropical Diseases. *World Hlth Stat, Q*, **45**, 257–266.

Wright, P. W., Avery, W. G., Ardill, W. D. and McLarty, J. W. (1993). Initial clinical assessment of the comatose patient: cerebral malaria vs meningitis. *Pediatr. Infect. Dis. J.*, **12**, 37–41.

Yen, L. M., Dao, L. M., Day, N. P. *et al.* (1994). Role of quinine in the high mortality of intramuscular injection tetanus [see comments]. *Lancet*, **344**, 786–787.

2

Neurological aspects of Lyme disease

Patricia K. Coyle

Introduction

Lyme disease is a bacterial infection due to a tick-borne spirochaete, *Borrelia burgdorferi* (Steere, 1989). With the exception of rare congenital cases, virtually all transmissions involve tick bite. The resulting infection targets specific body organs to cause characteristic skin, musculoskeletal, heart, eye, and nervous system syndromes. In the USA Lyme disease accounts for over 95% of vector-borne infections. It is routinely included in the differential diagnosis of many neurological conditions. Yet much misinformation exists about Lyme disease, with controversial diagnostic, management, and medical economic issues. Perhaps most importantly, Lyme disease provides a model to examine how a unique pathogen produces neurological disease. This chapter will review current information on this recently recognized infection, as well as areas that are likely to see advances in the next few years.

History

In retrospect, Lyme disease was recognized in Europe for more than a century (Coyle, 1997b). Acrodermatitis chronica atrophicans (ACA), a late stage skin lesion, was first described in 1883. Erythema migrans (EM), the skin lesion manifestation of early local infection, was first noted in 1909 (Dammin, 1989). Although known to be infectious, no organism could be identified. Some EM patients developed a painful lymphocytic meningoradiculoneuritis, referred to as Bannwarth s syndrome. Thus skin and neurological Lyme disease syndromes were described in the European literature well before the epidemic of arthritis cases in Lyme and Old Lyme, Connecticut, USA.

Between 1972 and 1976, 52 individuals living in the area of Lyme, Connecticut developed a relapsing and remitting arthritis misdiagnosed as juvenile rheumatoid arthritis (Steere *et al.*, 1977). Thirteen had had a prior rash, very similar to the EM reported from Europe. Subsequent epidemiological investigation recognized a new entity initially referred to as Lyme arthritis.

Once its multisystem involvement was appreciated, it was renamed Lyme disease.

In 1981 Dr Willy Burgdorfer at the Rocky Mountain Laboratories identified spirochaetes in *Ixodes scapularis* ticks harvested from Lyme-endemic areas (Burgdorfer, 1984). These new spirochaetes, named after their discoverer, were subsequently cultured from blood, cerebrospinal fluid (CSF), and skin of Lyme disease patients (Steere *et al.*, 1983; Benach *et al.*, 1983). Subsequent studies confirmed *B. burgdorferi* in European skin and neurological cases.

Initially, it was believed that *B. burgdorferi* was imported from Europe to North America. Subsequent data document that *B. burgdorferi* was present in North America long before the arthritis epidemic in the 1970s. EM occurred in a Wisconsin physician in 1969 (Burgdorfer, 1993). Montauk knee, a painless monoarticular arthritis, was noted on the eastern tip of Long Island in the 1940s. Archival data, using polymerase chain reaction (PCR), detect *B. burgdorferi* in samples dating back to the late 1800s in North America and Europe (Marshall *et al.*, 1994; Matuschka *et al.*, 1996).

Epidemiology

Lyme disease is widely distributed, but geographically restricted to regions inhabited by its vector, small hard body ticks of the *Ixodes ricinus* complex. In North America most cases occur in the northeast, mid-Atlantic, upper midwest, and upper Pacific coastal areas. Forty eight states and the District of Columbia have reported cases of Lyme disease. However, it is actually confined to approximately 100 counties in 10 states in the northeast and mid-Atlantic regions, upper northcentral region, and northern California. Over 90% of cases come from eight states (Connecticut, Delaware, Maryland, New Jersey, New York, Pennsylvania, Rhode Island, Wisconsin). *B. burgdorferi* or a similar spirochaete is present in the south as well, where it may show greater heterogeneity than in the north (Barbour, 1996; Oliver, 1996). In Canada, enzootic transmission is documented on the long point peninsula of Ontario. Most Canadian infections are from the provinces of Ontario and Manitoba, but cases have been reported from seven provinces and Ixodid ticks have been shown in six provinces. In Europe Lyme disease is a major problem in Germany, Austria, and Switzerland. In Sweden *B. burgdorferi* is the most common CNS bacterial pathogen. Cases of Lyme disease can be found in most European countries. In addition, Lyme disease occurs across a wide area of Asia, including Asiatic Russia, northeast China, and Japan.

The disease may be even more widespread (Olsen *et al.*, 1995). In the southern hemisphere PCR has been positive for *B. burgdorferi* DNA in *Ixodes* ticks. Suggestive cases are being investigated in Mexico, and apparent clinical cases are reported from Africa, Australia, and South America.

In the USA over 128 000 cases have been reported to the Centers for Disease Control and Prevention (CDC) since 1982, when formal surveillance began. In some endemic areas cases are increasing, and the organism is spreading to new regions. In 1998 there were 16 801 reported cases. This is probably too low, since there is significant under reporting (Orloski *et al.*, 1993). The incidence of Lyme disease approximates five cases per 100 000, and in very endemic areas the incidence rate is 1–3% a year. Lyme disease affects all ages and both sexes, but children up to age 14 and adults aged 30 or over are particular targets. Time spent out of doors is the most consistent risk factor.

Borrelia burgdorferi

B. burgdorferi is a helical, motile, Gram-negative bacterial spirochaete (Barbour and Hayes, 1986; Rosa, 1997). It consists of a central protoplasmic cylinder, with seven to twelve attached periplasmic flagella surrounded by an outer cellular membrane, and covered by a carbohydrate-containing slime layer. The organism requires specialized artificial medium for culture, grows best at a temperature between 30° and 37°C, and takes weeks to grow out. Organisms stain with Giemsa and special silver stains.

Recent molecular and genetic studies indicate that *B. burgdorferi* encompasses multiple genospecies. This probably has clinical significance (Table 2.1) (Balmetti and Piffaretti, 1995). The organism itself contains at least 105 lipoproteins. Some are unique, while others are shared with other pathogens. Shared antigenicity can lead to false positive antibody tests, and a positive Lyme serology occurs in approximately 25% of patients with significant bacterial infections such as endocarditis.

Recent studies also indicate that *B. burgdorferi* changes surface proteins in response to environmental stressors. During *in vitro* culture proteins are lost, which can lead to loss of pathogenicity. *In vitro* within the resting tick, organisms show marked expression of outer surface protein A (OspA), and minimal expression of OspC (Schwan *et al.*, 1995). In the feeding tick, OspA is

Table 2.1   *B. burgdorferi* sensu lato complex.

Genospecies	Features
B. burgdorferi sensu stricto	Isolated from North America, less so Europe and Asia Less genetic diversity Produces Lyme disease Associated with neurological, dermatological, and musculoskeletal disease
B. garinii	Isolated from Europe, Asia More genetic diversity Produces Lyme disease Associated with neurological disease
B. afzelii	Isolated from Europe, Asia More genetic diversity Produces Lyme disease Associated with dermatological disease
B. andersonii	Isolated from North America
B. japonica	Isolated from Asia

down-regulated and OspC up-regulated. By the time *B. burgdorferi* is inoculated into the host there is little expression of OspA and little host immune reactivity to this protein. In contrast, the early host immune response is directed against highly expressed OspC. Late in infection, however, and particularly in arthritis cases, there is a strong immune response to OspA. Higher temperatures (such as the 32–37°C found in the host) favour expression of OspC, while the 24°C of the tick does not. Once in the host certain proteins are known to be up-regulated, along with new expression of neoantigens. Thus the organism is quite heterogeneous (Mathiesen *et al.*, 1997). *B. burgdorferi* has nuclear genes, as well as extra-nuclear linear and circular plasmid genes. Plasmids may be lost, and there may be both point mutations and intragenic recombinations. Individual spiro-chaetes will differ in their protein expression, plasmids, and DNA, both between and within genospecies.

Other spirochaetal infections can serve as a model for Lyme disease. *Treponema pallidum* (syphilis), *Leptospira interrrogans* (leptospirosis), and *Borrelia recurrentis* and other *Borrelia* species (relapsing fever) are all spirochaetes which cause human disease. In all cases organisms enter through a skin or mucous membrane site, cause initial local infection, disseminate widely by early bacteraemia, cause persistent infection of target organs, and have vasculopathy as a common pathological feature. Clinical disease occurs in stages, with episodic reactivations. In relapsing fever the borreliae are known to undergo antigenic variation, with temporary immune escape. In the other infections, including Lyme disease, the mechanism for recurrent illness is not known.

Vectors and hosts

With the exception of two species of *Haemaphysalis* in China, all *B. burgdorferi* tick vectors belong to the genus *Ixodes* (Barbour, 1998). These small hard body ticks have a three-stage (larva, nymph, adult), two-year life cycle with only three blood meals (Anderson, 1989; Keirans *et al.*, 1996). Only ticks of the *I. ricinus* complex have transmitted infection to humans. They include *I. scapularis* (deer or black legged tick) in eastern and central USA and Canada, *I. pacificus* (western black legged tick) in the western USA and Canada, *I. ricinus* (sheep tick) in western and central Europe, and *I. persulcatus* (taiga tick) in eastern Europe and Asia. Other tick species, such as *I. uriae* in the north and south Atlantic, *I. hexagonus* in western and central Europe, and *I. spinipalpis* in the western USA, are helpful to monitor infection in various animal hosts. They can also transport spirochaetes to new locations.

One tick can carry several different genospecies or strains of *B. burgdorferi*. *Ixodes* requires a temperature between −10°C and 35°C to survive, and does not tolerate extreme cold or heat (Barbour, 1998). Relative humidity should be 80% or greater, so that ideally the soil is nearly saturated with water. Therefore *Ixodes* ticks are found in forests, damp soil with dense protective undergrowth, moist bushy areas, and tall grassy areas that border forests.

Ixodes ticks feed on dozens of hosts: large and small mammals, birds, and reptiles. The larval and nymphal ticks tend to feed on small mammals, ground feeding birds, and lizards. The white footed wild mouse is a particularly important host in North America. Adult ticks generally feed on larger mammals such as deer, and occasionally birds. Humans are completely accidental hosts. They are most likely to be bitten by questing nymphs, who feed in late spring and early summer.

Infected ticks probably need to feed for prolonged periods, perhaps 24–48 h, to transmit *B. burgdorferi* (Sood *et al.*, 1997). Spirochaetes in the midgut must be exposed to blood for a period of time to cause them to multiply, change outer surface proteins, and migrate to the salivary gland for injection into the skin. Thus there is a window of opportunity to remove a tick before it causes infection.

In hyperendemic areas, 30–70% of *Ixodes* ticks may be infected, and in highly localized pockets close to 100% are found to be infected. Tick infection rates can vary within short distances.

Clinical disease

The asymptomatic infection rate for *B. burgdorferi* is around 20–30%. This may reflect non-pathogenic strains, too small an inoculum, or an effective host immune response. Symptomatic infection can be divided into stages (Table 2.2) (Steere, 1989). Characteristic organ syndromes occur with local infection, early dissemination, and late stage infection. When spirochaetes are inoculated into skin at the tick bite site, they multiply locally. This is associated in at least 80% of patients with EM, an expanding erythematous skin lesion (Berger, 1997). EM is considered the only pathognomic marker for Lyme disease, but other

Table 2.2 Symptomatic Lyme disease.

Infection stage	Time from infection	Clinical syndromes
Early local infection	Up to 1 month	Skin (EM, LC) Systemic flu-like illness with seroconversion (? dissemination)
Early disseminated infection	Up to 3 months	Skin (multifocal EM) Musculoskeletal (arthralgias, myalgias, brief arthritis, myositis) Cardiac (conduction block, myopericarditis, pancarditis) Ocular (conjunctivitis) Neurological
Late stage infection	Over 3 months	Skin (ACA) Musculoskeletal (oligarticular arthritis, chronic arthritis) Ocular (keratitis, uveitis) Neurological

skin lesions can be mistaken for EM (Feder and Whitaker, 1995; Nadelman and Wormser, 1995). Skin punch biopsy of the leading edge of the EM lesion shows spirochaetes by silver stain, and *B. burgdorferi* DNA by PCR. Skin culture is positive in up to 80–90% of patients, but organisms take several weeks to grow out. Up to 68% of EM patients note constitutional features (fatigue, arthralgias, myalgias, headache, fever or chills, stiff neck) (Nadelman *et al.*, 1996). Up to 42% have systemic signs, including localized lymphadenopathy, fever, malar rash, meningismus, joint tenderness, joint swelling, or facial nerve palsy. Liver enzymes are abnormal in up to 37% and can suggest a viral hepatitis. EM is typically painless, although unusual cases are associated with pain, pruritus, diffuse urticarial eruptions, and even erythema multiforme (Schuttelaar *et al.*, 1997). A critical feature is enlargement over several days. EM occurs one to 30 days after the tick bite, typically within 7–10 days. Lesions that occur within 24 h reflect an allergic tick reaction.

Besides EM, early infection can also manifest as a flu-like syndrome with seroconversion. This probably reflects dissemination rather than local infection. A helpful negative feature is that less than 10% of patients have respiratory or gastrointestinal symptoms.

Spirochaetes disseminate within days to weeks into blood, and possibly lymphatics and peripheral nerves, to seed target organs. At its height, bacteraemia involves 1000 organisms per millilitre of blood. During early disseminated infection systemic complaints of fatigue may worsen. During early dissemination musculoskeletal involvement is most often migratory pains, cardiac involvement is heart block, and ocular involvement is conjunctivitis. Conjunctivitis occurs in up to 10% of patients. Overall, cardiac involvement occurs in 5–10% of patients (Nagi *et al.*, 1996). Most present with cardiac conduction abnormalities such as atrioventricular block. Patients may even develop complete heart block, and may require temporary pacing. Rarer manifestations are atrial or ventricular arrhythmias, and myocarditis. Neurological involvement is described below. Early dissemination syndromes spontaneously improve, but respond faster with appropriate antibiotics.

Late stage infection occurs months to years after the original inoculation. Again, characteristic target organ involvement can be seen. There is migratory oligoarticular or monoarticular large joint arthritis (tenosynovitis with joint swelling) (Steere, 1997). This most commonly involves the knees, and may be associated with formation of a Baker's cyst. Although any joint may be involved, small distal joints are unusual (less than 10%). Temporomandibular jaw pain is a particularly suggestive feature. Over time arthritis attacks become less severe, and attacks decrease. However, some 10% of patients develop a chronic antibiotic-refractory arthritis. Uveitis (Mikkila *et al.*, 1997), and characteristic neurological abnormalities are also seen in late stage infection.

There are several unusual skin manifestations which are virtually confined to European Lyme disease. Borrelia lymphocytoma cutis (LC), which consists of a collection of plasma cells within the earlobe, nipple, or scrotum, occurs in association with early infection. ACA is a late stage skin lesion more common in elderly women. It typically involves extensor surfaces of the distal lower extremities or occasionally the distal upper extremities. The skin becomes thin and sclerotic over infected areas. Other skin manifestations with a possible association to Lyme disease include eosinophilic fasciitis, lichen sclerosis, morphea, progressive hemifacial atrophy, and panniculitis.

Neurological involvement

Both the central (CNS) and peripheral (PNS) nervous systems are target organs in Lyme disease (Hansen, 1994; Haass, 1998). Neurological involvement can occur at any stages (Garcia-Monco and Benach, 1995). At the time of EM, dissemination may already have occurred. In one study, 10% of EM patients without neurological problems had evidence of CNS seeding (Kuiper et al., 1994). EM patients have had culture positive blood and CSF.

Early dissemination and late stage infections are associated with distinct neurologic syndromes (Table 2.3). Among the early dissemination syndromes, meningitis/encephalitis is the most common in adults. It can be quite subtle, and mimics an aseptic process rather than a typical bacterial meningitis. In Germany, Lyme meningitis accounts for 12–40% of childhood aseptic meningitis cases (Christen, 1996). Headache is the most common feature. It ranges from very mild to quite severe, is typically frontal or occipital, and may be accompanied by meningismus, nausea, vomiting, low grade fever, and photophobia. Headache is not uncommon in Lyme disease, and can mimic vascular or muscle contraction problems (Scelsa et al., 1995). Meningitis lasts for 4–8 weeks and then spontaneously resolves. In rare instances it can become chronic. Important clues to suggest Lyme meningitis are associated involvement of facial nerve, and spinal nerve roots. In CSF patients show a mononuclear pleocytosis of about 100–200 WBC/μl (range 5–4000 WBC/μl), which may include plasma cells and occasional atypical plasmocytoid cells. CSF protein is increased, while CSF glucose is normal. Opening pressure is generally normal. Intrathecal anti-B. burgdorferi antibody production is found in 50–100% of cases. In Europe oligoclonal IgG and IgM, and intrathecal IgG production are reported in virtually all cases. In contrast, in North America oligoclonal bands and intrathecal IgG production occur in 10% or less of cases. At the more severe end of this meningitis spectrum, there

Table 2.3 Neurological Lyme disease syndromes.

Infection Stage	Syndromes
Early local infection	Asymptomatic headache/meningismus (premeningitis CNS seeding)
Early disseminated infection	Meningitis, meningoencephalitis Cranial neuritis (facial nerve palsy) Acute painful radiculoneuritis
Late stage infection	Encephalopathy Chronic polyradiculoneuropathy Encephalomyelitis

are cases who present with a prominent encephalitic component. Patients may show acute confusional states, movement disorders, or transverse myelitis. Milder manifestations include cognitive, mood, and behavioural changes. CSF is almost always inflammatory, even when there is no obvious headache or meningismus.

Cranial neuritis is another neurological syndrome associated with early dissemination. The vast majority of cases involve the facial nerve. Involvement is bilateral in about one-third of patients. The nerves are usually asymmetrically affected, days to weeks apart. Important clues to suspect Lyme-related facial nerve palsy are occurrence during summer (in endemic areas which experience winter), and associated multisymptom complex (headache, stiff neck, arthralgias, myalgias, fatigue, concentration difficulties). Most cases of Lyme related facial nerve palsy have an occult meningitis, so that CNS seeding is present even when the facial nerve involvement is peripheral (Belman *et al.*, 1997.) Involvement of other cranial nerves (such as the optic nerve, nerves three to eight, and least often nine to twelve) is unusual, but has been reported in limited numbers of cases.

The third neurological syndrome associated with early dissemination is an acute painful radiculoneuritis referred to as Bannwarth's syndrome, or lymphocytic meningoradiculitis (Hansen and Lebech, 1992). Pain often starts between the scapulae, and may radiate down the spine or into the extremities. Asymmetric focal or multifocal dermatomal and myotomal abnormalities are seen. This neurological syndrome has the most inflammatory CSF changes of the early dissemination syndromes.

There are also three characteristic neurological syndromes associated with late stage infection (Logigian *et al.*, 1990). The most common, at least in North America, is a subtle encephalopathy characterized by memory, concentration, and mental processing disturbances. This syndrome probably reflects CNS infection, since CSF and cerebral blood flow studies are often abnormal. The most unusual neurological syndrome is a chronic progressive encephalomyelitis, which can mimic brain tumour, multiple sclerosis, or neurodegenerative disease. This is more common in Europe than North America. The third syndrome involves the PNS, and consists of a chronic axonal radiculoneuropathy (Halperin *et al.*, 1987; 1990). CSF is typically normal, unless patients also have encephalopathy. Unlike the early dissemination radicular syndrome, pain is not prominent. It may be absent, or confined to occasional brief shooting pains in the extremities. More commonly patients note intermittent paraesthesias, and complain of numbness in the extremities or restless legs. The clinical picture resembles a mild peripheral neuropathy or radiculoneuropathy. In Europe, symmetrical distal sensory polyneuropathy is often associated with the late infection ACA skin lesion (Kindstrand *et al.*, 1997).

Besides these six characteristic syndromes, a number of unusual syndromes have been reported (Table 2.4) (Coyle, 1997b). Vascular disease has included transient ischaemic attack, ischaemic infarction, intracranial aneurysm, and subarachnoid haemorrhage (Chehrenama *et al.*, 1997). An important clue in these cases is the associated CSF inflammatory changes. An apparently age-restricted intracranial hypertension syndrome has been seen in children and

Table 2.4 Unusual neurological Lyme disease syndromes.

Syndrome	Features
Cerebrovascular disease	Variety of manifestations (ischaemic, haemorrhagic strokes; vasculitis; transient ischaemic attack) Associated with abnormal CSF
Intracranial hypertension	Age restricted (children and adolescents) Associated with abnormal CSF No obesity, gender associations ? Immune mediated
Myositis/myopathy	Direct infection of muscle Isolated or multiple muscles involved
Psychiatric disease	Associated with abnormal CSF Variant of encephalomyelitis

adolescents. They are not obese, and typically show CSF abnormalities. There are over 15 cases of Lyme-related myositis, which most often follows an EM. Patients show isolated or multiple muscle involvement which can include limb, orbital, or oropharyngeal muscles. There have been unusual cases of psychiatric syndromes, dementia, and motor neuron disease-like syndromes attributed to Lyme disease (Fallon and Nields, 1994; Danek *et al.*, 1996). The psychiatric and dementia syndromes probably represent manifestations of parenchymal encephalitis, while the motor neuron syndrome may represent a CNS or PNS (motor nerve) involvement. With unusual cases, one would want seropositivity, confirming CSF abnormalities, and a response to antibiotic treatment before feeling reasonably comfortable that the syndrome was due to Lyme disease.

Diagnosis

For many reasons the diagnosis of Lyme disease, particularly neurological Lyme disease, is not always straightforward (Table 2.5) (Coyle, 1997a; Sigal, 1998). It remains a clinical diagnosis, ideally supported by laboratory data. Several formal criteria and consensus guidelines exist to guide diagnosis. The CDC epidemiological surveillance definition of Lyme disease is helpful, but too stringent for clinical practice (Table 2.6). The American Academy of

Table 2.5 Diagnostic problems encountered in neurological Lyme disease

No pathognomic neurological syndrome
No active infection assay
Inconsistent serologic assay results
Seronegative cases
Normal CSF (rare)
Infection with another tick pathogen
Delayed improvement after antibiotics
Continuing symptoms after antibiotics

Table 2.6   CDC surveillance definition for Lyme disease.

Infection stage	Clinical	Laboratory
Early (local)	Physician diagnosed EM (≥ 5 cm)	Not required (recommended when no known exposure)

Late (disseminated)	Musculoskeletal
	  joint swelling
	Cardiovasular
	  $-2°$, $3°$ AV block
	Neurological
	  meningitis
	  cranial neuropathy
	  radiculoneuropathy
	  encephalomyelitis (must have
	    intrathecal antibody
	    production)
		Required:
		  culture or
		  IgG or IgM antibodies in serum
		  or CSF or
		  paired acute and convalescent
		    serum antibodies (ideally using
		    two tier test system)

Neurology (AAN) has published a Practice Parameter for diagnosis of neurological Lyme disease (Table 2.7) (American Academy of Neurology Quality Standards Subcommittee 1996; Halperin *et. al.*, 1996). It distinguishes between unquestionable criteria for a cause and effect (this requires stringent criteria such as repeated isolation of organisms from CSF neural tissue, or rigorous epidemiological evidence), and criteria which justify treatment. When failure to treat has potential adverse consequences, it recommends to err on the side of overdiagnosis. The Practice Parameter indicates that a definitive diagnosis of neurological Lyme disease requires intrathecal organism-specific antibody production, demonstration of organisms by culture or histology, or detection of spirochaetal nucleic acid by PCR. Unlike the CDC case definition, the AAN Practice Parameter recognizes encephalopathy and peripheral neuropathy syndromes. It emphasizes that encephalomyelitis does not require

Table 2.7   American Academy of Neurology Practice Parameter for the diagnosis of neurological Lyme disease.

Requirements
1 Possible exposure to appropriate ticks in area where Lyme disease occurs
2 One or more of the following:
   EM, or histopathologically proven LC or ACA
   Immunological evidence of *B. burgdorferi* exposure
   Culture, histological, or PCR proof of detectable *B. burgdorferi*
3 Occurrence of one or more specified disorders; exclusion of other potential aetiologies; possible additional testing (CSF evaluation for suspected CNS infection)
   Causally related disease
     lymphocytic meningitis, with or without cranial neuropathy, painful radiculoneuritis, or both
     encephalomyelitis
     peripheral neuropathy
   Causally related syndrome
     encephalopathy

intrathecal antibody production, and that cranial neuropathy occurs in the setting of meningitis.

The cost of Lyme serology testing in the USA is staggering, and out of proportion to the number of cases (Strickland *et al.*, 1997; Fix *et al.*, 1998). Expert panels have provided guidelines for diagnosis based on diagnostic probabilities and cost-effective policies (Tugwell *et al.*, 1997; Nichol *et al.*, 1998). They recommend that patients with a high probability of Lyme disease, for example a characteristic EM-like skin lesion in someone with endemic area exposure, be diagnosed and treated without laboratory testing. Patients with a suggestive syndrome and reasonable probability of Lyme disease would undergo two-step laboratory testing (enzyme linked immunosorbent assay (ELISA), followed by Western immunoblot). Patients with a low probability of Lyme disease (non-specific symptoms) would undergo diagnostic testing only if they had other supportive clinical features.

Clinical features

There are certain diagnostically useful clinical clues (Table 2.8). Patients need endemic area exposure, but it can be as fleeting as a brief vacation or business trip. Perhaps half of patients give a history of tick bite. Since EM is almost a pathognomic clinical marker, neurological disease following an odd skin lesion should raise the suspicion for Lyme disease. ACA and LC, which are virtually confined to Europe, are other unusual skin lesions which diagnose Lyme disease. Lyme disease causes suggestive syndromes in both early and late stage infection. Neurological Lyme disease syndromes are often accompanied by multisystem complaints (arthralgias, myalgias, fatigue, palpitations, cognitive difficulties), but these complaints in isolation are rarely due to *B. burgdorferi* infection.

Table 2.8   Diagnostic clinical clues for neurological Lyme disease.

Endemic area exposure
  Outdoor activities
  Tick exposure
    strain
    presence of engorgement
    geographic origin of tick

EM prior to onset of preceding onset of neurological syndrome

Season appropriate flu-like illness, prior to onset of neurological syndrome

Suggestive extraneural involvement
  target organ disease (skin, musculoskeletal, cardiovascular, ocular)
  systemic symptoms (fatigue, arthralgias, myalgias, palpitations)

Characteristic early disseminated or late stage neurological syndrome

Laboratory

Culture is the gold standard test for infection, but it is not routinely performed in Lyme disease. Although *B. burgdorferi* can be cultured in various modifications of a complex solution (Barbour-Stoenner-Kelly broth), with perhaps an even greater yield using Kelly-Pettenkofer media (Picken *et al.*, 1997), the yield is low. Culture typically takes at least 2–8 weeks, and requires specific antibody stains or PCR for confirmation. The highest culture yield is punch biopsy or aspiration of the EM lesion, with positivity rates of 40–80%. Less than 10% of CSF cultures are positive. This poor yield probably reflects scarcity of tissue-tropic organisms in free CSF.

Serology

The major diagnostic laboratory test is detection of anti-*B. burgdorferi* antibodies, although this only confirms prior exposure rather than active infection (American College of Physicians, 1997). The vast majority of Lyme disease patients are seropositive. Seronegative Lyme disease occurs, but is unusual (less than 10%) (Dattwyler *et al.*, 1988) and is most often seen in the setting of early abortive antibiotics (Ledue *et al.*, 1996). For example, only 50% of EM patients are seropositive. With treatment, almost 30% never seroconvert (Luft *et al.*, 1996). IgM antibodies are detected as early as 2 weeks, peak by 3–6 weeks, then fall and generally become negative. IgM antibodies persist in a minority of patients (Hilton *et al.*, 1997). The significance of this finding is not known, since it can occur in successfully treated and recovered patients. IgM antibodies are sometimes found in patients with chronic problems, in the absence of IgG antibodies. The significance of this finding is also unknown, and the likelihood that an IgM reaction is a false positive is increased when it is associated with chronic problems. The early IgM response is directed mainly against the p23 OspC, P39 Bmp, and P41 flagellin proteins. IgG antibodies are detected by 4–6 weeks after inoculation, and will continue to rise unless there is early abortive antibiotic treatment.

The Association of State and Territorial Public Health Laboratory Directors (ASTPHLD) and the CDC currently recommend a two-tier system for serodiagnosis (Table 2.9). Screening ELISA or immunofluorescence assay (IFA) is performed first. Since IFA is technically more problematic and subjective, most laboratories use ELISA. Either indirect ELISA, which measures immunoglobulin binding to target spirochaetal antigens, or antibody capture ELISA, which first binds specific immunoglobulin isotype

Table 2.9   Current recommendations for serological testing in Lyme disease

Use first tier test to screen (ELISA, IFA)
Proceed to Western immunoblot if first test borderline or positive
Do IgM blot only in acute syndromes (lasting weeks)
  positive requires two of three possible bands (p23, 39, 41)
Positive IgG blot requires 5 of 10 possible bands (p18, 21, 28, 30, 39, 41, 45, 58, 66, 93)

then measures binding of spirochaetal antigens, can be used. Borderline (equivocal) and positive first tier tests are then examined by the more specific Western immunoblot. Although immunoblot is standardized for recommended bands to determine a positive IgM or IgG reaction, there is no standardization of either ELISA or immunoblot assays for antigen target. Typically whole organism sonicate is used, including specific and non-specific antigens. There is no standardized use of recombinant proteins and monoclonal antibodies, and a positive result depends on subjective assessment. In a best case scenario the false positive rate for a first tier test approximates 5% and can be even higher (Burkot *et al.*, 1997). Other infections (spirochaetal, rickettsial, bacterial), autoimmune diseases, and B-cell hyperreactivity states (such as Epstein-Barr virus infection) can all give false positive results. Lyme serology assays can show significant inter- and even intra-laboratory variability (Hofmann, 1996; Bakken *et al.*, 1997). IgM immunoblot use is recommended only for acute/subacute cases, and IgG immunblot is used for long standing complaints. One problem not addressed by the current system is that Western immunoblot can be positive despite negative screening ELISA (Nilsson and von Rosen, 1996). There has been some dissatisfaction with the current immunoblot criteria, and alternative criteria have been proposed but not accepted (Engstrom *et al.*, 1995; Hilton *et al.*, 1996; Norman *et al.*, 1996; Hauser *et al.*, 1997; Tilton *et al.*, 1997).

Current problems may be solved by second generation antibody assays, some of which are already in limited use (Magnarelli *et al.*, 1996; Ikushima *et al.*, 1998; Rauer *et al.*, 1998). They employ selected recombinant proteins or chimeric proteins (epitopes from selected recombinant proteins, strung together) as antigen target. The Food and Drug Administration (FDA) recently approved a rapid office-based immunostripe test (Prevue B, Chembio Diagnostics Systems), which provides a positive or negative single band readout for serum antibodies within 20 minutes. Optimal use of this point of service test has not been studied, however. Advances in immunoblot technology include complete automation, to remove interpreter bias and shorten assay time, and modification to a quantitative assay. At the current time development of commercial second generation assays is being hampered because a variety of sources hold patent rights on the major recombinant proteins.

Blood studies

In early infection there may be elevations in acute phase reactants and liver enzymes (Horowitz *et al.*, 1996). Neurological Lyme disease patients may show anticardiolipin IgM antibodies. Otherwise blood tests are used to rule out other conditions, including infections.

CSF

CSF is abnormal in most neurological Lyme disease patients (Smouha *et al.*, 1997). The main exceptions are pure PNS syndromes. Abnormalities are not as striking in late stage infection compared to early disseminated infection. In general, normal CSF rules out neurological Lyme disease, although there are always exceptions to the rule. Spirochaetes have been cultured from normal CSF. Intrathecal anti-*B. burgdorferi* antibody production is the single most helpful test. It requires paired CSF-serum samples. Paired immunoblot analysis may be helpful when there is a high suspicion of infection, but negative screening ELISA (Oschmann *et al.*, 1997). Lack of intrathecal antibody production does not rule out neurological Lyme disease, however (Albisetti *et al.*, 1997). In addition, intrathecal antibody production can persist months to years after successful treatment. False positive intrathecal antibody production is rare, but has occurred in conditions such as syphillis and immunoglobulin infusion (Treib *et al.*, 1997). It is very unusual to detect antibodies to *B. burgdorferi* in CSF of seronegative patients. CSF antibodies which are at a much lower concentration than serum antibodies probably reflect passive diffusion, and as an isolated finding in a seropositive patient should not be interpreted as proving CNS infection.

Intrathecal antibody production is indirect evidence of CNS infection. Direct evidence can be supplied by positive CSF culture or PCR (Schmidt, 1997). Unfortunately culture is rarely positive even in meningitis cases. PCR testing of CSF is very insensitive in Lyme disease. Less than one third of neurological patients are positive (Nocton *et al.*, 1996). PCR sensitivity may be improved in the future by sample concentration, primer selection, and other techniques (Priem *et al.*, 1997). A reliable positive PCR documents CNS infection, but the diagnostic laboratory must assure quality control since PCR is very susceptible to contamination (Schmidt, 1997). This is a particular problem in commercial laboratories which perform multiple PCR tests for many different organisms, and which also perform assays utilizing *B. burgdorferi* antigens. Aerosol contamination has led to false positive CSF PCR reactions.

Non-specific but supportive CSF findings include mononuclear pleocytosis (sometimes plasma cells are seen), increased protein, normal glucose, and negative VDRL. Research studies have reported abnormal matrix metallopro-teinase patterns (Perides *et al.*, 1998), increased levels of neurofilaments and glial fibrillary acidic proteins (Dotevall *et al.*, 1996), detection of *B. burgdorferi* antigens (Coyle *et al.*, 1993), and presence of immune complexes containing *B. burgdorferi*-reactive components (Coyle *et al.*, 1990). These CSF assays remain research tools at the current time, without a defined clinical role.

Other tests

Neuroimaging is normal in most neurological Lyme disease patients, but about 25% will show lesions on MRI. These are typically small or large T2-weighted hyperintensities, suggestive of vasculitis. Rare cases show grey matter lesions. Late stage encephalomyelitis is the neurological syndrome most likely to show brain MRI lesions. Unusual neuroimaging patterns include focal mass lesion, and there is a report of a large cerebellopontine angle lesion attributed to Lyme disease (Mokry *et al.*, 1990). Enhancement of cranial and spinal nerves are also reported. Single photon emission computer tomography (SPECT) can show reversible cerebral blood flow disturbances in late Lyme encephalopathy, with multifocal areas of cortical and subcortical hyperfusion (Logigian et al., 1997; Sumiya et al., 1997). The frontal and temporal lobes are particularly affected. This is a non-specific finding, however.

Electrophysiological studies (nerve conduction test, electromyography) help to document a suggestive pattern to PNS involvement. Typical findings are consistent with a sensorimotor axonal polyradiculoneuropathy, with reduction of distal component action potentials, mild conduction slowing, and denervation of both distal and paraspinal muscles (Halperin et al., 1990; Logigian and Steere, 1992). Facial nerve palsy patients frequently show evidence of a demyelinating nerve process.

Among other tests used to diagnose Lyme disease is the Lyme urine antigen test (LUAT). This is offered by a single commercial laboratory, and is not validated. The material being detected in urine, based on antibody reactivity, is not subjected to further tests to document presence of spirochaetal antigens, and urinary tract infections will produce false positive reactions. A positive LUAT should not be used in isolation to diagnose Lyme disease.

Although biopsy is rarely helpful except for skin lesions, there have been examples of spirochaetes identified in skeletal and cardiac muscle, synovium, brain, and a number of internal organs. The problem is that organisms are scarce within affected tissue, and visualized spirochaetes must be further identified as B. burgdorferi to distinguish them from commensal spirochaetes.

Research tests which have been used in the diagnosis of Lyme disease include the Borreliacidal antibody test (BAT) or Gundersen assay, which detects cytotoxic antibodies and is performed at a single centre (Callister et al., 1996; Agger and Case, 1997); CSF IgM to recombinant OspC, for diagnosis of early CNS infection (Schutzer et al., 1997); and analysis of B. burgdorferi-specific immune complexes in serum and CSF (Coyle et al., 1990; Schutzer et al., 1990; Zhong et al., 1997). Lymphocyte proliferative responses to B. burgdorferi have been positive in some antibody negative patients (Dattwyler et al., 1988b; Rutkowski et al., 1997), as have B. burgdorferi-specific immune complexes (Schutzer et al., 1990). Unfortunately cellular immune assays are cumbersome, not standardized, and detect reactions in healthy controls. The false positive rate can be as high as 67%. Only a small number of research laboratories currently analyse immune complexes.

Differential diagnosis

Neurological Lyme disease encompasses a variety of syndromes, and the differential diagnosis is broad. Lyme meningitis mimics aseptic meningitis. Suggestive features for Lyme disease include associated or prior EM skin lesion, and associated facial nerve or radicular involvement. Lyme-related facial nerve palsy can be distinguished from idiopathic Bell's palsy by seasonal occurrence, history of exposure, presence of suggestive features (EM, radicular or other cranial nerve involvement), associated multisystem complex, and seropositivity. Bilateral facial nerve involvement supports Lyme disease rather than idiopathic Bell's palsy. However, the differential diagnosis of bilateral seventh nerve palsy includes Guillain-Barré syndrome, neurosarcoidosis, Epstein Barr virus infection, Tangier disease, and human immunodeficiency type I infection. Acute radiculoneuritis can be seen with certain herpes virus infections (varicella zoster virus, cytomegalovirus, Epstein Barr virus) as well as neurosarcoidosis, vasculitic neuropathies, and proximal diabetic radiculoneuropathy. Late Lyme encephalopathy, which is typically subtle, can be confused with toxic and metabolic causes of encephalopathy, chronic fatigue syndrome, and fibromyalgia syndrome. Chronic Lyme polyradiculoneuropathy can be confused with polyneuropathy due to many causes. Lyme encephalomyelitis can be confused with multiple sclerosis, brain tumour, other structural lesions, or degenerative neurological disorders. As opposed to Lyme disease, multiple sclerosis is not associated with extraneural features and PNS involvement, is more likely to have abnormal brain MRI and CSF oligoclonal bands/intrathecal IgG production, and is less likely to have CSF pleocytosis, increased protein, or detectable *B. burgdorferi* antibodies (Coyle, 1989).

Treatment

Recommendations using cost-effective strategies have also been applied to treatment of Lyme disease (Shadick *et al.*, 1998). Lyme disease is a bacterial infection which responds to appropriate antibiotic therapy (Wormser, 1997). The sooner treatment is started, the better the response rate and outcome. Neurological Lyme disease is a disseminated infection. The CNS is an anatomically sequestered compartment with limited antimicrobial penetration. At the current time intravenous antibiotics are recommended for all neurological Lyme disease syndromes, with the possible exception of specific cranial nerve palsy patients with isolated peripheral nerve involvement (Table 2.10). In general, intravenous antibiotics penetrate the CNS compartment better than oral antibiotics. This recommendation for parenteral treatment of neurological

Table 2.10   Treatment of neurological Lyme disease.

Treatment	Comments
First line	
Ceftriaxone	Given once a day
2 g q.d.	Major concerns colitis, biliary disease
	Supplement with acidophilus, yoghurt
Second Line	
Cefotaxime	t.i.d. dosing not as convenient
2 g t.i.d.	
Penicillin G	Frequent dosing required
18–24 mU q.d.	CSF penetration not as good
(in divided doses)	Dose must be adjusted for abnormal renal function
Doxycycline	Oral or parenteral
200 mg b.i.d.	GI upset, photosensitivity major side-effects

disease is not true for other disseminated infection syndromes. Oral antibiotics (doxycycline 100 mg b.i.d.) seem to work as well as intravenous antibiotics for extraneural disseminated disease (Dattwyler *et al.*, 1997). The one exception is third degree atrioventricular heart block, where most experts advise initial intravenous antibiotics. These cardiac patients may also require temporary pacemaker insertion.

Early disseminated neurological syndromes improve without therapy, and most patients go on to clear or contain their infection. This is similar to asymptomatic neurosyphilis, where only a minority of patients develop late disease. Without assuring adequate antimicrobial therapy, however, untreated patients are at risk for late stage neurological disease. Although this risk is 10% or less for untreated patients, late stage infection does not respond as well to treatment, and there is a strong argument for instituting early appropriate antibiotics.

At the current time the preferred intravenous antibiotic agent is the third generation cephalosporin ceftriaxone (Rocefin). It is given at 2 g once a day, which is half the usual dose used for severe bacterial meningitis. The duration of treatment is 2–6 weeks. Once a day dosing, given over 30–60 minutes, is very convenient for outpatient (home) treatment. Treatment can be done through home infusion companies, with insertion of a midline which does not have to be replaced during the several weeks of therapy. Ceftriaxone is well tolerated, and no routine blood studies are indicated. In a minority of cases this broad spectrum antibiotic affects normal bowel flora to produce colitis, including *clostridium difficile* pseudomembranous colitis. Patients can take acidophilus (obtainable from health food stores), and yoghurt during the treatment course. Ceftriaxone is excreted in the bile, and in unusual cases is associated with gall bladder disease. This is a particular problem in children who are treated for more than a few weeks. In the majority of patients, treatment over several weeks is not associated with adverse events.

Alternative antibiotic agents include another third generation cephalosporin, cefotaxime (Claforan). Since this is dosed at 2 g t.i.d., it is not as convenient as ceftriaxone. Most of the experience with cefotaxime is from Europe. It is equivalent, but certainly not superior, to ceftriaxone. In Europe intravenous penicillin G (18 to 24 mU/day, in normal renal function patients, divided over four to six times daily) has been used successfully to treat neurological Lyme disease. Penicillin is an alternative agent to ceftriaxone, but it does not penetrate CSF well and has a much shorter serum half life. In small studies of late stage Lyme disease from North America, intravenous penicillin was inferior to intravenous ceftriaxone. In seven patients with neurological or musculoskeletal Lyme disease refractory to penicillin after ceftriaxone therapy, joint swelling resolved in five of seven and limb paraesthesias resolved in five of six patients (Dattwyler *et al.*, 1987). In a follow-up study, 23 patients with neurological disease or arthritis were randomized to intravenous penicillin (10 patients) or ceftriaxone (13 patients) (Dattwyler *et al.*, 1988a). Five of the 10 penicillin-treated patients continued to be symptomatic (fatigue, memory problems, arthritis). Four of the five resolved after ceftriaxone therapy. Of 13 patients who received ceftriaxone, none had objective disease after treatment, although three noted mild arthralgias and one noted fatigue and memory difficulties. In earlier studies of Lyme arthritis, the success rate with intramuscular benzathine penicillin was only 35%, while the success rate with intravenous penicillin was 55% (Steere *et al.*, 1983). In practice, an alternative regimen to treat neurological disease is high dose doxycycline (200 mg b.i.d. either orally or intravenously). Increased doses of doxycycline have better penetration into CSF (Dotevall and Hagberg, 1989; Karlsson *et al.*, 1996).

European studies report oral doxycycline at standard dosing (100 mg b.i.d.) to be adequate treatment for neurological Lyme disease, including meningitis (Karlsson *et al.*, 1994). Anecdotal data from North America however indicates that current oral antibiotics regimens are inadequate to treat established CNS infection. In a study of 40 adults and children with Lyme arthritis, randomized to 30 days of oral doxycycline or amoxicillin plus probenecid, five patients relapsed with neurological disease (Steere *et al.*, 1994). Four received amoxicillin with probenecid, and one received doxycycline. Probenecid is now largely abandoned, because it increases risk of allergic skin reactions and impairs penetration of beta lactam antibiotics into the brain (Wormser, 1997). All Lyme arthritis patients who developed neurological disease initially complained of paraesthesiae or memory problems, suggesting early neurological involvement. Patients responded to intravenous ceftriaxone, with the exception of one patient who failed 2 weeks of therapy and required 4 weeks.

It is argued that Lyme-related facial nerve palsy reflects PNS involvement, and therefore oral antibiotics are sufficient. Many patients have CSF abnormalities however, consistent with occult meninigitis and CNS seeding. PCR data also indicate that the CNS is seeded in facial nerve palsy patients with otherwise normal CSF (Luft *et al.*, 1992). In some endemic areas it is now common practice to examine CSF in all suspected Lyme-related facial nerve palsy patients, and to use intravenous antibiotics when there are CSF abnormalities or clinical features consistent with CNS seeding (headache, stiff neck, cognitive disturbances). In some endemic areas glucocorticoids are no longer used as initial treatment for Bell s palsy. Anecdotal data suggest that glucocorticoids used before antibiotics may lead to a more refractory syndrome and subsequent suboptimal antibiotic response (Coyle, 1997b).

Late infection neurological syndromes also respond to antibiotic therapy. Patients with late stage encephalopathy or polyneuropathy received 2 weeks of ceftriaxone (Logigian *et al.*, 1990). Six months later 63% had an excellent response, 22% showed initial improvement with subsequent relapse, and only 15% failed to respond. In a follow-up study of 18 late stage encephalomyelitis patients treated with ceftriaxone for 30 days, the response rate at 6 months was 93% in the 15 patients examined (Logigian *et al.*, 1990). In 10 patients with follow-up CSF analysis, protein levels decreased. Only one patient required retreatment after 8 months. More severe late encephalomyelitis cases sometimes require 4–6 weeks of antibiotic therapy.

All antibiotic treatment regimens for Lyme disease have treatment failures. This could reflect spirochaete or host factors, among other possibilities. *In vitro* studies indicate that *B. burgdorferi* can cause intracellular infection of synovial cells which is refractory to ceftriaxone therapy (Girschick *et al.*, 1996). Intracellular infection has never been shown *in vivo*, however. Approaches to treatment failure include use of higher drug doses, more prolonged treatment, or alternative antibiotics.

In addition to antibiotic treatment, symptomatic management of the assorted problems associated with Lyme disease (control of headache, arthralgias, myalgias; fatigue; sleep disturbances) are very important to decrease discomfort, and improve quality of life. Optimal symptomatic therapy is important to supplement antibiotic treatment, in order to maximize therapeutic response.

Prevention

The most definitive treatment of any infection is prevention. Preventive strategies for Lyme disease include exposure methods, prophylactic treatment, and immunoprophylaxis (Table 2.11). Infected *Ixodes* ticks must feed for a prolonged period of time to transmit infection, probably at least 24 h but perhaps as long as 72 h. Therefore removal of a tick early prevents infection, supporting the concept of daily body checks. Measures to avoid tick bite or exposure include personal protection (protective clothing), and use of tick repellants. Although tick control methods are difficult and often impractical, they can be useful practices to follow for individuals exposed to high endemic areas.

It is not uncommon for prophylactic antibiotics to be used following tick bite (Fix *et al.*, 1998). Yet prospective randomized double blind trials have failed to document a benefit of prophylactic therapy of tick bite vs. watchful waiting (Costello *et al.*, 1989; Shapiro *et al.*, 1992; Agre and Schwartz, 1993). In a recent meta-analysis involving over 600 patients with tick bite, antibiotic prophylaxis was not found to be beneficial (Warshafsky *et al.*, 1996). A single study suggests that when there is a high risk of Lyme disease after tick bite (>0.036), prophylactic doxycycline therapy should be considered (Magid *et al.*, 1992).

Table 2.11 Prevention measures for Lyme disease.

Environmental methods
Tick control
Host (deer, mouse) population control
Exfolients

Exposure methods
Avoid tick infested areas
Protective, light coloured clothing
Tick repellants
Routine body checks
Prompt removal of attached ticks

Prophylactic measures
Antibiotic treatment of high risk tick bites
Immunoprophylaxis

Table 2.12 Lyme disease vaccines.

Name	LYMErix (Smithkline Beecham)	ImuLyme (Pasteur Merieux Connaught)
Type	Monovalent, using 30 mcg recombinant Lipo-OspA (ZS7 strain) with adjuvant (aluminum hydroxide)	Monovalent, using 30 mcg recombinant OspA (B31 strain)
Schedule	3 i.m. injections: 0, 1, 12 months	3 i.m. injections: 0, 1, 12 months
Ages studied	15–70	18–92
Efficacy results	2 doses 49% 3 doses 76%	2 doses 68% 3 doses 92%
Asymptomatic infection	Screened for	Not screened for
FDA Status	Approved and available	Pending

Table 2.13 Potential problems with the Lyme disease vaccine.

Protection requires series of three injections, spaced over months
Protection based on development of specific type of OspA antibodies, which are not maintained over time
Booster vaccines required to maintain protection; frequency unclear
Vaccine may induce arthritis in genetically predisposed individuals
Vaccinated individuals become seropositive; new serological test needed for vacinees

The most definitive preventive therapy is effective immunoprophylaxis. Two vaccines, both based on recombinant OspA, have completed trials in thousands of patients (Table 2.12) (Sigal *et al.*, 1998; Steere *et al.*, 1998; Steigbigel and Benach, 1998). The FDA recently approved the Lymerix vaccine in late 1998. It works predominantly through antibody-mediated killing of spirochaetes within the feeding tick (Fikrig *et al.*, 1992). Although there are a number of concerns about the vaccine (Table 2.13), it provides reasonable (close to 80%) short-term protection against infection. Other vaccines are being developed with the goal of providing long-term protection, therapeutic benefit (to treat established infection), and no concern about disease induction.

Prognosis

Overall, Lyme disease has an excellent prognosis. There is virtually no mortality, with the exception of severe cardiac disease. Neurological syndromes associated with early dissemination spontaneously remit, although recovery is more rapid with treatment. Most patients with early disseminated neurological Lyme disease improve within 3–5 days of starting antibiotics, and radicular pain can improve within hours. The treatment response rate for EM and multifocal EM is close to 90%, while the response rate for disseminated syndromes other than multifocal EM is 70–80%. Perhaps

7% of patients do not improve during therapy, or even worsen. Facial nerve palsy, for example, can develop during antibiotic therapy. This does not seem to reflect therapeutic failure, and such patients typically do very well. Lyme related facial nerve palsy improves in 85% of patients, with 70% showing complete recovery (Smouha *et al.*, 1997).

In contrast, late stage infection neurological syndromes do not tend to improve or remit spontaneously. Outcome after antibiotic therapy is better in encephalopathy patients than encephalomyelitis patients. Three to 6 months after intravenous ceftriaxone, encephalopathy patients show improvements in their neuropsychiatric symptoms, cognitive measures, CSF abnormalities, and brain SPECT disturbances. Improvement may continue for months after antibiotics are stopped. In the rare patient who truly relapses following treatment, a second course of antibiotics may be helpful. Patients who relapse after 2 weeks of treatment can respond to 4 weeks.

European radiculoneuritis and encephalomyelitis patients are said to have an equally good long term outcome with or without antibiotic treatment (Krüger *et al.*, 1990).

Pathogenesis

Neuropathological findings in Lyme disease are not striking, with a low grade meningeal and perivascular mononuclear inflammation without marked structural changes (Table 2.14). Obliterative vasculopathy has been reported with late infection, and there are rare reports of prominent demyelination or granulomatous tissue (Oksi *et al.*, 1996; Coyle, 1997b). The occasionally noted spirochaete is always extracellular in CNS and muscle tissues. Organisms have never been visualized in peripheral nerve, although a recent study reported PCR reactivity in a sural nerve biopsy (Maimone *et al.*, 1997). Peripheral nerve changes involve axon damage, with perivascular inflammation (Vallat *et al.*, 1987). The fact that pathological changes are generally confined to focal inflammation, mild vasculopathy, and no significant tissue destruction suggests that indirect mechanisms may be more important than direct effects of spirochaetes on neural tissue.

In vitro studies indicate that *B. burgdorferi* has a variety of effects on host tissue and immune responses (Coyle, 1997a; Garcia-Monco and Benach, 1997; Hu and Klempner, 1997; Sigal, 1997). The spirochaete sheds pieces of outer surface membrane (so-called 'blebs'), which contain DNA and Osp proteins. These blebs induce an inflammatory response. In the rat, OspA-containing spirochaetal fractions cause an antigen-induced arthritis. *B. burgdorferi* is very tissue tropic (Coburn *et al.*, 1998; Leong *et al.*, 1998). It binds to endothelial cells, up-regulates adhesion molecules, and induces local chemokine production. Organisms cross blood vessels through intercellular openings or by transcytotic mechanisms, to penetrate multiple organs. *B. burgdorferi* also binds to platelets, red blood cells, plasminogen, and glycosphingolipids on the surface of neurons, astrocytes, oligodendrocytes, and Schwann cells. In culture, spirochaetes injure both astrocytes and oligodendrocytes. Individual organism

Table 2.14 Neuropathology of Lyme disease

General features
Mild vasculopathy
Mild inflammatory changes
Rare extracellular organisms
Limited tissue destruction

CNS
Meningeal inflammation (lymphocytes, plasma cells)
Scattered perivascular mononuclear (CD4$^+$ T cell) infiltrates
Perivascular inflammation
Focal microgliosis
Mild spongiform changes
Demyelinating lesions (rare)
Multifocal encephalitis (rare)
Vasculitis (rare)
Low numbers of spirochaetes

PNS (nerve)
Variable perivascular mononuclear (CD4$^+$ T cell, macrophage) infiltrates in epineurium, perineurium
Axon injury
Vasa nervorum angiopathy
No spirochaetes

PNS (muscle)
Focal myositis
Focal necrosis
Interstitial inflammation
Low numbers of spirochaetes

properties appear to play a role in determining pathogenicity as well as organotropism. Several different *B. burgdorferi* strains are neurotropic, and can invade the CNS (Wilske *et al.*, 1996).

Once *B. burgdorferi* disseminates, it is difficult to find spirochaetes in tissue. They may be truly absent, present in very low numbers, or present as fragments (e.g. DNA) rather than whole organisms. Among the early dissemination syndromes, meningitis and acute radiculoneuritis clearly reflect CNS invasion. Facial nerve palsy is often associated with an occult meningitis, and probably represents a sequelae of CNS invasion and inflammation in most cases. However, a minority of facial nerve palsy patients will have normal CSF, and electrophysiological changes consistent with PNS involvement. As is true for all spirochaetal infections, *B. burgdorferi* may persist within infected organs to cause late disease. Late stage infection syndromes undoubtedly represent neural tissue infection, since patients stabilize or improve with antibiotic treatment. It is likely that the limited number of organisms produce neurological problems through indirect mechanisms.

B. burgdorferi has a number of immune and inflammatory effects which could lead to disease (Table 2.15). The best example is chronic Lyme arthritis, which is now recognized as an immune-mediated syndrome (Gross *et al.*, 1998a). It occurs in approximately 10% of Lyme arthritis patients, who show

Table 2.15 Potential indirect mechanisms for damage due to *B. burgdorferi*.

Vasculopathy
Cytokine disturbance
pro-inflammatory cytokine induction
receptor changes
TH1 : Th2 imbalance
chemokine induction
Induction of toxin
nitric oxide
quinolinic acid
Humoral immunity
B cell mitogen
molecular mimicry, cross-reactive antibodies
immune complex formation
Cellular immunity
molecular mimicry
bystander damage
apoptosis

HLA-DR4 (DRB1*0401) positivity. They have an antibiotic unresponsive arthritis, with PCR negative synovial fluid (Gross *et al.*, 1998b). Patients show a strong cellular and humoral immune response to OspA. Within the joint CD4$^+$ T helper 1 (TH1) cells include OspA-reactive cells, which release high levels of damaging proinflammatory cytokines. The severity of the inflammatory arthritis parallels the TH1 : TH2 ratio within synovial fluid. OspA shows molecular mimicry with human lymphocyte functional antigen-type 1 (LFA-1). LFA-1 is an integrin receptor, and an adhesion molecule found primarily on T cells. It binds to intercellular adhesion molecule-1 (ICAM-1). Both LFA-1 and ICAM-1 are highly expressed in inflammatory tissue.

With regard to vascular effects, *B. burgdorferi* can cause a vasculopathy similar to endarteritis obliterans. Subsequent ischaemic changes could damage local tissue, blood–brain and blood–nerve barriers, and contribute to inflammation.

Cytokines have been implicated in the pathogenesis of Lyme disease. *B. burgdorferi* induces pro-inflammatory cytokines such as interleukin-1 (IL-1), IL-6, and tumour necrosis factor-α (TNF-α), and they are elevated in the joint of arthritis patients (Yin *et al.*, 1997). Cloned T cell lines from synovial fluid and blood of Lyme arthritis patients secrete interferon-γ (IFN-γ) when exposed to *B. burgdorferi*. The ratio of synovial fluid IL-1 to IL-1 receptor correlates with prognosis of Lyme arthritis. *B. burgdorferi* preferentially activates the IL-1 gene over the antagonist IL-1 receptor gene. Mononuclear cells collected from neurological patients preferentially secrete IFN-γ when exposed to *B. burgdorferi* Osp proteins (Ekerfelt *et al.*, 1997). CSF cells show a more striking preferential synthesis than peripheral blood cells, while an antagonistic anti-inflammatory/regulatory cytokine, IL-4, is down-regulated. CSF from neurological patients shows increased levels of IL-1 and TNF-α. Soluble IL-2 receptors are increased in both CSF and blood, and decrease after treatment (Nilsson *et al.*, 1994). IL-12 production is increased in monocytes collected from patients with long-standing Lyme disease (Pohl-Koppe *et al.*, 1998). This cytokine favours production of TH1 cells. Overall, the cytokine data suggests an imbalance of TH1 : TH2 CD4$^+$ T cell ratio in Lyme disease, with TH1 cells predominant in late infection. This would favour cell-mediated immunity and pro-inflammatory cytokine production. In contrast, humoral immunity appears to be protective in *B. burgdorferi* infection. *B. burgdorferi* also induces production of chemokines, small chemotactic cytokines which undoubtedly influence local inflammatory changes (Burns *et al.*, 1997; Sprenger *et al.*, 1997).

There is also evidence for toxic factors. *B. burgdorferi* induces nitric oxide production by CNS cells; quinolinic acid, an NMDA receptor antagonist and excitotoxin, is elevated in the CSF of neurological patients. Both are neurotoxins which disrupt cell function.

Although humoral immunity appears to be protective in this infection, antibodies and immune complexes may have a pathogenetic role as well. *B. burgdorferi* and its bleb material are B-cell mitogenic. Infection has been associated with autoreactive antibodies to cardiolipin and acidic ganglioside (GM1, asialo-GM1), anticardiolipin IgM, anti-axonal IgM, antibodies to myelin and myelin components, antineuronal antibodies, antibodies to heat shock protein, and antibodies to a 46kD protein which crossreacts with myosin (Coyle, 1997a; Sigal, 1997; Yu *et al.*, 1997). *B burgdorferi* specific immune complexes have been reported in both serum and CSF, and may correlate with disease activity (Coyle *et al.*, 1990; Schutzer *et al.*, 1990).

With regard to cell mediated immunity, CSF T cells in neurological patients react to cardiolipin as well as a variety of neural antigens, including myelin and galactocerebroside (Wang *et al.*, 1996). In the joint, antigen reactive T gamma delta cells are involved in apoptosis of CD4$^+$ T cells (Vincent *et al.*, 1996).

In summary, a number of indirect mechanisms may contribute, either alone or in combination, to neurological manifestations. One way to examine the role of diverse factors is in animal models, which have helped to advance the understanding of Lyme disease pathogenesis. However, the course of infection varies widely depending on the species, and no model completely mimics human infection. In some animals infection causes no obvious disease, while in others selected organs are involved. In some models infection spontaneously clears, in others infection clears with antibiotics, while in still others antibiotics contain but never clear infection (Goodman *et al.*, 1991; Foley *et al.*, 1995; Straubinger *et al.*, 1997). The mouse is excellent to study musculoskeletal and cardiac disease, but shows no nervous system involvement with the exception of skeletal muscle (Museteanu *et al.*, 1991). In this model cytokines play an important role in development of arthritis. The best animal model to study neurological Lyme disease is in rhesus monkey primates (Philipp *et al.*, 1993; Roberts *et al.*, 1995; Pachner *et al.*, 1995a, b; England *et al.*, 1997a, b). They can be infected by tick bite, and go on to develop EM, conjunctivitis, musculoskeletal and cardiac disease. Neurological involvement occurs both early and late, and involves both CNS and PNS. CSF pleocytosis occurs within 5 weeks of inoculation, and CSF is PCR positive. CSF pleocytosis and PCR positivity may wax and wane. Within 3 months of infection there is peripheral nerve involvement which persists at least 2 years. Infected monkeys show chronic meningeal inflammation. Unfortunately, it has not been possible to culture spirochaetes from CNS or PNS tissues. Nevertheless, ongoing studies may advance understanding of the human infection.

Specific issues

European versus North American Lyme disease

North America and Europe have distinct *B. burgdorferi* genospecies, with considerable strain heterogeneity between the two geographic regions. This seems to translate to a number of clinical and laboratory differences in Lyme disease (Table 2.16). This is probably relevant to interpreting published literature, since results may not be fully extrapolatable. Treatment of neurological infection with oral antibiotics was reported as successful in Europe, but has been associated with treatment failures in North America.

Paediatric Lyme disease

There may be age-related differences in Lyme disease. Children have the highest rate of infection. Most (90%) present with EM or multifocal EM. The major paediatric neurological syndrome is facial nerve palsy (Cook *et al.*, 1997; Shapiro and Seltzer, 1997). As opposed to adults PNS syndromes are unusual, and intracranial hypertension seems to be age-restricted to children and adolescents (Belman *et al.*, 1993). Sleep disturbance may be more common in children, while fatigue complaints are less common. Paediatric patients have

Table 2.16   North American versus European Lyme disease.

Lyme disease features	North America	Europe
Epidemiology	More restricted	More generalized
Genospecies	Limited to *B. burgdorferi sensu stricto*	*B. burgdorferi sensu stricto B. garinii B. afzelii*
Clinical	Skin manifestation limited to EM	Skin manifestations include EM, LC, ACA
	Arthritis common	Arthritis uncommon
	Acute painful radiculoneuritis	Acute painful radiculoneuritis very common
	Encephalopathy relatively common	Encephalopathy relatively uncommon
Laboratory	CSF inflammatory changes not striking	Striking CSF inflammatory changes
	Intrathecal antibody production variable	Intrathecal antibody production almost universal
	Oligoclonal band production, IgG unusual	Oligoclonal bands, IgG production very common

an excellent prognosis, and recover faster and with less sequelae than adults. In a recent study of 201 consecutive children (66% EM, 23% multifocal EM, 6% arthritis, 3% facial nerve palsy, 2% meningitis, 0.5% carditis), 94% were completely asymptomatic 1 month after presentation (Gerber *et al.*, 1996). At extended follow up an average of 25 months later, none had late or recurrent disease.

Congenital infection

There is no identifiable congenital Lyme disease syndrome, and the risk of congenital infection is very low (Silver, 1997). Although there are case reports of perinatal transmission resulting in preterm delivery, fetal death, and fetal malformations, epidemiological studies confirm a very low risk. In one study of 19 maternal infections, in whom only 13 received antibiotics, the transmission rate was zero (Markowitz *et al.*, 1986). In a European study of EM during pregnancy treated with ceftriaxone or penicillin, no adverse fetal outcome was documented (Maraspin *et al.*, 1996). Serological surveys indicate no difference in fetal outcomes between seropositive and seronegative mothers. Both oral amoxicillin or ceftriaxone can be used safely during pregnancy; with term pregnancies cefotaxime can be substituted for ceftriaxone, since it does not involve biliary excretion and does not carry a risk for jaundice in the newborn.

Persistent post-treatment symptoms/chronic Lyme disease syndrome

Up to half or more of patients with Lyme disease may note persistent problems 6 months or longer after completion of antibiotic therapy (Asch *et al.*, 1994; Shadick *et al.*, 1994; Benke *et al.*, 1995; Treib *et al.*, 1998). This is more likely to occur when patients are treated after dissemination. Most often patients note symptoms, with little in the way of signs. Problems include fatigue, arthralgias, myalgias, headache, cognitive problems, sleep disturbance, and depression or other mood disturbances (Bujak & Weinstein, 1996; Gaudino *et al.*, 1997). There are a number of possible explanations for persistent post-treatment problems (Table 2.17). Although there is always a concern about persistent infection, when patients receive adequate initial treatment this is unlikely to occur.

In some cases, such patients are diagnosed as having chronic Lyme disease or post Lyme syndrome. This diagnosis has never been defined, and is controversial. Patient groups are quite heterogeneous. In fact, both seropositive and seronegative patients with non-specific symptoms of fatigue, arthralgias, myalgias and other complaints are sometimes included in this group. There are no good data that such patients respond consistently to antibiotics (Fawcett *et al.*, 1997; Svenungsson and Lindh, 1997). In particular, patients with non-specific symptoms without laboratory support for *B. burgdorferi* infection should not be considered to have Lyme disease (Reid *et al.*, 1998). Chronic Lyme disease syndrome is a major clinical issue in certain areas, with patients being treated for prolonged periods of time with various combination

Table 2.17   Potential explanations for persistent post-treatment problems in Lyme disease.

Persistent *B. burgdorferi* infection
Postinfectious immune or inflammatory process
Coinfection by another tick pathogen
Slow recovery
Alternative diagnosis
Reinfection
Fixed damage
Hypochondriasis

antibiotics. Oral, intravenous, and intramuscular preparations are being used. Several ongoing studies are prospectively evaluating such patients. In the next few years it should become clearer whether this syndrome truly exists, and whether it is antibiotic-responsive.

Tick copathogens

Ixodid ticks can carry other pathogens (bacteria, parasites, viruses) besides *B. burgdorferi*, and patients can be coinfected with two or more pathogens through a tick bite (Table 2.18) (Mitchell *et al.*, 1996; Walker *et al.*, 1996; Nadelman *et al.*, 1997; Persing, 1997). Coinfection with a second agent produces more prolonged spirochaetaemia, more severe clinical illness, and a poorer therapeutic response. Perhaps 4–30% of Lyme disease patients are dually infected with a parasite or a rickettsia-like bacterium. *Babesia* is a parasite which typically causes a malaria-like illness. It was recently recognized to cause chronic infection, with fatigue, episodic fever, and chills (Krause *et al.*, 1998). Coinfected patients are more likely to experience fatigue, headache,

Table 2.18   Ixodid tick copathogens.

Agent	Comments
Babesia	Parasitic infection, causes babesiosis
	Acute illness involves malaria-like syndrome (at age extremes, asplenic individuals)
	Chronic infection associated with fatigue, fever, chills
	Treated with clindamycin plus quinine; possible alternatives atovaquone, azithromycin
Ehrlichia equi, or *E. phagocyophila*-like agent	Rickettsial-like bacterium, causes human granulocytic ehrlichiosis
	Infects neutrophils
	Acute illness is non-specific syndrome
	Helpful laboratory clue are ↓ platelets, ↓ WBC, ↑ liver enzymes (transaminases)
	Responds to doxycycline
Tick-borne flavivirus	No clinical syndrome recognized to date
	No specific therapy

sweats, chills, anorexia, emotional lability, nausea, conjunctivitis, and spleno-megaly (Krause *et al.*, 1996). They are thirteen times more likely to be symptomatic for months. They are three times more likely to be PCR positive in blood for circulating *B. burgdorferi* DNA. The antibiotic treatment for babesia is entirely different than that for *B. burgdorferi*.

Ehrlichiae are obligate intracellular Gram-negative like bacteria, which resemble rickettesiae. They show a marked tropism for leucocytes and platelets. Originally recognized as veterinary diseases, they are capable of producing chronic infection. The agent of human granulocyctic ehrlichiosis (HGE), an *E. equi-E. phagocyctophila*-like agent, infects Ixodid ticks (Dumler, 1997). It responds well to tetracycline agents such as doxycycline. Patients infected with Lyme disease and HGE also have worse clinical syndromes.

Coinfection may contribute to persistent post-treatment symptoms, and this is under current investigation. Both babesiosis and HGE increase alanine aminotransferase, and produce thrombobocytopenia. These are unusual in Lyme disease. Both infections appear to be immunosuppressive, which explains the more severe clinical illness. In endemic areas it is reasonable to consider tick copathogen exposure when evaluating for Lyme disease. The simplest way to screen for exposure is to look for an antibody response, but experimental PCR assay as well as culture are available for both agents.

Future directions

The next few years are likely to see advances in several areas. The basic biology of *B. burgdorferi* will be better understood, with regard to neurotropism, pathogenicity, and strain heterogeneity. The host immune and inflammatory response, and its impact on clinical disease manifestations, should be clarified. Improved and standardized antibody tests will be used, including an antibody test for vaccinees. It is hoped that an active infection assay, be it PCR, neoantigen detection, or some other test, can be developed. Improved vaccines will become available, and the role of dual infection will be further clarified. Finally, the bothersome clinical topic of chronic Lyme disease may be solved. Ultimately, however, the most important impact of Lyme disease may well be that lessons learned from dealing with this disorder will be applied to other infections of the nervous system, both old and new.

References

Agger, W. A. and Case, K. L. (1997). Clinical comparison of borrelicidal-antibody test with indirect immunofluorescence and enzyme-linked immunosorbent assays for diagnosis of Lyme disease. *Mayo Clin. Proc.*, **72**, 510–514.

Agre, F. and Schwarz, R. (1993). The value of early treatment of deer tick bite for the prevention of Lyme disease. *Am. J. Dis. Child.*, **147**, 945–947.

Albisetti, M., Schaer, G., Good, M., Boltshauser, E. and Nadal, D. (1997). Diagnostic value of cerebrospinal fluid examination in children with peripheral facial palsy and suspected Lyme borreliosis. *Neurology*, **49**, 817–824.

American Academy of Neurology Quality Standards Subcommittee (1996). Practice parameter: Diagnosis of patients with nervous system Lyme borreliosis (Lyme disease) – Summary statement. *Neurology*, **46**, 881–882.

American College of Physicians. (1997). Clinical guideline, Part 1. Guidelines for laboratory evaluation in the diagnosis of Lyme disease. *Ann. Intern. Med.*, **127**, 1106–1108.

Anderson, J. F. (1989). Epizootiology of *Borrelia* in *Ixodes* tick vectors and reservoir hosts. *Rev. Infect. Dis.*, **11** (suppl. 6), S1451–S1459.

Asch, E. S., Bujak, D.I., Weiss, M., Peterson, M. G. E. and Weinstein, A. (1994). Lyme disease: an infectious and postinfectious syndrome. *J. Rheumatol.*, **21**, 454–461.

Bakken, L. L., Callister, S. M., Wand, P. J. and Schell, R. F. (1997). Interlaboratory comparison of test results for detection of Lyme disease by 516 participants in the Wisconsin State Laboratory of Hygiene/College of American Pathologists Proficiency Testing. *J. Clin. Microbiol.*, **35**, 537–543.

Balmetti, T. and Piffaretti, J. C. (1995). Association between different clinical manifestations of Lyme disease and different species of *Borrelia burgdorferi sensu lato*. *Res. Microbiol.*, **146**, 329–340.

Barbour, A. G. (1996). Does Lyme disease occur in the south? A survey of emerging tick-borne infections in the region. *Am. J. Med. Sci.*, **311**, 34–40.

Barbour, A. G. (1998). Fall and rise of Lyme disease and other Ixodes tick-borne infections in North America and Europe. *Brit. Med. Bull.*, **54**, 647–658.

Barbour, A. G. and Hayes, S. F. (1986). Biology of species. *Microbiol. Rev.*, **50**, 381–400.

Belman, A. L., Coyle, P. K. and Dattwyler, R. (1993). Neurologic manifestations in children with neurologic Lyme disease. *Neurology*, **43**, 2609–2614.

Belman, A. L., Reynolds, L., Preston, T. *et al.* (1997). Cerebrospinal fluid findings in children with Lyme disease-associated facial nerve palsy. *Arch. Ped. Adolesc. Med.*, **151**, 1224–1228.

Benach, J. L., Bosler, E. M., Hanrahan, J. P. *et al.* (1983). Spirochetes isolated from the blood of two patients with Lyme disease. *N. Engl. J. Med.*, **308**, 740–742.

Benke, T.H., Gasse, T.H., Hittmair-Delazer, M. and Schmutzhard, E. (1995). Lyme encephalopathy: long term neuropsychological deficits years after acute neuro-borreliosis. *Acta Neurol. Scand.*, **91**, 353–357.

Berger, B. W. (1997). Current aspects of Lyme disease and other *Borrelia burgdorferi* infections. *Dermatol. Clin.*, **15**, 247–255.

Bujak, D. I. and Weinstein, A. (1996). Clinical and neurocognitive features of the post Lyme syndrome. *J. Rheumatol.*, **23**, 1392–1397.

Burgdorfer, W. (1983). Discovery of *Borrelia burgdorferi*. In: *Lyme Disease* (P. K. Coyle, ed.) St Louis: Mosby Year Book. pp. 3–7.

Burgdorfer, W. (1984). Discovery of the Lyme disease spirochete and its relation to tick vectors. *Yale J. Biol. Med.*, **57**, 515–520.

Burkot, T. R., Schriefer, M. E. and Larsen, S. A. (1997). Cross-reactivity to *Borrelia burgdorferi* proteins in serum samples from residents of a tropical country nonendemic for Lyme disease. *J. Infect. Dis.*, **175**, 466–469.

Burns, M. J., Sellati, T. J., Teng, E. I. and Furie, M. B. (1997). Production of interleukin-8 (IL-8) by cultured endothelial cells in response to *Borrelia burgdorferi* occurs independently of secreted IL-1 and tumor necrosis factor alpha and is required for subsequent transendothelial migration of neutrophils. *Infect. Immun.*, **65**, 1217–1222.

Callister, S. M., Jobe, D. A., Schell, R. F., Pavia, C. S. and Lovrich, S. D. (1996). Sensitivity and specificity of the borreliacidal–antibody test during early Lyme disease: A 'gold standard'? *Clin. Diag. Lab. Immunol.*, **3**, 399–402.

Chehrenama, M., Zagardo, M. T. and Koski, C. L. (1997). Subarachnoid hemorrhage in a patient with Lyme disease. *Neurology*, **48**, 520–523.

Christen, H. J. (1996). Lyme disease in children. *Ann. Med.*, **28**, 235–240.

Coburn, J., Magoun, L., Bodary, S. C. and Leong, J. M. (1998). Integrins alpha(v)beta3 and alpha5beta1 mediate attachment of Lyme disease spirochetes to human cells. *Infect. Immunol.*, **66**, 1946–1952.

Cook, S. P., Macartney, K. K., Rose, C. D. *et al.* (1997). Lyme disease and seventh nerve paralysis in children. *Am. J. Otolaryngol.*, **18**, 320–323.

Costello, C. M., Steere, A. C., Pinkerton, R. E. and Feder, H. M. JR. (1989). A prospective study of tick bite in an endemic area for Lyme disease. *J. Infect. Dis.*, **159**, 136–139.

Coyle, P. K. (1989). *Borrelia burgdorferi* antibodies in multiple sclerosis patients. *Neurology*, **39**, 760–761.

Coyle, P. K. (1997a). *Borrelia burgdorferi* infection: clinical diagnostic techniques. *Immunol. Invest.*, **26**, 117–128.

Coyle, P. K. (1997b). Lyme disease. In: *Central Nervous System Infectious Diseases and Therapy* (K. L. Roos, ed.) New York: Marcel Dekker. pp 213–236.

Coyle, P. K., Schutzer, S. E., Belman, A. L. *et al.* (1990). CSF immune complexes in patients exposed to *Borrelia burgdorferi*: detection of Borrelia specific and nonspecific complexes. *Ann. Neurol.*, **28**, 739–744.

Coyle, P. K., Deng, Z., Schutzer, S. E., Belman, A. L., Krupp, L. B. and Luft, B. (1993). Detection of *Borrelia burgdorferi* antigens in cerebrospinal fluid. *Neurology*, **43**, 1093–1097.

Dammin, G. J. (1989). Erythema migrans: a chronicle. *Rev. Infect. Dis.*, **11**, 142–151.

Danek, A., Uttner, I., Yoursry, T. and Pfister, H. W. (1996). Lyme neuroborreliosis disguised as normal pressure hydrocephalus. *Neurology*, **46**, 1743–1745.

Dattwyler, R. J., Halperin, J. J., Volkman, D. J. and Luft, B. J. (1988a) Treatment of late Lyme disease – randomised comparison of ceftriaxone and penicillin. *Lancet*, i, 1191–1194.

Dattwyler, R. J., Halperin, J. J., Pass, H. and Luft, B. J. (1987). Ceftriaxone as effective therapy for refractory Lyme disease. *J. Infect. Dis.*, **155**, 1322–1325.

Dattwyler, R. J., Luft, B. J., Kunkel, M. J. *et al.* (1997). Ceftriaxone compared with doxycycline for the treatment of acute disseminated Lyme disease. *N. Engl. J. Med.*, **337**, 289–294.

Dattwyler, R. J., Volkman, D. J., Luft, B. J. *et al.* (1988b) Seronegative Lyme disease. Dissociation of specific T- and B-lymphocyte responses to *Borrelia burgdorferi*. *N. Engl. J. Med.*, **319**, 1441–1446.

Dotevall, L. and Hagberg, L. (1989) Penetration of doxycycline into cerebrospinal fluid in patients treated for suspected Lyme neuroborreliosis. *Antimicrob. Agents Chemo.*, **33**, 1078–1080.

Dotevall, L., Rosengren, L. E. and Hagberg, L. (1996). Increased cerebrospinal fluid levels of glial fibrillary acidic protein (GFAP) in Lyme neuroborreliosis. *Infection*, **24**, 125–129.

Dumler, J. S. (1997). Is human granulocytic ehrlichiosis a new Lyme disease? Review and comparison of clinical, laboratory, epidemiological, and some biological features. *Clin. Inf. Dis.*, **25**, S43–S47.

Ekerfelt, C., Ernerudh, J., Bunikis, J. *et al.* (1997). Compartmentalization of antigen specific cytokine responses to the central nervous system in CNS borreliosis: secretion of IFN-gamma predominates over IL-4 secretion in response to outer surface proteins of Lyme disease Borrelia spirochetes. *J. Neuroimmunol.*, **79**, 155–162.

England, J. D., Bohm, R. P. jr, Roberts, E. D. and Philipp, M. T. (1997a) Lyme neuroborreliosis in the rhesus monkey. *Seminars Neurol.*, **17**, 53–56.

England, J. D., Bohm, R. P. jr, Roberts, E. D. and Philipp, M. T. (1997b). Mononeuropathy multiplex in rhesus monkeys with chronic Lyme disease. *Ann. Neurol.*, **41**, 375–384.

Engstrom, S. M., Shoop, E. and Johnson, R. C. (1995). Immunoblot interpretation criteria for serodiagnosis of early Lyme disease. *J. Clin. Microbiol.*, **33**, 419–427.

Fallon, H. and Nields, A. (1994). Lyme disease: a neuropsychiatric illness. *Am. J. Psychiatry*, **151**, 1571–1583.

Fawcett, P. T., Rose, C. D., Gibney, K. M. and Doughty, R. A. (1997). Correlation of seroreactivity with response to antibiotics in pediatric Lyme borreliosis. *Clin. Diagn. Lab. Immunol.*, **4**, 85–88.

Feder, H. M. jr and Whitaker, D. L. (1995). Misdiagnosis of erythema migrans. *Am. J. Med.*, **99**, 412–419.

Fikrig, E., Telford, S. R., Barthold, S. W. *et al.* (1992). Elimination of *Borrelia burgdorferi* from vector ticks feeding on OspA-immunized mice. *Proc. Natl. Acad. Sci.*, **89**, 5418–5421.

Fix, A. D., Strickland, T. and Grant, J. (1998). Tick bites and Lyme disease in an endemic setting: problematic use of serologic testing and prophylactic antibiotic therapy. *J. Am. Med. Assoc.*, **279**, 206–210.

Foley, D. M., Gayek, R. J., Skare, J. T., et al. (1995). Rabbit model of Lyme borreliosis: erythema migrans, infection-derived immunity, and identification of Borrelia burgdorferi proteins associated with virulence and protective immunity. J. Clin. Invest., 96, 965–975.

Garcia-Monco, J. C. and Benach, J. L. (1995). Lyme neuroborreliosis. Ann. Neurol., 37, 691–702.

Garcia-Monco, J. C. and Benach, J. L. (1997). Mechanisms of injury in Lyme neuroborreliosis. Seminars Neurol., 17, 57–62.

Gaudino, E., Coyle, P. K. and Krupp, L. (1997). Post-Lyme syndrome chronic fatigue syndrome. Neuropsychiatric similarities and differences. Arch. Neurol., 54, 1372–1376.

Gerber, M. A., Shapiro, E. D., Burke, G. S., Parcells, V. J. and Bell, G. L. (1996). Lyme disease in children in Southeastern Connecticut. N. Engl. J. Med., 335, 1270–1274.

Girschick, H. J., Huppertz, H. I., Russmann, H., Krenn, V. and Karch, H. (1996). Intracellular persistence of Borrelia burgdorferi in human synovial cells. Rheum., 16, 125–132.

Goodman, J. L., Jurkovich, P., Kodner, C. and Johnson, R. C. (1991). Persistent cardiac and urinary tract infections with Borrelia burgdorferi in experimentally infected Syrian hamsters. J. Clin. Microbiol., 29, 894–896.

Gross, D. M., Forsthuber, T., Tary-Lehmann, M. et al. (1998a). Identification of LFA-1 as a candidate autoantigen in treatment-resistant Lyme arthritis. Science, 281, 703–706.

Gross, D. M., Steere, A. C. and Huber, B. T. (1998b). T helper 1 reponse is dominant and localized to the synovial fluid in patients with Lyme arthritis. J. Immunol., 160, 1022–1028.

Haass, A. (1998). Lyme neuroborreliosis. Curr. Opinion Neurol., 11, 253–258.

Halperin, J. J., Little, B. W., Coyle, P. K. and Dattwyler, R. J. (1987). Lyme disease: cause of a treatable peripheral neuropathy. Neurology, 37, 1700–1706.

Halperin, J., Logogian, E. L., Finkel, M. F. and Pearl, R. A. (1996). Practice parameters for the diagnosis of patients with nervous system Lyme borreliosis (Lyme disease). Neurology, 46, 619–627.

Halperin, J. J., Luft, B. J., Volkman, D. J. and Dattwyler, R. J. (1990). Lyme neurologic Lyme disease: peripheral nervous system abnormalities. Brain, 113, 1207–1221.

Hansen, K. (1994). Lyme neuroborreliosis: improvements of the laboratory diagnosis and a survey of epidemiological and clinical features in Denmark 1985–1990. Acta Neur. Scand., 89S, 7–44.

Hansen, K. and Lebech, A.-M. (1992). The clinical and epidemiological profile of Lyme neurologic Lyme disease in Denmark 1985–1990. Brain, 115, 399–423.

Hauser, U., Lehnert, G., Lobentanzer, R. and Wilske, B. (1997). Interpretation criteria for standardized Western blots for three European species of Borrelia burgdorferi sensu lato. J. Clin. Microbiol., 35, 1433–1444.

Hilton, F., Devoti J. and Sood, S. K. (1996). Recommendation to include OspA and OspB in the new immunoblotting criteria for serodiagnosis of Lyme disease. *J. Clin Microbiol.*, **34**, 1353–1354.

Hilton, F., Tramontano, A., Devoti, J. and Sood, S. K. (1997). Temporal study of immunoglobulin M seroreactivity to *Borrelia burgdorferi* in patients treated for Lyme borreliosis. *J. Clin. Microbiol.*, **35**, 774–776.

Hofmann, H. (1996). Lyme borreliosis – problems of serological diagnosis. *Infection*, **24**, 470–472.

Horowitz, H. W., Dworkin, B., Forseter, G. *et al.* (1996). Liver function in early Lyme disease. *Hepatology*, **23**, 1412–1417.

Hu, L. T. and Klempner, M. S. (1997). Host-pathogen interactions in the immuno-pathogenesis of Lyme disease. *J. Clin. Immunol.*, **17**, 354–365.

Ikushima, M., Kawahashi, S., Ohzeki, Y. *et al.* (1998). A new specific serodiagnosis system for Lyme disease: use of synthetic peptides derived from outer surface protein C of *Borrelia burgdorferi*. *Opportunistic Pathogens*, **9**, 21–25.

Karlsson, M., Hammers-Berggren, S., Lindquist, L. *et al.* (1994). Comparison of intravenous penicillin G and oral doxycycline for treatment of Lyme neurologic Lyme disease. *Neurology*, **44**, 1203–1207.

Karlsson, M., Hammers, S., Nilsson-Ehle, I., Malmborg, A.-S. and Wretlind, B. (1996). Concentrations of doxycycline and penicillin G in sera and cerebrospinal fluid of patients treated for neuroborreliosis. *Antimicrob. Agents Chemo.*, **40**, 1104–1107.

Keirans, J. E., Hutcheson, H. J., Durden, L. A. and Klompen, J. S. H. (1996). *Ixodes (Ixodes) scapularis* (Acari: Ixodidae): Rediscription of all active stages, distribution, hosts, geographical variation, and medical and veterinary importance. *J. Med. Entomol.*, **33**, 297–318.

Kindstrand, E., Nilsson, B. Y., Hovmark, A., Pirskanen, R. and Asbrink, E. (1997). Peripheral neuropathy in acrodermitis chronica atrophicans – a late Borrelia manifestation. *Acta Neurol. Scand.*, **95**, 338–345.

Krause, P. J., Spielman, A., Telford, S. R. III, *et al.* (1998). Persistent parasitemia after acute babesiosis. *N. Engl. J. Med.*, **339**, 160–165.

Krause, P. J., Telford, S. R., Spielman, A. *et al.* (1996). Concurrent Lyme disease and Babesiosis. Evidence for increased severity and duration of illness. *J. Am. Med. Assoc.*, **275**, 1657–1660.

Krüger, H., Kohlehepp, W. and König S. (1990). Follow-up of antibiotically treated and untreated neuroborreliosis. *Acta Neurol. Scand.*, **82**, 59–67.

Kuiper, H., de Jongh, B. M., van Dam, A. P. *et al.* (1994). Evaluation of central nervous system involvement in Lyme borreliosis patients with a solitary erythema migrans lesion. *Eur. J. Clin. Microbiol. Infect. Dis.*, **13**, 379–387.

Lawrence, C., Lipton, R. B., Lowry, F. D. *et al.* (1995). Seronegative chronic relapsing neuroborreliosis. *Eur. Neurol.*, **35**, 113–117.

Ledue, T. B., Collins, M. F. and Craig, W. Y. (1996). New laboratory guidelines for serologic diagnosis of Lyme disease: evaluation of the two-test protocol. *J. Clin. Microbiol.*, **34**, 2343–2350.

Leong, J. M., Wang, H., Magoun, L. *et al.* (1998). Different classes of proteoglycans contribute to the attachment of *Borrelia burgdorferi* to cultured endothelial and brain cells. *Infect. Immunol.*, **66**, 994–999.

Logigian, E. L., Johnson, K. A., Kijewski, M. F. *et al.* (1997). Reversible cerebral hypoperfusion in Lyme encephalopathy. *Neurology*, **49**, 1661–1670.

Logigian, E. L., Kaplan, R. F. and Steere, A. C. (1990). Chronic neurologic manifestations of Lyme disease. *N. Engl. J. Med.*, **323**, 1438–1444.

Logigian, E. L. and Steere, A. C. (1992). Clinical and electrophysiologic findings in chronic neuropathy of Lyme disease. *Neurology*, **42**, 303–311.

Luft, B. J., Dattwyler, R. J., Johnson, R. C. *et al.* (1996). Azithromycin compared with amoxicillin in the treatment of erythema migrans: a double-blind, randomized controlled trial. *Ann. Int. Med.*, **124**, 785-791.

Luft, B. J, Steinman, C. R., Neimark, H. C. *et al.* (1992). Invasion of the central nervous system by *Borrelia burgdorferi* in acute disseminated infection. *J. Am. Med. Assoc.*, **267**, 1364–1367.

Magid, D., Schwartz, B., Craft, J. and Schwartz, J. S. (1992). Prevention of Lyme disease after tick bites. A cost-effective analysis. *N. Engl. J. Med.*, **327**, 534–541.

Magnarelli, L. A., Fikrig, E., Padula, S. J., Anderson, J. F. and Flavell, R. A. (1996). Use of recombinant antigens of *Borrelia burgdorferi* in serologic tests for the diagnosis of Lyme borreliosis. *J. Clin. Microbiol.*, **34**, 237–240.

Maimone, D., Villanova, M., Stanta, G. *et al.* (1997). Detection of *Borrelia burgdorferi* DNA and complement membrane attack complex deposits in the sural nerve of a patient with chronic polyneuropathy and tertiary Lyme disease. *Muscle Nerve*, **20**, 969–975.

Maraspin, V., Cimperman, J., Lotric-Furlan, S., Pleterski-Rigler, D. and Strle, F. (1996). Treatment of erythema migrans in pregnancy. *Clin. Inf. Dis.*, **22**, 788–793.

Markowitz, L. E., Steare, A. C., Benach, J. L., Slade, J. D. and Broome, C. V. (1986). Lyme disease during pregnancy. *J. Am. Med. Assoc.*, **225**, 3394–3396.

Marshall, W. F. III, Telford, S. R. III, Rys, P. N. *et al.* (1994). Detection of *Borrelia burgdorferi* DNA in museum specimens of *Peromyscus leucopus*. *J. Infect. Dis.*, **170**, 1027–1032.

Mathiesen, D. A., Oliver, J. H. JR, Kolbert, C.P. *et al.* (1997). Genetic heterogeneity of *Borrelia burgdorferi* in the United States *J. Infect. Dis.*, **175**, 98–107.

Matuschka, F. R., Ohlenbush, A., Eiffert, H., Richter, D. and Spielman, A. (1996). Characteristics of Lyme disease spirochetes in archived European ticks. *J. Infect. Dis.*, **174**, 424–426.

Mikkila, H., Seppala, I., Leirisalo-Repo, M., Immonen, I. and Karma, A. (1997). The etiology of uveitis: the role of infections with special reference to Lyme borreliosis. *Acta Ophthalmol. Scand.*, **75**, 716–719.

Mitchell, P. D., Reed, K. D. and Hofkes, J. M. (1996). Immunoserologic evidence of coinfection with *Borrelia burgdorferi, Babesia microti*, and human granulocytic Ehrlichia species in residents of Wisconsin and Minnesota. *J. Clin. Microbiol.*, **34**, 724–727.

Mokry, M., Flaschka, G., Kleinert, G. *et al.* (1990). Chronic Lyme disease with an expansive gratulomatous lesion in the cerebellopontine angle. *Neurosurgery*, **27**, 446–451.

Museteanu, C., Schaible, U. E., Stehle, T., Kramer, M. D. and Simon, M. M. (1991). Myositis in mice inoculated with *Borrelia burgdorferi*. *Am J Pathol.*, **139**, 11267–11271.

Nadelman, R. B., Horowitz, H. W., Hsieh, T.-C. *et al.* (1997). Simultaneous human granulocytic ehrlichiosis and Lyme borreliosis. *N. Eng. J. Med.*, **337**, 27–30.

Nadelman, R. B., Nowakowski, J., Forseter, G. *et al.* (1996). The clinical spectrum of early Lyme disease in patients with culture-confirmed erythema migrans. *Am. J. Med.*, **100**, 502–508.

Nadelman, R. B. and Wormser, G. P. (1995). Erythema migrans and early Lyme disease. *Am. J. Med.*, **98**, 15S–24S.

Nagi, K. S., Joshi, R. and Thakur, R. K. (1996). Cardiac manifestations of Lyme disease: a review. *Can. J. Cardiol.*, **12**, 503–506.

Nichol, G., Dennis, D. T., Steere, A. C. *et al.* (1998). Test-treatment strategies for patients suspected of having Lyme disease: a cost-effectiveness analysis. *Ann. Int. Med.*, **128**, 37–48.

Nilsson, I., Alves, M. and Nässberger, L. (1994). Response of soluble IL-2 receptor, interleukin-2 and interleukin-6 in patients with positive and negative *Borrelia burgdorferi* serology. *Infection*, **22**, 316–320.

Nilsson, I. and von Rosen, I. A. (1996). Serum antibodies against *Borrelia afzelii, Borrelia burgdorferi sensu stricto* and the 41-kiloDalton flagellin in patients from a Lyme borreliosis endemic area: analysis by EIA and immunoblot. *APMIS*, **104**, 907–914.

Nocton, J. J., Bloom, B. J., Rutledge, B. J. *et al.* (1996). Detection of *Borrelia burgdorferi* DNA by polymerase chain reaction in cerebrospinal fluid in Lyme neurologic Lyme disease. *J. Infect. Dis.*, **174**, 623–626.

Norman, G. L., Atig, G., Bigaigonon, G. and Hogrefe, W. R. (1996). Serodiagnosis of Lyme borreliosis by *Borrelia burgdorferi sensu stricto*, *G. garinii*, and *B. afzelii* Western blots (immunoblots). *J. Clin. Microbiol.*, **34**, 1732–1738.

Oksi, J., Kalimo, H., Marttila, R. J. *et al.* (1996). Inflammatory brain changes in Lyme borreliosis. A report on three patients and review of the literature. *Brain*, **119**, 2143–2154.

Oliver, J. H. JR (1996). Lyme borreliosis in the southern United States: a review. *J. Parasitol.*, **82**, 926–935.

Olsen, B., Duffy, D. C., Jaenson, T. G. T. *et al.* (1995). Transhemispheric exchange of Lyme disease spirochetes by seabirds. *J. Clin. Microbiol.*, **33**, 3270–3274.

Orloski, K. A., Campbell, G. L., Genese, C. A. *et al.* (1998). Emergence of Lyme disease in Hunterdon County, New Jersey, 1993: a case-control study of risk factors and evaluation of reporting patterns. *Am. J. Epidemiol.*, **147**, 391–397.

Oschmann, P., Wellensiek, H.-J., Dorndorf, W. and Pflughaupt, K. W. (1997). Intrathecal synthesis of specific antibodies in neuroborreliosis: comparison of immunoblotting, indirect immunofluorescence assay and enzyme-linked immunosorbent assay. *Lab. Med.*, **21**, 528–534.

Pachner, A. R., Delaney, E. and O'Neill, T. (1995a). Neuroborreliosis in the nonhuman primate: *Borrelia burgdorferi* persists in the central nervous systems. *Ann. Neurol.*, **38**, 667–668.

Pachner, A. R., Delaney, E., O'Neill, T. and Major, E. (1995b). Inoculation of nonhuman primates with the N40 strain of *Borrelia burgdorferi* leads to a model of Lyme neuroborreliosis faithful to human disease. *Neurology*, **45**, 165–172.

Perides, G., Charness, M. E., Tanner, L. M. *et al.* (1998). Matrix metalloproteinases in the cerebrospinal fluid of patients with Lyme neuroborreliosis. *J. Infect. Dis.*, **177**, 401–408.

Persing, D. H. (1997). The cold zone: a curious convergence of tick-transmitted diseases. *Clin. Infect. Dis.*, **25**, S35–S42.

Philipp, M. T., Aydintug, M. K., Bohm, R. P. JR *et al.* (1993). Early and early disseminated phases of Lyme disease in the rhesus monkey: a model for infection in humans. *Infect. Immun.*, **61**, 3047–3059.

Philipp, M. T., Lobet, Y., Bohm, R. P. *et al.* (1997). The outer surface protein A (OspA) vaccine against Lyme disease: efficacy in the rhesus monkey. *Vaccine*, **15**, 1872–1887.

Picken, M. M., Picken, R. N., Han, D. *et al.* (1997). A two year prospective study to compare culture and polymerase chain reaction amplification for the detection and diagnosis of Lyme borreliosis. *Molec. Pathol.*, **50**, 186–193.

Pohl-Koppe, A., Balashov, K. E., Steere, A. C., Logigian, E. L. and Hafler, D. A. (1998). Identification of a T cell subset capable of both IFN-gamma and IL-10 secretion in patients with chronic *Borrelia burgdorferi* infection. *J. Immunol.*, **160**, 1804–1810.

Priem, S., Rittig, M. G., Kamradt, T., Burmester, G. R. and Krause, A. (1997). An optimized PCR leads to rapid and highly sensitive detection of *Borrelia burgdorferi* in patients with Lyme borreliosis. *J. Clin. Microbiol.*, **35**, 685–690.

Rauer, S., Spohn, N., Rasiah, C., Neubert, U. and Vogt, A. (1998). Enzyme-linked immunosorbent assay using recombinant OspC and the internal 14-kDa flagellin fragment for serodiagnosis of early Lyme disease. *J. Clin. Microbiol.*, **36**, 857–861.

Reid, M. C., Schoen, R. T., Evans, J. *et al.* (1998). The consequences of overdiagnosis and overtreatment of Lyme disease: an observational study. *Ann. Intern. Med.*, **128**, 354–362.

Roberts, E. D., Bohm, R. P. JR, Cogswell, F. B. *et al.* (1995). Chronic Lyme disease in the rhesus monkey. *Lab. Invest.*, **72**, 146–160.

Rosa, P. A. (1997). Microbiology of *Borrelia burgdorferi*. *Seminars Neurol.*, **17**, 5–10.

Rutkowski, S., Busch, D. H. and Huppertz, H. I. (1997). Lymphocyte proliferation assay in response to *Borrelia burgdorferi* in patients with Lyme arthritis: analysis of lymphocyte subsets. *Rheumatol. Internat.*, **17**, 151–158.

Scelsa, S., Lipton, R., Sander, H. *et al.* (1995). Headache characteristics in hospitalized patients with Lyme disease. *Headache*, **35**, 125–130.

Schmidt, B. L. (1997). PCR in laboratory diagnosis of human *Borrelia burgdorferi* infections. *Clin. Microbiol. Rev.*, **10**, 185–201.

Schuttelaar, M. L., Laeijendecker, R., Heinhuis, R. J. and Van Joost, T. (1997). Erythema multiforme and persistent erythema as early cutaneous manifestations of Lyme disease. *J. Am. Acad. Dermatol.*, **37**, 873–875.

Schutzer, S. E., Coyle, P. K., Belman, A. L., Golightly, M. G. and Drulle, J. (1990). Sequestration of antibody to *Borrelia burgdorferi* in immune complexes in seronegative Lyme disease. *Lancet*, **335**, 312–315.

Schutzer, S. E., Coyle, P. K., Krupp, L. B. *et al.* (1997). Simultaneous expression of Borrelia OspA and OspC and IgM response in cerebrospinal fluid in early neurologic Lyme disease. *J. Clin. Inv.*, **100**, 763–767.

Schwan, T. G., Piesman, J., Golde, W. T. *et al.* (1995). Induction of an outer surface protein on *Borrelia burgdorferi* during tick feeding. *Proc. Nat. Acad. Sci.*, **92**, 2909–2913.

Shadick, N. A., Daltroy, L. H., Phillips, C. B. *et al.* (1998). Test-treatment strategies for patients suspected of having Lyme disease: a cost-effective analysis. *Ann. Int. Med.*, **128**, 37–48.

Shadick, N. A., Phillips, C. B., Logigian, E. L. *et al.* (1994). The long-term clinical outcomes of Lyme disease. A population-based retrospective cohort study. *Ann. Intern. Med.*, **121**, 560–567.

Shapiro, E. D., Gerber, M. A., Holabird, N. D. *et al.* (1992). A controlled trial of antimicrobial prophylaxis for Lyme disease after deer-tick bites. *N. Engl. J. Med.*, **327**, 1769–1773.

Shapiro, E. D. and Seltzer, E. G. (1997). Lyme disease in children. *Seminars Neurol.*, **17**, 39–44.

Sigal, L. H. (1997). Lyme disease: a review of aspects of its immunology and immunopathogenesis. *Ann. Rev. Immunol.*, **15**, 63–92.

Sigal, L. H. (1998). Pitfalls in the diagnosis and management of Lyme disease. *Arthr. Rheum.*, **41**, 195–204.

Sigal, L. H., Zahradnik, J. M., Lavin, P. *et al.* (1998). A vaccine consisting of recombinant *Borrelia burgdorferi* outer-surface protein A to prevent Lyme disease. *N. Eng. J. Med.*, **339**, 216–222.

Silver, H. M. (1997). Lyme disease during pregnancy. *Infect. Dis. Clin. N. Am.*, **11**, 93–97.

Smouha, E. E., Coyle, P. K. and Shukri, S. (1997). Facial nerve palsy in Lyme disease: Evaluation of clinical diagnostic criteria. *Am. J. Otol.*, **18**, 257–261.

Sood, S. K., Salzman, M. B., Johnson, B. J. *et al.* (1997). Duration of tick attachment as a predictor of the risk of Lyme disease in an area in which Lyme disease is endemic. *J. Infect. Dis.*, **175**, 996–999.

Sprenger, H., Krause, A., Kaufmann, A. *et al.* (1997). *Borrelia burgdorferi* induces chemokines in human monocytes. *Infect. Immunol.*, **65**, 4384–4388.

Steere, A. C. (1989). Lyme disease. *N. Engl. J. Med.*, **321**, 586–596.

Steere, A. C. (1997). Diagnosis and treatment of Lyme arthritis. *Med. Clin. Am.*, **81**, 179–194.

Steere, A. C., Grodzicki, R. L., Kornblatt, J. P. *et al.* (1983). The spirochetal etiology of Lyme disease. *N. Eng. J. Med.*, **308**, 733–740.

Steere, A. C., Malawista, S. E. and Snydman, D. R. (1977). Lyme arthritis: an epidemic of oligoarticular arthritis in children and adults in three Connecticut communities. *Arthritis Rheum*, **20**, 7–17.

Steere, A. C., Sikand, V. K., Meurice, F. *et al.* (1998). Vaccine against Lyme disease with recombinant *Borrelia burgdorferi* outer-surface lipoprotein A with adjuvant. *N. Eng. J. Med.*, **339**, 209–215.

Steigbigel, R. T. and Benach, J. L. (1998). Immunization against Lyme disease – an important first step. *N. Eng. J. Med.*, **339**, 263–264.

Straubinger, R. K., Summers, B. A., Chang, Y. F. and Appel, M. J. G. (1997). Persistence of *Borrelia burgdorferi* in experimentally infected dogs after antibiotic treatment. *J. Clin. Microbiol.*, **35**, 111–116.

Strickland, G. T., Karp, A. C., Mathews, A. and Pena, C. A. (1997). Utilization and cost of serologic tests for Lyme disease in Maryland. *J. Infect. Dis.*, **176**, 819–821.

Sumiya, H., Kobayashi, K., Mizukoshi, C. *et al.* (1997). Brain perfusion SPECT in Lyme neuroborreliosis. *J. Nucl. Med.*, **38**, 1120–1122.

Svenungsson, B. and Lindh, G. (1997). Lyme borreliosis – an overdiagnosed disease? *Infection*, **25**, 2140–2143.

Tilton, R. C., Sand, M. N. and Manak, M. (1997). The western immunoblot for Lyme disease: determination of sensitivity, specificity, and interpretive criteria with use of commercially available performance panels. *Clin. Inf. Dis.*, **25**, S31–34.

Treib, J., Fernandez, A., Haass, A. *et al.* (1998). Clinical and serologic follow-up in patients with neuroborreliosis. *Neurology*, **51**, 1489–1491.

Treib, J., Woessner, R., Dobler, G., Fernandez, A., Holzer, G. and Schimrigk, K. (1997). Clinical value of specific intrathecal production of antibodies. *Acta Virol.*, **41**, 27–30.

Tugwell, P., Dennis, D. T., Weinstein, A. *et al.* (1997). Clinical guideline, part 2. Laboratory evaluation in the diagnosis of Lyme disease. *Ann. Int. Med.*, **127**, 1109–1123.

Vallat, J. M., Hugon, J., Lubeau, M., Leboutet, M. J., Dumas, M. and Desproges-Gotteron, R. (1987). Tick-bite meningoradiculoneuritis: clinical, electrophysiologic, and histologic findings in 10 cases. *Neurology*, **37**, 749–753.

Vincent, M. S., Roessner, K., Lynch, D. *et al.* (1996). Apoptosis of Fashigh CD4$^+$ synovial T cells by borrelia-reactive Fas-ligand (high) gamma delta T cells in Lyme arthritis. *J. Exp. Med.*, **184**, 2109–2117.

Walker, D. H., Barbour, A. G., Oliver, J. H. *et al.* (1996). Emerging bacterial zoonotic and vector-borne diseases. Ecological and epidemiological factors. *J. Am. Med. Assoc.*, **275**, 463–469.

Wang, W.-Z., Fredikson, S., Xiao, B.-G., *et al.* (1996). Lyme neuroborreliosis: cerebrospinal fluid contains myelin protein-reactive cells secreting interferon-gamma. *Eur. J. Neurol.*, **3**, 122–129.

Warshafsky, S., Nowakowski, J., Nadelman, R. B. *et al.* (1996). Efficacy of antibiotic prophylaxis for prevention of Lyme disease. *J. Gen. Intern. Med.*, **11**, 329–333.

Wilske, B., Busch, U., Eiffert, H. *et al.* (1996). Diversity of OspA and OspC among cerebrospinal fluid isolates of *Borrelia burgdorferi sensu lato* from patients with neuroborreliosis in Germany. *Med. Microbiol. Imm.*, **184**, 195–201.

Wormser, G. P. (1997). Treatment and prevention of Lyme disease, with emphasis on antimicrobial therapy for neuroborreliosis and vaccination. *Seminars Neurol.*, **17**, 45–52.

Yin, Z., Braun, J., Neure, L. *et al.* (1997). T cell cytokine pattern in the joints of patients with Lyme arthritis and its regulation by cytokines and anticytokines. *Arthr Rheum.*, **40**, 69–79.

Yu, Z., Tu, J. and Chu, Y. H. (1997). Confirmation of cross-reactivity between Lyme antibody H9724 and human heat shock protein 60 by a combinatorial approach. *Anal. Chem.*, **69**, 4515–4518.

Zhong, W., Oschmann, P. and Wellensiek, H.-J. (1997). Detection and preliminary characterization of circulating immune complexes in patients with Lyme disease. *Med. Microbiol. Immunol.*, **186**, 153–158.

3

Postinfectious encephalomyelitis

Patricia K. Coyle

Introduction

There are a number of well described and characteristic postinfectious neurological syndromes (Table 3.1). These disorders can involve almost any region of the central (CNS) or peripheral nervous system (PNS). By definition, postinfectious syndromes are not due to direct neural invasion by a pathogen. Most have an acute onset, and are temporally linked either to a systemic infection or a vaccination. In addition to these acute/subacute disorders, there are several chronic postinfectious syndromes. Postpolio syndrome, which occurs years after the initial infection, is characterized by development of new muscle weakness, fatigue, pain and atrophy. Chronic fatigue syndrome (also called chronic immune dysfunction syndrome) is characterized by development of persistent debilitating fatigue and malaise accompanied by a number of multisystem complaints. Fibromyalgia syndrome, another chronic

Table 3.1 Postinfectious syndromes.

	Neurological area involved	Examples
Acute syndromes		
1 Encephalitis, encephalomyelitis	CNS	Acute disseminated encephalomyelitis, acute haemorrhagic leukoencephalitis
2 Encephalopathy	CNS	Acute toxic encephalopathy, Reye syndrome
3 Cerebellitis	Cerebellum	Acute cerebellar ataxia
4 Cranial neuropathy	Cranial nerve(s)	Postinfectious optic neuritis, facial nerve palsy
5 Myelitis	Spinal cord	Acute transverse myelitis or myelopathy
6 Brainstem encephalitis	Brainstem	Bickerstaff encephalitis, clinically isolated syndrome
7 Neuropathy	PNS	Guillain-Barré syndrome, plexopathy
Chronic syndromes		
8 Motor neuron disease	CNS motor neurons	Postpolio syndrome
9 Persistent fatigue	Unknown	Chronic fatigue syndrome
10 Chronic pain with muscle tender points	Unknown	Fibromyalgia syndrome

disorder, is characterized by development of generalized pain accompanied by multiple discrete muscle tender points. With the exception of postinfectious encephalopathy, which is non-inflammatory, all acute postinfectious syndromes are believed to be immune-mediated. The aetiology of the chronic postinfectious syndromes is much less clear.

The major postinfectious CNS syndrome is postinfectious encephalitis or encephalomyelitis. This disorder is estimated to account for at least 20% of acute encephalitis cases (Johnson, 1998), and in some series has been responsible for as many as one third of cases (Kennard and Swash, 1981). The remainder of the chapter will focus on the syndrome of postinfectious encephalomyelitis.

Definition

Postinfectious encephalomyelitis is an acute monophasic disorder of CNS white matter. It is characterized by multifocal inflammatory and demyelinating lesions. The first case, described in 1790, was a 23-year-old woman who developed neurological problems one week after measles (Lucas, 1790). Interestingly enough, she had noted similar problems after being vaccinated for smallpox 10 years earlier. Postinfectious encephalomyelitis shows a very characteristic pathology (see below). It affects both sexes and all ages, but is most common in children and young adults. It is rare in very young children under age 3, however. These young children are more likely to develop a toxic encephalopathy following infection. This age-related distinction between developing an inflammatory versus non-inflammatory postinfectious process may relate to a differential effect on immature myelin (Tselis and Lisak, 1998).

Over the years postinfectious encephalomyelitis has been described under many different names. It has been called allergic, immune-mediated, hyperergic, parainfectious, postexanthematous and post-vaccinal encephalomyelitis, as well as disseminated vasculomyelinopathy (Johnson and Griffin, 1987; Johnson 1998). Postinfectious encephalomyelitis can be divided into moderate and severe forms. Each has a distinctive pathology, and they are probably part of a continuum. Both forms may follow natural infection or vaccination. Acute disseminated encephalomyelitis (ADEM) is a milder disorder, characterized neuropathologically by perivenular mononuclear inflammation and demyelination. Acute haemorrhagic leukoencephalitis (AHLE) is a hyperacute and fulminant disorder, characterized pathologically by necrosis and haemorrhage. These two forms of postinfectious encephalomyelitis differ on a number of features besides their neuropathology (Table 3.2). Although it has been suggested that they are separate conditions (Behan and Curriels, 1978), the weight of evidence does not support this notion. It is known that ADEM can progress to AHLE (Dangond et al., 1991). In addition, either form can be recreated fairly closely in animal models with a simple adjustment of the triggering stimulus (see below). The incidence of postinfectious encephalomyelitis after measles is particularly high. It is estimated that

Table 3.2   Spectrum of postinfectious encephalomyelitis.

Feature	Acute disseminated encephalomyelitis	Acute haemorrhagic leukoencephalitis
Age	Most common in children	Most common in young adults
Trigger	Exanthematous virus (historically) or vaccination	Respiratory tract virus
Course	Acute	Hyperacute, fulminant
Blood studies	Normal	Leucocytosis, ↑ acute phase reactants
CSF cell count	↑ Mononuclear cells	↑ Neutrophils, red blood cells
Neuroimaging	Multifocal white matter lesions	Large cerebral lesions
Pathology	Perivenular inflammation with demyelination	Blood vessel (vein, arteriole) necrosis, intense neutrophil inflammation, multiple small haemorrhages superimposed on demyelination
Mortality rate	Lower	Higher

Table 3.3   Frequency of postinfectious encephalomyelitis following exanthematous virus (Johnson, 1998).

Agent	Case rate	Mortality (%)	Morbidity
Vaccinia	1 : 63 to 1 : 200 000	10	Rare
Measles	1 : 1000	25	Frequent
Varicella	1 : 10 000	5	10%
Rubella	1 : 20 000	20	Very rare

one in 1000 cases of natural measles will develop this postinfectious syndrome, although the rate is much lower for very young children (Table 3.3).

Classic postinfectious encephalomyelitis is always a generalized CNS process. However, one can also see focal syndromes after infection, with clinical involvement limited to the optic nerve, brainstem, cerebellum, or spinal cord. These so-called clinically isolated syndromes can be considered restricted forms of encephalomyelitis, but they can also represent the first attack of multiple sclerosis (MS). In such patients there is always an issue as to whether they have a monophasic and self-limited postinfectious process, or MS. The risk of MS in this setting is predictable, based on the presence or absence and extent of suggestive abnormalities on brain magnetic resonance imaging (MRI), as well as the presence or absence of immune disturbances in cerebrospinal fluid (CSF) (O'Riordan et al., 1998; Sailer et al., 1999). The issue of restricted syndromes is discussed further below.

There are also exceptions to the rule that postinfectious encephalomyelitis is an acute monophasic process (Mizutani et al., 1994; Khan et al., 1995; Tsai and Hung, 1996). In rare cases onset can occur over weeks (Kesselring et al., 1990). There are also examples of patients who experience one or more relapses. This is true for both the milder ADEM (Alcock and Hoffman 1962;

Durston and Milnes, 1970; Yahr and Lobo-Antunes, 1972; Poser *et al.*, 1978; Hemachudha *et al.*, 1988), as well as the more severe AHLE (Lamarche *et al.*, 1972) forms of the disease.

Repeated attacks have occurred up to 18 months, without subsequent development of MS during extended follow-up periods (Miller and Evans, 1953; Alcock and Hoffman 1962). There has been a recommendation that patients be followed for a minimum of 6 months, before determining that new neurological problems indicate MS rather than a protracted postinfectious encephalomyelitis. In the case of unusual features, observation for up to 2 years has been suggested (Kesselring *et al.*, 1990).

TRIGGERING EVENTS

Although postinfectious encephalomyelitis can occur spontaneously, most often it follows a precipitating event (Table 3.4). The major preceding event is viral infection. Historically most cases of ADEM, the milder form of postinfectious encephalomyelitis, have followed infection by an exanthematous virus such as measles, varicella, rubella, or vaccinia (Griffith *et al.*, 1970; Johnson, 1998). Mumps, influenza A and B, Epstein-Barr virus and hepatitis A are other viruses which have been associated with CNS pathology consistent with ADEM (Miller *et al.*, 1956; Hoult and Flewett, 1960; Schwartz *et al.*, 1964; Wells, 1971; Hart and Earle, 1975; Davis and Kornfield, 1980; Davis *et al.*, 1993; Paskavitz *et al.*, 1995; Johnson, 1998). The other major inciting event is vaccination, particularly for smallpox or rabies (Warren, 1956; Woods and Ellison, 1964; Rosenberg, 1970; Cherington, 1977; Gross *et al.*, 1978; Fenichel, 1982; Hemachudha *et al.*, 1987a, b; Johnson, 1987; Trevisani *et al.*, 1993; Kaplanski *et al.*, 1995). In general, the vaccines which are most likely to produce a postinfectious syndrome involve enveloped viruses; vaccine that contains neural antigens. The rate of post-vaccinal encephalomyelitis following rabies vaccines is said to range from one in 7000 to one in 50 000 (Hemachudha *et al.*, 1987b). The Semple rabies vaccine, an old vaccine that uses phenol-inactivated homogenate of virus grown in sheep or goat brain, has an incidence of postvaccinal encephalomyelitis that approximates to one in 220 (Hemachudha *et al.*, 1987b). Intercurrent illness increases the risk of developing a post-vaccinal problem.

Besides viral infection and vaccination, other associations include mycoplasma infection (Decaux *et al.*, 1980; Fisher *et al.*, 1983; Fernandez *et al.*, 1993; Kornips *et al.*, 1993; Nishimura *et al.*, 1996), certain bacterial infections (Kopp *et al.*, 1978; Shakir *et al.*, 1987), serum and drug reactions (Russell, 1937; Fisher and Gilmour, 1939; Marsh, 1952; Williams and Chaffee, 1961; Cohen *et al.*, 1985), and insect stings (Means *et al.*, 1973).

Neurological problems typically begin within 3 weeks of the precipitating infection or vaccination. On rare instances they can even precede or occur during the triggering infection. Postinfectious encephalomyelitis most often presents within 2–13 days of exanthematous illness, and within 8–15 days of

Table 3.4 Potential precipitating factors for postinfectious encephalomyelitis

Viral infection
  measles
  varicella
  rubella
  vaccinia (in smallpox vaccine)
  mumps
  influenza A, B
  hepatitis A, B
  non-specific upper respiratory tract pathogens
  coxsackie virus
  Epstein-Barr virus

Bacterial infection
  Borrelia burgdorferi
  brucella
  Mycobacterium tuberculosis
  Streptococcus pyogenes

Mycoplasma infection

Insect sting

Vaccination
  hepatitis B vaccine
  tetanus antitoxin
  rabies
  smallpox
  Japanese B
  influenza
  pertussis
  hog cholera vaccine (accidental injection)
  measles
  rubella

Drug
  gold
  arsphenical
  sulphanilamide
  streptomycin/PAS
  serum

vaccination. Rubella has been associated with a shorter interval (1–5 days), measles an intermediate interval (2–7 days), and influenza, mumps and varicella zoster virus a longer interval between infection and onset of neurological involvement.

AHLE is invariably associated with respiratory pathogens. It tends to follow influenza (particularly influenza A), or non-specific respiratory infection (Hoult and Flewett, 1960; Hart and Earle 1975), and has only rarely been associated with exanthematous agents such as measles or varicella zoster virus (Pearl *et al.*, 1990).

With the institution of effective vaccine programmes for measles, rubella, and mumps, as well as the elimination of smallpox and the need for vaccination, postinfectious complications from these precipitating factors have fallen dramatically. World-wide, in areas where vaccination is not practised, measles continues to be a significant cause of postinfectious encephalomyelitis. Overall, however, most current cases, including the milder ADEM form, now occur after a non-specific upper respiratory tract infection.

Clinical presentation

The clinical features of postinfectious encephalomyelitis are those of a diffuse cerebral disturbance, with superimposed multifocal involvement. Symptoms begin abruptly and are generally accompanied by some degree of depressed level of consciousness. Patients can progress to frank stupor or even coma. They experience severe headache, vomiting, and stiff neck, with or without fever. Perhaps half of patients develop generalized or focal seizure activity. There can be accompanying spinal cord involvement (myelitis), cranial nerve involvement (such as optic neuritis), and focal parenchymal abnormalities. These include hemiparesis, paraparesis, visual field cuts, aphasia, sensory deficits, and movement disorders (such as ataxia, choreoathetosis, myoclonus) which reflect involvement of basal ganglia or other pertinent regions (Gollomp and Fahn, 1987). In the case of rabies vaccine-induced encephalomyelitis, PNS involvement with radiculitis accompanies the CNS involvement in up to 82% of cases (Swamy et al., 1984).

The clinical presentation of AHLE often mimics that of an expanding mass lesion. There is abrupt onset of high fever, stiff neck, headache, seizures and stupor going on to coma. The whole course is fairly fulminant over days to 1–2 weeks, but rarely can be subacute over 6–12 weeks (Huang et al., 1988). In these unusual cases the subacute course has been characterized by slow progression of symptoms, and biopsy was required to make the diagnosis. On occasion AHLE has been confined to the posterior fossa (Michaud and Helle, 1982).

Atypical presentations of postinfectious encephalomyelitis have included acute psychosis without focal findings (Nasr et al., in press), and solitary mass lesion mimicking brain tumour (Youl et al., 1991; Miller et al., 1993).

The mortality rate of postinfectious encephalomyelitis is at least 10–20%, and can reach 30% (Miller et al., 1956; Epperson et al., 1988). It ranges from 10% to 40% for post-measles encephalomyelitis (Johnson and Griffin 1987), and is even higher in the AHLE form, where death typically occurs within the first week. Recovery from postinfectious encephalomyelitis can begin within days, but often takes weeks to months. Complete recovery is seen in at least 50% of cases, and can occur in patients who were comatose. Significant morbidity is reported in about 19% of survivors; the rest do quite well. A worse prognosis has been associated with hyperacute onset, coma, and complicating seizures (Miller et al., 1956; Tyler, 1957).

Diagnosis

The diagnosis of postinfectious encephalomyelitis involves a compatible clinical picture, supplemented by supportive laboratory data (Table 3.5). The primary laboratory studies are neuroimaging and CSF evaluation; these can be supplemented by secondary blood and electrophysiological studies. Blood cultures should be negative in postinfectious patients. Other blood studies are generally not useful, although acute phase reactants (erythrocyte sedimentation rate, C reactive protein) may be elevated in AHLE. This more acute illness may also be associated with a peripheral leucocytosis of up to 30 000 white blood cells (WBC), and with proteinuria (Lisak, 1994).

Neuroimaging is a key diagnostic laboratory test, since MRI is invariably abnormal and generally shows a suggestive pattern. CT is not sensitive and may be normal in almost 40% of cases. When abnormal, CT findings include patchy hypodense lesions in cortex, subcortex, or basal ganglia which often do not enhance. Alternatively, they may be associated with focal or diffuse enhancement. Oedema is unusual but can occur in association with lesions, or more diffusely and even involving the brainstem (Lukes and Norman, 1983). CT lesions are said not to correspond well with the extent or pattern of clinical disease.

MRI is much more sensitive than CT, and can be used to make an early diagnosis (Dunn *et al.*, 1986; Shaw and Cohen, 1993; Al Tahan *et al.*, 1997). T2-weighted and proton density imaging show multiple hyperintense lesions, while T1-weighted imaging may be normal or show hypointense lesions.

Table 3.5 Diagnostic features of postinfectious encephalomyelitis.

Clinical features
Acute to subacute onset
Compatible syndrome (headache, fever, abnormal level of consciousness, seizures, multifocal findings)
Prior triggering event

Laboratory features
Blood and urine studies
  negative cultures
  leucocytosis (AHLE)
  ↑ acute phase reactants (AHLE)
  proteinuria (AHLE)
Neuroimaging
  brain, spinal MRI lesions
  brain CT lesions (less sensitive)
Cerebrospinal fluid
  mild pleocytosis (mononuclear ADEM, neutrophils with red blood cells AHLE)
  increased protein (mild ADEM, moderate/marked AHLE)
  myelin basic protein
  variable immunoglobulin disturbances
  negative nucleic acid, antigen, culture and stain studies
Electrophysiology
  EEG abnormalities (generalized slow activity, high voltage)
  evoked potential abnormalities (somatosensory, visual)

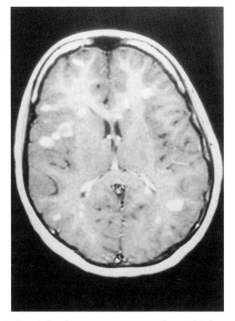

Figure 3.1 On the T1-weighted post-contrast study multiple enhancing lesions are noted without significant mass effect.

Contrast enhancement is common, and most of the lesions may enhance (Figure 3.1). This does not have to be the case, however, and the simultaneous presence of enhancing and non-enhancing lesions cannot be used to rule out a diagnosis of postinfectious encephalomyelitis. MRI lesions typically involve white matter but can also involve grey matter, basal ganglia, thalamus, and brainstem (Atlas *et al.*, 1986; Kubota *et al.*, 1995; Kimura *et al.*, 1996; Pellegrini *et al.*, 1996; Matsushita *et al.*, 1997; Menor, 1997). MRI patterns include multifocal lesions within white matter and basal ganglia, single or multifocal grey matter lesions, and localized brainstem, basal ganglia or cerebellar lesions (Donovan and Lenn, 1989; Baum *et al.*, 1994; Kimura *et al.*, 1996). Unusual patterns have included multiple ring enhancing lesions (DeRecondo and Guichard, 1997). In the case of AHLE, MRI lesions tend to be larger and to show a haemorrhagic component.

CSF examination is used to exclude active CNS infection, as well as to support the diagnosis with compatible abnormalities. The abnormalities reported with postinfectious encephalomyelitis are non-specific. They include mild to moderate mononuclear pleocytosis, mildly increased protein, and detectable myelin basic protein (MBP). Approximately two thirds of patients have abnormal CSF (Miller *et al.*, 1956). Most common is a modest increase in CSF cell count and protein concentration. In one study of post measles encephalomyelitis, 72% of patients had a mononuclear pleocytosis of 6–100 WBC/μl, and 13% had a cell count of over 100 WBC/μl (Johnson *et al.*, 1984). CSF protein levels were elevated in 44%, and 10% of patients had protein levels above 100 mg/dl. Myelin basic protein was detected in 60%, while intrathecal IgG production was noted in less than 10%.

In AHLE the CSF is under increased pressure. The pleocytosis contains neutrophils and total white blood cell counts can range up to 3000 WBC/µl. Red blood cells are often noted as well. Consistent with a more intense pathological process, the majority of patients have increased CSF protein levels. In 25% CSF protein is greater than 200 mg/dl, and it can be as high as 1 g/dl (Byers, 1975). CSF is normal in only 10% of patients with AHLE.

With regard to neurophysiological tests, EEG is often abnormal. The most frequent disturbance is moderate to severe diffuse high voltage asymmetric theta-delta activity (Ziegler, 1966). The extent of the EEG abnormalities correlate somewhat with disease activity. Other abnormalities include a spindle coma pattern, as well as an alternating pattern (Bortone et al., 1996). In patients with spinal cord or optic nerve involvement, somatosensory and visual evoked potentials are abnormal.

Restricted syndromes

If postinfectious encephalomyelitis is considered to encompass a broad spectrum of conditions, then localized involvement of optic nerve, spinal cord, brainstem or cerebellum may represent restricted forms of encephalo-myelitis (Al Deeb et al., 1997; Tselis and Lisak, 1998). Such focal disorders can follow infection or vaccination, and at least a proportion of patients with a restricted syndrome turn out to have a postinfectious aetiology (Adams and Armstrong, 1990). After MS, a postinfectious process is the most common cause of optic neuritis (Miller, 1982). Children seem to be particularly vulnerable to this disorder, and their optic nerve involvement can follow systemic infection or vaccination (Selbst et al., 1983; Hamed et al., 1993). The optic neuritis can be anterior (this form is particularly associated with vaccination) or retrobulbar, and is frequently bilateral. Although vision loss may be severe, it is usually temporary.

Transverse myelitis is an intramedullary spinal cord syndrome which is classically characterized by motor and sensory leg deficits, sensory level, and sphincter disturbance, with or without back pain. It may be complete or incomplete. Incomplete transverse myelitis with asymmetric findings carries a high risk for MS (Jeffery et al., 1993; Scott et al., 1998). Part of the requirements to diagnose postinfectious transverse myelitis requires that there is no obvious alternative diagnosis, such as cord compression, trauma, tumour, primary infection of spinal cord, or relevant disease which can cause a spinal cord lesion, such as MS or systemic lupus erythematosus. Parainfectious transverse myelitis accounts for about 37–46% of cases. There is often a history of preceding febrile illness. A parainfectious aetiology is more likely under the age of 40 years, and with a presentation involving either severe persistent back pain and weakness, or spinal shock (Knebusch et al., 1998). MRI may show acute cord swelling and abnormal signal intensity over several levels (Bakshi et al., 1997). Three distinct patterns for parainfectious myelitis have been described, involving focal lesions, continuous multisegment lesions, or scattered lesions (Pradhan et al., 1997). CSF is abnormal in up to 94% of patients with findings of pleocytosis, increased protein, or both (Al Deeb et al., 1997). The thoracic region is referentially involved. Transverse myelitis in rare instances can recur repeatedly, without leading to more generalized disease (Pandit and Rao, 1996; Ungurean et al., 1996).

Bickerstaff brainstem encephalitis is a localized encephalitis characterized by ophthalmoplegia, ataxia, lower cranial nerve palsies, and hypo- or areflexia (Derakshan et al., 1979; Fargas et al., 1998). Typically the outcome is excellent. This focal syndrome has features reminiscent of the Miller-Fisher variant of the Guillain-Barré syndrome/acute inflammatory demyelinating polyradiculoneuropathy. Bickerstaff encephalitis and the Miller-Fisher syndrome may represent CNS and PNS ends of an immune-mediated spectrum disorder.

Most cases of postinfectious cerebellitis involve children between the ages of 6 and 12 years. Approximately 75% give a history of recent infection, either varicella (the reported incidence rate is one in 4000) or a non-specific infection in the rare case in a very young child under the age of 2 years. Patients present with prominent nausea, vomiting, headaches, and dramatic ataxia, particularly of the lower extremities. Less commonly there may be significant dysarthria, tremor, and nystagmus. Seizures are rare, there is no corticospinal tract involvement, and the level of consciousness is either normal or only minimally affected. CSF and EEG studies are normal in up to 67% of patients. In this restricted syndrome neuroimaging is either normal, or the lesions are confined to the cerebellum and pons. There is an excellent prognosis for recovery within weeks, with a negligible mortality rate related to extra-neural problems.

Differential diagnosis

Once the initial evaluation is completed, the differential diagnosis of post-infectious encephalomyelitis involves a limited number of conditions (Table 3.6). One major consideration is acute encephalitis or encephalomyelitis due to an alternative aetiology. Most cases of acute encephalitis reflect CNS invasion by a pathogen. Most pathogens turn out to be viruses, although a handful of bacterial, parasitic, rickettsial and other agents can also produce acute enceph-alitis. Infectious encephalomyelitis is an important differentiation to make, because the optimal management involves starting the appropriate antimicro-bial treatment regimen. These cases are typically diagnosed based on docu-menting presence of the organism by culture, polymerase chain reaction, antigen or stain studies. A limited number of conditions cause a non-infectious encephalitis, including infectious endocarditis with secondary CNS involve-ment due to vascular lesions.

Metabolic or toxic encephalopathy also causes diffuse cerebral disturbances, but without focal deficits. Both brain MRI and CSF studies are generally normal.

Table 3.6   Differential diagnosis of postinfectious encephalomyelitis.

Acute infectious encephalitis/encephalomyelitis
  viral
  bacterial
  parasitic
  rickettsial

Acute non-infectious encephalitis/encephalomyelitis
  Behçet disease
  collagen vascular disease
  drug reaction
  endocarditis
  gliomatosis cerebri
  vasculitis

Acute metabolic/toxic encephalopathy

Multiple sclerosis
  initial clinical attack
  Marburg variant

The first clinical relapse of MS can sometimes be difficult to distinguish from postinfectious encephalomyelitis. However, there are a number of features that can be used to differentiate these two conditions (Table 3.7). Postinfectious encephalomyelitis shows a much more abrupt onset than a first attack of MS. It is more likely to affect children, and to have a clear precipitating event. The typical clinical syndrome is much more severe and frequently involves abnormal level of consciousness, bad headache, fever, and seizures. All of these features would be unusual in a first attack of MS. MRI abnormalities tend to be much more extensive, to involve grey matter, and to show more contrast enhancement than in MS. CSF patterns are quite different in the two diseases. Although oligoclonal bands and intrathecal IgG production can occur in postinfectious encephalomyelitis, these abnormalities are not as common as in MS. In contrast to MS they are transient, and clear over time.

A specific form of MS, called acute variant Marburg disease, is a more fulminant process in which the clinical picture may mimic postinfectious encephalomyelitis (Johnson *et al.*, 1990). It usually takes a monophasic and fairly malignant course with rapid worsening leading to death within a year or two, but occasionally over weeks to months. For most patients this is the presentation of their MS, although in unusual cases this aggressive course may be superimposed on known MS which has shown a more typical course. Marburg variant disease most often affects young people, but not children. At least one case has been associated with a post translational change in myelin basic protein (MBP), to produce an immature form which is extensively citrullinated and poorly phosphorylated (Wood *et al.*, 1996). It has been postulated that Marburg variant occurs in genetically susceptible hosts with unstable MBP.

In summary, a careful analysis of the history and examination, along with MRI and CSF findings, can generally distinguish postinfectious encephalomyelitis from MS and direct infection syndromes.

Table 3.7   Differentiating features between postinfectious encephalomyelitis and MS.

Factor	Postinfectious encephalomyelitis	MS
Time course	Monophasic, rarely relapsing	Multiphasic, 85% relapsing
Onset	Abrupt	Subacute
Preceding event	Preceding infection or vaccination in 70%	Preceding infection in 33%
Demographic features	More common in children No gender preference	More common in young adults Female gender preference (70–75%)
Clinical syndrome	More severe with ↓ level of consciousness, seizures (50%), multifocal abnormalities Bilateral optic neuritis Complete transverse myelitis with areflexia	Rarely severe with normal level of consciousness, seizures ≤5% Clinically isolated syndromes more common than multifocal abnormalities Unilateral optic neuritis Incomplete transverse myelitis with hyperreflexia
Mortality rate	10–25%	Rare
Neuroimaging	Bilateral extensive symmetric lesions Asymmetric lesions are not periventricular Many enhancing lesions Basal ganglia involvement common Serial MRI shows partial resolution of existing lesions without new lesions	Scattered asymmetric lesions Periventricular lesions Occasional enhancing lesions Basal ganglia involvement uncommon (≤25) Serial MRI shows new lesion development
CSF	Mild to moderate pleocytosis common Increased protein Oligoclonal bands, intrathecal IgG production uncommon and transient	Mild pleocytosis uncommon (≤33%) Normal protein Oligoclonal bands, intrathecal IgG production common and persistent

Management

The most effective way to treat any disorder is to prevent it. Vaccination programmes for pathogens that can trigger postinfectious encephalomyelitis, by eliminating natural infection, prevent the disorder. Measles is the best example, and post-measles encephalomyelitis is now essentially eliminated in countries that have an effective vaccine programme. The same could be expected to occur for all of the recognized pathogen triggers: effective immunoprophylaxis, with elimination of the natural infection, should prevent the postinfectious syndrome.

Vaccines which contain CNS tissue or enveloped viruses are associated with the greatest risk of postinfectious complications. With the switch to rabies vaccines which do not use brain or spinal cord of infected rabbits, sheep, or

Table 3.8   Supportive care for postinfectious encephalomyelitis.

Assure access; monitor vital signs and fluid balance
Control body temperature
Control seizures
Control increased intracranial pressure
Monitor for/treat hyponatraemia
Assisted ventilation if necessary
Avoid skin breakdown
Avoid/early treatment of secondary infections

Table 3.9   Agents which have been used to treat postinfectious
encephalomyelitis.

Glucocorticoids
Adrenocorticotropin
Intravenous immune globulin
Plasma exchange
Cyclosporine
Glatiramer acetate
Polyinosine- polycytidylic acid polylysine

goats, rabies vaccine complications have decreased. Newer vaccines, such as
the human diploid cell strain vaccine, use embryonated eggs and cell cultures.

Those who survive the acute insult of postinfectious encephalomyelitis
generally recover and do quite well. This is true even for those who have
been very ill and in coma. Therefore, aggressive supportive care during the
illness is a mandatory and key component of management (Table 3.8). Fever is
reduced, sodium is monitored to detect development of the syndrome of
inappropriate antidiuretic hormone, and any complicating features (such as
seizures or increased intracranial pressure) are managed aggressively.

With regard to disease-specific therapeutic strategies, there are no controlled
trials and no proven treatment. A number of agents have been tried either alone
or in combination (Table 3.9). Probably the most commonly used therapy
involves glucocorticoids. These drugs have potent anti-inflammatory and
immunosuppressant effects, including shutting down gene transcription for
pro-inflammatory cytokine production. They can also temporarily repair a
damaged blood–brain barrier. A number of studies suggest a benefit of
treatment with oral and intravenous glucocorticoids (Pasternak et al., 1980;
Tenorio and Whitaker, 1991; Straub et al., 1997; Hauley, 1998). In addition,
there are reports of patients who improved with glucocorticoids, worsened
when they were discontinued, and then regained a response when they were
reinstituted (Ziegler, 1966). Glucocorticoids are also reported to benefit the
more severe AHLE form of postinfectious encephalomyelitis (Byers, 1975).
However, there are also examples where glucocorticoids had no apparent effect
(Swanson, 1956; Karelitz and Eisenberg, 1961; Ziegna, 1961). In a
retrospective Norwegian study, the group which received glucocorticoids
actually showed increased mortality and sequelae (Boe et al., 1965). Adrenocorticotropin (ACTH) has been used both alone and in combination with

glucocorticoids (Applebaum and Abler, 1951; Miller and Gibbons, 1953; Allen, 1957; Karelitz and Eisenberg, 1961; Ziegler, 1966). Presumably the rationale for use is based on its use in MS. The major action of ACTH is to stimulate glucocorticoid production. Other theoretic beneficial actions remain unproven, and there are no convincing data to support its use.

There are case reports suggesting that intravenous immune globulin, when used early in the disease course, is helpful (Kleiman and Brunquell, 1995; Finsterer et al., 1998). This treatment was also said to be helpful in a patient who showed glucocorticoid responsive relapsing disease (Hahn et al., 1996).

Plasma exchange has also been used as therapy, often in conjunction with glucocorticoids and immunosuppressive agents (Newton, 1981; Cotter et al., 1983; Seales and Greer, 1991; Stricker et al., 1992; Dodick et al., 1998). There are reports of patients responding to plasma exchange after failing glucocorticoids (Kanter et al., 1995). A recent small study suggested this therapy could be helpful in patients with MS or other CNS inflammatory demyelinating conditions who experienced severe attacks which were steroid-unresponsive (Weinshenker et al., 1999).

With regard to other treatments, immunosuppressive agents have been used in a very small number of cases (Belendiuk and Solch, 1988; Seales and Greer, 1991). Glatiramer acetate (copaxone), a biophysical analogue of MBP, is a disease modifying therapy used to treat relapsing MS. It also ameliorates experimental allergic/autoimmune encephalomyelitis (EAE), a model of postinfectious encephalomyelitis (see below). This treatment was reported to benefit three patients with postinfectious encephalomyelitis, who recovered within 3 weeks (Abramsky et al., 1977). However, the data from MS indicate that glatiramer acetate takes several months to show clinical and MRI benefit. That suggests that the rapid recovery of these patients was probably independent of their treatment. Polyinosinic-polycytidylic acid – polylysine stabilized with carboxymethyl cellulose (poly ICLC) – was reported to benefit a single patient with an unusually protracted 5-month course (Salazar et al., 1981). Poly ICLC induces interferon with concomitant immunomodulatory effects, but this remains a single case report in which the diagnosis of postinfectious encephalomyelitis is somewhat questionable.

In summary, based on anecdotal data, patients with postinfectious encephalomyelitis are often treated with high dose glucocorticoid protocols. The most commonly used protocol involves several days of intravenous methylprednisolone with or without an oral taper. This is identical to how a severe MS relapse would be treated. Glucocorticoid therapy remains unproven in any definitive trial, and to date no treatment can be considered as established for postinfectious encephalomyelitis.

Pathogenesis

Postinfectious encephalomyelitis is believed to be immune mediated. Several lines of evidence support this contention (Table 3.10). There is a lag phase between the infection itself and the onset of the postinfectious syndrome, as

Table 3.10   Evidence to support an immune pathogenesis for postinfectious encephalomyelitis

Lag phase between inciting event and disease

Inciting event (infection, vaccination) stimulate host immune system

Pathogens are not present within neural tissue/intrathecal compartment

Neuropathology (perivascular mononuclear cells with adjacent demyelination)

Animal models
   experimental allergic/autoimmune encephalomyelitis (EAE)

Studies on human disease
   measles
   rabies vaccine
   other aetiologies

though certain immune responses (such as delayed type hypersensitivity) need to be generated. There has been a consistent failure to demonstrate infectious agents in neural tissue or within the intrathecal compartment. There are also supporting neuropathological and immunologic data. These data are based primarily on studies of patients with postinfectious encephalomyelitis, who show findings which parallel those in specific animal models.

The neuropathology of postinfectious encephalomyelitis involves perivenular mononuclear cell infiltration with demyelination. These pathological features mimic those of a recognized autoimmune disease produced by inoculating animals with brain tissue (particular white matter myelin proteins) in complete Freund's adjuvant. EAE is known to be a cell-mediated process, although humoral factors amplify the disease. It can also be produced by inoculating with myelin components such as MBP, proteolipid protein, and myelin oligodendrocyte glycoprotein (MOG). In particular, antibodies to MOG accentuate myelin damage. EAE can also be produced by passive transfer of sensitized T cells, or T cell lines or clones. The pathological features of EAE are duplicated not only in cases of postinfection encephalomyelitis, but in the neuroparalytic disease which occurs after rabies vaccine prepared in CNS tissue.

Extensive studies of post measles encephalomyelitis in humans have found no evidence that measles virus is present in the CNS. Intrathecal measles antibody production is absent, but there are high levels of soluble CD8 in the CSF, a sign of intrathecal immune activation (Griffin et al., 1989). Patients show a vigorous immune response to CNS white matter, in particular MBP. MBP is released into the CSF, particularly early in the disease course, consistent with it being the target of an immune attack. Almost half of patients have demonstrable lymphoproliferative responses to MBP. This observation is not unique to post measles encephalomyelitis. Similar MBP proliferative responses are reported for encephalomyelitis cases following varicella zoster virus or rubella infections (Lisak and Zweiman, 1977; Johnson, 1998). Increased T-cell reactivity to MBP is noted in both blood and CSF lymphocytes from postinfectious encephalomyelitis (Lisak et al., 1974). Neurological complications after Semple rabies vaccine are also associated with elevated levels of serum antibodies to brain white matter and to MBP, as well as intrathecal MBP antibody production. In addition, there is a partial correlation with antibodies to cerebroside and ganglioside, and other CNS white matter antigens (Hemachudha *et al.*, 1987a; Piyasirisilp *et al.*, 1999). This suggests that they are amplifying the immune response to MBP, the presumptive primary antigen.

Although the above immune disturbances have been noted in patients with postinfectious CNS syndromes, patients who develop polyneuritis after rabies vaccination also show an immune response to CNS white matter and particularly MBP. It has been postulated that postinfectious or post vaccinal PNS neuropathies are actually dual-antigen induced autoimmune processes, and that they require two complementary infections, viral and bacterial (Westall and Root-Bernstein, 1986). The two agents must interact before they are immunologically-processed. One infection must be an agent with sequence homology to MBP or P2 protein (such as measles, Epstein-Barr virus, influenza A and B, hepatitis B), or another CNS or PNS component. The second infection must be a chemically complementary component analogous to a bacterial adjuvant (such as muramyl peptides). This dual infection hypothesis might explain the clinical observations that vaccines should be avoided in patients with acute infections because they are more likely to produce complications, that vaccines have resulted in increased paralysis in acute polio patients, and that most patients who develop post vaccinal neuritis have a concomitant complicating illness.

In animal models of autoimmune disease triggered by measles, passive transfer of non-encephalitogenic T cells sensitized to MBP can induce EAE in animals with measles infection of the CNS (Liebert and Ter Meulen, 1993). This implies a synergistic reaction between the virus and MBP reactive T cells, and supports the importance of cell-mediated immunity in this postinfectious syndrome.

Recent studies have reported increased frequency of T helper 2 (TH2) MBP reactive T cells during the recovery phase in patients with postinfectious encephalomyelitis (Pohl-Koppe *et al.*, 1998). These cells produce high amount of interleukin-4 but not interferon gamma. The authors postulate that these cells are related to recovery, and attempts to boost autoreactive TH2 cells might be a reasonable therapeutic strategy.

As is true for all immune mediated disorders, it is likely that there is an element of genetic susceptibility involved. Patients who develop encephalomyelitis after Semple rabies vaccine are more likely to be HLA-DR9 and HLA-DR17 positive, and are less likely to be HLA-DQ7 positive, than vaccinated or unvaccinated healthy controls (Piyasirisilp *et al.*, 1999). Patients with post-measles encephalomyelitis are more likely to be HLA-DR4 and HLA-DR5 positive (Lebon *et al.*, 1986).

A histopathological picture more consistent with AHLE can be induced, in place of EAE, by modifying the adjuvant with addition of pertussis vaccine (Levine and Wenk, 1965). This hyperacute EAE can be considered an animal model of AHLE (Ravkina *et al.*, 1979).

Only a minority of postinfectious encephalomyelitis cases actually occur following vaccination with neural tissue. In most cases it is clear that there is no

Table 3.11 Potential mechanisms for induction of postinfecti
encephalomyelitis.

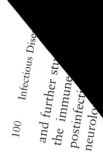

Molecular mimicry
Superantigen induction
Immune dysregulation
Direct sequelae of infection

inoculation with myelin antigens. Somehow
induce CNS autoimmune disease. A number of poten...
explain how a virus or other pathogen could trigger postinfectious enc..
lomyelitis (Table 3.11). Molecular mimicry has been documented between
certain epitopes expressed by pathogens and by myelin components (Fujinami
and Oldstone, 1985; Jahnke *et al.*, 1985; Wucherpfennig and Strominger,
1995). It is now known that the T-cell recognition response is much more
degenerate than previously realized, making it easier to see how infection by an
agent containing antigenic epitopes similar to myelin or other CNS tissue
epitopes could induce autoreactive cells (Gran *et al.*, 1999). Conceivably an
immune response triggered against a shared epitope could be the link between
infection and subsequent CNS disease. Alternatively, there are viral and
bacterial superantigens which can activate massive numbers of CD4$^+$ T cells,
including myelin reactive T cells (Zhang *et al.*, 1995). Activated T cells traffic
into the CNS compartment, and if they were being generated in sufficient
numbers these autoreactive cells could lead to disease. Infection might lead to
immune dysregulation, with loss of supresor cell activity and consequent
upregulation of existing autoreactive cells. Although direct infection of CNS
has never been shown in these postinfectious patients, it is possible that there is
an occult infection which has simply not been detected. Infection of CNS cells
such as oligodendrocytes, or barrier cells such as endothelium, could lead to
local CNS immune activation and damage.

Summary

The diagnosis of postinfectious encephalomyelitis rests on a characteristic
neurological picture, prodromal infection or vaccination, consistent CSF and
MRI picture, and lack of ability to isolate a CNS infectious agent. Treatment
requires full supportive care, since complete recovery is possible despite severe
acute illness. High dose glucocorticoids are an unproven but commonly used
therapy, while plasma exchange or intravenous immune globulin are
sometimes added for more severe illness. Case numbers of this postinfectious
disorder are likely to decrease in the future, as natural infections are eradicated
and better vaccines are developed. Nevertheless, postinfectious encephalomyelitis provides an excellent model to examine how interactions between the
environment and the host immune system lead to disease. The pathogenesis of
this infection related immune-mediated disease remains poorly understood,

...dies are needed. With the increasing appreciation of the role of ... system in many different disorders, lessons learned from this ...ous illness are likely to have wide applicability to a broad range of ...gical and systemic diseases.

References

Abramsky, O., Teitelbaum, D. and Arnon, R. (1977). Effect of a synthetic polypeptide (cop-1) on patients with multiple sclerosis and with acute disseminated encephalomyelitis. *J. Neurol. Sci.*, **31**, 433–438.

Adams, C. and Armstrong, D. (1990). Acute transverse myelopathy in children. *Can. J. Neurol. Sci.*, **17**, 40–45.

Al Deeb, S. M., Yaqub, B. A., Bruyn, G. W. and Biary, N. M. (1997). Acute transverse myelitis. A localized form of postinfectious encephalomyelitis. *Brain*, **120**, 1115–1122.

Al Tahan, A., Arora, S., Alzeer, A., Al Tahan, F., Malabarey, T. and Daif, A. (1997). Acute disseminated encephalomyelitis: the importance of early magnetic resonance imaging. *Eur. J. Neurol.*, **4**, 52–58.

Alcock, N. and Hoffman, H. (1962). Recurrent encephalomyelitis in childhood. *Arch. Dis. Child.*, **37**, 40.

Allen, J. E. (1957). Treatment of measles encephalitis with adrenal steroids. *Pediatrics*, **20**, 87–91.

Applebaum, E. and Abler, C. (1951). Treatment of measles encephalitis with corticotropin. *Am. J. Dis. Child.*, **92**, 147–150.

Atlas, S. W., Grossman, R. I., Goldberg, H. I., Hackney, D. B., Bilaniuk, L. T. and Zimmerman, R. A. (1986). MR diagnosis of acute disseminated encephalomyelitis. *J. Comp. Ass. Tom.*, **10**, 798–801.

Bakshi, R., Kinkel, P. R., Mechtler, L. L. *et al.* (1997). Magnetic resonance imaging findings in 22 cases of myelitis: comparison between patients with and without multiple sclerosis. *Eur. J. Neurol.*, **5**, 35–48.

Baum, P. A., Barkovich, A. J., Koch, T. K. and Berg, B. O. (1994). Deep gray matter involvement in children with acute disseminated encephalomyelitis. *Am. J. Neuroradiol.*, **15**, 1275–1283.

Behan, P. O. and Curriels., L. S. (1978). *Clinical Neuroimmunology*. London: WB Saunders.

Belendiuk, G. and Solch, S. (1988). Cyclosporine in neurological autoimmune disease. *Clin. Neuropharm.*, **11**, 291–302.

Boe, J., Solberg, C. O. and Saeter, T. (1965). Corticosteroid treatment of acute meningoencephalitis: retrospective study of 346 cases. *Br. Med. J.*, **1**, 1094–1095.

Bortone, E., Bettoni, L., Buzio, S., Delsoldato, S., Giorgi, C. and Mancia, D. (1996). Spindle coma and alternating pattern in the course of measles encephalitis. *Clin. Electroenceph.*, **27**, 210–214.

Byers, R. K. (1975). Acute hemorrhagic leukoencephalitis: report of 3 cases and a review of the literature. *Pediatrics*, **56**, 727–735.

Cherington, C. (1977). Locked-in syndrome after 'swine flu' vaccination. *Arch. Neurol.*, **34**, 258.

Cohen, M., Day, C. P. and Day, J. L. (1985). Acute disseminated encephalomyelitis as a complication of treatment with gold. *Br. Med. J.*, **290**, 1170–1180.

Cotter, F. E., Bainbridge, D. and Newland, A. C. (1983). Neurological deficit associated with *Mycoplasma pneumoniae* reversed by plasma exchange. *Br. Med. J.*, **286**, 22.

Dangond, F., Lacomis, D., Schwartz, R. B. *et al.* (1991). Acute disseminated encephalomyelitis progressing to hemorrhagic encephalitis. *Neurology*, **41**, 1697–1698.

Davis, L. E., Brown, J. E., Robertsen, B. H., Khanna, B. and Polish, L. B. (1993). Hepatitis A post-viral encephalitis. *Acta Neurol. Scand.*, **87**, 67–69.

Davis, L. E. and Kornfeld, M. (1980). Influenza A virus and Reye's syndrome in adults. *J. Neurol. Neurosurg. Psych.*, **43**, 516–521.

De Recondo, A. and Guichard, J. P. (1997). Acute disseminated encephalomyelitis presenting as multiple cystic lesions. *J. Neurol. Neurosurg. Psych.*, **63**, 15.

Decaux, G., Szyper, M., Ectors, M. *et al.* (1980). Central nervous system complications of *Mycoplasma pneumoniae*. *J. Neurol. Neurosurg. Psych.*, **43**, 883–887.

Derakshan, I., Lotfi, J. and Kaufman, B. (1979). Ophthalmoplegia, ataxia and hyporeflexia (Fisher's syndrome). *Eur. Neurol.*, **18**, 361–366.

Dodick, D. W., Silber, M. H., Noseworthy, J., Wilbright, W. A. and Rodriguez, M. (1998). Acute disseminated encephalomyelitis after accidental injection of a hog vaccine: successful treatment with plasmapheresis. *Mayo Clin. Proc.*, **73**, 1193–1195.

Donovan, M. K. and Lenn, N. J. (1989). Postinfectious encephalomyelitis with localized basal ganglia involvement. *Pediatr Neurol.*, **5**, 311–313.

Dunn, V., Bale, J. F., Zimmerman, R. A., Perdue, Z. and Bell, W. E. (1986). MRI in children with postinfectious disseminated encephalomyelitis. *Mag. Res. Imaging.*, **4**, 25–32.

Durston, J. H. J. and Milnes, J. N. (1970). Relapsing encephalomyelitis. *Brain*, **93**, 715–730.

Epperson, L. W., Whitaker, J. N. and Kapila, A. (1988). Cranial MRI in acute disseminated encephalomyelitis. *Neurology*, **38**, 332–334.

Fargas, A., Roig, M., Vazquez, E. and Fito, A. (1998). Brainstem involvement in a child with ophthalmoplegia, ataxia, areflexia syndrome. *Pediatr. Neurol.*, **18**, 73–75.

Fenichel, G. M. (1982). Neurological complications of immunization. *Ann. Neurol.*, **12**, 119–128.

Fernandez, C. V., Bortolussi, R., Gordon, K. *et al.* (1993). *Mycoplasma pneumoniae* infection associated with central nervous system complications. *J. Child. Neurol.*, **8**, 27–31.

Finsterer, J., Grass, R., Stollberger, C. and Mamoli, B. (1998). Immunoglobulins in acute, parainfectious, disseminated encephalomyelitis. *Clin. Neuropharm.*, **21**, 258–261.

Fisher, J. H. and Gilmour, J. R. (1939). Encephalomyelitis following administration of sulphanilamide. *Lancet*, ii, 301–305.

Fisher, R. S., Clark, A. W., Wolinsky, J. S. *et al.* (1983). Postinfectious leukoencephalitis complicating *Mycoplasma pneumoniae* infection. *Arch. Neurol.*, **40**, 109–113.

Fujinami, R. S. and Oldstone, M. B. A. (1985). Amino acid homology between the encephalitogeneic site of myelin basic protein and virus: mechanism for autoimmunity. *Science*, **230**, 1043–1045.

Gollomp, S. M. and Fahn, S. (1987). Transient dystonia as a complication of varicella. *J. Neurol. Neurosurg. Psych.*, **50**, 1228–1229.

Gran, B., Hemmer, B., Vergelli, M., McFarland, H. F. and Martin, R. (1999). Molecular mimicry and multiple sclerosis: degenerate T-cell recognition and the induction of autoimmunity. *Ann. Neurol.*, **45**, 559–567.

Griffin, D. E., Ward, B. J., Jauregui, E. *et al.* (1989). Immune activation in measles. *N. Engl. J. Med.*, **320**, 1667–1672.

Griffith, J. F., Salam, M. V. and Adams, R. D. (1970). The nervous system diseases associated with varicella. *Acta Neurol. Scand.*, **46**, 279–300.

Gross, W. L., Ravens, K. G. and Hansen, H. W. (1978). Meningoencephalitis syndrome following influenza vaccination. *J. Neurol.*, **217**, 219–222.

Hahn, J. S., Siegler, D. J. and Enzmann, D. (1996). Intravenous gammaglobulin therapy in recurrent acute disseminated encephalomyelitis. *Neurology*, **46**, 1173–1174.

Hamed, L. M., Silbiger, J., Guy, J. *et al.* (1993). Parainfectious optic neuritis and encephalomyelitis. *J. Clin. Neuro-Ophthalmol.*, **13**, 18–23.

Hart, M. N. and Earle, K. M. (1975). Hemorrhagic and perivenous encephalitis: a clinico-pathological review of 38 cases. *J. Neurol. Neurosurg. Psych.*, **38**, 585–591.

Hauley, R. J. (1998). Early high-dose methylprednisolone in acute disseminated encephalomyelitis. *Neurology*, **51**, 644–645.

Hemachudha, T., Griffin, D. E., Giffels, J. J., Johnson, R. T., Moser, A. B. and Phanuphak, P. (1987a). Myelin basic protein as an encephalitogen in encephalomyelitis and polyneuritis following rabies vaccination. *N. Engl. J. Med.*, **316**, 369–374.

Hemachudha, T., Phanuphak, P., Johnson, R. T., Griffin, D. E., Katanavongsriri, J. and Siriprasomsup, W. (1987b). Neurologic complications of Semple-type rabies vaccine: clinical and immunologic studies. *Neurology*, **37**, 550–556.

Hemachudha, T., Griffin, D. E., Johnson, R. T., Giffels, J. J. (1988). Immunologic studies of patients with chronic encephalitis induced by post-exposure Semple rabies vaccine. *Neurology.* **38**, 42–44.

Hoult, J. G. and Flewett, T. H. (1960). Influenza encephalopathy and post influenzal encephalitis: histological and other observations. *Br. Med. J.*, **1**, 1847–1850.

Huang, C. L., Chu, N. S., Chen, T. J. and Shaw, C. M. (1988). Acute hemorrhagic leukoencephalitis with a prolonged clinical course. *J. Neurol. Neurosurg. Psych.*, **51**, 870–874.

Jahnke, U., Fischer, E. H. and Alvord, E. C. jr (1985). Sequence homology between certain viral proteins and proteins related to encephalomyelitis and neuritis. *Science*, **229**, 282–284.

Jeffery, D. R., Mandler, R. N. and Davis, L. E. (1993). Transverse myelitis. Retrospective analysis of 33 cases, with differentiation of cases associated with multiple sclerosis and parainfectious events. *Arch. Neurol.*, **50**, 532–535.

Johnson, M. D., Lavin, P. and Whetsell, W. O. jr (1990). Fulminant monophasic multiple sclerosis, Marburg's type. *J. Neurol. Neurosurg. Psych.*, **53**, 918–921.

Johnson, R. T. (1987). The pathogenesis of acute viral encephalitis and postinfectious encephalomyelitis. *J. Infect. Dis.*, **155**, 359–364.

Johnson, R. T. (1998). Postinfectious demyelinating diseases. In: *Viral Infections of the Nervous System*, 2nd edn (R. T. Johnson ed.) Philadelphia: Lippincott-Raven. pp 181–210.

Johnson, R. T., Griffin, D. E., Hirsch, R. L. *et al.*(1984). Measles encephalomyelitis – clinical and immunological studies. *N. Engl. J. Med.*, **310**, 137–141.

Johnson, R. T. and Griffin, D. E. (1987) Postinfectious encephalomyelitis. In: *Infections of the Nervous System* (P. G. E. Kennedy and R. T. Johnson, eds). London: Butterworth. pp 209–226.

Kanter, D. S., Horensky, D., Sperling, R. A. *et al.* (1995). Plasmapheresis in fulminant acute disseminated encephalomyelitis. *Neurology*, **45**, 824–827.

Kaplanski, G., Retornaz, F., Durand, J. M. and Soubeyrand, J. (1995). Central nervous system demyelination after vaccination against hepatitis B and HLA haplotype. *J. Neurol. Neurosurg. Psych.*, **58**, 758–759.

Karelitz, S. and Eisenberg, M. (1961). Measles encephalitis: evaluation and treatment with adrenocorticotropin and adrenal corticosteroids. *Pediatrics*, **27**, 811–818.

Kennard, C., Swash, M. (1981). Acute viral encephalitis. Its diagnosis and outcome. *Brain*, **104**, 129–148.

Kesselring, J., Miller, D. H., Robb, S. A. *et al.*, (1990). Acute disseminated encephalomyelitis. MRI findings and the distinction from multiple sclerosis. *Brain*, **113**, 291–302.

Khan, S., Yaqub, B. A., Boser, C. M., Al Deeb, S. M. and Bohlega, S. (1995). Multiphasic disseminated encephalomyelitis presenting as alternating hemiplegia. *J. Neurol. Neurosurg. Psych.*, **58**, 467–470.

Kimura, S., Nezu, A., Ohtsuki, N., Kobayashi, T., Osaka, H. and Uehara, S. (1996). Serial magnetic resonance imaging in children with postinfectious encephalitis. *Brain Devel.*, **18**, 461–465.

Kleiman, M. and Brunquell, P. (1995). Acute disseminated encephalomyelitis: response to intravenous immunoglobulin? *J. Child. Neurol.*, **10**, 481–483.

Knebusch, M., Strassburg, H. M. and Reiners, K. (1998). Acute transverse myelitis in childhood: Nine cases and review of the literature. *Dev. Med. Child. Neur.*, **40**, 631–639.

Kopp, N., Groslambert, R., Pasquier, B. *et al.* (1978). Leucoencephalite aigue hemorrhagique au cours d'une tuberculose. *Rev. Neurol. (Paris)*, **134**, 313–323.

Kornips, H. M., Verhagen, W. I. and Prick, M. J. (1993). Acute disseminated encephalomyelitis probably related to a *Mycoplasma pneumoniae* infection. *Clin. Neurol. Neurosurg.*, **95**, 59–63.

Kubota, K., Kobayashi, M., Nakamoto, N. *et al.* (1995). A case of acute disseminated encephalomyelitis with lesions in the cerebral gray matter on MRI in the acute phase. *Br. Devel.*, **27**, 226–230.

Lamarche, J. B., Behan, P. O., Segarra, J. M. and Feldman, R. G. (1972). Recurrent acute necrotizing hemorrhagic encephalopathy. *Acta Neuropathol. (Berl.)*, **22**, 79–87.

Lebon, P., Ponsot, G., Gony, J. and Hors, J. (1986). HLA antigens in acute measles encephalitis. *Tissue Antigens*, **27**, 75–77.

Levine, S and Wenk, E. J. (1965). A hyperacute form of allergic encephalomyelitis. *Am. J. Pathol.*, **47**, 61–88.

Liebert, U. G. and Ter Meulen, V. (1993). Synergistic interaction between measles virus infection and myelin basic protein peptide specific T cells in the induction of experimental allergic encephalomyelitis in Lewis rats. *J. Neuroimmunol.*, **46**, 217–223.

Lisak, R. (1994). Immune-mediated parainfectious encephalomyelitis. In: *Handbook of Neurovirology* (R. McKendall and W. Stroop, eds). New York: Dekker. pp. 173–186.

Lisak, R. P., Behan, P. O., Zweiman, B. and Shetty, T. (1974). Cell-mediated immunity to myelin basic protein in acute disseminated encephalomyelitis. *Neurology*, **24**, 560–564.

Lisak, R. P. and Zweiman, B. (1977). In vitro cell-mediated immunity of cerebrospinal fluid lymphocytes to myelin basic protein in primary demyelinating diseases. *N. Engl. J. Med.*, **297**, 850–853.

Lucas, J. (1790). An account of uncommon symptoms succeeding the measles; with additional remarks on the infection of measles and smallpox. *London Med. J.*, **11**, 325–331.

Lukes, S. A. and Norman, D. (1983). Computed tomography in acute disseminated encephalomyelitis. *Ann. Neurol.*, **13**, 567–572.

Marsh, K. (1952). Streptomycin-PAS hypersensitivity treated with ACTH. *Lancet*, ii, 606–608.

Matsushita, E., Takita, K. and Shimada, A. (1997). Suspected acute encephalopathy with symmetrical abnormal signal areas in the basal ganglia, thalamus, midbrain and pons diagnosed by magnetic resonance imaging. *Acta Paed. Jap.*, **39**, 454–458.

Means, E. D., Barron, K. D. and Van Dyne, B. J. (1973). Nervous system lesions after sting by yellow jacket. A case report. *Neurology*, **23**, 881–890.

Menor, F. (1997). Demyelinating diseases in childhood. Diagnostic contribution of magnetic resonance. *Rev. Neurol.*, **25**, 966–969.

Michaud, J. and Helle, T. L. (1982). Acute hemorrhagic leukoencephalitis localized to the brainstem and cerebellum: a report of two cases. *J. Neurol. Neurosurg. Psych.*, **45**, 151–157.

Miller, D. H., Scaravilli, F. Thomas, D. C. T., Harvey, P. and Hirsh, N. P. (1993). Acute disseminated encephalomyelitis presenting as a solitary brainstem mass. *J. Neurol. Neurosurg. Psych.*, **56**, 920–922.

Miller, H. G. and Evans, M. J. (1953). Prognosis in acute disseminated encephalomyelitis: with a note on neuromyelitis optica. *Quart. J. Med.*, **22**, 347–479.

Miller, H. G. and Gibbons, J. L. (1953). Acute disseminated encephalomyelitis and acute disseminated sclerosis: results of treatment with ACTH. *Br. Med. J.*, **2**, 1345–1348.

Miller, H. G., Stanton, J. B. and Gibbons, J. L. (1956). Parainfectious encephalomyelitis and related syndromes. A critical review of the neurological complications of certain specific fevers. *Q. J. Med.*, **25**, 427–505.

Miller, N. R. (1982). Optic neuritis. In: *Walsh and Hoyt's Clinical Neuro-Ophthalmology*, 4th edn. Baltimore: William and Wilkins. pp. 227–248.

Mizutani, K., Atsuta, J., Shibata, T., Azuma, E., Ito, M. and Sakurai, M. (1994). Consecutive cerebral MRI findings of acute relapsing disseminated encephalomyelitis. *Acta Pediatr. Jao*, **36**, 709–712.

Nasr, J. T., Andriola, M. R. and Coyle, P. K. (2000). ADEM: Literature review and case report of acute psychosis presentation. *Ped. Neurol.*, **22**, 8–18.

Newton, R. (1981). Plasma exchange in acute post-infectious demyelination. *Dev. Med. Child. Neurol.*, **23**, 538–543.

Nishimura, M., Saida, T., Kunoki, S. *et al.* (1996). Postinfectious encephalitis with anti-galactocerebroside antibody subsequent to mycoplasma pneumoniae infection. *J. Neurol. Sci.*, **140**, 91–95.

O'Riordan, J. I., Thompson, A. J., Kingsley, D. P. E. *et al.* (1998). The prognostic value of brain MRI in clinically isolated syndromes of the CNS. A 10-year follow-up. *Brain*, **121**, 495–503.

Ohtaki, E., Murakami, Y., Komori, H. *et al.* (1992). Acute disseminated encephalomyelitis after Japanese B encephalitis vaccination. *Pediatr. Neurol.*, **8**, 137–139.

Pandit, L. and Rao, S. (1996). Recurrent myelitis. *J. Neurol. Neurosurg. Psych.*, **60**, 336–338.

Paskavitz, J. F., Anderson, C. A., Filley, C. M., Kleinschmidt-DeMasters, B. K. and Tyler, K. L. (1995). Acute arcuate fiber demyelinating encephalopathy following Epstein-Barr virus infection. *Ann. Neurol.*, **38**, 127–131.

Pasternak, J. F., De Vivo, D. C. and Prensky, A. L. (1980). Steroid-responsive encephalomyelitis in childhood. *Neurology*, **30**, 481–486.

Pearl, P. L., Hussam, A.-F., Starke, J. R., Dreyer, Z., Louis, P. T. and Kirkpatrick, J. B. (1990). Neuropathology of two fatal cases of measles in the 1988–1989 Houston epidemic. *Pediatr. Neurol.*, **6**, 126–130.

Pellegrini, M., O'Brien, T. J., Hoy, J. and Sedal, L. (1996). *Mycoplasma pneumoniae* infection associated with an acute brainstem syndrome. *Acta Neurol. Scand.*, **93**, 203–206.

Piyasirisilp, S., Schmeckpeper, B. J., Chandanayinyong, D., Hemachudha, T. and Griffin, D. E. (1999). Association of HLA and T-cell receptor gene polymorphisms with Semple rabies vaccine-induced autoimmune encephalomyelitis. *Ann. Neurol.*, **45**, 595–600.

Pohl-Koppe, A., Burchett, S. K., Thiele, E. A. and Hafler, D. A. (1998). Myelin basic protein reactive Th2 T cells are found in acute disseminated encephalomyelitis. *J. Neuroimmunol.*, **91**, 19–27.

Poser, C., Roman, G. and Emery, E. (1978). Recurrent disseminated vasculomyelinopathy. *Arch. Neurol.*, **35**:166.

Pradhan, S., Gupta, R. K. and Ghosih, D. (1997). Parainfectious myelitis: three distinct clinico-imagiological patterns with prognostic implications. *Acta Neurol. Scand.*, **95**, 241–247.

Ravkina, L., Harib, I., Manovitch, Z. *et al.* (1979). Hyperacute experimental allergic encephalomyelitis in rhesus monkeys as a model of acute necrotizing hemorrhagic encephalomyelitis. *J. Neurol.*, **221**, 113–125.

Rosenberg, G. A. (1970). Meningoencephalitis following an influenza vaccination. *N. Engl. J. Med.*, **283**, 1209.

Russell, D. S. (1937). Changes in the central nervous system following arsphenamine medication. *J. Pathol. Bacteriol.*, **45**, 357–366.

Sailer, M., O'Riordan, J. I., Thompson, A. J. *et al.* (1999). Quantitative MRI in patients with clinically isolated syndromes suggestive of demyelination. *Neurology*, **52**, 599–606.

Saito, H., Endo, M., Takase, S. and Itahara, K. (1980). Acute disseminated encephalomyelitis after influenza vaccination. *Arch. Neurol.*, **37**, 564–566.

Salazar, A. M., Engel, W. K. and Levy, H. B. (1981). Poly ICLC in the treatment of postinfectious demyelinating encephalomyelitis. *Arch. Neurol.*, **38**, 382–383.

Schwartz, G. A., Yang, D. C. and Noone, E. L. (1964). Meningoencephalomyelitis with epidemic parotitis. *Arch. Neurol.*, **11**, 453–462.

Scott, T. F., Bhagavatula, K., Snyder, P. J. and Chieffe, C. (1998). Transverse myelitis. Comparison with spinal cord presentations of multiple sclerosis. *Neurology*, **50**, 429–433.

Seales, D. and Greer, M. (1991). Acute hemorrhagic leukoencephalitis: a successful recovery. *Arch. Neurol.* **48**, 1086–1088.

Selbst, R. G., Selhorst, J. B., Harbison, J. W. and Myer, E. C. (1983). Parainfectious optic neuritis: report and review following varicella. *Arch. Neurol.*, **40**, 347–350.

Shakir, R. A., Al-Din, A. S. N., Araj, G. F. *et al.* (1987). Clinical categories of neurobrucellosis. *Brain*, **110**, 213–223.

Shaw, D. W. W. and Cohen, W. A. (1993). Viral infections of the CNS in children: imaging features. *Am. J. Roentgen.*, **160**, 125–133.

Straub, J., Chofflon, M. and Delavelle, J. (1997). Early high dose intravenous ethylprednisolone in acute disseminated encephalomyelitis. A successful recovery. *Neurology*, **49**, 1145–1147.

Stricker, R. B., Miller, R. G. and Kiprov, D. D. (1992). Role of plasmapheresis in acute disseminated (postinfectious) encephalomyelitis. *J. Clin. Apheresis*, **7**, 173–179.

Swamy, H. S., Shankar, S. K., Chandra, P. S., Aroor, S. R., Krishna, A. S. and Perumal, V. G. K. (1984). Neurological complications due to beta-propiolactone (BPL)-inactivated antirabies vaccination. *J. Neurol. Sci.*, **63**, 111–128.

Swanson, B. E. (1956). Measles meningoencephalitis. A summary of 24 cases treated at Grasslands over a 10 year period. *Am. J. Dis. Child.*, **12**, 272–275.

Tenorio, G. and Whitaker, J. N. (1991). Steroid dependent postvaricella encephalomyelitis. *J. Child. Neurol.*, **6**, 45–48.

Trevisani, F., Gattinari, G. C., Caraceni, P. *et al.* (1993). Transverse myelitis following hepatitis B vaccination. *J. Hepatol.*, **19**, 317–318.

Tsai, M.-L. and Hung, K.-L. (1996). Multiphasic disseminated encephalomyelitis mimicking multiple sclerosis. *Brain Devel.*, **18**, 412–414.

Tselis, A. C. and Lisak, R. P. (1998). Acute disseminated encephalomyelitis. In: *Clinical Neuroimmunology* (J. Antel, G. Birnbaum and H. P. Hartung, eds). Boston, Massachusetts: Blackwell Science. pp. 116–147.

Tyler, H. R. (1957). Neurological complications of rubeola (measles). *Medicine*, **36**, 147–167.

Ungurean, A., Palfi, S., Dibo, G., Tiszlavicz, L. and Vecsei, L. (1996). Chronic recurrent transverse myelitis or multiple sclerosis. *Funct. Neuro.*, **11**, 209–214.

Warren, W. B. (1956). Encephalopathy due to influenza vaccine. *Arch. Intern. Med.*, **97**, 803–805.

Weinshenker, B. G., O'Brien, P. C., Peterson, T. M. *et al.* (1999). Plasma exchange reverses severe neurologic disability in corticosteroid refractory attacks of idiopathic inflammatory demyelinating disease of the CNS. *MS*, **5**(S1), S12.

Wells, C. E. C. (1971). Neurological complications of so-called 'influenza'. A winter study in Southeast Wales. *Br. Med. J.*, **1**, 369–373.

Westall, F. C. and Root-Bernstein, R. (1986). Cause and prevention of postinfectious and postvaccinal neuropathies in light of a new theory of autoimmunity. *Lancet*, **2**, 251–252.

Williams, H. W. and Chafee, F. H. (1961). Demyelinating encephalomyelitis in a case of tetanus treated with antitoxin. *N. Engl. J. Med.*, **264**, 489–491.

Wood, D. D., Bilbao, J. M., O'Connors, P. and Moscarello, M. A. (1996) Acute multiple sclerosis (Marburg type) is associated with developmentally immature myelin basic protein. *Neurology*, **40**, 18–24.

Woods, C. A. and Ellison, G. W. (1964). Encephalopathy following influenza immunization. *J. Pediatr.*, **65**, 745–748.

Wucherpfennig, K. W. and Strominger, J. L. (1995). Molecular mimicry in T cell mediated autoimmunity: viral peptides activate human T cell clones specific for myelin basic protein. *Cell*, **80**, 695–705.

Yahr, M. D. and Lobo-Antunes, J. (1972). Relapsing encephalomyelitis following the use of influenza vaccine. *Arch. Neurol.*, **27**, 182–183.

Youl, B. D., Kermode, A. G., Thompson, A. J. *et al.* (1991). Destructive lesions in demyelinating disease. *J. Neurol. Neurosurg. Psych.*, **54**, 288–292.

Zhang, J., Vandevyver, C., Stinissen, P., Mertens, N., van den berg Loonen, E. and Raus, J. (1995). Activation and clonal expansion of human myelin basic protein reactivate T cells by bacterial superantigens. *J. Autoimmun.*, **8**, 615–632.

Ziegler, D. K. (1966). Acute disseminated encephalomyelitis. Some therapeutic and diagnostic considerations. *Arch. Neurol.*, **14**, 476–488.

Ziegna, S. R. (1961). Corticosteroid treatment for measles encephalitis. *J. Pediatr.*, **59**, 322–323.

4

Cytomegalovirus infection of the adult nervous system

Alex Tselis and Ehud Lavi

Introduction

Cytomegalovirus is a member of the herpesvirus family and causes both acute and latent or persistent infections of humans. It is transmitted in the normal population through saliva, milk, genital secretions, semen, blood transfusions, and organ transplants. The prevalence of cytomegalovirus (CMV) infection is high in all human populations studied. The seroprevalence is higher in groups of poor socioeconomic background, increases with age in all groups and is very high (>90%) in homosexual men (Drew *et al.*, 1981; Ho, 1985).

CMV is an uncommon cause of encephalitis and therefore its clinical picture is not well delineated. (Arribas *et al.*, 1996). During severe, prolonged immunosuppression, CMV becomes an important opportunistic organism, and diseases caused by CMV are common. CMV disease is a well-known complication of bone marrow and solid organ transplantation, although CMV encephalitis is rare in transplant recipients. A few patients with other forms of immunosuppression have been reported to have CMV encephalitis ((Kauffman *et al.*, 1979; Koeppen *et al.*, 1981). Patients with AIDS have numerous CNS complications, including viral opportunistic infections. CMV infection is one of the opportunistic infections of the CNS in late stage AIDS patients (Peters *et al.*, 1991), when there is severe immunosuppression and a very low CD4 count, almost universally less than 100 cells/mm^2 (Gallant *et al.*, 1992). In early studies, CMV was seen so commonly in the brains of demented patients that it was speculated that CMV was the main cause of the subacute encephalitis in AIDS patients (Nielsen *et al.*, 1984). In a neuropathological autopsy series (Kure *et al.*, 1991), it was found that CMV infection of the brain occurred in 16% of patients, making it the second most common finding in the brains of AIDS patients, after HIV encephalitis, and more common than toxoplasmosis or cryptococcal meningitis. In another older autopsy series, approximately 25% of patients were found to have CMV infection of the brain at autopsy (Navia *et al.*, 1986). With the advent of aggressive antiretroviral therapy, however, there has been a decline in the incidence of opportunistic infections in patients with advanced HIV disease. Three important indicators of immunodeficiency (pneumocystis pneumonia, *Mycobacterium avium* complex disease, and CMV retinitis) have become much less common in the age of combination antire-troviral therapy (Palella *et al.*, 1998). Furthermore, partial reconstitution of immunity by the use of antiretroviral therapy can arrest cytomegalovirus retinitis, without the use of specific anticytomegaloviral therapy (Reed *et al.*, 1997).

Acute primary CMV infection is usually asymptomatic, but can manifest as a mononucleosis-like syndrome (Cheeseman, 1992). This is followed by a latent or persistent infection in the normal host, which may be reactivated during times of stress or immunosuppression. Reactivation is usually asymptomatic in the immunocompetent host, but can be detected as a transient viruria or an asymptomatic viraemia (Weller, 1971). Latency is defined as the presence of viral nucleic acid with limited expression of viral genes and no replication. Persistent infection occurs with low level, usually chronic, replication of virus, but few or no pathological consequences. For CMV, there is evidence for latency in lymphocytes and monocytes (Jordan, 1983; Rice *et al.*, 1984; Schrier *et al.*, 1989). However, solid organs have also been implicated as sites of latency (or persistence), since kidneys transplanted from asymptomatic seropositive donors to seronegative recipients have apparently transmitted the disease (Ho *et al.*, 1975). Similar observations have been made for other viscera, including the heart, lungs and liver (Ho, 1993). Furthermore, in studies of autopsies of trauma victims, immediate early antigen of CMV was found in visceral tissues by immunocytochemistry, with no other changes (such as expression of late antigens, cytomegalic cells or inflammation) attributable to CMV (Toorkey and Carrigan, 1989). Some of the organs with cells staining positively were brain, kidney, spleen, lung and liver. The specific types of cells that were infected were not identified.

CMV encephalitis

Clinical presentation

CMV encephalitis appears to be exceedingly uncommon in the normal host beyond the neonatal age period. There are only a few case reports in the literature. In the non-immunocompromised host, CMV encephalitis often develops in the context of systemic disease, beginning with a relatively prolonged prodrome of malaise, fever, sore throat, lethargy, and lymph-adenopathy. (Perham *et al.*, 1971). Occasionally, there is an accompanying hepatitis or myocarditis (Waris *et al.*, 1972). The encephalitis is characterized by any combination of lethargy, headache, photophobia, neck stiffness, aphasia, focal weakness and spasticity, upgoing toes, and seizures (Perham *et al.*, 1971; Waris *et al.*, 1972; Dorfman, 1973; Back *et al.*, 1977; Siegman-Igra *et al.*, 1984). Focal deficits may be superimposed on mild confusion (Phillips *et al.*, 1977). Occasionally, there is a more restricted presentation of myelopathy, with a paraplegia, quadriplegia, respiratory distress due to weakness of the respiratory musculature, broad-based gait, spinal sensory level and urinary urgency (Chin *et al.*, 1973; Tyler *et al.*, 1986; Miles *et al.*, 1993). One immunocompetent patient presented with a brainstem encephalitis (Kanzaki *et al.*, 1995).

CMV encephalitis in the transplant patient presents as a non-specific febrile encephalopathy, and may or may not have focal features (Dorfman, 1973; Schober and Herman, 1973; Hotson and Pedley, 1976).

AIDS-associated CMV encephalitis presents in two forms: one is a microglial nodule encephalitis, characterized by acute onset, confusion, delirium and a relatively bland CSF formula, and the other is a ventriculoencephalitis, characterized by a slow progressive apathy, confusion and cranial nerve palsies, and occasionally a CSF formula of pleocytosis (with a neutrophilic predominance) and hypoglycorrhachia (Kalayjian *et al.*, 1993; Grassi *et al.*, 1997). (See below.) CMV encephalitis can be difficult, in some cases, to distinguish from HIV dementia. In a retrospective case-control study, in which 14 autopsy-confirmed CMV cases were characterized and compared to 17 controls with HIV dementia (Holland *et al.*, 1994), CMV encephalitis patients were found to have relatively more confusion, disorientation, apathy, withdrawal, and focal neurological signs and relatively less primitive reflexes than the HIV dementia controls. Furthermore, there is often other disease in the brain (in 50% of the brains in the series of Vinters *et al.*, 1989) which can complicate clinical-pathological correlation. Thus, in many cases, the effects of CMV in the brain are obscured by the presence of fulminant systemic disease (Hawley *et al.*, 1983) or other coexisting CNS disease (Vinters *et al.*, 1989). It is possible that a few isolated inclusion-bearing cells or a few microglial nodules do not have much clinical effect (Navia *et al.*, 1986). Indeed, in seven cases of microglial nodule encephalitis in which clinical data were available (Morgello *et al.*, 1987), two were apparently without cognitive dysfunction, while five were demented. Further, one patient (case 3 of Moskowitz *et al.*, 1984), developed lethargy, confusion and a poor memory over several months. He was found to have a pure CMV microglial nodule encephalitis, with a few cytomegalic cells and no perivascular infiltrates.

Other presentations include hemispheral signs with heminumbness (Masdeu *et al.*, 1988), seizures (Fuller *et al.*, 1989), hallucinations (Fuller *et al.*, 1989), prominent brainstem involvement (Fuller *et al.*, 1989) and multiple cranial neuropathies (Kenyon *et al.*, 1998).

Abnormalities in serum electrolytes and osmolarity have been noted to occur in AIDS-associated CMV encephalitis. In the study of Holland *et al.* (1994), these were the rule in CMV encephalitis patients, with 53% hyponatraemic, 30% hypernatraemic and 15% normonatraemic. The HIV dementia controls all had normal electrolytes. Serum electrolytes are rarely reported in the literature, but abnormal electrolytes or osmolarity were reported in two of the seven cases by Kalayjian *et al.* (1993). It is of note that CMV adrenalitis, which can cause serum electrolyte abnormalities, is very commonly described in autopsy series. Thus, in the series of Morgello *et al.* (1987), 26 out of 29 patients with CMV encephalitis had CMV adrenalitis.

Diagnosis

Diagnosis of CMV encephalitis can be difficult and in the older case reports, the diagnosis was made by a significant increase in anti-CMV antibodies between acute and convalescent phase sera in the context of a febrile encephalopathic illness (Perham *et al.*, 1971; Chin *et al.*, 1973; Back *et al.*, 1977; Duchowny *et al.*, 1979).

Viral isolation

Isolation of CMV from blood or urine is common in systemic CMV infection, but is non-specific, since this can occur in asymptomatic reactivation (Weller, 1971). The virus can be isolated from the brain or CSF in immunocompetent CMV encephalitis patients (Phillips *et al.*, 1977).

In AIDS-associated CMV encephalitis, the virus often cannot be cultured from the CSF (Berman and Kim, 1994: none of five patients; Cohen, 1996: none of seven patients; Kalayjian *et al.*, 1993: none of four patients). Only rare isolations have been reported in individual case reports (Edwards *et al.*, 1985; Belec *et al.*, 1990).

Serology

Anti-CMV antibody levels for the diagnosis of CMV encephalitis can be misleading, since CMV antibody titres can fluctuate spontaneously. In one study, serial complement-fixing (CF) antibody titres from healthy donors were shown to fluctuate between 'significant' and 'non-detectable' titres in 22%, without known external cause (Waner *et al.*, 1973). Two patients with biopsy-proven CMV encephalitis had no changes in the level of anti-CMV antibody (Phillips *et al.*, 1977). Neutralizing antibodies are more stable, and can be used more reliably to demonstrate previous exposure to CMV. Commercially, most CMV antibody tests nowadays measure binding of antibody to whole CMV virus, rather than using functional assays (such as neutralization or complement-fixation) as before. Nevertheless, while serology can prove past or recent infection, it is of little use in proving the diagnosis of encephalitis.

A different approach to diagnosis would be to look for a specific intrathecal immune response, by measuring the cerebrospinal fluid (CSF)-to-serum ratio of CMV antibody. However, in the one study in which this was examined, only three patients with presumed AIDS-associated CMV encephalitis (only one confirmed by autopsy) and five HIV positive patients with other neurological disease (none with autopsy) had such CSF tests done (Fiala *et al.*, 1993). The results showed a trend towards slightly higher CSF/serum ratios for the CMV cases, but with a two-sided P-value of 0.05. This approach clearly requires more work for validation. Furthermore, as discussed above, the interpretation of CMV antibody titres is problematic.

Brain imaging

There is a paucity of data on the imaging findings in CMV encephalitis in the non-immunocompromised host and transplant patients.

In the AIDS patient, CMV encephalitis can give a wide range of imaging results, from normal to generalized atrophy, periventricular abnormalities, and focal, discrete lesions. CT of the brain can be normal or show only mild atrophy (Kalayjian *et al.*, 1993). In a series of 10 patients with autopsy-proven CMV encephalitis, all had abnormal CT scans, but only three had abnormalities specific for CMV, and the pathology was often more extensive than the CT would indicate (Post *et al.*, 1986). MRI scans are more sensitive but can still be normal or show only atrophy (Kalayjian *et al.*, 1993; Holland *et al.*, 1994; Arribas *et al.*, 1995). The most common specific MRI finding in CMV encephalitis is periventricular increased signal on T2-weighted images and ependymal enhancement on T1-weighted images (Kalayjian *et al.*, 1993) (Figures 4.1 and 4.2). On CT scan and MRI, CMV encephalitis can result in discrete white matter lesions (Post *et al.*, 1986). In one CT scan, a hypodensity was noted in a cerebellar hemisphere, which was shown to be a necrotizing leucoencephalopathy at autopsy (Figure 4.3). In another (Laskin *et al.*, 1987), small right frontal lobe lucencies were noted. These were found to contain cytomegalic cells, as well as cells staining with herpes simplex virus 1 (HSV-1) antigens. In an MRI scan (Masdeu *et al.*, 1988), lesions were noted in the right internal capsule, right basis pontis and left pontine tegmentum, with the first lesion showing necrosis with admixed cytomegalic cells on biopsy.

In one immunocompetent patient with probable CMV myelitis, MRI of the spinal cord was normal (Miles *et al.*, 1993).

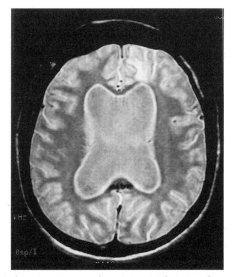

Figure 4.1   An MRI showing increased periventricular signal on a T2-weighted image

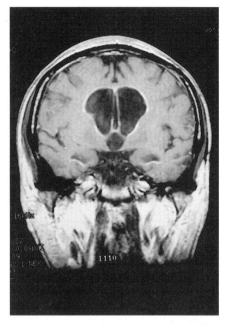

Figure 4.2   A T1-weighted MRI image showing prominent ependymal enhancement in a case of CMV ventriculoencephalitis

EEG

The electroencephalogram in CMV encephalitis is non-specific. In a 52-year-old man with sudden onset of headache, nausea and lethargy, the EEG showed slow left temporal activity. In a 20-year-old woman with rapid onset of severe headache and confusion, followed by a seizure, serial EEGs showed an initial diffuse slowing evolving to left sided focal 'changes' and right temporal spikes (Phillips *et al.*, 1977).

Cerebrospinal fluid findings

There are no pathognomonic CSF finding in CMV encephalitis in the immunocompetent host. There may be no (Waris *et al.*, 1972; Dorfman, 1973; Back *et al.*, 1977) or only a mild pleocytosis. In one report, two patients had seven and 18 white blood cells (WBCs) (Phillips *et al.*, 1977). One patient with lethargy and headache had a moderate pleocytosis of 96 WBCs (mostly lymphocytes) (Perham *et al.*, 1971). The CSF of a patient with a myelopathy showed 202 WBCs (68% neutrophils, 32% lymphocytes), 17 RBCs, and a protein of 46 mg/dl. A repeat CSF examination a week later showed only six WBCs and a protein of 22 mg/dl (Chin *et al.*, 1973).

The CSF findings in AIDS-associated CMV encephalitis reported in the literature are highly variable. In one study, two out of 13 CMV encephalitis patients had a pleocytosis, with 25 and 3179 cells/µm (Holland *et al.*, 1994). In another study, two CMV ventriculoencephalitis patients had CSF pleocytosis,

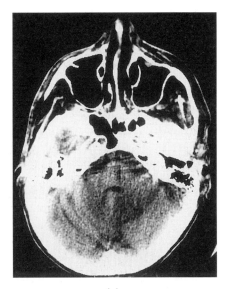

(a)

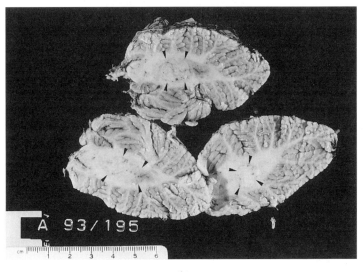

(b)

Figure 4.3 (a) An unenhanced CT scan of the brain showing a prominent lucency in the left cerebellar hemisphere. (Courtesy of R. Howard, MD, Division of Neuroradiology, University of Pennsylvania). (b) Macroscopic sections of the lesion shown in (a) outlined by arrowheads

with cell counts of 10 and 50. A substantial proportion of these cells were neutrophils. None of the CSFs from patients with microglial nodule encephalitis had pleocytosis (Grassi *et al.*, 1998). Four out of nine patients with ventriculoencephalitis in another study had pleocytosis, which was greater than

800 cells in two of them (Arribas *et al.*, 1995). It is noteworthy that neutrophilic pleocytosis can be seen in CMV encephalitis in both the normal and severely immunocompromised host.

Detection of CMV genome in CSF using PCR

Recently, the polymerase chain reaction (PCR) to detect CMV DNA in CSF has been proposed as a means of diagnosing CMV encephalitis ante-mortem. Two recent reports document the use of PCR amplification of CMV DNA in the diagnosis of CMV encephalitis in four immunocompetent hosts (Studahl *et al.*, 1992; Kanzaki *et al.*, 1995).

In AIDS-associated CMV encephalitis, PCR methods have been more extensively studied. The sensitivity of PCR is high, but results are difficult to compare across studies due to the marked differences both in the population of patients studied in each series and in the PCR assay employed (Cinque *et al.*, 1992; Gozlan *et al.*, 1992; Wolf and Spector, 1992; Clifford *et al.*, 1993; Fillet *et al.*, 1993; Achim *et al.*, 1994; Holland *et al.*, 1994). Some remarks and caveats follow.

Severity of disease
The severity of disease varies from widespread ventriculoencephalitis to focal microglial nodules or isolated cytomegalic cells. Arribas *et al.* (1995) have hypothesized that the level of CMV DNA in the CSF of AIDS patients might correlate with the extent of CMV infection of the CNS. By subjecting serial dilutions of CSF to PCR, Arribas *et al.* found that only patients with ventriculoencephalitis had levels of CMV DNA higher than 10^3 genomes per µl of CSF. Only one sample was available from a patient with isolated cytomegalic cells obtained shortly (3 days) before death. This specimen had a level of CMV DNA of 10–100 genomes per 8 µl of CSF. Quantity of virus (measured in genomes per cell) appears to correlate with the presence of disease (Wildemann *et al.*, 1998).

Pre-mortem versus Post-mortem CSF samples
Four studies (Cinque *et al.*, 1992; Gozlan *et al.*, 1992; Fillet *et al.*, 1993; Holland *et al.*, 1994) used only pre-mortem CSF samples, one study used only post-mortem CSF samples (Achim *et al.*, 1994), and one study used both pre- and post-mortem samples (Wolf and Spector, 1992). The study in which only post-mortem samples were used showed a low specificity and differs from the other studies which used pre-mortem samples and had much higher specificities. Results of CMV CSF PCR in samples obtained post-mortem are probably not comparable with results obtained with pre-mortem samples.

Specimen preparation and assay sensitivity
Analytic sensitivity of the different PCR assays varied between one (Achim *et al.*, 1994) and 40 CMV genome copies (Gozlan *et al.*, 1992). These differences in the analytic sensitivity are likely related to differences in CSF preparation, PCR target, PCR protocol and method of detection of amplified products. This will affect the clinical sensitivity of the PCR assay.

A potential pitfall of CMV CSF PCR as a diagnostic test is that, due to its extreme sensitivity, it might detect CMV DNA in the CSF of AIDS patients with only minimal focal involvement (such as isolated cytomegalic cells within areas of normal brain parenchyma) (Cinque *et al.*, 1992; Wolf and Spector, 1992). This should be considered when interpreting the results of CMV CSF PCR.

CMV radiculomyelitis and peripheral neuropathy

CMV also infects the peripheral nerves, nerve roots and spinal cord in patients with advanced HIV disease. There is only a single report of CMV polyradiculo-pathy, identical in presentation to that in advanced HIV disease, in an apparently immunocompetent patient (Kabins *et al.*, 1976).

CMV polyradiculopathy generally presents with pain and paraesthesias in the lower extremities, followed by a subacute hypotonic weakness and areflexia in the legs, urinary retention, and sensory loss (Eidelberg *et al.*, 1986; Behar *et al.*, 1987; Mahieux *et al.*, 1989; Cohen *et al.*, 1993). CSF examination usually, but not always, shows a neutrophilic pleocytosis and hypoglycorrhachia (deGans *et al.*, 1990; Miller *et al.*, 1996). CMV PCR is positive in the CSF, while virus only occasionally can be cultured. Electro-myography generally shows diffuse denervation in the lower extremities. Imaging studies show enhancement of the conus medullaris, cauda equina and nerve roots as well as diffuse meningeal enhancement of the lumbar thecal sac (Bazan *et al.*, 1991; Talpos *et al.*, 1991).

CMV mononeuropathy multiplex generally presents with numbness and painful paraesthesias in a multifocal distribution, followed weeks to months later by progression to a severe sensorimotor neuropathy. Most patients have CMV detectable in the CSF by PCR. The EMG findings are typical of a mononeuropathy multiplex with multifocal axonopathy (Roullet *et al.*, 1994). Occasionally, there is a relative dominance of demyelination in the roots and peripheral nerves in CMV neuropathy (Morgello and Simpson, 1994).

Differential diagnosis

CMV encephalitis in the normal host usually presents as an encephalopathy (possibly with focal features), occurring in the context of a subacute febrile illness. The differential is broad, but one would have to consider the possibility of herpes simplex encephalitis, bacterial meningitis, tuberculous meningitis, and other treatable diseases. Occasionally, restricted forms of the disease, such as a transverse myelopathy, can occur in such a setting. The diagnosis is made most easily by recovery of CMV genome from the CSF by PCR.

In the transplant patient, the diagnosis is difficult to make since there are a number of complications that can cause a febrile encephalopathy, especially encephalopathy due to systemic sepsis and that due to the effects of drugs such as cyclosporine, which may be particularly common early in the post-transplant period. Systemic CMV disease usually occurs between 1 and 4 months after a transplant, and CMV encephalitis would be expected in this time scale. Other complications occurring in the transplant patient include aspergillosis, listeria meningitis, and CNS nocardiosis.

In the AIDS patient with progressive encephalopathy, the differential diagnosis is broad, and includes HIV-associated dementia, progressive multi-focal leucoencephalopathy, primary CNS lymphoma and cerebral toxoplas-mosis. In a patient with subacute encephalopathy and cranial nerve palsies or nystagmus, neutrophilic pleocytosis, increased CSF protein and hypoglycor-rhachia, CMV ventriculoencephalitis is very likely, and can be confirmed by PCR detection of CMV DNA in the CSF.

Practical diagnostic points

There are no specific clinical or CSF or imaging findings characteristic of CMV infection of the CNS, except perhaps for the ventriculoencephalitis (or polyradiculopathy forms) discussed above. Thus, the picture of a patient with advanced HIV disease who presents with a subacute encephalopathy, coarse nystagmus, neutrophilic pleocytosis with hypoglycorrhachia, and abnormal periventricular signal on MRI is virtually pathognomonic for CMV encephalitis.

CSF CMV PCR is most reliable when it is positive in the context of a compatible clinical illness, such as a subacutely progressive encephalopathy or lumbosacral radiculopathy in an AIDS patient, or in a transplant patient in whom there is no other obvious cause of encephalopathy or in an immuno-competent host with an otherwise undiagnosed encephalitis. In such cases, it is reasonable to initiate anti-CMV therapy (see below under practical therapeutic points), although the specificity of this test is best established for AIDS-associated CMV encephalitis. The significance of positive CSF PCR in an otherwise asymptomatic person is not known.

Pathology and pathogenesis

The neuropathology of CMV encephalitis in the normal host is not fully known because of the rarity of the disease. However, studies in the immunocompro-mised host (see below) and in animal models augment the limited data available in the intact human host. The only tissue samples described were from two cases (case 2 of Phillips et al., 1977; case 4 of Dorfman, 1973). Case 2 of Phillips et al. (1977) was from biopsy tissue, and subject to sampling error; it showed microgliosis ('rod cell proliferation'), astrocytosis and neuronal degeneration. A patient of Waris et al. (1972) with systemic CMV disease characterized by myocarditis, hepatitis and adrenal insufficiency had a single, 2-week episode of encephalopathy which resolved completely. The histopathol-ogy had likely resolved along with the clinical disease, so that the autopsy findings may not reflect the pathologic process during the acute stage of the encephalitis. Finally, in case 4 of Dorfman (1973), an apparently normal host

Cytomegalovirus infection of the

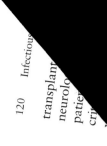

120

Infectiou

transplan

neurolo

patie

cri

died in the course of acute CMV disease with enceph̵
given steroids for an unclear period during her initial
ogy consisted of diffusely scattered microglial nodu
bearing cells. Thus, the pathology of CMV enceph
appears to be a microglial nodule encephalitis, with
such as perivascular cuffing, much less prominent. T̵
with the pathological results in a guinea-pig mode̵
which scattered microglial nodules predominate, v
again less prominent (Booss et al., 1989; Booss and Kim, 1989). ̵̵ ̵̵
that higher viral loads are required for the encephalitis to display necrosis (see
below).

The pathology of CMV encephalitis in transplant patients is better known.
In a classic study (Schneck, 1965), the brains of 11 renal transplant patients
were examined for evidence of an 'unusual viral infection' in the brain. All 11
had microglial nodules in the brain, particularly concentrated in the cortex and
deep gray matter. Only rarely were perivascular lymphocytic cuffs noted. Only
two patients had cells with intracellular inclusions, all of which were at the
centres of microglial nodules. Four patients had 'rod cell proliferation', one of
whom had no microglial nodules. Four other patients had Alzheimer's type II
astrocytes. Viral isolation (from lung) was accomplished in only two patients,
although nine of the patients had evidence of CMV infection of the lungs. The
neuropathological findings were not correlated with the patients' clinical status
and no details of the patients' clinical illness were given. This was the first
paper to relate CMV encephalitis to a microglial nodule picture. The author
argued that a tentative identification of the microglial nodule encephalitis with
CMV could be made, because this pathology was seen only in patients with
systemic CMV and no other pathogens were present to account for it. The
microglial nodules resembled those seen in other viral encephalitides. Finally,
an occasional cytomegalic cell (pathognomonic of CMV infection) was present
at the centre of a microglial nodule.

In a later study of the neuropathology of 31 cardiac transplant patients who
expired for various reasons, 18 were found to have central nervous system
(CNS) pathology and 10 of these had scattered microglial nodules, in all cases
mainly in the central grey structures (Schober and Herman, 1973). In one
patient, toxoplasma encephalitis was found, which can also be associated with
microglial nodules. In the other nine, the microglial nodule encephalitis was
believed to be due to CMV, although three of these patients had concurrent
fungal CNS infection. In seven of the patients, pulmonary cytomegalovirus
infection was demonstrable. Of the brains with microglial nodules, only in two
were cells with inclusions seen. It was not completely clear to the authors what
the impact of the viral encephalitis on the clinical course was, since the diffuse
encephalopathy in these patients could be from several causes, such as uraemia,
systemic bacterial or fungal infection, electrolyte abnormalities, and medication
effects.

In another series (Hotson and Pedley, 1976), CNS infections were the most
common neurological complication of heart transplantation, and CMV was
the second most likely pathogen (along with HSV). In that series, 83 heart

patients were reviewed and 45 (54%) were found to have ...gical complications, 20 of which had CNS infection. Of these, three ...ts had CMV encephalitis, for an overall incidence of 3/83 (4%). The ...eria for viral encephalitis in that study were (1) diffuse encephalopathy, (2) ...iral isolation from the brain, or CSF, or a fourfold elevation in CMV antibody titre and (3) pathological demonstration of microglial nodule formations or nuclear inclusions. As discussed above, some of these criteria are not very specific. Clinically, all three patients were encephalopathic, but in two patients, Gram-negative sepsis was present and may have been responsible for some of the patients' symptoms. In all three cases, disseminated microglial nodules were noted, but there was only scant evidence of perivascular cuffs, neuronophagia, necrosis, or haemorrhage.

Three other renal transplant patients with immunosuppression were reported by Dorfman (1973), who noted microglial nodules in the brain, and a lack of perivascular cuffing. Of interest is that the CMV microglial nodule encephalitis occurred during a rejection crisis in two of the patients, with a systemic immune response activated by the presence of the foreign organ.

The 'typical' histopathological picture of CMV encephalitis we have discussed so far is a microglial nodule encephalitis, with much less of the pathology usually associated with other encephalitides, such as lymphocytic perivascular cuffing, neuronophagia or astrocytosis (Leestma, 1991). It is possible that this may not be an accurate picture of the disease and may be due to observational bias in that almost all of the patients reported with CMV encephalitis have had severe suppression of cell-mediated immunity.

Disseminated CMV infection and CMV encephalitis appear to affect patients with defects in cell-mediated immunity. Indeed, clearance of systemic CMV is associated with the onset of cell-mediated immunity rather than with the presence of antibodies (van den Berg et al., 1992).

Humoral immunity seems to be less important in CMV disease. Disseminated CMV disease is not commonly seen in patients with agammaglobulinaemia or hypogammaglobulinaemia, in which infections with bacteria (Buckley, 1986) or mycoplasma (Roifman et al., 1986) occur. Also, apart from chronic enterovirus meningoencephalitis (McKinney et al., 1987), viral infections in hypo- and agammaglobulinaemic patients are not different from normal (Buckley, 1986). Very rarely such patients have had encephalitis ascribed to measles virus and herpes simplex virus (Lederman and Winkelstein, 1985), although most encephalitis has been due to enteroviruses. Systemic infections (but not encephalitis) with a few other viruses have been described in patients with hypogammaglobulinaemia, but not CMV (Lederman and Winkelstein, 1985). Therefore, hosts with deficits in humoral immunity appear to handle CMV as do intact hosts.

However, there are subtleties in the relative effectiveness of the two arms of immunity against CMV. For example, in one patient with thymoma and immunoglobulin deficiency (Kauffman et al., 1979), there was a noticeable inflammatory response in the brain, with perivascular haemorrhages and lymphocytic cuffs, even though microglial nodules were not seen. The patient had immunoglobulin deficiency and a selective non-responsiveness of lymphocytes to CMV antigens, but with other T-cell functions (formation of rosettes, and mitogenic responsiveness to non-specific and specific activators) normal. Furthermore, CMV immune globulin has been useful in the prevention of CMV opportunistic infection in transplant patients (Emanuel, 1991), so humoral immunity may be subtly involved (see below).

In a guinea-pig CMV encephalitis model, the histopathology is predominantly that of a microglial nodule encephalitis, with some perivascular cuffing (Booss et al., 1989), as seen in almost all of the reported human cases. It appears that, with a few exceptions, CMV encephalitis manifests similarly in normal hosts and immunosuppressed patients, although it is extremely rare in the former and quite uncommon in the latter. However, this statement is uncertain, given the paucity of autopsy studies. Furthermore it is possible that the so-called 'normal' hosts were immunosuppressed in some way that was not superficially evident.

It is interesting that periventricular necrosis was not especially prominent in any of the immunosuppressed or transplant patients. This is in contrast to CMV encephalitis in the AIDS patient as well as in the neonate. In general, the end-organ patterns of CMV disease differ in transplant and AIDS patients. In transplant patients CMV mononucleosis syndrome is the most common manifestation of CMV disease, but occasionally organ-specific CMV disease occurs. The pattern of this organ-specific CMV disease is intriguing. Clinically important CMV pneumonia is seen most often in lung, heart-lung and bone marrow transplants (although the precise pathogenetic mechanism may not be identical in each) and CMV hepatitis is seen most often in liver transplantation (Ho, 1993). CMV retinitis is quite uncommon in bone marrow transplant (Winston, 1993) and heart-lung transplant (Smyth et al., 1993) patients. On the other hand, CMV retinitis and encephalitis are quite common in AIDS patients (Schober and Herman, 1973; Hotson and Pedley, 1976; Peters et al., 1991). The reason for this difference in end-organ disease between AIDS and transplant patients is unclear, but almost certainly involves differing pathogenetic mechanisms.

Some CMV end-organ disease in transplant patients is immunopathologically mediated (Grundy et al., 1987). Thus, treatment of CMV pneumonia with antiviral agents is successful in AIDS but not in bone marrow transplant patients (Grundy et al., 1987; Frank and Friedman, 1988). However, an impressive response to combination therapy with ganciclovir and CMV immune globulin has been noted in two independent trials in bone marrow transplant patients with CMV pneumonia (Frank and Friedman, 1988; Reed et al., 1988; Emanuel et al., 1988). Also, in a series of 100 bone marrow transplants between syngeneic identical twin pairs, no CMV pneumonia was seen (Applebaum et al., 1982), while in a concurrent series of allogeneic bone marrow transplant patients, 20% had the disease, a statistically significant difference. The rates for other pneumonias were the same in the two groups. Further, in a murine model of CMV pneumonia, ganciclovir will clear the virus from the lungs but not affect disease progression (Grundy et al., 1987).

In AIDS, on the other hand, it is likely that CMV causes disease through different mechanisms (Hirsch, 1991). First, CMV can be directly cytolytic to cells. Second, it has immunosuppressive effects by itself, and can therefore further depress an already-depressed immune system. Finally, CMV can coinfect cells with HIV, and each genome can induce up-regulation of protein synthesis and replication by the other (Ho *et al.*, 1990; Skolnik *et al.*, 1988; Nelson *et al.*, 1988).

There is a broad pathological spectrum of CMV infection of the brain in AIDS, ranging from the presence of isolated scattered cytomegalic cells, to scattered microglial nodules (with and without inclusions), to widespread necrotizing ependymitis with periventricularly distributed cytomegalic cells, microglial nodules and perivascular infiltrates, to vasculitis, and to necrotizing leukoencephalopathy (Vinters *et al.*, 1989) (Figure 4.4) In an autopsy study of 30 AIDS patients with CMV encephalitis, Morgello *et al.* (1987) distinguished five types of neuropathological findings: microglial nodules ($n = 30$), isolated inclusion-bearing cells ($n = 15$), focal parenchymal necrosis ($n = 4$), necrotizing ventriculoencephalitis ($n = 3$), and necrotizing radiculomyelitis ($n = 3$).

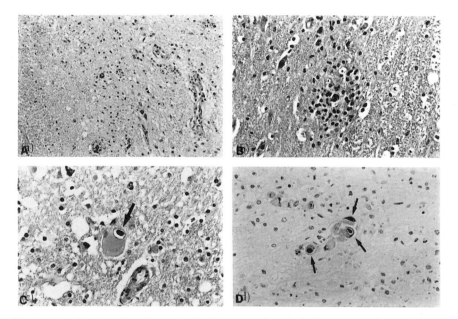

Figure 4.4 (a) A section from the border zone of a cerebellar necrotic lesion demonstrating necrotic debris and 'ghost' cells on the left with gliovascular and mild perivascular inflammatory reaction on the right. This section is from the patient in Figure 4.3. (H&E × 100). (b) A section of spinal cord exhibiting a microglial module surrounding a cell with an intranuclear inclusion body. (H&E × 100). (c) A section from the periphery of a microscopic necrotic lesion in the striatum exhibiting a cytomegalic astrocyte with eccentric nucleus containing a typical CMV intranuclear inclusion body. (H&E × 100). (d) Immunoperoxidase staining of a section from the periphery of a cerebellar lesion demonstrating positive immunostaining (arrows) of several endothelial cell nuclei with antibodies specific for CMV antigen. From the cerebellar lesion in Figure 4.3. (DAB with slight haematoxylin counterstaining × 400).

The pathology of CMV radiculomyelitis usually consists of inflammation and necrosis, with typical cytomegalic inclusion cells in the lumbosacral roots (especially the ventral roots) and motor neurons, conus medullaris and cauda equina (Behar *et al.*, 1987; Mahieux *et al.*, 1989). CMV inclusion bodies may be found in both endothelial and endoneurial cells in the roots. Focal areas of vasculitis in the nerve roots are also seen (Eidelberg *et al.*, 1986). CMV infection can simultaneously affect nerve roots and peripheral nerves (Grafe and Wiley, 1989).

The pathology of CMV neuropathy consists of multifocal inflammatory infiltrates (mostly with mononuclear cells and neutrophils) in the nerves, with associated necrosis. Cells with cytomegalic inclusions are seen (Said *et al.*, 1991). Cases with disproportionate loss of myelin relative to axonal dropout have been described (Morgello and Simpson 1994). Schwann cells have also been shown to be infected with CMV (Grafe and Wiley, 1989).

This broad spectrum of observed disease is likely related to the immuno-suppression in AIDS allowing relatively greater replication of CMV and therefore a broader range of viral load. Different viral loads may induce qualitatively different pathologies. In animal models, lower viral loads led to microglial nodules and cells with inclusions, while higher viral loads led to perivascular infiltrates and necrosis (Booss *et al.*, 1989). Another explanation for the unique pathological manifestations of CMV encephalitis in AIDS could stem from increased CMV load due to synergistic interactions between CMV and HIV. Coinfection of cell lines with HIV and CMV can enhance the replication of both viruses (Skolnik *et al.*, 1988; Ho *et al.*, 1990). Both HIV and CMV may infect the brain simultaneously (Nelson *et al.*, 1988) and brain cells have been found coinfected *in vivo* (Nelson *et al.*, 1988). This is not unprecedented. A possible transactivation of a papovavirus promoter by HIV proteins has been suggested in cases with a combination of enhanced progressive multifocal leukoencephalopathy (PML) and HIV infection (Tada *et al.*, 1990; Vazeux *et al.*, 1990).

Pathogenetic model of the disease

We propose the following heuristic model of CMV infection in the central nervous system. From our discussion above, the following concepts emerge.

There are three basic pathological forms of nervous system involvement in CMV disease, each of which has a hierarchy of severity of pathology:

1   Diffuse multifocal CMV encephalitis (DMCE)
    a. isolated inclusion-bearing cells
    b. microglial nodule encephalitis
    c. focal parenchymal necrosis
2   CMV ventriculoencephalitis (CVE)
    a. ependymitis
    b. ependymitis and subependymitis
    c. CVE with necrotizing periventricular lesions

3   CMV radiculomyelitis (CRM)
    a. CMV polyradiculitis
    b. necrotizing radiculomyelitis

CMV encephalitis can present in different degrees of severity with a spectrum of clinical, pathological, virological and radiological manifestations associated with each one of the forms. Morgello *et al.* (1987) suggested five distinct entities, as mentioned above. However, it seems to us that some of the pathological entities are part of the spectrum of the same process. For example, the mildest form of multifocal encephalitis is that of isolated inclusion-bearing cells. In the microglial nodule form, there are usually inclusion-bearing cells in addition to the scattered microglial nodules. Focal parenchymal necrosis is the most advanced form of this spectrum since it usually contains microglial nodules and inclusion-bearing cells in addition to areas of necrosis. DMCE is different from CVE and CRM because these can be seen in isolated forms although occasionally more than one form is seen in one patient.

In normal individuals and in non-AIDS immunosuppressed patients usually only DMCE is seen, mostly in its non-necrotizing forms. The last two (CVE and CRM), in addition to DMCE, are usually associated with the AIDS population. The reason for that is not entirely clear, but as previously discussed, it may be related to viral load.

The severity of CSF abnormalities can be roughly correlated with the pathological picture. Microglial nodule encephalitis usually presents with normal or slightly abnormal CSF. Pleocytosis, increased protein and decreased glucose are usually correlated with diffuse multifocal necrotizing lesions or with CVE and CRM. It would be interesting to correlate viral quantity with type of disease process.

We speculate that the precise distribution of CMV CNS infection depends on the mode of entry of the virus into the brain and that the degree of disease depends on viral dose. It is known from the literature on guinea pig models that infection with a low viral dose of CMV results in inclusion-bearing cells and microglial nodule encephalitis, while infection with a high viral dose results in more exuberant inflammation and necrosis (Booss *et al.*, 1989; Booss and Kim, 1989). There are two possible modes of entry into the brain. One is through the choroid plexus, when CMV choroid plexitis allows virus to diffuse through the CSF. The other is by passage through the blood–brain barrier, either through infection of endothelial cells or by passage of infected, activated lymphocytes or monocytes through the endothelium or through other, as yet poorly understood, means (Petito and Cash, 1992). There is no evidence that CMV can reach the CNS by transneuronal and interneuronal propagation, so that this mode of entry which is commonly used by rabies and HSV, probably does not apply to CMV encephalitis. We suggest that the choroid plexus mode of entry results in periventricular disease. The haematogeneous-endothelial mode of entry is postulated to lead to diffuse disease. A low trans-choroid plexus viral dose will result in a mild ependymitis, while a large dose causes necrotizing periventricular lesions. A small trans-blood–brain barrier (BBB) viral dose will cause scattered inclusion-bearing cells and some microglial nodules, while a large trans-BBB viral dose will result in focal parenchymal necrosis, microglial nodules and inclusion-bearing cells. In addition, infection of endothelial cells by CMV may lead to vascular thrombosis and parenchymal necrosis and infarction which may be a factor in the pathogenesis of the focal necrotizing forms of the disease (Wiley and Nelson, 1988). Similar mechanisms have been documented in CNS disease in mice caused by a murine leukemia virus (Park *et al.*, 1993, 1994).

Therapy

Presently available antiviral therapy clinically effective against CMV consists of three drugs: ganciclovir, foscarnet and cidofovir. Two non-immunocompromised CMVE patients had an apparent response to vidarabine. (Phillips *et al.*, 1977)

Ganciclovir, a nucleoside analogue, is active against many members of the herpesvirus family in addition to CMV and has good CSF penetration (Fletcher *et al.*, 1986). Ganciclovir is toxic to bone marrow, and causes significant neutropenia in one-third of patients receiving it for CMV retinitis (Jabs *et al.*, 1989). The clinical response of CMV encephalitis to ganciclovir is not impressive (Price *et al.*, 1992; Arribas *et al.*, 1996) and several cases of CMV encephalitis developing during maintenance ganciclovir treatment of CMV retinitis have been described (Berman and Kim, 1994).

Foscarnet is an analogue of inorganic pyrophosphate which, at therapeutic concentrations, binds to the pyrophosphate-binding site on viral DNA polymerases and reverse transcriptase, but not cellular DNA polymerases. It inhibits replication not only of all known herpesviruses, but HIV as well (Chrisp and Clissold, 1991). Foscarnet has good CSF penetration, being found in concentrations of about 25% of those found in serum (Raffi *et al.*, 1993). The CSF concentration was found to be higher when the meninges were inflamed in one study (Raffi *et al.*, 1993), but not in another (Hengge *et al.*, 1993). The main toxicity is renal and significant in one-half of treated patients (Chrisp and Clissold, 1991).We discuss separately (see below) the issues of pharmacokinetics and viral sensitivity to these agents.

Both ganciclovir and foscarnet have efficacy in treating CMV retinitis, a complication of AIDS. In one two-armed study of AIDS patients with CMV retinitis, foscarnet and ganciclovir were compared according to the time to progression of the CMV retinitis and time to death. The drugs had equal efficacy in increasing time to progression, but survival was significantly better in the foscarnet group and led to suspension of the trial 19 months after it began. The median survivals were 8.5 months in the ganciclovir group and 12.6 months in the foscarnet group. The reason for the improved survival is not clear, but may be because of foscarnet's greater anti-CMV efficacy or because of the anti-HIV activity of foscarnet (Studies of Ocular Complications of AIDS Research Group 1992; Dieterich *et al.*, 1993).

Combination therapy with ganciclovir and foscarnet may have greater efficacy since the drugs have synergistic antiviral effects *in vitro* (Freitas *et al.*, 1989; Manischewitz *et al.*, 1990; Enting *et al.*, 1992). In an open label study, AIDS patients with systemic CMV disease (retinitis, colitis, oesophagitis) who had progressed on both monotherapies were put on a combination of ganciclovir and foscarnet. Out of a total of 10 patients, nine had an objective response, and all patients tolerated the combination acutely (Dieterich *et al.*, 1993). In a phase I trial of ganciclovir and foscarnet given either concurrently or on alternate days to patients with CMV retinitis who had just completed a 14 day induction course of ganciclovir, those on concurrent therapy had more toxicity than the others, but less than those in previous studies (Jacobson *et al.*, 1994). Survival and median time to progression were not statistically significantly different in the two arms of the study, although these were not primary outcome variables. The doses of the drugs in this study were less than those usually given for maintenance.

Cidofovir is a new anti-CMV drug which is licensed for use in cytomegalovirus retinitis (Polis *et al.*, 1995). It is highly nephrotoxic (Fletcher *et al.*, 1986) and can cause ocular hypotony. There is one report of its successful use in AIDS-associated CMVE with both clinical improvement and reversion of CSF to CMV negative by PCR (Sadler *et al.*, 1997). Etoposide, an inhibitor of topoisomerase II, irreversibly inhibits replication of human CMV (which induces host topoisomerase II and appears to require the activity of this enzyme for replication) in tissue culture (Huang *et al.*, 1992). The drug is used in cancer chemotherapy, but there have been no trials in AIDS patients with CMV.

The clinical response of CMV encephalitis to antiviral drugs is not known since there has been no study in which patients with CMVE were treated and followed in a systematic and organized way. Anecdotal experience suggests that it is not dramatic. A survey of cases reported in the literature shows that the median survival of those treated compared with those not treated was not much different (Tucker *et al.*, 1985; Vital *et al.*, 1985; Belec *et al.*, 1990; Kalayjian *et al.*, 1993; Fiala *et al.*, 1993; Singh *et al.*, 1993), although there are individual cases of dramatic response to therapy.

Therapy of AIDS-associated CMV neuropathy and radiculopathy appears to be more efficacious, with some response (which can take months) to therapy with ganciclovir and foscarnet, although failure of therapy has also been described (Cohen *et al.*, 1993; Kim and Hollander, 1993). Painful peripheral neuropathy due to CMV appears to be much more responsive to anti-CMV drugs with 14 out of 15 patients showing 'marked improvement' in one series (Roullet *et al.*, 1994).

Pharmacokinetics and anti-viral activity

Two important considerations in the use of these medications are the degree of CNS penetration of the drugs, and the antiviral activity of the levels typically reached in the CNS.

The published data are meagre. Only one study examined CSF levels of ganciclovir (Huang *et al.*, 1992) and four studies examined CSF levels of foscarnet (Sjovall *et al.*, 1989; Raffi *et al.*, 1993; van den Berg *et al.*, 1992; Hengge *et al.*, 1993). The level of drug necessary for suppression of viral replication varies widely, depending upon CMV strain and what cell lines were used to study the drug. In most such studies, the determination is made of the drug concentration necessary to decrease plaque titre by 50%, the 50% inhibitory concentration (IC50). CSF levels of foscarnet roughly overlap the IC50s of various established viral strains as well as CMV clinical isolates (Smee et al., 1983; Mar et al., 1983; Rasmussen et al., 1984; Freitas et al., 1985, Plotkin et al., 1985, Andrei et al., 1991, Wahren and Oberg, 1980; Eriksson et al., 1982). However, ganciclovir may not reach CSF levels (based on five samples) adequate to suppress most strains of CMV at the doses used (Wiley and Nelson, 1988). For foscarnet, on the other hand, it appears that drug levels readily achievable in the CSF tend to be considerably higher than IC50, and one might therefore expect foscarnet to be quite effective. This is based on 31 CSF samples (Raffi et al., 1993; van den Berg et al., 1992; Hengge et al., 1993).

Furthermore, it is difficult to determine the sensitivity of the virus to the antiviral drugs since isolation of virus from CSF is uncommon, so that measurement of IC50 by plaque reduction assays cannot be done.

Practical therapeutic points

Since there are no systematic data on the treatment of CMV encephalitis and radiculomyelitis in the AIDS patient, treatment of neurological CMV disease most reasonably follows that of CMV retinitis, in which an initial induction phase is followed by a lifelong maintenance phase, given the high risk of relapse (Whitley et al., 1998). The induction phase dosing consists of ganciclovir 5 mg/kg every 12 h intravenously for 14–21 days to be followed by ganciclovir 5 mg/kg/day. The dose of foscarnet is 90 mg/kg every 12 h, for 2 or 3 weeks, to be followed by 90 mg/kg/day intravenously. Cidofovir, with which there has been even less experience, is started at a dose of 5 mg/kg intravenously once a week for 2 weeks, to be followed by 5 mg/kg once every 2 weeks thereafter. Many neurologists experienced in the care of such patients would use ganciclovir and foscarnet in combination. Bone marrow and renal function must particularly be monitored when these drugs are used. For cidofovir, because of the potential adverse effects of ocular hypotony and uveitis, tonometry and slit lamp monitoring are mandatory.

In the immunocompetent patient, there are even fewer data to guide therapy but a single drug is probably sufficient. A maintenance phase is not necessary, since clear relapses of CMV encephalitis have not been described in the immunocompetent host.

For the transplant patient, the expected benefit from a two drug combination must be balanced against the toxicity of ganciclovir (bone marrow) and foscarnet (nephrotoxicity). Given the lack of data on the natural history of CMV encephalitis in transplant patients, therapy must be individualized.

Prognosis

Prognosis of CMV encephalitis in non-immunocompromised hosts is difficult to state, given the paucity of well-characterized cases. Several patients recovered with no or minimal residual deficits several weeks to months after the acute illness (Perham *et al.*, 1971; Chin *et al.*, 1973; Back *et al.*, 1977). Recovery to normal can take 2 years (Duchowny *et al.*, 1979). Two patients treated with vidarabine returned to work within a few weeks (Phillips *et al.*, 1977). Another patient had permanent residual right hemiparesis, aphasia and seizures, which prevented an independent existence (Siegman-Igra *et al.*, 1984). Death from CMVE has been reported (Dorfman, 1973) but this appears to be uncommon.

A review of the published literature suggests that the prognosis of AIDS patients with CMVE is grim. The median survival time is about 49 days (Tucker *et al.*, 1985; Vital *et al.*, 1985; Belec *et al.*, 1990; Fiala *et al.*, 1993; Singh *et al.*, 1993; Kalayjian *et al.*, 1993; Cohen, 1996). A similar figure was arrived at in a short case-control study (Holland *et al.*, 1994). The prognosis for AIDS patients with any kind of CMV infection is very poor, but appears to be better for patients who do not have CNS involvement. In studies of AIDS patients with CMV infection (of all types), the median survival time is between 4 and 9 months (Harb *et al.*, 1991; Gallant *et al.*, 1992). The figure we have derived of 1.5 months is suggestive of a worse prognosis of CMVE in AIDS patients than other types of CMV infection. However, a proper natural history study of CMV encephalitis has not been done, and at least one AIDS patient with CMV encephalitis appears to have improved spontaneously (Edwards *et al.*, 1985).

Conclusion

Cytomegalovirus infection is nearly universal among AIDS patients. Systemic CMV is an important cause of death in AIDS patients. CMV encephalitis is likely to become clinically significant as it becomes more common, with increasing survival. It is clear that CMV encephalitis has a broad clinical spectrum, which has not been adequately characterized, because of the absence of a standard diagnostic tool. In the classical case of progressive dementia, cranial nerve palsies, a CSF with neutrophilic pleocytosis and hypoglycorrhachia, and ependymal enhancement on MRI, the diagnosis is not difficult. Most cases are not so distinctive. It is clear from the above that PCR is the best test we have for CMVE, although there may be subtleties in its interpretation.

Systemic and retinal CMV infections are known to respond very well to ganciclovir and foscarnet either alone or in combination, at least initially (Whitley *et al.*, 1998). The clinical response of AIDS-associated CMV encephalitis to antiviral drugs appears to be poor, however (Arribas *et al.*, 1996). The response of peripheral nerve infection with CMV appears to be better.

Acknowledgements

This work was supported in part by PHS Grant Numbers PO1-NS32228-01 (ACT), T32-NS-01780 (ACT), P01-NS27405-06 (EL). Some of the work described herein arose from clinical questions encountered while one of the authors (ACT) was at the University of Pennsylvania AIDS Clinical Trials Unit.

References

Achim, C. L., Nagra, R. M., Wang, R., Nelson, J. A. and Wiley, C. A. (1994) Detection of cytomegalovirus in cerebrospinal fluid autopsy specimens from AIDS patients. *J. Infect. Dis.*, **169**, 623–627.

Andrei, G., Snoeck, R., Schols, D. *et al.* (1991). Comparative activity of selected antiviral compounds against clinical isolates of HCMV. *Eur. J. Clin. Microbiol. Infect. Dis.*, **10**, 1026–1033.

Applebaum, F. R., Meyers, J. D., Fefer, A. *et al.* (1982). Nonbacterial nonfungal pneumonia following bone marrow transplantation in 100 identical twins. *Transplantation*, **33**, 265–268.

Arribas, J., Clifford, D. B., Fichtenbaum, C. J. *et al.* (1995) Level of cytomegalovirus (CMV) DNA in cerebrospinal fluid of subjects with AIDS and CMV infection of the central nervous system. *J. Infect. Dis.*, **172**, 527–531.

Arribas, J., Storch, G. A., Clifford, D. B. and Tselis, A. C. (1996). Cytomegalovirus encephalitis. *Ann. Intern. Med.*, **125**, 577–587.

Back, E., Hoglund, C. and Malmlund, H. O. (1977). Cytomegalovirus infection associated with severe encephalitis. *Scand. J. Infect. Dis.*, **9**, 141–143.

Bazan, C., Jackson, C., Jinkins, J. R. and Barohn, R. J. (1991). Gadolinium enhanced MRI in a case of cytomegalovirus polyradiculopathy. *Neurology*, **41**, 1522–1523.

Behar, R., Wiley, C. A. and McCutchan, J. A. (1987). Cytomegalovirus polyradiculo-pathy in acquired immune deficiency syndrome. *Neurology*, **37**, 557–561.

Belec, L., Gray, F., Mikol, J. *et al.* (1990). CMV encephalomyeloradiculitis and HIV encephalitis: presence of HIV and CMV coinfected multinucleated giant cells. *Acta Neuropathol.*, **81**, 99–104.

Berman, S. M. and Kim, R. C. (1994). The development of cytomegalovirus encephalitis in AIDS patients receiving ganciclovir. *Am. J. Med.*, **96**, 415–419.

Booss, J., Winkler, S. R., Griffith, B. P. and Kim, J. H. (1989). Viremia and glial nodule encephalitis after experimental systemic cytomegalovirus infection. *Lab. Invest.*, **61**, 644–649.

Booss, J. and Kim, J. H. (1989). Cytomegalovirus encephalitis: neuropathological comparison of the guinea pig model with the opportunistic infection in AIDS. *Yale J. Biol. Med.*, **62**, 187–195.

Buckley, R. (1986) Humoral Immunodeficiency. *Clin. Immunol. Immunopathol.*, **40**, 13–24.

Cheeseman, S. H. (1992). Cytomegalovirus infection. In: *Infectious Diseases* (S. L. Gorbach, J. G. Bartlett, and N. R. Blacklow, eds). Philadelphia: WB Saunders, pp. 1359–1365.

Chin, W., Magoffin, R., Frierson, J. G. and Lennette, E. H. (1973). Cytomegalovirus infection: a case with meningoencephalitis. *J. Am. Med. Assoc.*, **225**, 740–741.

Chrisp, P. and Clissold, S. P. (1991), Foscarnet: a review of its antiviral activity, pharmacokinetic properties and therapeutic use in immunocompromised patients with cytomegalovirus retinitis. *Drugs*, **41**, 104–129.

Cinque, P., Vago, L., Brytting, M. *et al.* (1992). Cytomegalovirus infection of the CNS in patients with AIDS: diagnosis by DNA amplification from CSF. *J. Infect. Dis.*, **166**, 1408–1411.

Clifford, D. B., Buller, J. E., Mohammed, R. K. *et al.* (1993). Use of polymerase chain reaction to demonstrate cytomegalovirus DNA in CSF of patients with human immunodeficiency virus infection. *Neurology*, **43**, 75–79.

Cohen, B. A. (1996). Prognosis and response to therapy of cytomegalovirus encephalitis and meningomyelitis in AIDS. *Neurology*, **46**, 444–450.

Cohen, B. A., McArthur, J. C., Grohman, S., Patterson, B. and Glass, J. D. (1993). Neurologic prognosis of cytomegalovirus polyradiculomyelopathy in AIDS. *Neurology*, **43**, 493–499.

deGans, J., Tiessens, G., Portegies, P., Tutuarima, H. A. and Troost, D. (1990). Predominance of polymorphonuclear leukocytes in cerebrospinal fluid of AIDS patients with cytomegalovirus polyradiculomyelitis. *J. AIDS*, **3**, 1155–1158.

Dieterich, D. T., Poles, M. A., Low, E. A. *et al.* (1993). Concurrent use of ganciclovir and foscarnet to treat cytomegalovirus infection in AIDS patients. *J. Infect. Dis.*, **167**, 1184–1188.

Dorfman, L. J. (1973). Cytomegalovirus encephalitis in adults. *Neurology* 23, 136–144.

Drew, W. L., Mintz, L., Miner, R. C., *et al.* (1981). Prevalence of cytomegalovirus in homosexual men. *J. Infect. Dis.*, **143**, 188–192.

Duchowny, M., Caplan, L. and Siber, G. (1979). Cytomegalovirus infection of the adult nervous system. *Ann. Neurol.*, **5**, 458–461.

Edwards, R. H., Messing, R. and McKendall, R. R. (1985). Cytomegalovirus meningoencephalitis in a homosexual man with Kaposi's sarcoma: Isolation of CMV from CSF cells. *Neurology*, **35**, 560–562.

Eidelberg, D., Sotrel, A., Vogel, H. *et al.* (1986). Progressive polyradiculopathy in acquired immune deficiency syndrome. *Neurology*, **36**, 912–916.

Emanuel, D., Cunningham, I., Jules-Elyse, K. *et al.* (1988). Cytomegalovirus pneumonia after bone marrow transplant successfully treated with the combination of ganciclovir and high dose intravenous immune globulin. *Ann. Int. Med.*, **109**, 777–782.

Emanuel, D. J. (1991). Uses of immunotherapy for control of human cytomegalovirus-associated diseases. *Transplant. Proc.*, **23**, 144–146.

Enting, R., de Gans, J., Reiss, P. *et al.* (1992). Ganciclovir/foscarnet for cytomegalovirus meningoencephalitis in AIDS. *Lancet*, **340**, 559–560.

Eriksson, B., Oberg, B. and Wahren, B. (1982). Pyrophosphate analogues as inhibitors of DNA polymerases of cytomegalovirus, herpes simplex virus and cellular origin. *Biochim. Biophys. Acta*, **696**, 115–123.

Fiala, M., Singer, E. J., Graves, M. C. *et al.* (1993). AIDS-dementia complex complicated by cytomegalovirus encephalopathy. *J. Neurol.*, **240**, 223–231.

Fillet, A. M., Katlama, C., Visse, B. *et al.* (1993). Human CMV infection of the CNS; concordance between PCR detection in the CSF and pathological examination. *AIDS*, **7**, 1016–1018.

Fletcher, C., Sawchuck, R., Chinnock, B. *et al.* (1986). Human pharmacokinetics of the antiviral drug DHPG. *Clin. Pharmacol Ther.*, **40**, 281–286.

Frank, I. and Friedman, H. M. (1988). Progress in the treatment of cytomegalovirus pneumonia. *Ann. Int. Med.*, **109**, 769–771.

Freitas, V. R., Smee, D. R., Chernow, M. *et al.* (1985). Activity of 9-(1,3-dihydroxy-2-propoxymethyl) guanine compared with that of acyclovir against human, monkey and rodent cytomegalovirus. *Antimicrob. Agents Chemother.*, **28**, 240–245.

Freitas, V. R., Fraser-Smith, E. and Matthews, T. R. (1989). Increased efficacy of ganciclovir in combination with foscarnet against cytomegalovirus and herpes simplex virus type 2 in vitro and in vivo. *Antiviral Res.*, **12**, 205–212.

Fuller, G. N., Guilloff, R. J., Scaravilli, F. and Harcourt-Webster, J. N. (1989). Combined HIV–CMV encephalitis presenting with brainstem signs. *J. Neurol. Neurosurg. Psych.*, **52**, 975–979.

Gallant, J. E., Moore, R. D., Richman, D. D. *et al.* (1992). Incidence and natural history of cytomegalovirus disease in patients with advanced HIV disease treated with zidovudine. *J. Infect. Dis.*, **166**, 1223–1227.

Gozlan, J., Salord, J.-M., Roullet, E. *et al.* (1992). Rapid detection of CMV DNA in CSF of AIDS patients with neurologic disorders. *J. Infect. Dis.*, **166**, 1416–1421.

Grafe, M. R. and Wiley, C. A. (1989). Spinal cord and peripheral nerve pathology in AIDS: the roles of cytomegalovirus and human immunodeficiency virus. *Ann. Neurol.*, **25**, 561–566.

Grassi, M. P., Clerici, F., Perin, C. *et al.* (1998). Microglial nodular encephalitis and ventriculoencephalitis in patients with AIDS: two distinct clinical patterns. *Clin. Infect. Dis.*, **27**, 504–508.

Grundy, J. E., Shanley, J. D. and Griffiths, P. D. (1987). Is cytomegalovirus pneumonitis in transplant patients an immunopathological condition? *Lancet*, **2**, 996–998.

Harb, G, E,, Bacchetti, P. and Jacobson, M. (1991). Survival of patients with AIDS and cytomegalovirus disease treated with ganciclovir or foscarnet. *AIDS*, **5**, 959–965.

Hawley, D. A., Schaeffer, J. F., Schalz, D. M. and Muller, J. (1983). Cytomegalovirus encephalitis in acquired immunodeficiency syndrome. *Am. J. Clin. Pathol.*, **80**, 874–877.

Hengge, U. R., Brockmeyer, N. H., Malessa, R. *et al.* Foscarnet penetrates the blood–brain barrier: rationale for therapy of cytomegalovirus encephalitis. *Antimicrob. Agents Chemother.*, **37**, 1010–1014.

Hirsch, M. S. (1991). Cytomegalovirus and its role in the pathogenesis of acquired immune deficiency syndrome. *Transplant. Proc.*, **23** (suppl. 3), 118–121.

Ho, M. (1985). Cytomegalovirus. In: *Principles and Practice of Infectious Diseases*, (G. L. Mandell, R. G. Douglas ᴊʀ and J. E. Bennett, eds). New York: J Wiley, pp. 960–970.

Ho, M. (1993). Cytomegalovirus infection after solid organ transplantation. In: *Molecular Aspects of Human Cytomegalovirus Diseases*. (Y. Becker, G. Darau and E.-S. Huang, eds). New York: Springer-Verlag.

Ho, M., Suwansirikul, S., Dowling, J. N., Youngblood, L. A. and Armstrong, J. A. (1975). The transplanted kidney as a source of cytomegalovirus infection. *N. Engl. J. Med.*, **293**, 1109–1112.

Ho, W.-Z., Harouse, J. M., Rando, R. F. *et al.* (1990). Reciprocal enhancement of gene expression and viral replication between human cytomegalovirus and human immunodeficiency virus-1. *J. Gen. Virol.*, **71**, 97–103.

Holland, N. R., Power, C., Mathews, V. P. *et al.* (1994). CMV encephalitis in acquired immunodeficiency syndrome. *Neurology*, **44**, 507–514.

Hotson, J. and Pedley, T. (1976). The neurological complications of cardiac transplantation. *Brain*, **99**, 673–694.

Huang, E.-S., Benson, J. D., Huong, S.-M., Wilson, B. and van der Horst, C. (1992). Irreversible inhibition of human cytomegalovirus replication by topoisomerase II inhibitor, etoposide: a new strategy for the treatment of human cytomegalovirus infection. *Antiviral Res.*, **17**, 17–32.

Jabs, D. A., Enger, C. and Bartlett, J. G. (1989). Cytomegalovirus retinitis and acquired immunodeficiency syndrome. *Arch. Ophthalmol.*, **107**, 75–80.

Jacobson, M. A., Kramer, F., Bassiakos, Y. *et al.* (1994). Randomized phase I trial of two different combination foscarnet and ganciclovir maintenance therapy regimens for AIDS patients with cytomegalovirus retinitis: AIDS Clinical Trials Group Protocol 151. *J. Infect. Dis.*, **170**, 189–193.

Jordan, M. C. (1983). Latent infection and the elusive cytomegalovirus. *Rev. Infect. Dis.*, **5**, 205–215.

Kabins, S., Keller, R., Naraqi, S. and Peitchel, R. (1976). Viral ascending radiculomyelitis with severe hypoglycorrhachia. *Arch. Intern. Med.*, **136**, 933–935.

Kalayjian, R. C., Cohen, M. L., Bonomo, R. A. and Flanigan, T. P. (1993) Cytomegalovirus ventriculoencephalitis in AIDS: a syndrome with distinct clinical and pathological features. *Medicine*, **72**, 67–77.

Kanzaki, A., Yabuki, S. and Yuki, N. (1995). Bickerstaff's brainstem encephalitis associated with cytomegalovirus infection. *J. Neurol Neurosurg Psych.*, **58**, 260–261.

Kauffman, C. A., Linnemann, C. C. JR and Alvira, M. M. (1979). Cytomegalovirus encephalitis associated with thymoma and immunoglobulin deficiency. *Amer. J. Med.*, **67**, 724–728.

Kenyon, L. C., Goldberg, H. I., Kolson, D. L., Collman, R. G. and Lavi, E. (1998). Case of the month: May 1998: A patient with HIV infection and multiple cranial neuritis. *Brain Pathol.*, **8**, 815–816.

Kim, Y. S. and Hollander, H. (1993). Polyradiculopathy due to cytomegalovirus: report of two cases in which improvement occurred after prolonged therapy and review of the literature. *Clin. Infect. Dis.*, **17**, 32–37.

Koeppen, A., Lansing, L. S., Peng, S.-K. and Smith, R. S. (1981). Central nervous system vasculitis in cytomegalovirus infection. *J. Neurol. Sci.*, **51**, 395–410.

Kure, K., Llena, J. F., Lyman, W. D. *et al.* (1991). HIV-1 Infection of the nervous system: an autopsy study of 268 adult, pediatric and fetal brains. *Hum. Pathol.*, **22**, 700–710.

Laskin, O. L., Stahl-Bayliss, C. M. and Morgello, S. (1987). Concomitant herpes simplex virus type 1 and cytomegalovirus ventriculoencephalitis in acquired immunodeficiency syndrome. *Arch. Neurol.*, **44**, 843–847.

Lederman, H. M. and Winkelstein, J. A. (1985). X-linked agammaglobulinemia: an analysis of 96 patients. *Medicine*, **64**, 145–156.

Leestma, J. E. (1991). Viral infections of the nervous system. In: *Textbook of Neuropathology* 2nd edn, (R. L. Davis and D. M. Robertson, eds) Baltimore: Williams and Wilkins.

McKinney, R., Katz, S. L. and Wilfert, C. M. (1987). Chronic enteroviral meningoencephalitis in agammaglobulinemic patients. *Rev. Infect. Dis.*, **9**, 334–356.

Mahieux, F., Gray, F., Fenelon, G. *et al.* (1989). Acute myeloradiculitis due to cytomegalovirus as the initial manifestation of AIDS. *J. Neurol. Neurosurg. Psych.*, **52**, 270–274.

Manischewitz, J. F., Quinnan, G. V., Lane, H. C. and Wittek, A. E. (1990). Synergistic effect of ganciclovir and foscarnet on cytomegalovirus replication in vitro. *Antimicrob. Agents Chemother.*, **34**, 373–375.

Mar, E.-C., Cheng, Y.-C. and Huang, E.-S. (1983). Effect of 9-(1,3-dihydroxy-2-propoxymethyl) guanine on human cytomegalovirus replication in vitro. *Antimicrob. Agents Chemother.*, **24**, 518–521.

Masdeu, J. C., Small, C. B., Weiss, L. *et al.* (1988). Multifocal cytomegalovirus encephalitis in AIDS. *Ann. Neurol.*, **23**, 97–99.

Miles, C., Hoffman, W., Lai, C.-W. and Freeman, J. W. (1993). Cytomegalovirus-associated transverse myelitis. *Neurology*, **43**, 2143–2145.

Miller, R. F., Fox, J. D., Thomas, P. *et al.* (1996). Acute lumbosacral polyradiculopathy due to cytomegalovirus in advanced HIV disease: CSF findings in 17 patients. *J. Neurol. Neurosurg. Psych.*, **61**, 456–460.

Morgello, S., Cho, E.-S., Nielsen, S., Devinsky, O. and Petito, C. K. (1987). Cytomegalovirus encephalitis in patients with acquired immunodeficiency syndrome: an autopsy study of 30 cases and a review of the literature. *Hum. Path.*, **18**, 289–297.

Morgello, S. and Simpson, D. M. (1994). Multifocal cytomegalovirus demyelinative polyneuropathy associated with AIDS. *Muscle and Nerve*, **17**, 176–182.

Moskowitz, L. B., Gregorios, J. B., Hensley, G. T. and Berger, J. B. (1984). Cytomegalovirus-induced demyelination associated with acquired immunodeficiency syndrome. *Arch. Pathol. Lab. Med.*, **108**, 873–877.

Navia, B. A., Cho, E.-S., Petito, C. K. and Price, R. W. (1986). The AIDS dementia complex: II. Neuropathology. *Ann. Neurol.*, **19**, 525–535.

Nelson, J. A., Reynolds-Kohlewr, C., Oldstone, M. B. A. and Wiley, C. A. (1988). HIV and CMV coinfect brain cells in patients with AIDS. *Virology*, **165**, 286–290.

Nielsen, S. L., Petito, C. K., Urmacher, C. D. and Posner, J. B. (1984). Subacute encephalitis in acquired immune deficiency syndrome: a postmortem study. *Amer. J. Clin. Pathol.*, **82**, 678–682.

Palella, F. J., Delaney, K. M., Moorman, A. C. *et al.* (1988). Declining morbidity and mortality among patients with advanced human immunodeficiency virus infection. *N. Engl. J. Med.*, **338**, 853–860.

Park, B. H., Lavi, E., Blank, K. J. and Gaulton, G. N. (1993) Intracerebral hemorrhages and syncytia formation induced by endothelial cell infection with a murine leukemia virus. *J. Virol.*, **67**, 6015–6024.

Park, B. H., Lavi, E., Stieber, A. and Gaulton, G. N. (1994). Pathogenesis of cerebral infarction and hemorrhage caused by a murine leukemia virus. *Lab. Invest.*, **70**, 78–85.

Perham, T. G. M., Caul, E. O., Clarke, S. K. R. and Gibson, A. G. F. (1971). Cytomegalovirus meningoencephalitis. *Brit. Med. J.*, **2**, 50.

Peters, B. S., Beck, E. J., Coleman, D. G. *et al.* (1991). Changing disease patterns in patients with AIDS in a referral centre in the United Kingdom: the changing face of AIDS. *Brit. Med. J.*, **302**, 203–207.

Petito, C. K. and Cash, K. S. (1992). Blood-brain barrier abnormalities in the acquired immune deficiency syndrome: immunohistochemical localization of serum proteins in postmortem brain. *Neurology*, **32**, 658–666.

Philips, C. A., Fanning, L., Gump, D. W. and Phillips, C. F. (1977). Cytomegalovirus encephalitis in immunologically normal adults: successful treatment with vidarabine. *J. Am. Med. Assoc.*, **238**, 2299–2300.

Plotkin, S. A., Drew, W. L., Felsenstein, D. and Hirsch, M. (1985). Sensitivity of clinical isolates of human cytomegalovirus to 9-(1,3-dihydroxy-2-propoxymethyl) guanine. *J. Infect. Dis.*, **152**, 833–834.

Polis, M., Spooner, K. M., Baird, B. F. *et al.* (1995). Anticytomegaloviral activity and safety of cidofovir in patients with human immunodeficiency virus infection and cytomegalovirus viruria. *Antimicrob. Agents Chemother.*, **39**, 882–886.

Post, M. J. D., Hensley, G. T., Moskowitz, L. B. and Fischl, M. (1986). Cytomegalic inclusion virus encephalitis in patients with AIDS: CT, clinical and pathologic correlation. *Am. J. Neuroradiol.*, **7**, 275–280.

Price, T. A., Digioia, R. A. and Simon, G. L. (1992). Ganciclovir treatment of cytomegalovirus ventriculitis in a patient infected with human immunodeficiency virus. *Clin. Infect. Dis.*, **15**, 606–608.

Raffi, F., Taburet, A.-M., Ghaleh, B. *et al.* (1993). Penetration of foscarnet into cerebrospinal fluid of AIDS patients. *Antimicrob. Agents Chemother.*, **37**, 1777–1780.

Rasmussen, L., Chen, P. T., Mullenax, J. G. and Merigan, T. C. (1984). Inhibition of human cytomegalovirus replication by 9-(1,3-dihydroxy-2-propoxymethyl) guanine alone and in combination with human interferons. *Antimicrob. Agents Chemother.*, **26**, 441–445.

Reed, E., Bowden, R. A., Dandliber, P. *et al.* (1988). Treatment of cytomegalovirus pneumonia with ganciclovir and intravenous cytomegalovirus immune globulin in patients with bone marrow transplants. *Ann. Int. Med.*, **109**, 783–788.

Reed, J. B., Schwab, I. R., Gordon, J. and Morse, L. S. (1997). Regression of cytomegalovirus retinitis associated with protease-inhibitor treatment in patients with AIDS. *Amer. J. Ophthalmol.*, **124** 199–203.

Rice, G. P. A., Schrier, R. D. and Oldstone, M. B. A. (1984). Cytomegalovirus infects human lymphocytes and monocytes: Virus expression is restricted to immediate-early gene products. *Proc. Natl Acad. Sci.* (USA), **81**, 6134–6138.

Roifman, C. M., Rao, C. P., Lederman, H. M. *et al.* (1986). Increased susceptibility to mycoplasma infection in patients with hypogammaglobulinemia. *Am. J. Med.*, **80**, 590–594.

Roullet, E., Assuerus, V., Gozlan, J. *et al.* (1994). Cytomegalovirus multifocal neuropathy in AIDS: analysis of 15 consecutive cases. *Neurology*, **44**, 2174–2182.

Sadler, M., Morris-Jones, S., Nelson, M. and Gazzard, B, G. (1997). Successful treatment of cytomegalovirus encephalitis in an AIDS patient using cidofovir. *AIDS*, **11**, 1293–1294.

Said, G., Lacroix, C., Chemouilli, P. *et al.* (1991). Cytomegalovirus neuropathy in acquired immunodeficiency syndrome: a clinical and pathological study. *Ann. Neurol.*, **29**, 139–146.

Schneck, S. A. (1965). Neuropathological features of human organ transplantation. I Probable cytomegalovirus infection. *J. Neuropath. Exp. Neurol.*, **24**, 415–429.

Schober, R. and Herman, M. M. (1973). Neuropathology of cardiac transplantation. Survey of 31 cases. *Lancet*, **1**, 962–967.

Schrier, R. D., Nelson, J. A. and Oldstone, M. B. A. (1989). Detection of human cytomegalovirus in peripheral blood lymphocytes in a natural infection. *Science* **230**, 1048–1051.

Siegman-Igra, Y., Michaeli, D., Doron, A., Weinberg, M. and Heilbrun, Y. (1984). Cytomegalovirus encephalitis in a noncompromised host. *Isr. J. Med. Sci.*, **20**, 163–166.

Singh, N., Anderegg, K. A. and Yu, V. L. (1993). Significance of hypoglycorrhachia in patients with AIDS and CMV encephalitis. *Clin. Infect. Dis.*, **17**, 283–284.

Sjovall, J., Bergdahl, S., Movin, G., *et al.* (1989). Pharmacokinetics of Foscarnet and Distribution to CSF after iv infusion in patients with human immunodeficiency virus infection. *Antimicrob. Agents Chemother.*, **33**, 1023–1031.

Skolnik, P. Bozloff, B. R. and Hirsch, M. S. (1988). Bidirectional interactions between human immunodeficiency virus type 1 and cytomegalovirus. *J. Infect. Dis.*, **157**, 508–514.

Smee, D. F., Martin, J. C., Verheyden, J. P. H. and Matthews, T. R. (1983). Antiherpesvirus activity of the acyclic nucleotide 9-(1,3-dihydroxy-2-propoxy-methyl) guanine. *Antimicrob. Agents Chemother.*, **23**, 676–689.

Smyth, R. L., Higenbottom, T. W., Scott, J. P. and Wallwork, J. (1993) The management of cytomegalovirus infection in heart-lung transplant recipients. In: *Molecular Aspects of Human Cytomegalovirus Diseases*. (Y. Becker, G. Darai, and E.-S. Huang, eds). New York: Springer-Verlag.

Studahl, M., Ricksten, A., Sandburg, T. and Burgstrom, T. (1992). Cytomegalovirus encephalitis in four immunocompetent patients. *Lancet*, **340**, 1045–1046.

Studies of Ocular Complications of AIDS Research Group. (1992). Mortality in patients with the acquired immunodeficiency syndrome treated with either foscarnet or ganciclovir for cytomegalovirus retinitis. *N. Engl. J. Med.*, **326**, 213–220.

Tada, H., Rappaport, J., Lashgari, M., Amini, S., Wong-Staal, F. and Khalili, K. (1990). Transactivation of the JC virus late promoter by the tat protein of type 1 human immunodeficiency virus in glial cells. *Proc. Natl Acad. Sci.*, **87**, 3479–3483.

Talpos, D., Tien, R. D. and Hesselink, J. R. (1991). Magnetic resonance imaging of AIDS-related polyradiculopathy. *Neurology*, **41**, 1996–1997.

Toorkey, C. B. and Carrigan, D. B. (1989). Immunohistochemical detection of an immediate early antigen of human cytomegalovirus in normal tissues. *J. Infect. Dis.*, **160**, 741–751.

Tucker, T., Dix, R. D., Katzen, C., Davis, R. L. and Schmidley, J. W. (1985). CMV and HSV ascending myelitis in a patient with AIDS. *Ann. Neurol.*, **18**, 74–79.

Tyler, K. L., Gross, R. A. and Cascino, G. D. (1986). Unusual viral causes of transverse myelitis: hepatitis A and cytomegalovirus. *Neurology*, **36**, 855–858.

van den Berg, A. P., van Son, W. J., Janssen, R. A. J. *et al.* (1992). Recovery from cytomegalovirus infection is associated with activation of peripheral blood lymphocytes. *J. Infect. Dis.*, **166**, 1228–1235.

Vazeux, R., Cumont, M., Girard, P. M. *et al.* (1990). Severe encephalitis resulting from coinfection with HIV and JC virus. *Neurology*, **40**, 944–948.

Vinters, H. V., Kwok, M. K., Ho, H. W. *et al.* (1989). Cytomegalovirus in the nervous system of the aquired immunodeficiency syndrome patient. *Brain*, **112**, 245–268.

Vital, C., Vital, A., Vignoly, B. *et al.* (1985). CMV encephalitis in a patient with acquired immunodeficiency syndrome. *Arch. Pathol. Lab. Med.*, **109**, 105–106.

Wahren, B. and Oberg, B. (1980). Reversible inhibition of cytomegalovirus replication by phosphonoformate. *Intervirology*, **14**, 7–15.

Waner, J. L., Weller, T. H. and Kevy, S. V. (1973). Patterns of cytomegaloviral complement-fixing antibody activity: a longitudinal study of blood donors. *J. Infect. Dis.*, **127**, 538–543.

Waris, E., Rasanen, O., Kreus, K.-E. and Kreus, R. (1972). Fatal cytomegalovirus disease in a previously healthy adult. *Scand. J. Infect. Dis.*, **4**, 61–67.

Weller, T. H. (1971). The cytomegaloviruses: ubiquitous agents with protean clinical manifestations. *N. Engl. J. Med.*, **285**, 203–214, 267–274.

Whitley, J. R., Jacobson, M. A., Friedberg, D. N. *et al.* (1998). Guidelines for the treatment of cytomegalovirus diseases in patients with AIDS in the era of potent antiretroviral therapy. Recommendations of an international panel. *Arch. Intern. Med.*, **158**, 957–969.

Wildemann, B., Haass, J., Lynen, N., Stingele, K. and Storch-Hagenlocher, B. (1998). Diagnosis of cytomegalovirus encephalitis in patients with AIDS by quantitation of cytomegalovirus genomes in cells of cerebrospinal fluid. *Neurology*, **50**, 693–697.

Wiley, C. A. and Nelson, J. A. (1988). Role of human immunodeficiency virus and cytomegalovirus in AIDS encephalitis. *Am. J. Pathol.*, **133**, 73–81.

Winston, D. J. (1993). Cytomegalovirus infection in bone marrow transplants. In: *Molecular Aspects of Human Cytomegalovirus Diseases*. (Y. Becker, G. Darai and E.-S. Huang, eds) New York: Springer-Verlag.

Wolf, D. G. and Spector, S. A. (1992). Diagnosis of human CMV CNS disease in AIDS patients by DNA amplification from CSF. *J. Infect. Dis.*, **166**, 1412–1415.

5

Herpes simplex virus encephalitis

J. Richard Baringer

Introduction

Herpes simplex virus types 1 and 2 are members of the herpes virus family, a group of DNA-containing viruses that are ubiquitous in nature. The currently recognized members of the virus family are herpes simplex viruses type 1 and type 2, the subject of this discussion; varicella zoster virus, the virus responsible for chicken pox and for zosteriform skin lesions; Epstein-Barr virus, the virus responsible for mononucleosis; cytomegalovirus, a virus which causes severe disease in newborns and in immunosuppressed individuals; and human herpes viruses types 6, 7 and 8. Types 6 and 7 cause roseola infantum. Type 8 has been associated with Kaposi's sarcoma (Hall, 1997). Many of the herpes viruses are known to establish latency within humans and have the capability to cause recurrent disease or to produce disease when the host becomes immunosuppressed. Herpes simplex virus types 1 and 2 and varicella zoster establish latency in sensory ganglion cells in humans. In the case of herpes simplex virus type 1, the ganglion cells may serve as the reservoir for recurrent cutaneous eruptions. These take the form of the commonly recognized cold sore or the less frequent episodes of recurrent herpetic keratitis, presumed related to the latency of this virus in trigeminal ganglia. Latency of herpes simplex virus type 2 is established in human sacral ganglia after a primary genital infection, resulting in recurrent episodes of genital herpes (Baringer, 1974). Varicella zoster virus establishes latency in numerous cranial and spinal sensory ganglia after the initial episode of chicken pox, and it may erupt in a segmental fashion later in life to produce shingles (Mahalingam *et al.*, 1992). Latency of cytomegalovirus is presumed to be the basis for severe nervous system infections in the immunosuppressed. Lymphomas of the brain in AIDS patients can be shown in most cases to harbour Epstein-Barr virus genomes within the tumour tissue. Human herpes virus-6 is the cause of roseola in children and is associated with a large percentage of cases of febrile seizures. There is recent and somewhat controversial information that this virus may be related in some way to multiple sclerosis (Rand *et al.*, 1998).

The ability of herpes simplex viruses types 1 and 2 to travel from a peripheral site of inoculation to the sensory ganglion cells and more centrally into the brain or spinal cord has been recognized since the pioneering work of Goodpasture and Teague (1923). He inoculated herpes simplex virus obtained from the lips of patients with cold sores into the cornea of rabbits. The virus travelled centripetally within nerves to infect the sensory ganglion cells and then proceeded more centrally into the associated areas of the brainstem. Many subsequent studies have shown that herpes simplex viruses types 1 and 2 produce an encephalitic process in experimental animals involving the central nervous system after inoculation at the periphery.

Pathophysiology of herpes simplex virus encephalitis in humans

Since the 1940s, herpes simplex viruses (HSV) types 1 and 2 have been implicated in the causation of acute necrotizing encephalitis in infants, children and adults. Early work by Nahmias and Dowdle (1968) distinguished the two antigenically distinctive variants of HSV and called attention to the fact that the type 1 virus is commonly associated with recurrent cold sores or with ocular infection or cutaneous infections above the waist, while the type 2 virus is commonly associated with recurrent genital infections. The two viruses differ not only antigenically but in their DNA composition and in their cytopathic effect in tissue culture.

Both HSV 1 and 2 have the capability to establish latent infections in sensory ganglia after inoculation at the periphery. The latency of HSV in sensory ganglion cells was initially demonstrated by Stevens and Cook (1971). Using *in situ* hybridization, he demonstrated viral DNA and RNA transcripts in latently infected ganglia. Subsequent investigations utilizing the polymerase chain reaction (PCR) technique have demonstrated that HSV DNA sequences can be readily amplified from ganglia that are latently infected. HSV also can establish a latent state in the central nervous system of animals inoculated at the periphery (Cabrera *et al.*, 1980; Rock and Fraser, 1983).

The mechanism by which recurrent HSV eruptions are induced at the periphery (e.g. recurrent lip herpes or recurrent genital herpes) remains unknown. Recurrent episodes of lip herpes may be provoked by fever, exposure to sunlight, or menstruation. The factors that may provoke recurrent genital herpes to activation are less well known. Neurosurgeons have observed that when the trigeminal sensory root is manipulated, herpetic eruptions occur in the mouth and/or on the face in a very large proportion of individuals, suggesting that mechanical trauma can provoke recurrent herpes lesions (Carton and Kilbourne, 1952). This has been confirmed in animal studies. The precise mechanisms for this remain obscure.

Studies in humans have shown that HSV 1 genomes are present in trigeminal sensory ganglia of humans in 85–90% of unselected individuals coming to autopsy (Baringer and Swoveland, 1973). The data for the prevalence of HSV type 2 infections in sacral ganglia are less secure, but it is probable that these are present in 10–15% of an unselected population (Baringer, 1974).

With respect to the latency of HSV in the central nervous system of humans, autopsy studies using PCR have suggested the presence of HSV genomes in the central nervous system of patients without known neurological disease (Baringer and Pisani, 1994). The greatest frequency of isolates are from the medulla, pons and olfactory bulb, although HSV genomes can be demonstrated in other areas of the brain with lesser frequency. The relationship of HSV genomic material in human brain to disease processes is problematical. It has been conjectured by some that HSV might be responsible for diseases such as multiple sclerosis (MS). The rationale for such a suggestion involves the fact that HSV type 1 is, in all likelihood, acquired at an early age, it is known to be latent for decades, certainly within human sensory ganglia and perhaps within brain, and the virus has a tendency to cause recurrent disease in the form of recurrent cold sores, ophthalmic infections, or genital lesions. Similar cases have been made for Epstein-Barr virus (Rand *et al.*, 1998) and human herpes virus-6 (Challoner *et al.*, 1995; Mayne *et al.*, 1998). These phenomena fit with current concepts that MS may result from an infection in childhood with disease production some years later and the known tendency of the disease to become recurrent. However, the evidence for the association with MS is not convincing at the moment, and further work is clearly needed to explore this possibility.

The relationship of latent herpes simplex virus to herpes simplex virus encephalitis is also not well understood. Encephalitis due to HSV 2 in newborn infants is a widespread disease in the brain and commonly involves a variety of other organs in the body including the skin, eyes, and lungs. In contrast, HSV 1 infection in children and adults is a much more circumscribed form of encephalitis with a characteristic localization that is limited to the inferior portion of the frontal lobes, the medial temporal and subjacent insular structures and the cingulate gyrus, sparing the parietal and occipital lobes, and the cerebellum. There is frequent involvement of the olfactory bulbs and tracts where that has been investigated (Twomey *et al.*, 1979). This characteristic localization in children and adults suggests a close association with the limbic structures in brain. This has led to the conjecture that the encephalitic process may be the result of infection in the olfactory mucosa which might then spread through the olfactory system resulting in the typical distribution of lesions. Whether this is related to the latency of virus in the olfactory system or an acute exogenous infection is uncertain. Studies by Whitley and associates comparing the DNA obtained from the brain and from the cold sores on the lip in patients with herpes simplex virus encephalitis demonstrated identity of the two isolates in about 50% of the cases but non-identity in the remainder (Whitley *et al.*, 1982a).

An alternative suggestion has been put forth by Davis and Johnson (1979) that herpes simplex virus might spread from trigeminal ganglia into the subjacent medial temporal and frontal cortex along the nerves innervating the dura; however, this hypothesis has not received confirmation.

While HSV 1 can readily be cultured from the brain of patients with herpes simplex virus encephalitis, it can be cultured from the cerebrospinal fluid only on rare occasions. It is the author's impression that in the instances where the virus can be cultured from the spinal fluid, the patient usually has an overwhelming infection. Attempts to demonstrate the presence of viral antigen in the spinal fluid have met with only limited success, but recent studies from a number of institutions have suggested that, using PCR, viral genomes can be amplified from the cerebrospinal fluid in the majority of cases of herpes simplex virus encephalitis during the acute phase of the disease (Anderson *et al.*, 1993; Aurelius *et al.*, 1991; Lakeman and Whitley, 1995). One presumes that this discrepancy arises from the ability of PCR to detect fragments of viral genomes which may be present in the absence of complete replicating virus.

Clinical features

In neonatal infants, herpes simplex virus appears to arise from maternal genital infection with the virus. A small percentage of such infections appear to be due to intrauterine infections prior to the time of birth, but the majority appear to arise from infection acquired as the newborn infant passes through the birth canal. The infection in newborns may present in a variety of forms, from an infection limited to the skin, eyes, and mouth, to more severe processes with involvement of brain or generalized herpetic infection of many organ systems.

The disease affecting children or adults is considered to be the most frequent cause of an acute necrotizing encephalitis occurring on a non-epidemic basis. The clinical presentation is quite similar to that of encephalitis produced by a variety of other viruses. Patients develop an acute or subacute onset of headache, fever, alteration in personality or behaviour, progressing over a period of hours to days. Seizures may be focal or generalized and may assume the characteristic of a partial complex or generalized seizure. Often the patients develop dysphasia if there is involvement of the dominant hemisphere, or focal signs such as hemiparesis, signifying involvement of the deep structures of the brain. All of these clinical symptoms and signs are similar to those that could be seen in an acute case of arbovirus encephalitis or encephalitis due to other causes, and it is difficult on the basis of clinical features alone to make a diagnosis of herpes simplex virus encephalitis (Whitley *et al.*, 1982b). Occasionally, patients complain of olfactory or gustatory hallucinations during the evolution of the encephalitic process, but this phase is usually transient, superceded by the development of impaired consciousness and communication. Such phenomena in the setting of a developing picture of encephalitis might hint strongly at the possibility of a herpetic aetiology since the olfactory system is so characteristically involved. Fodor *et al.* (1998) and Klapper *et al.* (1984) have recently called attention to milder or more slowly evolving patterns of disease in herpes simplex virus encephalitis, often in immunocompromised hosts.

While herpetic infection on the lip may be seen from time to time in patients with herpes simplex virus encephalitis, it is present with equal frequency in encephalitis due to other causes.

The electroencephalogram has traditionally been used as an aid in suggesting the diagnosis of herpes simplex virus encephalitis. The most characteristic electroencephalographic pictures are those of periodic high voltage discharges predominating in one or both temporal lobes on a background of generalized slowing. Unlike the case in other structural lesions of the temporal lobe, such as tumours or abscesses, the electroencephalographic pattern may change rapidly from day to day. The changes, however, are often less specific and, thus, less helpful in arriving at a definite diagnosis. It would be extremely unusual for the electroencephalogram to be normal in a patient with herpes simplex virus encephalitis, and a normal EEG should prompt a consideration of other diagnoses.

Diagnostic imaging studies have contributed greatly to our ability to recognize herpes simplex virus encephalitis and to distinguish it from other processes in the brain. The characteristic affection of the medial temporal lobe structures, subfrontal structures, and deep insular structures with sparing of parietal and occipital lobes and cerebellum is a typical pattern that should raise one's index of suspicion of herpes simplex virus encephalitis. These changes can be seen on computerized tomographic scanning of the brain when the lesions are of sufficient intensity; they may enhance after intravenous administration of contrast material. Late in the course of the process, the lesions may become haemorrhagic, and this change also can be appreciated by CT scanning. However, it is now well recognized that CT scans are relatively insensitive to the early changes in herpes simplex virus encephalitis (Schroth *et al.*, 1987) and can appear virtually normal within the first several days of the illness. In contrast, MRI scans are almost always abnormal when the patient first presents. The changes consist of the early appearance of hypointensity on T1 weighted images in the medial temporal and subjacent insular and inferior frontal regions of the brain and the occasional appearance of a seemingly independent lesion in the cingulate gyrus. These areas of involvement show increased signal on T2-weighted images and often enhance conspicuously after the administration of gadolinium contrast (Figures 5.1–5.5) Often there is a moderate to marked amount of brain oedema associated with these lesions. Haemorrhagic changes, if they occur, tend to appear later on in the disease process and conspicuously involve the cortical ribbon. Advances in MRI technology and skill in interpretation have greatly enhanced our ability to discriminate herpes simplex virus encephalitis from other conditions which may mimic it.

Studies some years ago by Whitley and associates (1989), prior to the widespread utilization of MRI technology, indicated a substantial range of other processes that could be confused with herpes simplex virus encephalitis including cerebrovascular lesions, brain abscesses, infections due to bacteria, fungi, or other viruses, and tumours. The distinction of these processes from herpes simplex virus encephalitis is far easier with currently available MRI technology and interpretation by experienced radiologists. The changes that are seen on the MRI closely approximate those recognized in pathological studies of brains of patients with herpes simplex virus encephalitis. Early changes consist of increased signal on T2-weighted images in the medial and anterior temporal lobes, extending anteriorly into the subfrontal region and medially into the insular region. Cingulate involvement is common (Demaerel

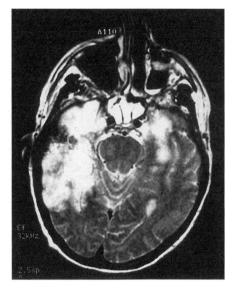

Figure 5.1 T2-weighted MRI showing extensive area of increased signal in right temporal lobe and lesser involvement of the right.

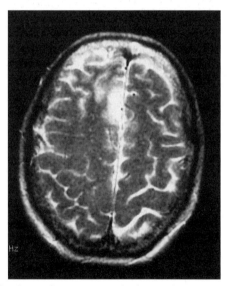

Figure 5.2 T2-weighted scan from same study depicted in Figure 5.1, showing involvement of cingulate gyrus.

et al., 1992). Involvement of parietal, occipital or cerebellar structures is distinctly rare and should raise suspicion of some other process. Contrast enhancement usually follows the appearance of the T2 lesions with striking enhancement in the cortical ribbon. Cystic lesions as late residua are seen in the medial temporal regions. In our experience, the most common conditions

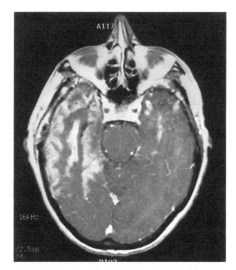

Figure 5.3   Same patient as shown in Figure 5.1, 17 days later, showing contrast enhancement in same areas.

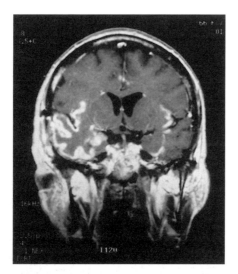

Figure 5.4   Coronal contrast enhanced MRI scan showing enhancement of cortical ribbon of temporal lobal on right, with bilateral lesions in insular cortex.

which may still be confused with herpes simplex virus encephalitis are vascular lesions involving the posterior cerebral arteries which can cause lesions in the medial temporal lobes and mitochondrial encephalopathies which can produce patchy areas of tissue damage in the same area.

The analysis of cerebrospinal fluid has been of considerable help in the approach to cases of suspected herpes simplex virus encephalitis. The general findings on CSF examination are those that might be expected in any acute

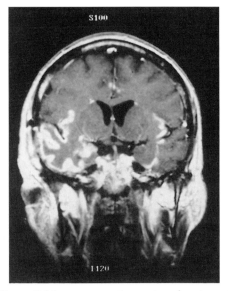

Figure 5.5   Same as Figure 5.4 in more anterior section showing subfrontal localization and involvement of cingulate gyrus.

viral encephalitic or meningitic process. Cases have been reported in which the initial cerebrospinal fluid findings are normal, but such cases are quite unusual. In the majority of cases, the cerebrospinal fluid typically contains 20–200 lymphocytes/μl. Polymorphonuclear leucocytes may be present but usually are outnumbered by lymphocytes and monocytes. The CSF protein is usually elevated in the range from 50–200 mg/dl, and the CSF glucose is usually normal. All of these findings are relatively non-specific. There is a widespread assumption that the presence of red cells in the CSF is of help either in suggesting the diagnosis of herpes simplex virus encephalitis or excluding it if they are absent. The presence or absence of red blood cells or xanthochromia is of virtually no use in discriminating herpes simplex virus encephalitis from encephalitis due to other causes and should not be used as a diagnostic feature (Whitley *et al.*, 1982b).

Testing for the presence of antibody to HSV in the spinal fluid can be of diagnostic help, but unfortunately detectable antibody levels in CSF develop only late in the process, usually after the first week. Thus, these are of little or no help within the first few days of the illness when prompt diagnosis and treatment are imperative. Antibody levels tend to persist in the cerebrospinal fluid for many weeks or months, so that they may be of use in retrospectively establishing the diagnosis of herpes simplex virus encephalitis. Attempts to detect HSV antigen in the CSF have offered some better promise because antigen, when detectable, may be present earlier in the process. However, there is great variability in the presence of antigen in the CSF, particularly within the first 2 or 3 days, and it is not generally useful in confirming the diagnosis.

The application of the PCR technique to CSF has provided a significant advance in our ability to make a specific and early diagnosis of herpes simplex virus encephalitis. Data from several laboratories (Rowley *et al.*, 1990; Aurelius *et al.*, 1991; Lakeman and Whitley, 1995) have suggested that herpes virus genomes can be amplified from the CSF at very early stages of the development of the encephalitic process. Furthermore, in large numbers of controls with other neurological diseases, PCR testing for HSV genomes has been negative. The test is thus both highly sensitive and specific. This would suggest that even though HSV genomes may be present in latent fashion in normal human ganglia and brain, they are not reactivated during other disease processes in brain and, thus, they do not cause diagnostic confusion (Mitchell *et al.*, 1997).

There are several advantages of the PCR technique. The technique is exquisitely sensitive to the presence of HSV genomes in spinal fluid. Falsely negative PCR tests appear to be confined to samples obtained on the first day or two of the illness and after 10–14 days. The failure to detect HSV genomes by the PCR technique in an experienced laboratory should raise considerable doubts about the diagnosis of herpes simplex virus encephalitis. Further advantages of the test are that it now can be accomplished within 6–8 h, requires only a very small volume of CSF, and is highly specific for herpes simplex virus since the primers, if appropriately chosen, will not amplify DNA sequences from other herpes viruses.

With the development of both MRI scanning of brain and PCR studies of the CSF, the need for brain biopsy in patients with suspected herpes simplex virus encephalitis has been greatly reduced. Brain biopsy has, for many years, been considered the gold standard for the diagnosis of herpes simplex virus encephalitis. The affected tissue undergoes marked tissue necrosis combined with an inflammatory reaction in the perivascular space and in the brain parenchyma associated with viral inclusions in the nuclei of astrocytes, neurons and other cells in the brain. While the presence of inclusions is relatively insensitive and, in the author's experience, often lacking in patients with herpes simplex virus encephalitis, viral antigen can usually be readily demonstrated by immunofluorescence or immunoperoxidase tests using appropriate antibodies to HSV 1, and virus can frequently be recovered by cultivation. The presence of large amounts of DNA in the lesions should make detection by PCR extremely easy from biopsy tissue and, in fact, it has been possible to demonstrate DNA genomes in paraffin embedded archival tissue from patients with herpes simplex virus encephalitis (Nicoll *et al.*, 1993). Thus, if biopsy is performed, the tissue should be subjected to PCR analysis as well as the other studies listed above. Biopsy of suspected herpes simplex virus encephalitis should now be confined to cases where the nature of the disease process after appropriate MRI and CSF studies remains in doubt, and alternative diagnoses must be entertained.

Differential diagnosis

There is a broad range of conditions which may mimic herpes simplex encephalitis at the onset (Table 5.1), but a thorough history together with

Table 5.1   Difrrential diagnosis of herpes simplex virus encephalitis.

Viral deseases	
Arbovirus encephalitis	Summer/fall occurrence
	Community outbreaks
Enterovirus encephalitis	Often as aseptic meningitis
	Chronic encephalopathy in immunosuppressed
Varicella zoster virus and CMV Encephalitis	Common in AIDS or immunosuppressed
HHV-6 Encephalitis	May mimic HSV encephalitis
	Consider in younger patients
EBV Encephalitis	Association with acute mononucleosis common
	Positive IgM VCA titer
	PCR of CSF
Bacterial diseases	
Mycoplasma	Antecedent respiratory infection
	Positive CF antibodies
Listeria monocytogenes	Immunocompromised patient
	Brainstem signs
Cat scratch disease	Children; history of contact with kittens; adenopathy
Tuberculoma	Patient from developing country or with AIDS
Lyme disease	Exposure in endemic area; rash; arthralgia
Rickettsial diseases	
Rocky Mountain spotted fever	Children in eastern seaboard; tick bite; rash beginning distally
	Thrombocytopenia, disseminated intravascular coagulation
Q fever	Contact with sheep, goats, cattle
Parasitic disease	
Cysticercosis	Patient from Latin America; seizures; calcified cystic lesions on CT; positive ELISA test on CSF
Schistosomiasis	Travel to Asia, Africa, South or Central America; contaminated water exposure
MELAS syndrome	History of prior episodes; diabetes; deafness; short stature; ophthalmoparesis; increased lactate in CSF; point mutation in mitochondrial DNA
Cerebrovascular disease	Sudden onset of deficit, underlying cardiovascular disease, other lesions in posterior circulation
Miscellaneous	OKT 3 induced encephalopathy
	Pseudomigraine with CSF pleocytosis

careful examination of the cerebrospinal fluid and detailed imaging studies will usually permit accurate diagnosis (Whitley, 1988).

Given a patient with the acute or subacute development of fever, headache, alteration in consciousness with or without seizures, an abnormal CSF with lymphocytic pleocytosis and some elevation of the protein, a variety of other processes may have to be considered. These can be grouped into viral encephalitides, bacterial or rickettsial encephalitides, encephalitides due to fungal or parasitic organisms and a variety of other processes including central nervous system lymphomas, mitochondrial disease, vascular disease, and acute postinfectious inflammatory processes.

Many of the diseases that mimic herpes simplex virus encephalitis are eminently treatable. Thus, confronted with a patient with suspected herpes simplex virus encephalitis, it is not appropriate after obtaining a PCR for HSV in the CSF and initiating treatment with acylovir to adopt a 'wait and see' attitude without promptly considering other treatable entities.

Viral diseases

The acute viral encephalitides that may be confused with herpes simplex virus encephalitis, such as eastern and western equine encephalitis, St Louis encephalitis and California virus encephalitis, have to be considered. Because these processes depend upon mosquito vectors for their transmission, they tend to occur in mid and late summer. They also tend to occur in localized outbreaks in somewhat characteristic geographic locations. Eastern equine encephalitis, which is perhaps the most malignant of the processes, occurs sporadically in outbreaks along the entire east coast of the USA. It is characterized by a rapidly progressive encephalitic process with disseminated lesions within the basal ganglia and brainstem on MRI scanning and a very high mortality and morbidity rate (Deresiewicz et al., 1997). In some cases, involvement of the medial temporal lobes has caused the diagnosis of herpes simplex virus encephalitis to be considered. Prominent lesions in basal ganglia and thalamus are, however, unusual in herpes simplex virus encephalitis. Western equine encephalitis occurs, as its name implies, mainly in the western and midwestern states and has a much lower mortality and morbidity rate than eastern equine encephalitis. It appears to be particularly severe in infants and children.

St Louis encephalitis has occurred in a rather wide region in the midwestern USA but has occasionally been reported in states along the eastern or western seaboard. It is the most frequent cause of epidemics of viral encephalitis in the USA. California encephalitis virus, a member of the bunyavirus family, is transmitted by mosquitoes. The encephalitis occurs principally east of the Mississippi River and with highest incidence in Minnesota, Wisconsin, Ohio and adjacent states. It is much more frequent in children than adults. The similarity in clinical findings in patients with herpes simplex virus encephalitis may be a source of diagnostic confusion. Currently, the diagnosis of California group encephalitis rests on a rise in serum antibody titre or presence of IgM antibody in the CSF. Antigen can be demonstrated in cerebral tissue.

Enteroviruses, including the echoviruses and coxsackieviruses, are frequent causes of aseptic meningitis. The difficulty in culturing virus from the CSF has probably caused the frequency of enteroviral infections to be greatly under-estimated. Although enteroviruses usually cause a self-limited meningitis, they also are occasional causes of focal or generalized encephalitis in immunocompetent hosts (Rotbart, 1995; Tong et al., 1997). Again, the frequency of this process has probably been underestimated. PCR analysis of CSF will add greatly to our understanding of the frequency and range of encephalitides due to enteroviruses. Enteroviruses are also recognized to cause chronic meningitis or meningoencephalitis in children with hypogammaglobulinaemia (Rudge *et al.*, 1996).

In each of the above conditions, the patients may present with an encephalitic process marked by fever, alteration of consciousness, seizures, and focal deficits together with an abnormal cerebrospinal fluid containing an excessive number of lymphocytes and an elevated protein value. The differential diagnosis rests upon the epidemiological features of the illness. They usually occur in the late summer or early fall, often in clusters within a community or within a given locale. Serological studies must be utilized for verification of the causative agent. Treatment in these cases is purely supportive. However, if herpes simplex virus encephalitis is in the differential, treatment for this condition should be added until confirmatory tests serve to indicate the diagnosis.

Varicella zoster virus and cytomegalovirus each can cause an acute necrotizing and demyelinative encephalitic process (Kleinschmidt-DeMasters *et al.*, 1996). In adults, it is quite unusual for either of these viruses to produce encephalitis in the immunocompetent host. They are, however, always to be considered in patients with AIDS or who are undergoing immunosuppressive treatment for transplantation. Cytomegalovirus encephalitis may be accompanied by an acute viral retinopathy which is only rarely seen in herpes simplex virus encephalitis. In the immunocompromised host, the distribution of lesions in varicella zoster virus or cytomegalovirus encephalitis is more random within the cerebral hemispheres than the typical inferior frontal, medial temporal and inferior insular localization that is so highly characteristic of herpes simplex virus encephalitis.

Human herpes virus 6 (HHV-6) is the cause of roseola infantum and is frequently associated with febrile seizures in children. Recent retrospective studies from Whitley's group have indicated that approximately 6% of a series of children and adults with encephalitis have HHV-6 genomes demonstrable in the CSF by PCR analysis. (McCullers *et al.*, 1995). Although the average age of the patients positive for HHV-6 (18 years) was somewhat younger than the remainder of the group (27 years), there were no clinical features that characterized those with encephalitis due to HHV-6.

Epstein-Barr (EBV) virus infection of the nervous system can produce a variety of clinical neurological syndromes including meningitis, encephalitis, transverse myelopathy, and the Guillain-Barré syndrome (Ross and Cohen, 1997). Most of these infections occur in young individuals and in the wake of either a clinically evident picture of acute mononucleosis or in the absence of such a picture, with serological evidence of recent EBV infection. Cases of encephalitis resulting from acute infectious mononucleosis are uncommon, especially considering the very great frequency of infectious mononucleosis in children and young adults. The infectious process in the brain does not have the characteristic localization that is seen in herpes simplex virus encephalitis but may cause focal disturbances in any portion of the brain. In our own limited experience, cases with severe encephalopathy may be associated with minimal parenchymal changes in the brain as judged by MRI. Patients suspected of having EBV neurological disease should have a serum assay for

IgM antibodies to viral capsid antigen. These are uncommonly seen in the general population and can be seen in a majority of cases of acute infectious mononucleosis. Epstein-Barr nuclear antigens (EBNA) persist for the lifetime of the individual and are useful as a marker of past infection. A PCR assay for Epstein Barr virus DNA is now available. Experience with this assay in patients with encephalitis is limited. A positive PCR on CSF would be strongly suggestive of viral causation, but whether PCR testing of the CSF will be invariably, or even frequently, positive in EBV-induced neurological syndromes has not been well studied. The treatment of EBV infections is symptomatic. Acyclovir is not efficacious in treatment of EBV infections.

Bacterial diseases

A variety of bacterial organisms may cause an acutely or subacutely developing illness that potentially may be confused with herpes simplex virus encephalitis. Mycoplasma infection must be considered if there has been an antecedent upper respiratory or pneumonic infection. In most cases, the mycoplasma-induced upper respiratory infection presents with cough, sore throat, and influenza-like symptoms (Bayer *et al.*, 1981). Often, other family members have been affected. A wide variety of neurological complications have been described including aseptic meningitis, meningoencephalitis, transverse myelitis, or Guillain-Barré syndrome. The plethora of neurological syndromes that may result from mycoplasma infection (Hodges *et al.*, 1972) makes it important to be cognizant of this possibility and to carry out appropriate serological tests including the presence of cold haemagglutinins and the measurement of serum complement fixing antibodies against *M. pneumoniae*. Treatment for mycoplasma infection consists of tetracycline or erythromycin.

Listeria monocytogenes has emerged in recent years as an important cause of meningitis in the neonate. However, in the immunocompromised or elderly or alcoholic adult, *Listeria monocytogenes* has been recognized with increasing frequency as a cause of meningitis or encephalitis (Calder, 1997). It is increasingly recognized that improperly processed and contaminated food-stuffs, particularly dairy products, may be the source of *Listeria* infection in many cases. The neurological process in adults can present as a meningitis with CSF pleocytosis, but the organism seems to have a particular predilection for causing an infection in the brainstem in addition to the meninges and, thus, has been characterized as producing a 'rhombencephalitis'. The differential diagnosis between *Listeria* involving the brainstem and the rare case of herpes simplex virus encephalitis involving the brainstem may be quite difficult and rest upon careful attempts to culture *Listeria* from the CSF and the utilization of PCR to detect HSV genomes in the spinal fluid. Treatment is initiated with ampicillin or penicillin with the addition of gentamicin.

The development of an encephalitic picture on a background of fatigue, headache, lymphadenopathy and conjunctivitis should suggest the possibility of cat scratch disease, especially if there has been contact with kittens (Case records of Massachusetts General Hospital, 1998). This disease, recently recognized to result from infection by *Bartonella henselae* is usually a self-limited disease involving fever, lymphadenopathy and conjunctivitis, often in young children who are scratched or bitten by kittens. However, occasional patients develop an encephalitic picture with seizures and variable degrees of CSF pleocytosis. In some, the CSF is acellular. Abnormal MRI signals, especially on T2-weighted images, can be seen in the grey matter of the thalami or the posterior parietal and occipital lobes. Serological tests for *B. henselae* are available to confirm the diagnosis. Treatment consists of administration of trimethoprim-sulphamethoxazole intravenously.

Central nervous system tuberculosis, and specifically tuberculomas, have in the past presented diagnostic confusion with herpes simplex virus encephalitis. Certainly tuberculosis involving the nervous system must be suspected in any patient from a developing country, and with its resurgence in the USA, must be suspected particularly in patients who are HIV positive or suffering from AIDS. The patient need not have evidence of tuberculosis elsewhere in the body, and a sizeable proportion of patients have a negative tuberculin skin test. Patients with intraparenchymal tuberculomas may present with seizures and focal signs with varying degrees of confusional states attended by increased intracranial pressure and by CSF pleocytosis. The distinction between herpes simplex virus encephalitis and intracranial tuberculoma is, in most cases, easily made by the appearances of the lesions on CT scans or by MR scanning (Vengsarkar *et al.*, 1986). The pattern of lesions seen on either technique is that of solid or ring enhancing lesions which are often rather spherical in outline, associated with moderate to marked degrees of brain oedema and often with ventricular obstruction, particularly if the lesions are located in the posterior fossa.

Although Lyme disease often produces a radiculopathy commonly involving the seventh cranial nerve, it may also present as an aseptic meningitis and rarely as an encephalitic syndrome (Reik *et al.*, 1979) characterized by headache, fever, stiff neck and occasional focal signs. However, the course of such processes is usually subacute or even chronic, and diagnostic confusion with herpes simplex virus encephalitis would be unusual.

Rickettsial disease

Rocky Mountain spotted fever must be considered in the differential diagnosis. Although initially identified in Montana, this disease is now prevalent along the eastern seaboard of the USA, particularly in the middle and southern portions. It tends to affect children far more frequently than adults (Bell and Lascari, 1970). The disease, caused by *R. rickettsii* is transmitted by the dog tick, and a history of a tick bite is frequent. Fever, headache, and conjunctivitis are associated with a rash which begins on the distal portion of the extremities and migrates centripetally. The rash, which may be haemorrhagic in character, can be mistaken for the rash of meningococcaemia. The nervous system process is part of a systemic vasculitis (Case records of Massachusetts General Hospital, 1997) which prominently infects not only the skin but the lungs and may result in pulmonary oedema. Thrombocytopenia, anaemia, and disseminated intravascular coagulation are frequent features of the disorder.

The nervous system involvement consists of headache admixed with variable focal signs and a CSF formula with a mild pleocytosis and an elevated protein. The infection of endothelial cells and the resulting vasculitis produces widespread cerebral oedema which may be reflected in retinal venous engorgement and papilloedema. Hyponatraemia is common. Prompt institution of antibiotic therapy consisting of tetracycline or chloramphenicol is important, and in addition, measures to lower intracranial pressure may be important in determining the outcome. The diagnosis rests upon suspicion of the disease in a person who resides in or who has travelled in the eastern seaboard, inquiry into the possibility of a tick bite, and the observation of the clinical syndrome taking place in the presence of a rash on the extremities.

Q fever may have to be considered in the differential diagnosis. This rickettsial infection, which most often presents as a self-limited febrile illness, occasionally can involve the nervous system, either because it may cause endocarditis or it may directly produce an encephalitis. The organism is commonly present in cattle, sheep and goats and it often causes disease in meat packers, abattoir workers or in individuals who work in animal research facilities. However, a number of cases have been described in which the contact with animals is either remote or non-existent (Brooks *et al.*, 1986). Unpasteurized milk can be a source of infection. When the disease process is that of an encephalitis, the patients may develop focal signs such as an aphasia or hemiparesis; often a CSF pleocytosis with an elevated protein level is found (Case records of Massachusetts General Hospital, 1996a). Antibodies against *Coxiella burnetii* can be detected by indirect fluorescent antibody technique. The disease is to be highly suspected in a patient presenting with an encephalitic process whose work brings them into contact with animals and particularly if they are involved with the slaughter of animals or exposed to placenta or fetal membranes. Tetracycline compounds should be employed in the treatment of the disease.

Parasitic disease

Cysticercosis must be considered in individuals who have come from or resided in Mexico, Central, or South America. The disease results most often from the accidental ingestion of fertilized eggs of *Taenia solium* and subsequent penetration of the larvae through the gastrointestinal wall into the blood with establishment of the embryos in muscle, eye, and brain. The condition may present primarily as a syndrome of an intracranial tumour or as a diffuse encephalitic picture or as an arachnoiditis with hydrocephalus or combinations of these features. Seizures and headache are common. The spinal fluid may show a pleocytosis with a normal glucose; eosinophilia may be present but this is not uniform. The diagnosis is most easily suspected on CT or MRI scanning. CT reveals single or multiple calcified lesions which may be either solid or cystic and which may show ring-like or nodular enhancement after administration of contrast. Alternatively, if the disease is present mainly in the subarachnoid space, hydrocephalus is seen. MRI scanning frequently reveals a mural nodule within the cystic lesions representing the larvae of the cysticercus. The ELISA test for the presence of IgM antibodies in the CSF is highly sensitive and specific in establishing the diagnosis in problematic cases.

Schistosomiasis must be considered in individuals residing in or having travelled in Asia, Africa, the Caribbean, and South America. It results from contact with water containing cercariae which penetrate the skin of swimmers and migrate to the heart, lungs, liver, and to the nervous system. Although the spinal cord is involved most frequently, eggs may migrate to the cerebrum where they may produce focal deficits combined with seizures. The cerebrospinal fluid may show a lymphocytic pleocyotosis, occasionally with a disproportionate number of eosinophils. A recently published case demonstrated involvement of the temporal lobe in a pattern compatible with that seen in herpes simplex virus encephalitis (Case records New England Journal of Medicine, 1996b). Praziquantal is the drug of choice for the treatment of cerebral schistosomiasis.

Mitochondrial encephalopathy

MELAS syndrome (mitochondrial encephalopathy, lactic acidosis and stroke-like episodes) has occasionally presented as a source of diagnostic confusion with herpes simplex virus encephalitis (Johns et al., 1993; Kimata et al., 1998; Sharfstein et al., 1999). This syndrome may present acutely with appearance of focal deficits, confusional states, headache, and seizures. These often relate to involvement of the posterior parietal or occipital lobes, but sometimes the medial or lateral temporal areas. A variety of clinical features may point to the possibility of MELAS syndrome. A history of prior episodes of stroke-like events, or the findings of progressive external ophthalmoplegia, diabetes, deafness, myopathy, pigmentary retinopathy, short stature, or ataxia should raise consideration of MELAS syndrome. Often there is a history of diabetes, hearing loss, or stroke-like events in close relatives. The diagnosis can be suspected on the basis of an MRI scan which shows lesions involving the grey matter, both of the cortex and the basal ganglia not respecting vascular territories. Magnetic resonance spectroscopy shows an increase in the lactate in the affected region of the brain and may be used to monitor the effect of treatment (Pavlakis et al., 1998) The CSF lactate is often elevated. The diagnosis is established by the demonstration of a point mutation in the mitochondrial DNA, most often at the 3243 locus. While the mitochondrial DNA mutation may be demonstrated in blood, it is more frequently present in muscle, and in some cases muscle biopsy may be required. Ragged red fibres characteristic of excess mitochondrial deposition may be seen, and the typical point mutation in the mitochondrial DNA can be identified.

Cerebrovascular disease occasionally can mimic herpes simplex virus encephalitis, particularly if emboli shower branches of the posterior cerebral artery that supplies the medial and undersurface of the temporal lobe. Patients with such lesions may exhibit memory disorder combined with field deficits and a confusional state. The CSF is usually normal in such cases. Medial temporal lobe lesions with increased signal in the cortex on T2-weighted MRI images can mimic, to some degree, the lesions seen in herpes simplex virus encephalitis. In such case, the extreme abruptness of the disorder, the presence of a source of emboli from underlying heart disease, and the occasional evidence of lesions in other areas of the brain supplied by the posterior circulation may point to the diagnosis of embolic vascular disease.

Miscellaneous conditions

Immunosuppressive medications, notably the monoclonal anti-CD3 antibody (OKT3) given to prevent transplant rejection have been associated with development of fever, headache, seizures, confusion and CSF pleocytosis (Adair *et al.*, 1991). Herpes simplex virus encephalitis might enter into the differential diagnosis of such patients, as would other infections in transplant patients such as aspergillosis, candidiasis, cryptococcosis, listeriosis and bacterial endocarditis. The syndrome of OKT3 induced encephalopathy resolves spontaneously.

The syndrome of pseudomigraine with lymphocytic pleocytosis has been recently reviewed (Gomez-Aranda *et al.*, 1997). The patients, usually young adult males, present with focal neurological deficits (hemisensory deficits, dysphasia, hemiparesis) and headache usually contralateral to the focal symptoms, often in repeated episodes. Frequently there is an antecedent viral-like illness. The CSF when examined shows a lymphocytic pleocytosis with 10–700 cells/µl with mild elevation of the CSF protein and normal glucose concentration. While the EEG is frequently slow on the affected side, CT and MRI scans are normal. Single positron emission computed tomography (SPECT) scans in three patients showed reduced (^{99m}Tc) HMPAO (hexamethylene propylene amine oxime) uptake on the affected side. The aetiology of this syndrome remains controversial. The clinical characteristics may cause initial diagnostic consideration of herpes simplex virus encephalitis, usually ruled out by the normal MRI scan.

As illustrated by the above, there is a wide variety of other conditions which, even in the era of improved modalities for the diagnosis of herpes simplex virus encephalitis, may be confused with this disease. Careful attention must be given to the patient's country of origin or travel history, residence in areas where mosquitoes or ticks are common, contact with animals, occupation, underlying disease processes, occurrence of encephalitis in the region, and past medical and family history. Often careful enquiry will enhance one's suspicion of alternative disease processes which have to be considered in the differential diagnosis and which may merit entirely different forms of treatment.

How to establish the diagnosis

The diagnosis of herpes simplex virus encephalitis must be suspected in any patient presenting with the acute or subacute evolution of fever, headache, seizures, behavioural change and/or focal signs. The chief element in establishing the diagnosis is the presence of a CSF which usually shows a mild to moderate pleocytosis with some elevation of the protein and a normal glucose concentration. The MRI scan, even early in the disease, will often demonstrate involvement of the medial temporal, insular, and subfrontal structures of the brain with a necrotizing process which shows a high signal on T2 weighted images (Schroth *et al.*, 1987). Sometimes there is an independent small lesion in the cingulate gyrus. Extensive lesions in the basal ganglia, the parietal or occipital areas or the cerebellum weigh against the diagnosis of herpes simplex virus encephalitis and should immediately turn one's attention to other diagnostic possibilities as listed in the differential diagnosis.

An electroencephalogram may be helpful if it demonstrates a pattern of periodic lateralized epileptiform discharges (PLEDS) in one or both temporal lobes, but the pattern is often less specific than this, and the lack of a typical pattern of PLEDS should not mitigate the diagnosis. The combination of the clinical picture, the CSF findings and the MRI findings mandates the institution of treatment with acyclovir as soon as possible. It is probably best not to delay treatment pending the results of PCR testing for HSV in the CSF.

The diagnosis can be firmly established by the PCR test on the CSF. In accumulated series of patients with herpes simplex virus encephalitis and controls, it has become evident that the PCR test for HSV often becomes positive on the first or second day of the illness, remaining positive through the first 10–20 days of the illness, after which it again becomes negative (Aurelius *et al.*, 1991; Anderson *et al.*, 1993; Guffond *et al.*, 1994; Lakeman and Whitley, 1995). Thus, in suspected cases, the PCR test should be done on the first spinal fluid specimen. The test has two inherent advantages. Because it depends upon the annealing of HSV specific primers to HSV-DNA in the spinal fluid, it has the advantage of great specificity, since annealing will not occur to other DNAs that do not have the same nucleotide sequences. Secondly, the test involves the serial annealing, primer extension and amplification of herpes genomes through 30 or more cycles resulting in enormous amplification of genomic material which may be present in picogram amounts. The assay is, thus, exquisitely sensitive to the presence of small amounts of HSV genomic material. This extreme specificity and sensitivity does mean that the laboratory must exert stringent measures to avoid contamination of specimens by herpes virus DNA because picogram amounts as contaminants can result in false positive tests (Landry, 1995). Nevertheless, in the hands of capable personnel, the test has proven to be positive in over 90% of confirmed cases of herpes simplex virus encephalitis and is uniformly negative in control specimens from patients with other neurological diseases.

A negative PCR test on the first or second day of illness should, if the clinical suspicion is high enough, be repeated in 24–48 h. If a second test is negative, one should seriously consider alternative diagnoses. It should be noted, as well, that blood in the CSF may inhibit the PCR reaction with the potential to cause a false negative test.

In rare cases, it may be necessary to resort to brain biopsy to establish the diagnosis of herpes simplex virus encephalitis when the clinical picture, the MR findings, or the findings on CSF examination are equivocal or confusing. While it seems obvious, biopsy of the inferior portion of the temporal lobe on the involved side will provide the highest diagnostic yield. Biopsies on occasion have been performed at other sites (e.g. frontal convexity) and have provided false negative results because of the fact that herpes simplex virus encephalitis is often highly localized to the inferior frontal and temporal regions. The biopsy tissue should be processed for routine histology but additionally should be processed for demonstration of herpes simplex virus antigen by immunoperoxidase or other technique, viral culture and PCR analysis for HSV. Obviously the fact that HSV genomes can be found rarely in amygdala or hippocampus of normal brain by PCR must be taken into account. A positive assay for HSV by PCR in biopsy temporal lobe tissue that shows a necrotizing and inflammatory process should probably be interpreted as significant. Antigen detection or culture of HSV, although less sensitive, would obviously be of greater importance in establishing the presence of an active infection. Fungal and bacterial cultures should also be established. Because the circumstances in which one must resort to biopsy are most often those in which the clinical diagnosis is in considerable doubt, it is always wise to save a portion of the biopsy tissue frozen at −70 degrees for later assay. Finally, one should not neglect to send an acute serum specimen to the laboratory early in the clinical course so that this may be compared with later convalescent sera to assess antibodies against HSV or other viruses.

Management

The management of patients with herpes simplex virus encephalitis requires general measures for care of patients with any encephalitic process that may cause seizures or obtundation. The patient should be treated initially in an intensive care unit where nursing personnel are accustomed to managing patients who are obtunded and may have seizures and raised intracranial pressure. Careful attention must be given to fluid and electrolyte balance with careful measurement of intake and output in order to maintain adequate hydration and kidney function. It is often helpful to weigh the patients daily as an additional measure of net fluid retention or loss which sometimes is not reflected in input and output data.

The patient's skin must be watched carefully to avoid the development of decubitus ulcers. The patients are often immobile, and because of impaired consciousness, heparin should be administered subcutaneously to avoid the possibility of venous thrombosis in the lower extremities and the development of pulmonary emboli.

The management of raised intracranial pressure may be particularly vexing. It is important to avoid the use of intravenous fluids containing only glucose because the hypo-osmolarity of such fluids contributes to increased intracranial pressure. The cerebral oedema that is frequently present in the temporal lobe in patients with herpes simplex virus encephalitis is likely due to cytotoxic oedema from the death of cells in the involved area and the fact that they imbibe water. However, there is also a component of vasogenic oedema from the inflammatory process that involves cerebral vessels. To the extent that vasogenic oedema is an important component of the overall swelling, the use of dexamethasone is indicated to reduce raised intracranial pressure. Data are lacking about the extent to which dexamethasone may impair the clearance of virus from the brain of patients with herpes simplex virus encephalitis, but studies from experimental animals (Baringer *et al.*, 1976) would suggest that the magnitude of this effect is modest. Confronted with the immediate and serious consequences of raised intracranial pressure and possible transtentorial herniation, one should not hesitate to use dexamethasone to reduce intracranial pressure when this appears to be an important element in the overall process. The use of mannitol has not been studied in any systematic way. Because considerable portions of the brain in patients with herpes simplex virus encephalitis would appear to have an intact blood–brain barrier, mannitol potentially could be beneficial because of its ability to shrink the brain where the blood–brain barrier is intact. However, to the extent that mannitol may leak into the portions of the brain that were affected by the encephalitic process because of the increased vascular permeability, the overall benefits of mannitol might be lessened. Thus, administration of dexamethasone would seem to be preferred initially to control increased intracranial pressure reserving mannitol for use in situations in which the effect of dexamethasone seems insufficient. One must be alert to the occasional development of hyponatraemia. It should be managed by careful adjustment of fluid and sodium intake.

Seizures are perhaps best treated by the use of intravenously administered phenytoin (Dilantin) or phenobarbital. It is unusual in this author's experience for seizures to remain uncontrolled in patients with herpes simplex virus encephalitis when adequate amounts of phenytoin are employed. There are no data concerning duration of phenytoin therapy. The author's personal bias would be to continue therapy for at least 6–12 months in patients who have had a seizure.

Acyloguanosine (Acyclovir) should be administered intravenously at a dose of 10 mg/kg every 8 h beginning as soon as the presumptive diagnosis can be made based upon the clinical picture, the presence of a CSF pleocytosis, and appropriate findings on MRI scan (Skoldenberg *et al.*, 1984; Whitley and Lakeman, 1995). Acyclovir administered in this fashion is usually well tolerated with few side-effects. (Whitley *et al.*, 1986). One of the advantages of acyclovir is that the initial conversion to the monophosphate form is principally due to the virus-encoded thymidine kinase. Cellular thymidine kinases are less efficient in this conversion; thus, the compound is converted selectively to its monophosphate form in infected cells. Acyclovir is subsequently converted intracellularly to the triphosphate form which inhibits viral DNA polymerase. The triphosphate form inhibits viral DNA polymerases more completely than cellular DNA polymerases. These two steps, which are highly selective, result in a favourable therapeutic ratio for the medication and mitigate any deleterious effect on uninfected cells (Whitley, 1988; Elion, 1993). The development of resistant strains seems to be a problem only rarely, and only in patients who are immunosuppressed and who are treated repeatedly with acyclovir. Acyclovir is excreted by glomerular filtration and may precipitate in the renal tubules if it is administered too rapidly. Thus, the blood urea nitrogen (BUN) and creatinine concentrations should be monitored in patients receiving acyclovir, and measures should be taken to administer it slowly. Also, the rate of administration of acyclovir must be modified in patients with impaired creatinine clearance. Ayclovir toxicity usually arises in patients with impaired renal function. In these patients, the toxicity presents as an encephalopathy which can cause considerable confusion in the clinical assessment. It is recommended that for patients with creatinine clearances of $25-50$ ml/min/1.73 M^2, the dosing interval be increased to 12 h and for patients with creatinine clearances of $10-25$, the dosing interval be increased to 24 h. The recommended duration of administration of acyclovir intravenously for patients with herpes simplex virus encephalitis is 10 days. However, personal and anecdotal experience would suggest that occasional cases treated with a 10-day course of acyclovir undergo a relapse of the disease after a short interval, necessitating re-treatment. Our own experience suggests that most relapses are due to inadequate treatment, but it may be that some relapses are due to other mechanisms (Dennett *et al.*, 1996). Many authorities now recommend that the treatment with intravenous acyclovir be extended to $14-21$ days in order to assure complete killing of the virus, thus avoiding the risk of recurrent encephalitis. The PCR test for HSV usually becomes negative at $10-14$ days after treatment. A CSF PCR that remains positive after 2 weeks of treatment would raise consideration of inadequate treatment or resistant virus (Cinque *et al.*, 1996). The latter circumstance is quite rare. The cost of the prolonged intravenous administration may be lessened if the patient's clinical status permits the continued administration of the medication at home or in a convalescent facility, but many patients with herpes simplex virus encephalitis are not appropriate candidates for home care at this stage of the illness, and a longer in-hospital stay may be required.

Prognosis

In confirmed cases of herpes simplex virus encephalitis, the prognosis is extremely poor with a high mortality and severe morbidity in those who survive. Data derived from the studies of Whitley and associates (1982b) suggest that in patients treated with placebo or with drugs now known to be ineffective, mortality rates are in the range of 70%. Fewer than 10% of untreated patients return to normal function. In a retrospective analysis by Kennedy (1988) only 16% of those patients untreated survived. In a study comparing acyclovir with its predecessor vidarabine (Whitley *et al.*, 1986), vidarabine reduced mortality to 54% and acyclovir reduced it further to 28%. Similar reductions were noted in a study from Norway (Skoldenberg *et al.*, 1984), although the criteria for the diagnosis in the latter series were less stringent than in the series reported by Whitley. Approximately half of those treated with acyclovir in the series in the USA returned to normal function.

A number of factors appeared to be important in determining outcome, the most important of which were the age of the individual and the Glasgow coma scale at the time that treatment was administered. The prognosis for recovery of function was markedly better in the patients under 30 years of age and whose Glasgow coma scale was over six at the time of admission; conversely, patients over 30 years of age who had a Glasgow coma scale of under six had the highest mortality, whether treated with Vidarabine or acyclovir. Additionally, there was a trend towards lower survival in those patients whose duration of disease was longer than 4 days before the initiation of treatment with acyclovir compared with those whose treatment was instituted less than 4 days from the development of symptoms. In patients whose Glasgow coma scale was under six at the time of institution of treatment, not only was the mortality high, but severe morbidity, even with acyclovir treatment, was the rule. In a recent study, Domingues *et al.* (1998) found using quantitative PCR that patients with over 100 copies of HSV DNA per microlitre of CSF had poorer prognosis than those with lower amounts. There are occasional and pleasing exceptions to the observations from these series. We have had occasional elderly patients who have made quite satisfactory recoveries, although not from deep stages of coma. We have also encountered a small number of patients in whom it is clear on the basis of MRI studies and CSF antibodies that they have made a spontaneous and satisfactory recovery from herpes simplex virus encephalitis without the application of any treatment. Others have reported similar experience (Klapper *et al.*, 1984). Despite these anecdotal observations, the general principles derived from the observations of Whitely and others strongly suggest that the early recognition and early treatment of herpes simplex virus encephalitis with acyclovir is crucial to optimize the outcome.

Even in patients who are treated early in the course of their disease with acyclovir and who have relatively high Glasgow coma scales, neuropsychological testing may reveal residual changes which are of sufficient degree to impair the return of patients to normal functioning. These changes are usually in the areas of dysphasia and memory difficulty but also may involve difficulty with calculation and visualization. Mood and behavioural distrubances are frequent sequelae, impairing social and professional adjustment (Caparros-Lefebvre *et al.*, 1996).

It is evident from the above that one of the major factors determining outcome in herpes simplex virus encephalitis is the delay in the recognition of the disease, either because the patient fails to get to medical attention or because of the failure of physicians to recognize the early signs and to proceed promptly with diagnostic studies. Additionally, it is clear that while acyclovir represents a significant advance in the treatment of herpes encephalitis, a considerable amount of tissue destruction is usually present at the time patients are first seen, and that no amount of acyclovir will repair such damage.

References

Adair, J. C., Woodley, S. L., O'Connell, J. B., *et al.* (1991). Aseptic meningitis following cardiac transplantation: Clinical characteristics and relationship to immunosuppressive regimen. *Neurology*, 4, 249–252.

Anderson, N. E., Powell, K. F. and Croxson, M. C. (1993). A polymerase chain reaction assay of cerebrospinal fluid in patients with suspected herpes simplex encephalitis. *J. Neurol. Neurosurg. Psych.*, **56**, 520–525.

Aurelius, E., Johansson, B., Skoldenberg, B. *et al.* (1991). Rapid diagnosis of herpes simplex encephalitis by nested polymerase chain reaction assay of cerebrospinal fluid. *Lancet*, **337**, 189–192.

Baringer, J. R. (1974). Recovery of herpes simplex virus from human sacral ganglions. *N. Engl. J. Med.*, **291**, 828–830.

Baringer, J. R. and Pisani, P. (1994). Herpes simplex virus genomes in human nervous system tissue analyzed by polymerase chain reaction. *Ann. Neurol.*, **36**, 823–829.

Baringer, J. R. and Swoveland P. (1973). Recovery of herpes-simplex virus from human trigeminal ganglions. *N. Engl. J. Med.*, **288**, 648–650.

Baringer, J. R., Klassen, T. and Grumm, F. (1976). Experimental herpes simplex virus encephalitis. *Arch. Neurol.*, **33**, 442–446.

Bayer, A. S., Galpin, J. E., Argyrios, N. *et al.* (1981). Neurologic disease associated with mycoplasma pneumoniae. *Ann. Intern. Med.*, **94**, 15–20.

Bell, W. E. and Lascari, A. D. (1970). Rocky Mountain spotted fever. *Neurology*, **20**, 841–847.

Brooks, R. G., Licitra, C. M. and Peacock, M. G. (1986). Encephalitis caused by *Coxiella burnetii. Ann. Neurol.*, **20**, 91–93.

Cabrera, C. V., Wholenberg, C., Openshaw, H. *et al.* (1980). Herpes simplex virus DNA sequences in the CNS of latently infected mice. *Nature*, **288**, 288–290.

Calder, J. A. M. (1997). Listeria meningitis in adults. *Lancet*, **350**, 307.

Caparros-Lefebvre, D., Girard-Buttaz, L., Reboul, S. *et al.* (1996). Cognitive and psychiatric impairment in herpes simplex virus encephalitis suggests involvement of the amygdalo-frontal pathways. *J. Neurol.*, **243**, 248–256.

Carton, I. A. and Kilbourne, E. D. (1952). Activation of latent herpes simplex by trigeminal sensory root section. *N. Engl. J. Med.*, **246**, 172–176.

Case Records of the Massachusetts General Hospital. (1996a). *N. Engl. J. Med.*, **335**, 1829–1834.

Case Records of the Massachusetts General Hospital. (1996b). *N. Engl. J. Med.*, **335**, 1906–1914.

Case Records of the Massachusetts General Hospital. (1997). *N. Engl. J. Med.*, **337**, 1149–1156.

Case Records of the Massachusetts General Hospital. (1998). *N. Engl. J. Med.*, **338**, 112–119.

Challoner, P. B., Smith, K. T., Parker, J. D. *et al.* (1995). Plaque-associated expression of human herpesvirus 6 in multiple sclerosis. *Proc. Natl Acad. Sci. USA*, **92**, 7440–7444.

Cinque, P., Cleator, G. M., Weber, T. *et al.* (1996). The role of laboratory investigation in the diagnosis and management of patients with suspected herpes simplex encephalitis: a consensus report. *J. Neurol. Neurosurg. Psych.*, **61**, 339–345.

Davis, L. E. and Johnson, R. T. (1979). An explanation for the localization of herpes simplex encephalitis? *Ann. Neurol.*, **5**, 2–5.

Demaerel, P. H., Wilms, G., Robberecht, W. *et al.* (1992). MRI of herpes simplex encephalitis. *Neuroradiology*, **34**, 490–493.

Dennett, C., Klapper, P. E. and Cleator, G. M. (1996). Polymerase chain reaction in the investigation of 'relapse' following herpes simplex encephalitis. *J. Med. Virol.*, **48**, 129–132.

Deresiewicz, R. L., Thaler, S. J., Hsu, L. *et al.* (1997). Clinical and neuroradiographic manifestations of eastern equine encephalitis. *N. Engl. J. Med.*, **336**, 1867–1874.

Domingues, R. B., Lakeman, F. D., Mayo, M. S. *et al.* (1998). Application of competitive PCR to cerebrospinal fluid samples from patients with herpes simplex encephalitis. *J. Clin. Microbiol.*, **36**, 2229–2234.

Elion, G. B. (1993). Acyclovir: discovery, mechanism of action, and selectivity. *J. Med. Virol. suppl.*, **1**, 2–6.

Fodor, P. A., Levin, M. J., Weinberg, M. D. *et al.* (1998). Atypical herpes simplex virus encephalitis diagnosed by PCR amplification of viral DNA from CSF. *Neurology*, **51**, 554–559.

Gomez-Aranda, F., Canadillas, F., Marti-Masso, J. F. *et al.* (1997) Pseudomigraine with temporary neurological symptoms and lymphocytic pleocytosis: a report of 50 cases. *Brain*, **120**, 1105–1113.

Goodpasture, E. W. and Teague, O. (1923). Transmission of the virus of herpes febrilis along nerve in experimentally infected rabbits. *J. Med. Res.*, **44**, 139–184.

Guffond, T., Dewilde, A., Lobert, P. E. *et al.* (1994). Significance and clinical relevance of the detection of herpes simplex virus DNA by the polymerase chain reaction in cerebrospinal fluid from patients with presumed encephalitis. *Clin. Infect. Dis.*, **18**, 744–749.

Hall, C. B. (1997). Human herpesviruses at sixes, sevens, and more. *Ann. Intern. Med.*, **127**, 481–483.

Hodges, G. R., Fass, R. J. and Saslaw, S. (1972). Central nervous system disease associated with mycoplasma pneumoniae infection. *Arch. Intern. Med.*, **130**, 277–282.

Johns, D. R., Stein, A. G. and Wityk, R. (1993). MELAS syndrome masquerading as herpes simplex encephalitis. *Neurology*, **43**, 2471–2473.

Kennedy, P. G. E. (1988). A retrospective analysis of forty-six cases of herpes simplex encephalitis seen in Glasgow between 1962 and 1985. *Q. J. Med.*, **255**, 533–540.

Kimata, K. G., Gordan, L., Ajax, E. T. *et al.* (1998). A case of late-onset MELAS. *Arch. Neurol.*, **55**, 722–725.

Klapper, P. E., Cleator, G. M. and Longson, M. (1984). Mild forms of herpes encephalitis. *J. Neurol. Neurosurg. Psych.*, **47**, 1247–1250.

Kleinschmidt-DeMasters, B. K., Amlie-Lefond, C. and Gilden, D. H. (1996). The patterns of varicella zoster virus encephalitis. *Hum. Pathol.*, **27**, 927–938.

Lakeman, F. D. and Whitley, R. J. (1995). Diagnosis of herpes simplex encephalitis: application of polymerase chain reaction cerebrospinal fluid from brain-biopsied patients and correlation with disease. *J. Infect. Dis.*, **171**, 857–863.

Landry, M. L. (1995). False-positive polymerase chain reaction results in the diagnosis of herpes simplex encephalitis. *J. Infect. Dis.*, **172**, 1641–1643.

Mahalingam, R., Wellish, M. C., Dueland, A. N. *et al.* (1992). Localization of herpes simplex virus and varicella zoster virus DNA in human ganglia. *Ann. Neurol.*, **31**, 444–448.

Mayne, M., Krishnan, J., Metz, L. *et al.* (1998). Infrequent detection of human herpesvirus 6 DNA in peripheral blood mononuclear cells from multiple sclerosis patients. *Ann. Neurol.*, **44**, 391–394.

McCullers, J. A., Lakeman, F. D. and Whitley, R. J. (1995). Human herpesvirus 6 is associated with focal encephalitis. *Clin. Infect. Dis.*, **21**, 571–576.

Mitchell, P. S., Espy, M. J., Smith, T. F. *et al.* (1997). Laboratory diagnosis of central nervous system infections with herpes simplex virus by PCR performed with cerebrospinal fluid specimens. *J. Clin. Microbiol.*, **35**, 2873–2877.

Nahmias, A. J. and Dowdle, W. R. (1968). Antigenic and biologic differences in herpes virus hominis. *Prog. Med. Virol.*, **10**, 110–159.

Nicoll, J. A. R., Love, S. and Kinrade, E. (1993). Distribution of herpes simplex virus DNA in the brains of human long-term survivors of encephalitis. *Neurosci. Lett.*, **157**, 215–218.

Pavlakis, S. G., Kingsley, P. B., Kaplan, G. P. *et al.* (1998). Magnetic resonance spectroscopy. Use in monitoring MELAS treatment. *Arch. Neurol.*, **55**, 849–852.

Rand, K. H., Houck, H., Denslow, N. D. and Heilman, K. M. (1998). Molecular approach to find target(s) for oligoclonal bands in multiple sclerosis. *J. Neurol. Neurosurg. Psych.*, **65**, 48–55.

Reik, L., Steere, A. C., Bartenhagen, N. H. *et al.* (1979). Neurologic abnormalities of Lyme disease. *Medicine*, **58**, 281–294.

Rock, D. L. and Fraser, N. W. (1983). Detection of HSV 1 genome in central nervous system of latently infected mice. *Nature*, **302**, 523–525.

Ross, J. P. and Cohen, J. I. (1997). Epstein Barr virus. In: *Infections of the Central Nervous System*, 2nd edn. (W. M. Scheld, R. J. Whitley and D. T. Durack, eds). Philadephia: Lippincott-Raven. pp. 117–127.

Rotbart, H. A. (1995). Enteroviral infections of the central nervous system. *Clin. Infect. Dis.*, **20**, 971–981.

Rowley, A., Lakeman, F., Whitley, R. *et al.* (1990). Rapid detection of herpes simplex virus DNA in cerebrospinal fluid of patients with herpes simplex encephalitis. *Lancet*, **335**, 440.

Rudge, P., Webster, A. D. B., Revesz, T. *et al.* (1996). Encephalomyelitis in primary hypogammaglobulinaemia. *Brain*, **119**, 1–15.

Schroth, G., Gawehn, M. D., Thron, A. *et al.* (1987). Early diagnosis of herpes simplex encephalitis by MRI. *Neurology*, **37**, 179–183.

Sharfstein, S. R., Gordon, M. F., Libman, R. B. *et al.* (1999). Adult-onset MELAS presenting as herpes encephalitis. *Arch. Neurol.*, **56**, 241–243.

Skoldenberg, B., Forsgren, M., Alestig, K. *et al.* (1984). Acyclovir versus vidarabine in herpes simplex encephalitis: randomised multicentre study in consecutive Swedish patients. *Lancet*, **2**, 707–712.

Stevens, J. G. and Cook, M. L. (1971). Latent herpes simplex virus in spinal ganglia of mice. *Science*, **173**, 843–845.

Tong, C. W., Potter, F. A., Pang, K. A. *et al.* (1997). Severe encephalitis with rapid recovery. *Lancet*, **349**, 470.

Twomey, J. A., Barker, C. M., Robinson, G. *et al.* (1979). Olfactory mucosa in herpes simplex encephalitis. *J. Neurol. Neurosurg. Psych.*, **42**, 983–987.

Vengsarkar, U. S. Pisipaty, R. P., Parekh, B. *et al.* (1986). Intracranial tuberculoma and the CT scan. *J. Neurosurg.*, **64**, 568–574.

Whitley, R. J. (1988). Herpes simplex virus infections of the central nervous system: a review. *Am. J. Med.*, **85**, 61–67.

Whitley, R. J. and Lakeman, F. (1995). Herpes simplex virus infections of the central nervous system: therapeutic and diagnostic considerations. *Clin. Infect. Dis.*, **20**, 414–420.

Whitley, R., Lakeman, A. D., Nahmias, A. J. *et al.* (1982a). DNA restriction-enzyme analysis of herpes simplex virus isolates obtained from patients with encephalitis. *N. Engl. J. Med.*, **307**, 1060–1062.

Whitley, J. R., Soong, S. J., Linneman, C. JR *et al.* (1982b). Herpes simplex encephalitis: Clinical assessment. *J. Am. Med. Assoc.*, **247**, 317–320.

Whitley, R. J., Alford, C. A., Hirsch, M. S. *et al.* (1986). Vidarabine versus acyclovir therapy in herpes simplex encephalitis. *N. Engl. J. Med.*, **314**, 144–149.

Whitley, R. J., Cobbs, C. G. and Alford, C. A. JR. (1989). Diseases that mimic herpes simplex encephalitis. *J. Am. Med. Assoc.*, **262**, 234–239.

6

HIV-associated dementia

Justin C. McArthur

Introduction

In the 19 years since the first cases of AIDS were recognized in 1981, this pandemic has spread to involve every continent. Our concept of the biology of HIV infection has changed radically to a model of continuous active HIV replication throughout both asymptomatic and symptomatic stages of HIV infection (Ho *et al.*, 1995). In addition, recent work indicates that resting memory CD4+ T lymphocytes may serve as a reservoir for latent HIV infection (Finzi *et al.*, 1997; Wong *et al.*, 1997). Neurological complications usually develop only in advanced infection, with immunodeficiency. HIV-associated neurological disorders include dementia, myelopathy, and sensory neuropathy, and represent a substantial source of morbidity and mortality for people with AIDS (Janssen *et al.*, 1992).

Encouraging declines have been observed in the USA in the incidence rates for various opportunistic infections, including cytomegalovirus disease, atypical mycobacterial infections, and toxoplasmosis (Moore *et al.*, 1997). These are attributable to improved antiretroviral regimens and prophylactic therapies. Downward trends in the incidence rates for HIV dementia have also been observed in cohort studies, and from surveillance by the CDC (Figure 6.1) (Brodt *et al.*, 1997). Despite these advances, HIV-associated dementia (HIV-D) will eventually develop in about 15% of individuals with AIDS.

The results of clinical trials of combination antiretroviral therapy, and the subsequent widespread introduction of highly active antiretroviral therapy (HAART) have produced a new optimism for HIV-infected patients. Current guidelines include early initiation of combination antiretrovirals which may result in virological suppression and some immune reconstitution. However, progress in developing an effective vaccine has been slow, and for at least 90% of HIV-infected persons worldwide, any treatment is unaffordable.

Therapeutic failures with combination antiretroviral regimens occur in about 50% of patients (Deeks *et al.*, 1997), and it remains uncertain whether HAART will provide a durable suppression of CNS HIV replication. There is concern that the brain might also serve as a reservoir for latent or inadequately-suppressed HIV infection. This is in part because of the unique characteristics of the blood–brain barrier which prevent CNS penetration of many available antiretrovirals. It is also partly because the principal target cells

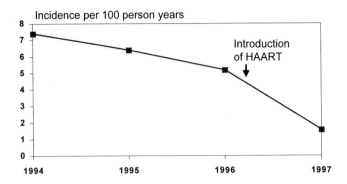

Figure 6.1 Johns Hopkins University AIDS Service: declining incidence of HIV dementia in last few years. Note that the prevalence of dementia may, in fact, rise as survival after AIDS increases. (From McArthur JC, Sacktor N, Selnes OA. HIV-associated dementia. *Seminars in Neurology* (in press)).

within the CNS – macrophages and microglia – may represent sequestered sites of HIV untouched by even potent combination antiretrovirals.

Epidemiology of the AIDS epidemic

On a worldwide scale, the World Health Organization (WHO) has estimated that approximately 42 million people have been infected with the HIV-1 virus (Mertens and Low-Beer, 1996), and that 16 000 new infections occur each day. There have been 11.7 million deaths from AIDS and in 1998 one in 100 people worldwide is infected with HIV-1. By the year 2000 the number of infections will reach 54 million.

Though the disease was originally recognized in the USA among homosexual men and injection drug users, people infected through heterosexual contact now constitute the most rapidly growing group. *In utero* transmission from mother to infant has been significantly reduced through the use of antiretrovirals during pregnancy (Connor *et al.*, 1994). Since the initial descriptions of cases of unusual pneumonia among homosexual men in Los Angeles, AIDS has expanded to become a global pandemic which is now the leading cause of death among some segments of the population. New infections are occurring at high rates among adolescents and young adults of both sexes. Heterosexual transmission is the most common mode of infection of HIV worldwide. Blood products are now an infrequent source of HIV infection in the USA, with the risk of HIV infection estimated at one in 493 000 units of blood (Schreiber *et al.*, 1996). Asia represents an area which has seen an explosive growth in the number of new infections, largely by heterosexual transmission. In some areas of world, for example Australia, downward trends in the number of new infections have been seen, probably because of intensive public education efforts. In 1995, AIDS surpassed cancer as the predominant cause of death in young Americans (25–44 years) in the USA (Centers for Disease Control and

Prevention, 1995). From the beginning of the epidemic up to December 31, 1997, there have been 641 086 cases of AIDS and 390 692 AIDS deaths in the USA (Centers for Disease Control and Prevention, 1997). A 40% fall in AIDS death rates has been seen in the USA since 1996, attributable to the use of combination antiretrovirals. Most of the dramatic change in death rates in the USA, however, was seen among white homosexual males, and women and minorities continued to show increases in AIDS death rates. The factors explaining this discrepancy probably reflect restricted access for these groups to medical care, and particularly to the newer and more potent antiretroviral therapies. Several surveys have confirmed that women of colour are least likely to be able to access the system of specialized clinics that has developed in the USA (Chaisson *et al.*, 1995; Haverkos and Quinn, 1995; Rosenberg, 1995; Quinn, 1996), although female gender *per se* is not a risk factor for more rapid disease progression (Melnick *et al.*, 1994). AIDS rates among women, children, and injecting drug users (IDUs) and HIV infection acquired through heterosexual contact have continued to rise, although the largest proportion of reported cases continues to be among homosexual men. AIDS cases among women have increased from 8 to 13% with proportional decreases in cases among homosexual men (Figure 6.2).

The most frequent disease manifestations of AIDS are listed in Table 6.1. Since the Centers for Disease Control (CDC) revised the case definition of AIDS in 1993 to include severe HIV-related immunosuppression, this is now the most common AIDS-indicator condition, accounting for 85% of cases in the USA (Centers for Disease Control and Prevention, 1995). The only AIDS-defining illness specific to women is invasive cervical carcinoma. Oesophageal candidiasis and recurrent bacterial pneumonia have higher incidence rates among women than men, while Kaposi sarcoma is far more common among homosexual males.

HIV infection has been defined, staged, and classified in a variety of different ways since the beginning of the epidemic. The currently-used system, proposed by the CDC in 1993 is used primarily for epidemiological purposes, and

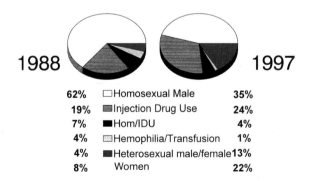

Figure 6.2   Changing epidemiology of HIV infection: risk behaviours in AIDS cases in USA. (From McArthur, J. C., Sacktor, N. and Selnes, O. A. HIV-associated dementia. *Seminars in Neurology* (in press)).

Table 6.1 Frequency of AIDS-defining illnesses in the USA, 1997 (excluding low CD4 counts) (Centers for Disease Control and Prevention, 1997).

Condition	%
Pneumocystis carinii pneumonia	38
Candida oesophagitis	14
HIV wasting syndrome	18
HIV-associated encephalopathy (HIV-associated dementia)	5
Cerebral toxoplasmosis	4
Cytomegalovirus infection	7
Mycobacterium avium or *M. kansasii*, disseminated or extrapulmonary	5
Cryptococcosis, extrapulmonary	5
Herpes simplex infection, with oesophagitis, pneumonitis or chronic mucocutaneous ulcers	4
Extrapulmonary tuberculosis	2
Cryptosporidiosis	1
Lymphoma, primary in brain	1
Kaposi sarcoma	7

categorizes infection into asymptomatic (stage A), symptomatic but without AIDS-defining illnesses (stage B), and AIDS-defining illnesses (stage C). Further classification by the level of CD4 count is made.

The early diagnosis of HIV infection is particularly important in women to permit treatment and to decrease the risk of both sexual and vertical transmission (mother to child). An NIH-funded trial showed that the use of zidovudine during pregnancy and intravenously during labour, with continued use in the infant for 6 weeks cut the transmission risk from 26% to 8% (Connor *et al.*, 1994; Sorell and Kesson, 1995; Mijch *et al.*, 1997). This is now the standard of care, with use of HIV RNA polymerase chain reaction (PCR) in the newborn to assess the state of infection.

The results of clinical trials of combination antiretroviral therapy, and the subsequent widespread introduction of highly active antiretroviral therapy (HAART) have produced a new era of optimism for the care of HIV-infected patients. However, for at least 90% of HIV-infected persons worldwide, these expensive treatments are out of reach, and progress on an effective vaccine has been slow.

Biology of HIV infection

The virus

There are important parallels between the human infection and the animal lentivirus infections, because all lentiviruses cause an encephalitis (Johnson *et al.*, 1988). The lentiviruses or 'slow viruses,' of which HIV-1 is a member, share certain pathogenic similarities, including mechanisms by which they evade host defences and immune clearance and cause persistent infection. They typically have long incubation periods and are associated with chronic diseases occurring in nature. They comprise: visna virus, with which HIV-1 shares

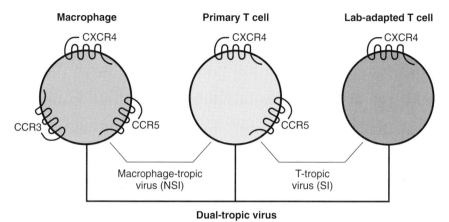

Figure 6.3   Coreceptor use by HIV.

morphological and genomic characteristics; caprine arthritis encephalitis virus; equine infectious anaemia virus; bovine immunodeficiency virus; and feline immunodeficiency virus. Human infection with HIV-2 and simian disease with SIV-1, which produces an AIDS-like syndrome after experimental inoculation in macaques, complete the currently recognized list. HIV-2 is a retrovirus distinct from HIV-1, which is prevalent in part of Western Africa (De-The *et al.*, 1989). Although there have been some reports of neurological disease associated with HIV-2, it is not frequent in the West.

HIV is a non-transforming retrovirus that produces a cytopathic or lytic effect on T-cells, although the precise mechanisms for T-cell depletion are uncertain. The CD4 receptor is the principal target site for HIV; however, specific chemokine receptors appear to serve as important secondary cellular receptors for HIV (Premack and Schall, 1996; He *et al.*, 1997). HIV-1 strains have been divided into T-tropic (preferring to replicate in T lymphocytes) and M-tropic (macrophages) on the basis of *in vitro* experiments. The chemokine receptor usage is different for each with T-tropic viruses making use of CD4 and CXR4 (or fusin, the receptor for SDF-1), and M-tropic making use of CCR5 (receptor for RANTES) (Figure 6.3). A genetic variant of CCR5, Delta32, has been found to be protective against HIV infection and to delay disease progression.

HIV structure and life cycle

The retrovirus family, retroviridae, is composed of three major subfamilies: lentivirus, to which HIV belongs (lenti : slow); oncovirus, to which HTLV-l belongs (onco : tumour); and spumavirus (spuma : foam). Of these three subfamilies, members of the lentivirus and oncoviruses have been linked to neurological disease in humans, but to date, spumaviruses do not appear to cause human disease. The retroviruses share genomic and morphological similarities and may have originally derived from an ancestral virus. The

Table 6.2   Common properties of lentiviruses.

Contain RNA genome and reverse transcriptase
Host specific
Prolonged incubation period
Persistent infections in natural hosts
Restricted viral replication
Cytopathic effects *in vitro*
Infect cells of the immune system

retroviruses include a number of RNA viruses which replicate in a unique manner; their other distinguishing characteristics are listed in Table 6.2.

The viruses are distinguished from other viruses because they carry a unique pair of enzymes; first, an RNA-dependent DNA polymerase (reverse transcriptase), which uses RNA as a template to make a complementary DNA strand, and a second enzyme (a ribonuclease) which breaks down the original RNA strand, thus allowing a complementary DNA strand to be synthesized on the remaining DNA strand. After the double-stranded DNA has been synthesized, it is incorporated by the enzyme integrase into the host cell DNA and replicates with it. Once integrated into the host cell genome, it is termed a provirus, and may remain latent for months or years, without affecting cellular function. Alternatively, the provirus may separate from the host cell DNA to produce retrovirus mRNA, which directs viral protein synthesis.

The HIV virion is a relatively large, icosahedral structure with numerous external spikes (Figure 6.4). The envelope spikes are composed of gp120 with a transmembrane component, gp41. The lipid bilayer is derived from host proteins during viral budding. The core is formed from four nucleic capsid proteins: p24 (the major component), p17, p9, and p7. Genomic structure of HIV includes genes that code for structural proteins and several genes that code for regulatory proteins (Figure 6.5). The three groups of structural proteins are coded for by the *gap*, *pol*, and *env* regions of the HIV gene. The *env* gene encodes for the two major envelope proteins, gp120 and gp41; gp120 is a large glycoprotein that forms the surface spikes of the virion, while gp41 is a transmembrane glycoprotein. The two envelope proteins are critical for viral binding and cell fusion. The *pol* region codes for reverse transcriptase, a protease and an endonuclease. Endonuclease is critical for the integration of DNA into the host genome and the protease cleaves the polyproteins encoded for by *gag* and *pol* into their active forms. The *gag* region encodes for the core proteins, including p24, the nucleoid shell and several smaller proteins. Additional information is available in two reviews (Levy, 1989; Greene, 1991). At least five genes (*tat*, *rev*, *nef*, *vif*, and *vpr*) are involved in the regulation of HIV-1 replication (Figure 6.6).

Initially it was thought that infection and integration of HIV DNA into the host cell genome was followed by a long period of virological and clinical latency. Recent work has shown that even during the period of clinical latency, there is very active viral replication and release of active virions (Michael *et al.*, 1992; Ho *et al.*, 1995). Current concepts of HIV infection include a very rapid

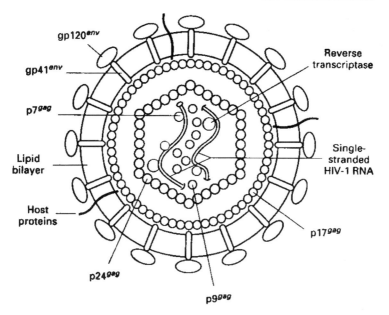

Figure 6.4   Structure of the HIV-1 virion (From Harrison, M. J. G. and McArthur, J. C. (1995) *AIDS and Neurology*, Edinburgh: Churchill Livingstone., after Greene 1991)

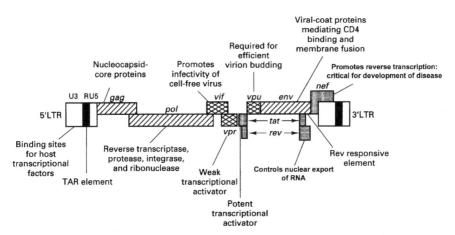

Figure 6.5   Genome of HIV-1 (from Harrison and McArthur 1995, after Greene 1991).

turnover of CD4 lymphocytes (approximately 2 billion daily), with release of approximately 10 billion new virions daily. The half-life of virions in plasma is about 6 h, and in actively infected CD4 lymphocytes, about 1.4 days (Coffin, 1996; Saag, 1997). A new generation of HIV is produced in 2.6 days, yielding 140 generations in a year. With millions of replicative cycles daily, and a relatively high error rate in RNA transcription, resistant mutants can arise readily unless HIV replication is suppressed. This rapid replication leads to the establishment of a *swarm* of related HIV quasispecies within an individual.

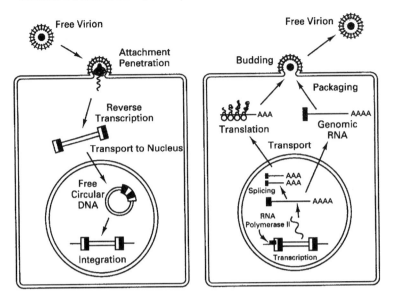

Figure 6.6 Retrovirus replication (from Harrison and McArthur 1995, after Hasaltine 1989).

Differences among HIV strains may account for biological differences in tropism or virulence. Other compartments, including tissue macrophages, and resting memory lymphocytes harbour HIV, although the dynamics of HIV replication are more attenuated in these cellular compartments. Resting memory CD4+ T lymphocytes may serve as a reservoir for latent HIV infection (Finzi *et al.*, 1997; Wong *et al.*, 1997), and seminal fluid cells may contain replication competent proviruses in individuals receiving HAART (Zhang *et al.*, 1998). In infected persons with high viral loads the capacity for CD4 cell regeneration becomes exhausted sooner, leading to the earlier onset of immunodeficiency and AIDS. Several studies have now shown the strong predictive value of plasma viral load, and CD4 count also has an independent predictive value (Mellors *et al.*, 1995, 1997). As an example, Mellors indicates that an individual with plasma HIV levels > 30 000 copies/ml has about a 60% risk of developing AIDS over 5 years, compared to a risk of < 10% if plasma level is < 4000. Coffin has used the analogy of a speeding train, with plasma load indicating the *velocity* of the train and CD4 count the *distance* travelled down the track towards AIDS (Coffin, 1996).

Most patients show a slow decline in CD4 counts during the asymptomatic period, with an average annual drop of 50–100 cells/mm^3. Some HIV-infected individuals, however, show remarkable stability in CD4 levels for many years, suggesting that their infection is held under closer control, through uncertain mechanisms. Eventually the virus 'escapes', overwhelming the lymphoreticular system, and a rapid increase in HIV RNA levels is associated with the onset of symptomatic disease (Figure 6.7) (Pantaleo *et al.*, 1993). The development of reliable, commercially available tests to measure plasma HIV RNA levels has

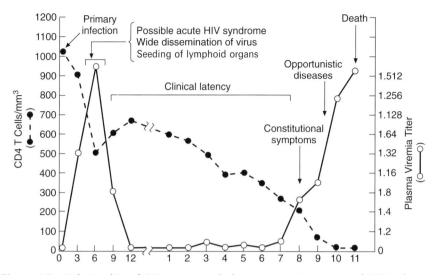

Figure 6.7   Relationship of CD4 count and plasma viraemia to stage of HIV infection and clinical consequences (From Harrison and McArthur 1995, after Pantaleo 1993).

significantly altered the management of HIV infection. Although plasma HIV RNA levels represent only about 2% of total body levels, they reflect the turnover of HIV within lymph nodes. Several studies, using either quantitative polymerase chain reaction (PCR) or branched DNA (bDNA) techniques, have shown that viral load monitoring is a powerful predictor of disease progression and clinical outcomes (Schooley, 1995). Mellors *et al.* (1995) showed that plasma HIV-1 RNA was a strong CD4-independent predictor of rapid progression to AIDS. Studies of plasma viral load have determined that decreases in plasma RNA confer significant reduction in the risk of disease progression in the controlled clinical trials (Merigan and Schooley, 1995; O'Brien *et al.*, 1996; Saag *et al.*, 1996). Plasma HIV RNA levels are now monitored regularly, with CD4 counts, to monitor the response of the infection to HAART. Rising plasma HIV levels indicate therapeutic failure, in many indicating the development of resistance mutations, in some reflecting poor medication adherence.

The major effect of HIV infection on the immune system is the profound and progressive loss of CD4 lymphocytes. Proposed mechanisms include CD4 killing associated with viral budding, cell fusion with syncytia formation, and virus-specific immune responses. This loss of the regulatory CD4 subset appears to lead to a dysregulation of macrophages, with the overproduction of a variety of pro-inflammatory cytokines and chemokines. This may be particularly important for the development of HIV dementia and sensory neuropathy, as is discussed in other sections (Tyor *et al.*, 1995).

HIV enters the nervous system early after infection, but at this time point, before immunosuppression has developed, it is uncertain that a persistent infection is established. It is more likely that CNS reseeding occurs later, after immunosuppression has developed. The monocyte/macrophage appears to play a critical role in carrying HIV into the brain. The ingress of infected monocytes may be dependent on the presence of circulating activated monocytes. Recently, Pulliam and colleagues showed that patients with HIV dementia had higher levels of circulating activated monocytes bearing CD14 +/ CD69 + (Pulliam *et al.*, 1997).

Clinical and pathological features of HIV-associated dementia

Epidemiology of HIVD

Within the first year or two of clinical experience with AIDS it became apparent that many patients developed cognitive impairment (Snider *et al.*, 1983; Levy *et al.*, 1985). At first, this psychomotor slowing and mental dulling was mistakenly attributed to 'depression' or 'delirium' or confused with opportunistic infections of the nervous system.

Risk factors for HIVD include anaemia, low weight, and constitutional symptoms, i.e. dementia develops in 'sicker' patients (McArthur *et al.*, 1993). Higher plasma HIV RNA levels and lower CD4 counts are predictive, both of dementia and sensory neuropathy (Childs *et al.*, 1998). Recently, one study has suggested that individuals with the E4 isoform of apolipoprotein E are at higher risk for development of dementia. This is an important observation which requires confirmation and shows that gene–viral interactions may be important.

In adults, only 3% of AIDS cases *present* initially with dementia as their first AIDS defining illness; more typically, dementia develops *after* constitutional symptoms, immune deficiency and systemic opportunistic processes (McArthur, 1987; Navia and Price, 1987; Janssen *et al.*, 1992). Typically, the onset of dementia is relatively insidious, developing over months. In antiretroviral naive patients, however, dementia can develop over weeks. By contrast, the CNS opportunistic infections, like CMV encephalitis and toxoplasmosis have a more rapid course (see Table 6.3). In children, progressive dementia occurs more commonly than opportunistic infections (Epstein *et al.*, 1985; Mintz *et al.*, 1989). Belman estimated that 62% of children developed dementia in the years before effective antiretrovirals (Belman *et al.*, 1988).

Table 6.3 Differentiation of HIV dementia from opportunistic infections.

Disorder	HIV dementia	CMV encephalitis	PML
Features	Memory, mental slowing, gait	Delirium, seizures, brainstorm signs	Focal neurosigns
Course	Several months	Days–weeks	Weeks–months
Typical CD4 range	< 500	< 100	< 100
MRI	Diffuse atrophy/deep WM diffuse hyperintensity	Normal or periventriculitis	Subcortical WM lesions
CSF	Non-specific; immune activation	PCR + 90%	PCR + 60%

Since the introduction of HAART in developed countries, around 1996, the incidence of HIV-D in patients with good medication compliance has been decreasing. However, cognitive impairment eventually develops in about 30% of people with AIDS and frank dementia in about 15%, with an annual incidence after AIDS of approximately 5% (McArthur *et al.*, 1993; Moore *et al.*, 1998).

Terminology

The neurological literature has developed several different terms over the past decade to describe the encephalopathy which we now term HIV-associated dementia or HIV dementia. HIV dementia was originally termed 'subacute encephalitis' (Snider *et al.*, 1983). Later, Navia *et al.* (1986b) used the phrase 'AIDS dementia complex' to indicate the association with AIDS, the predominance of cognitive impairment and dementia in the syndrome, but the additional term 'complex' to indicate the prevalence of motor deficits and myelopathy. 'HIV encephalopathy' was added to the list of AIDS-defining illnesses in 1987 (Centers for Disease Control, 1987) and in 1991, the American Academy of Neurology AIDS Task Force (Janssen *et al.*, 1991) developed terminology and definitional criteria for AIDS dementia, myelopathy, neuropathy, and minor forms of cognitive impairment. These definitional criteria have improved clinicopathological correlations and helped to define the natural history and response to antiretroviral therapy.

The terms AIDS dementia complex, HIV dementia, HIV encephalopathy, and the more recently introduced term, *HIV-associated dementia complex*, are synonymous. Minor degrees of cognitive, motor, and functional impairment which are not sufficient to diagnose dementia are termed '*HIV-associated minor cognitive/motor disorder*'. Because it is uncertain whether this minor impairment always progresses to frank dementia, it is reasonable to maintain this as a separate term. The term 'HIV encephalitis' should be reserved for the pathological features of multinucleated giant cell encephalitis with HIV identified in the brain and *not* used to describe the clinical syndrome. Similarly, while HIV-associated dementia complex can develop concurrently with other HIV-associated neurological disorders such as myelopathy and neuropathy, it appears that these are all discrete disorders with different manifestations, courses, and treatments.

Price and colleagues (1988) have developed a staging scheme for dementia severity that is useful both in clinical practice and for research studies (Table 6.4).

Frequency of neurocognitive deficits in different stages of HIV infection

Several groups have described high rates of neuropsychological test abnormalities in healthy HIV-1-infected homosexual men (Grant *et al.*, 1987; Janssen *et al.*, 1988) and in injecting drug users (Silberstein *et al.*, 1987). Mayeux *et al.* (1993) found that new cognitive abnormalities in symptomatic HIV infection predicted reduced survival. Cognitive decline on tests of psychomotor speed,

Table 6.4   Clinical staging of HIV associated dementia

Stage	Clinical description
Stage 0 (normal)	Normal mental and motor function
Stage 0.5 (equivocal/subclinical)	Absent, minimal, or equivocal symptoms without impairment of work or capacity to perform ADL. Mild signs (snout response, slowed ocular or extremity movements) may be present. Gait and strength are normal.
Stage 1 (mild)	Able to perform all but the more demanding aspects of work or ADL but with unequivocal evidence (signs or symptoms that may include performance on neuropsychological testing) of functional intellectual or motor impairment. Can walk without assistance.
Stage 2 (moderate)	Able to perform basic activities of self-care but cannot work or maintain the more demanding aspects of daily life. Ambulatory, but may require a single prop.
Stage 3 (severe)	Major intellectual incapacity (cannot follow news or personal events, cannot sustain complex conversation, considerable slowing of all outputs) or motor disability (cannot walk unassisted, requiring walker or personal support, usually with slowing and clumsiness of arms as well).
Stage 4 (end stage)	Nearly vegetative. Intellectual and social comprehension and output are at a rudimentary level. Nearly or absolutely mute. Paraparetic or paraplegic with urinary and a faecal incontinence.

Developed at Memorial Sloan Kettering Center (Price and Brew, 1988).

that is sustained at a subsequent visit, is also predictive of poor survival (Sacktor *et al.*, 1996). The clinical significance of new cognitive symptoms or test impairment in *asymptomatic* HIV infection is uncertain because the reported neuropsychological abnormalities do not necessarily progress and may reflect the effects of low education, age, and alcohol and drug use. For example, among several hundred homosexual HIV-1 seropositive men without AIDS, the prevalence of HIV dementia was less than 1% and the frequency of neuropsychological impairment was no higher than in HIV-1 seronegatives (McArthur *et al.*, 1989). Similar results have been described in injecting drug users (Royal *et al.*, 1991). From longitudinal neuropsychological evaluation in cohorts of homosexual men and injecting drug users, no evidence for cognitive decline was found during the asymptomatic phase of infection (Selnes *et al.*, 1990, 1992).

Earlier reports of frequent neuropsychological abnormalities among asymptomatic seropositives provoked concern that dementia might be a very early event (Grant *et al.*, 1987). Subsequent studies have suggested that these findings more likely reflect other confounding factors rather than the effects of CNS HIV infection, as reviewed by Newman and Harrison (1995).

In summary, it appears that dementia is rare during the asymptomatic phase of HIV infection. In later stages of HIV infection, however, progression of neurocognitive deficits to frank dementia is more common. The Dana cohort is a cohort of subjects at high risk for dementia (with a CD4 count <200 or a CD4 count <300 with cognitive symptoms) (The Dana Consortium on Therapy for HIV Dementia and Related Cognitive Disorders, 1996). Among subjects in the Dana cohort who were not impaired at baseline, over one year 17% went on to develop HIV-associated minor cognitive/motor disorder and 9% developed HIV-D (Marder *et al.*, 1998).

Clinical features of HIV dementia

In adults, the clinical manifestations of HIV dementia suggest early and predominant subcortical involvement (Navia *et al.*, 1986b). Typical symptoms of HIV-D include increasing forgetfulness, difficulty with concentration, loss of libido, apathy, inertia, and waning interest in work and hobbies resulting in social withdrawal (Figure 6.8). Patients complain of losing track of conversations and the plots of books and films and of taking longer to complete more complex daily tasks. Impaired short-term memory causes difficulty with remembering appointments, medications, and telephone numbers. Motor complaints include poor handwriting, insecure balance, and a tendency to drop things easily. Gait difficulty is a relatively early symptom. Friends and partners report change in personality with apathy and social withdrawal and blunting of emotional responsiveness. Considerable variability in presentation has been reported, and in 5% agitation or mania may be the initial manifestation (Navia *et al.*, 1986b). The early symptoms are often subtle and may be overlooked or confused with psychiatric complaints, the effects of substance abuse, or delirium (Table 6.5). This reinforces the need for screening of individuals at highest risk: those with unsuppressed plasma HIV RNA and CD4 <200. Screening is recommended in those individuals (see below). Neuropsychological features of HIV dementia reflect the prominence of

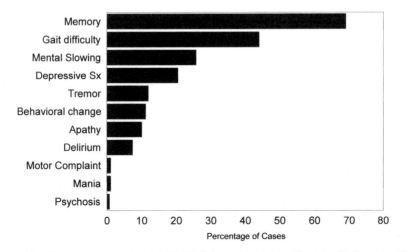

Figure 6.8 Symptoms associated with HIV dementia. Johns Hopkins University AIDS Service.

Table 6.5   Differential diagnosis of mild HIV dementia.

Anxiety
Depression
Alcohol
Recreational drugs
Medication side-effects
Metabolic encephalopathy
Vitamin B_{12} deficiency
Drug interactions with protease inhibitors

subcortical involvement initially and are characterized by memory loss selective for impaired retrieval; impaired manipulation of acquired knowledge; and a general slowing of psychomotor speed and thought processes. Neuropsychological testing adds to the neurological evaluation of suspected HIV dementia by virtue of being sensitive to mild or early symptoms of HIV-related cognitive impairment. In addition to quantifying the severity of any cognitive symptoms, it can also provide information regarding the overall pattern of cognitive impairment.

For example, attention, calculations, and language are usually not affected in HIV dementia, at least initially, fitting with the subcortical pattern of involvement. Memory impairments, both verbal and non-verbal, and deficits in psychomotor speed are characteristic of HIV dementia and are typically more severe than deficits in other cognitive domains (Figure 6.9). As with other neurodiagnostic tests, the neuropsychological test results are not specific and thus not sufficient by themselves to establish a diagnosis of HIV dementia.

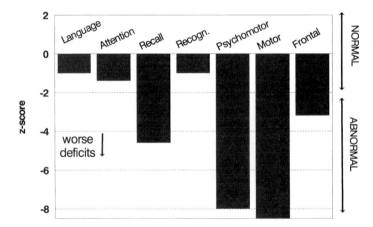

Figure 6.9   Typical neuropsychological profile from 53-year-old homosexual man with moderate HIV dementia. Vertical axis indicates z score of performance (standard deviation units). Note relatively preserved language, attention, and recognition memory, but severely impaired recall memory and test of psychomotor speed. (From McArthur, J. C., Sacktor, N. and Selnes, O. A. HIV-associated dementia. *Seminars in Neurology* (in press))

Neuropsychological testing, therefore, should be an adjunct to the neurological examination, and any abnormalities should be interpreted in the context of the clinical history and other laboratory findings. The influence of premorbid conditions, including previous head trauma, learning disability, as well as the effects of systemic illness and substance abuse need to be considered carefully when interpreting results from neuropsychological testing. Age and education are particularly critical variables which influence neuropsychological test performance independently. The most useful tests for screening for HIV dementia are those which examine psychomotor speed – Trailmaking, Grooved Pegboard, Symbol-Digit. The HIV Dementia Scale is a modification of the Mini Mental Status Exam (Power *et al.*, 1995). It has the advantage of being extremely simple and rapid, and can be easily used by non-neurologists (Figure 6.10).

With advancing dementia, new learning and memory deteriorate, there is a further slowing of mental processing, and abulia with reduced output of spontaneous speech (Table 6.6). The terminal phases of the syndrome are characterized by a global impairment with severe psychomotor retardation and mutism. Many of these patients are very sensitive to the effects of sedatives, which may provoke delirium, or to neuroleptics, to which there appears to be a heightened sensitivity (Hriso *et al.*, 1991).

Neurological examination is often normal in the early stages of HIV dementia, although there may be impairments of rapid eye and limb movements and diffuse hyperreflexia. As HIV dementia progresses, increased tone develops, particularly in the lower extremities, and is usually associated with tremor, clonus, release signs, and hyperactive reflexes. Some of these signs may reflect the effects of an accompanying HIV-related myelopathy (Petito *et al.*, 1985). In some patients myelopathy is the predominant neurological problem, with severe paraparesis but only mild cognitive involvement. The clinical features include the progressive development of a spastic paraparesis, with variable sensory ataxia and bladder involvement. No sensory level is evident, and the arms are usually spared. Sensory neuropathy may develop

Table 6.6 Features of HIV-associated dementia.

	Early	*Late*
Behaviour	Apathy 'Depression' Agitation/mania	Mutism Abulia Hallucinations
Cognition	Memory loss Concentration Mental slowing Reading comprehension	Global impairment Severe psychomotor slowing Reduced insight

Neurological symptoms/signs	Unsteady gait
	Poor coordination
	Tremor
		Hyperreflexia, hypertonia
		  release signs
		Myelopathy, neuropathy
		Sensitivity to neuroleptic
		  agents

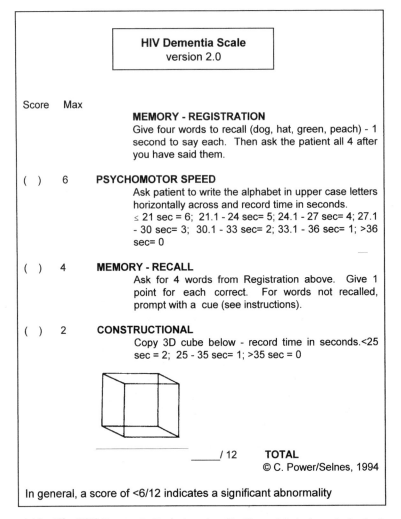

HIV Dementia Scale
version 2.0

Score   Max

MEMORY - REGISTRATION
Give four words to recall (dog, hat, green, peach) - 1 second to say each. Then ask the patient all 4 after you have said them.

( )   6   **PSYCHOMOTOR SPEED**
Ask patient to write the alphabet in upper case letters horizontally across and record time in seconds.
≤ 21 sec = 6; 21.1 - 24 sec= 5; 24.1 - 27 sec= 4; 27.1 - 30 sec= 3; 30.1 - 33 sec= 2; 33.1 - 36 sec= 1; >36 sec= 0

( )   4   **MEMORY - RECALL**
Ask for 4 words from Registration above. Give 1 point for each correct. For words not recalled, prompt with a cue (see instructions).

( )   2   **CONSTRUCTIONAL**
Copy 3D cube below - record time in seconds.<25 sec = 2; 25 - 35 sec= 1; >35 sec = 0

_____ / 12   **TOTAL**
© C. Power/Selnes, 1994

In general, a score of <6/12 indicates a significant abnormality

Figure 6.10   The HIV Dementia Scale (version 2). (From McArthur, J. C., Sacktor, N. and Selnes O. A. HIV-associated dementia. *Seminars in Neurology* (in press))

concurrently. *Focal* neurological signs usually point to CNS opportunistic processes rather than HIV dementia. Retinal 'cotton-wool' spots occur in 60% of patients with AIDS, but are not pathognomonic for HIV dementia (Pomerantz *et al.*, 1987). Myoclonus and other involuntary movements are not common features, but generalized seizures may occur (So *et al.*, 1990). Without treatment, the dementia is typically rapidly progressive, with a mean survival of about 6 months, less than half the average survival of non-demented AIDS patients (McArthur, 1987; Rothenberg *et al.*, 1987). However, the progression of HIV dementia can be quite variable, some patients having a 'typical' progression with worsening neurological deficits over 3–6 months, while others remain only mildly demented and cognitively stable right up until

Table 6.7 Clinical features useful for diagnosis of HIV-1 related dementia.

HIV-1 seropositivity

History of *progressive* cognitive/behavioral decline with apathy, memory loss, slowed mental processing

Neurological exam: diffuse CNS signs including slowed rapid eye/limb movements, hyperreflexia, hypertonia, and release signs

Neuropsychological assessment: impairment in at least two areas including frontal lobe, motor speed, and non-verbal memory

CSF analysis: exclusion of neurosyphilis and cryptococcal meningitis

Imaging studies: diffuse cerebral atrophy with ill-defined white matter hyperintensities on MRI, exclusion of opportunistic processes

Absence of major psychiatric disorder or intoxication

Absence of metabolic derangement, e.g. hypoxia, sepsis

Absence of active CNS opportunistic processes

death. The cause of this variability is determined partly by the degree of immunodeficiency at onset of dementia. Those with CD4 counts less than 100 tend to progress more quickly (Bouwman *et al.*, 1998). Survival after diagnosis of AIDS has improved significantly over the past few years with the advent of HAART, and this is likely to extend the survival of patients with HIV-D.

Differentiation from infections such as CMV encephalitis, cerebral toxo-plasmosis, neurosyphilis, and cryptococcal or tuberculous meningitis is critical. Table 6.7 lists features that may be helpful in establishing the diagnosis of HIV dementia. Table 6.3 indicates the clinical features which distinguish HIV dementia from other CNS processes. One frequent CNS opportunistic infection which is easily mistaken for HIV dementia is CMV encephalitis. This was relatively common, occurring in up to 5% of patients with AIDS as a rapidly developing encephalopathy. In the last few years, however, incidence rates of CMV disease have dropped considerably under the influence of HAART. Features distinguishing CMV encephalitis from HIV dementia include: co-existing CMV infection (retinitis, colitis, etc); hyponatraemia reflecting CMV adrenalitis; and periventricular abnormalities on MRI con-sistent with a periventriculitis (Holland *et al.*, 1994).

Clinical features in children include microcephaly, progressive motor dysfunction and developmental delay, leading to loss of milestones, with death occurring within the first few years of life.

Laboratory findings

1 CSF findings

The majority of patients with HIV dementia will have abnormalities of routine constituents; however, identical CSF abnormalities are frequently found in neurologically *normal* HIV seropositives. Lumbar puncture is important to exclude opportunistic infections in the patient with suspected HIV dementia who has fever or other atypical features. In a typical case, however, screening of peripheral blood for cryptococcal antigen, vitamin B_{12} and RPR (rapid plasma reagin) is adequate. The CSF is usually acellular, or shows a mild lymphocytic pleocytosis. Elevated total protein is found in about 65% of cases and increased total immunoglobulin (IgG) fraction in up to 80% (McArthur, 1987). Oligoclonal bands are found in up to 35%, but myelin basic protein is usually not elevated. The immune activation marker, $\beta 2$ micro-globulin, is useful in diagnosis, particularly in mild dementia in the absence of opportunistic infections, and a value ≥ 3.8 mg/dl has a positive predictive value of 88% (McArthur *et al.*, 1992). In an individual patient, the absolute levels of CSF HIV RNA are not diagnostic of HIV-D. However, CSF HIV RNA levels correlate with the severity of dementia (Figure 6.11), and it might be useful to measure CSF levels if dementia develops despite systemic virological suppression.

Pialoux *et al.* (1997) report a patient with undetectable plasma HIV RNA and CSF HIV RNA greater than 1 million copies/ml. This scenario of progressive HIV-D with high CSF HIV RNA when plasma HIV RNA is suppressed would be termed 'CNS escape'. We anticipate that it may be seen more frequently, especially in patients who have received HAART for prolonged periods of time, and where compliance may be less than adequate. The CNS and other sequestered sites such as the semen may become sites of viral replication (Zhang *et al.*, 1998). Even with successful suppression of plasma HIV, there might be viral sequestration within the central nervous system, with 'escape' of HIV replication. Resistant strains of HIV-1 that are no longer susceptible to HAART can develop from incomplete adherence, the underdosing of antiretroviral medications, or the concomitant administration of other medications.

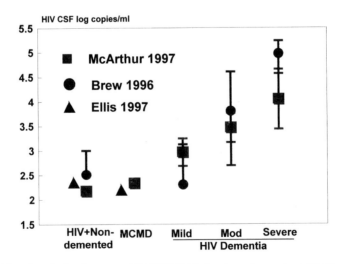

Figure 6.11   Correlation between CSF HIV RNA levels and severity of HIV-associated dementia. (From McArthur, J. C. Understanding measurement of CSF HIV levels. *HIV Neurology Newsletter*, 1998; 1:1–8.

Table 6.8 Radiological pattern of HIV-related CNS disease.

Disorder	Number	Pattern	Enhancement	Location
HIV encephalitis	Diffuse	Ill-defined	0	Deep white
Toxoplasmosis	1 – many	Ring mass	++	Basal ganglia
1° lymphoma	1 – several	Solid mass	+++	Periventricular
PML	1 – several	No mass effect	0	Subcortical white
Cryptococcus	1 – many	'Lacunar'	0	Basal ganglia
CMV encephalitis	1 – several	Confluent	++	Periventricular

Modified from Price, R. W. American Academy of Neurology Course 1991.

2 Imaging studies

Imaging studies are critical in the evaluation of suspected HIV dementia to exclude opportunistic processes. Table 6.8 contrasts the different radiological patterns. Radiological features of HIV dementia include both central and cortical atrophy and white matter abnormalities. In children, calcifications of the basal ganglia are commonly seen on CT scan. Diffuse cerebral atrophy can sometimes be observed to progress in parallel with clinical deterioration, however, some studies have shown no relationship between the degree of atrophy and cognitive impairment (Di Sclafani et al., 1997). White matter hyperintensities (on MRI) or attenuation (on CT) correlate with HIV leukoencephalitis, and are helpful diagnostically. MRI demonstrates white matter abnormalities better than CT (Levy et al., 1986; Price and Navia, 1987). These often evolve from small ill-defined hyperintensities seen in deep white matter in patients with early HIV dementia to more diffuse abnormalities in severely demented individuals (Figure 6.12). Perturbation of the blood–brain barrier has been shown with contrast MRI quantitation (Berger et al., 1996), but contrast enhancement is not typically overt. Quantitative MRI studies have shown that selective caudate region atrophy occurs in HIV dementia (Dal Pan et al., 1992), and that there is loss of grey matter volume diffusely (Aylward et al., 1993). Proton MR spectroscopy (MRS) may be sensitive to changes in markers of neuronal viability such as NAA (N-acetylaspartate) even in areas that appear normal on standard MR images (Menon et al., 1990). This is particularly relevant with the recent observations of neuronal loss in cortical areas (Everall et al., 1991; Masliah et al., 1992b). Myoinositol may be an even earlier marker of CNS damage reflecting glial turnover (Chang L, personal communication). Proton MRS is being used as an outcome measure in an ongoing trial of memantine for HIV dementia as specific biochemical markers of brain injury correlate with the degree of neurological deficits (Navia et al., 1998). Over the course of the trial with memantine it is hoped that normalization of these biochemical deficits will be seen. MRS may become another method to assess brain damage reliably, and to measure treatment response.

Both single positron emission computed tomography (SPECT) and positron emission tomography (PET) have been used in small numbers of individuals with HIV dementia. Using PET, Rottenberg and colleagues demonstrated subcortical hypermetabolism in the early stages of HIV dementia, with later

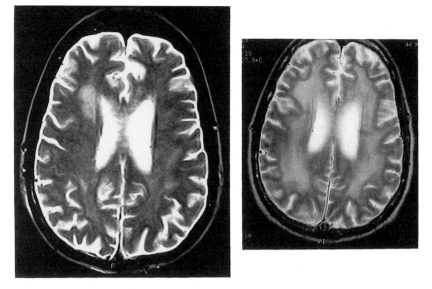

Figure 6.12   Serial T2-weighted MRI scans revealing evolution of visible white matter changes over 6 months. (From Harrison and McArthur, 1995)

progression to cortical and subcortical hypometabolism (Rottenberg *et al.*, 1987). Normalization of PET abnormalities has also been shown with administration of antiretrovirals (Yarchoan *et al.*, 1987). With SPECT, abnormalities in cerebral blood flow are frequently identified (LaFrance *et al.*, 1988), however, some of these changes may represent the effects of cocaine (Handelsman *et al.*, 1992). Neither PET nor SPECT are useful in detection of HIV dementia or in assessing treatment effects.

3 EEG

Minor EEG abnormalities have been reported in asymptomatic HIV sero-positives (Koralnik *et al.*, 1990), but not confirmed by others (Nuwer *et al.*, 1992). As with the neuropsychological tests, their clinical significance is uncertain. EEG has not been systematically studied in either the diagnosis or staging of HIV dementia. In the late stages of HIV dementia a diffuse slowing is frequently noted (Navia *et al.*, 1986b), however, in less advanced stages of dementia the EEG may be normal in 50% of patients (McArthur, 1987). The specificity of EEG in differentiating psychiatric disorders from early dementia is uncertain and in general neither standard EEG nor computerized spectral analysis adds significant information.

Pathological features

1 Pathology: *macroscopic and microscopic*

Cerebral atrophy is common in patients with HIV dementia, often occurring in a frontotemporal distribution. The pathology of HIV-D is that of a chronic encephalitis with marked macrophage activation, and has been well summarized by others (Budka *et al.*, 1991; Navia *et al.*, 1986a). Multiple small nodules containing macrophages, lymphocytes and microglia (termed microglial nodules) are scattered throughout both grey and white matter of the brain, appearing more commonly in white matter and the subcortical grey matter of the thalamus, basal ganglia, and brainstem (de La Monte *et al.*, 1987). These inflammatory nodules are not specific for HIV-1 infection and occur in other infections, including toxoplasmosis and cytomegalovirus encephalitis. The number of nodules does not correlate with the severity of the dementia (Navia *et al.*, 1986a). Multinucleated giant cells are also characteristically seen (Sharer *et al.*, 1985; Budka, 1986; Rhodes, 1987) and their presence correlates both with the degree of dementia and the detection of HIV-1 DNA (Figure 6.13) (Price *et al.*, 1988). These giant cells are thought to reflect HIV-1 replication, since giant multinucleated cells form in HIV-infected macrophage cultures (Gartner *et al.*, 1986). Perivascular infiltrations of lymphocytes and monocyte/macrophages are also frequently seen (Navia *et al.*, 1986a; Wiley *et al.*, 1986; de la Monte *et al.*, 1987; Rhodes, 1987). The inflammatory infiltrates, multinucleated giant cells and endothelial cells have been demonstrated to contain viral nucleic acid sequences (Wiley *et al.*, 1986). Other neuropathological changes include myelin pallor, which corresponds to perturbation of the blood–brain barrier (Power *et al.*, 1993), neuronal loss (Ketzler *et al.*, 1990) and dendritic changes (Masliah *et al.*, 1992a). A large number of correlative studies have been completed examining the association between macro- and microscopic abnormalities and the presence of neurological disease (clinical dementia) or the neuropathological abnormalities characteristic of HIV infection (encephalitis: multinucleated giant cells, microglial nodules, and expression of HIV antigens). Interpretation of some of these studies is difficult because of differences in the terminology and definitional criteria used. As Mucke and Buttini (1998) have summarized, cortical atrophy and neuronal loss are frequent in AIDS, but does not correlate well with clinical

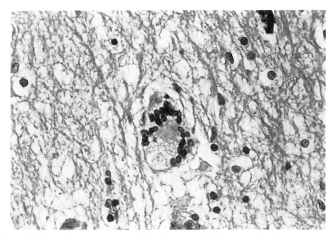

Figure 6.13   Multinucleated giant cell in focus of HIV encephalitis.

dementia or the presence of HIV encephalitis (Weis *et al.*, 1993; Everall *et al.*, 1994). Apoptosis of neurons, astrocytes, and endothelial cells has been demonstrated (Shi *et al.*, 1996), but does not correlate particularly well with the severity of neurological disease. On the other hand, dementia is associated with an increased clustering of neurons (Asare *et al.*, 1996) and encephalitis correlates with decreased dendritic and synaptic density (Masliah *et al.*, 1992b) and a loss of specific neuronal subpopulations, including calbindin-positive, parvalbumin-positive and somatostatin-positive neurons (Fox *et al.*, 1997; Masliah *et al.*, 1992c, 1995). These observations suggest that HIV dementia is associated with relatively localized and specific damage to particular subpopulations of neurons, rather than massive, widespread neuronal death.

The neuropathological features of HIV dementia in children differ somewhat from those in adults. Vascular mineralization of the basal ganglia and white matter are common (Belman *et al.*, 1986). Perivenular infiltrates and multi-nucleated giant cells are seen both in adults and children, but white matter pallor is difficult to identify in the developing brain.

2 Terminology of pathological changes

The combination of multinucleated giant cells, microglial nodules and periven-ular inflammation has been termed *HIV encephalitis* (Snider *er al.*, 1983; Sharer and Kapila, 1985; Navia *et al.*, 1986a; Budka *et al.*, 1991) and has been identified in 30–90% of patients dying with AIDS (de La Monte *et al.*, 1987). There is frequently a diffuse pallor of the myelin, particularly in deep areas of the centrum semiovale, with microscopic evidence of macrophage activation, astrocytosis and productive HIV infection. This is termed *HIV leukoencephalo-pathy* and appears to correlate with the white matter changes noted on MRI (Budka *et al.*, 1991). This probably represents perturbation of the blood–brain barriers rather than demyelination (Power *et al.*, 1993). Recent quantitative MRI and morphometric studies have identified changes in grey matter (Everall *et al.*, 1991; Wiley *et al.*, 1991), with a loss of neuronal numbers particularly in frontal and temporal areas (Ketzler *et al.*, 1990; Everall *et al.*, 1991; Wiley *et al.*, 1991). Other neuronal changes including a loss of dendritic arborization and synaptic simplifications have also been identified (Masliah *et al.*, 1992a). These cortical changes have been termed diffuse poliodystrophy (Budka *et al.*, 1991; Power *et al.*, 1993).

3 Correlation with clinical features

The original description of the 'AIDS dementia complex' (Navia *et al.*, 1986a) showed an association between the presence of multinucleated giant cells, myelin pallor, and the severity of dementia. However, in some patients the pathological changes may be very bland. For example, we completed a prospective analysis of HIV dementia (Glass *et al.*, 1993) and found that only 25% of cases with HIV dementia had multinucleated giant cells, and 50% showed neither multinucleated giant cells nor white matter pallor. The brain levels of HIV RNA correlate with the pathological features of encephalitis

(Wiley *et al.*, 1998), but do not clearly distinguish demented from non-demented subjects (McArthur *et al.*, 1997). In fact, the intensity of macrophage activation correlates best with dementia severity (Glass *et al.*, 1995), suggesting that this pathological change is critical in the development of HIV dementia. Correlation between HIV-associated dementia and the presence of HIV within the CNS (Wiley and Achim, 1994; Wiley *et al.*, 1994), dendritic pathology (Masliah *et al.*, 1992a), neuronal loss (Ketzler *et al.*, 1990; Everall *et al.*, 1991), spatial pattern of neurons (Asare *et al.*, 1996), increased numbers of macrophages in the brain (Glass *et al.*, 1995), and elevated levels of isoform of Nitric Oxide Synthase (iNOS) (Adamson *et al.*, 1996) has been shown. Evidence of productive HIV replication has consistently been localized to macrophages and microglia within CNS parenchymal and perivascular infiltrates.

4 Vacuolar myelopathy

The pathology of the vacuolar myelopathy includes a patchy vacuolation in the spinal white matter, particularly in the lateral and posterior columns of the thoracic spinal cord (Figure 6.14). The vacuoles develop from splitting of the myelin lamellae by intramyelinic oedema and from macrophage infiltration between myelin and axon. There appears to be a gradation of severity of lesions, perhaps reflecting their temporal development. Early lesions have small numbers of vacuoles with intramyelinic macrophages. Later or more severe lesions showed complete demyelination with astrocytic gliosis and some evidence of remyelination. The final or most severe stage included necrosis and replacement by foamy macrophages and astrocytic processes. A similar type of vacuolar myelopathy develops in other conditions not associated with HIV-1 infection including B_{12} deficiency with subacute combined degeneration of the cord and in other immune deficiency states (Kamin and Petito, 1988).

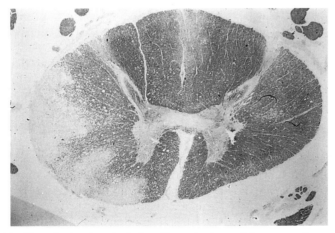

Figure 6.14   Vacuolation (particularly of lateral columns) in a case of vacuolar myelopathy.

5 Cellular targets of HIV infection

Initially cytomegalovirus (CMV) was suspected to be the cause of the progressive dementia (Snider *et al.*, 1983). The evidence for HIV-1 as the causative agent rests on morphological identification of the virus (Gyorkey *et al.*, 1987), intrathecal synthesis of antibody (Elovaara *et al.*, 1987), virus isolation (Stoler *et al.*, 1986), immunocytochemical staining for viral antigens (Wiley *et al.*, 1986), and *in situ* hybridization (Wiley *et al.*, 1986).

The majority of studies have consistently shown that HIV-1 infection is frequent in macrophages and multinucleated giant cells and that the deep white matter and basal ganglia contain higher concentrations of HIV than the cortical grey matter (Kure *et al.*, 1990). Fujimura *et al.* (1997) also detected high levels of HIV DNA in medial temporal lobe in demented individuals. Endothelial cells, oligodendrocytes or neurons contain replicating virus only rarely, if ever, however, recent studies using the sensitive technique of PCR *in situ* hybridization have demonstrated HIV DNA (latent provirus) in a proportion of astrocytes (Takahashi *et al.*, 1996).

6 Entry of HIV into the CNS

HIV-1 probably gains access to the central nervous system from the blood stream, either by direct infection of capillary endothelial cells (Johnson *et al.*, 1988), or more likely by ingress of infected monocytes/macrophages (Figure 6.15). The triggering mechanisms for initial monocyte/macrophage recruitment to the brain during HIV infection are unknown, but are likely to involve the up-regulation of chemoattractant β-chemokines such as MCP-1 (Conant *et al.*, 1998) and the expression of adhesion molecules on endothelial cells. Experimental studies using an artificial blood–brain barrier demonstrated that up-regulation of adhesion molecules and pro-inflammatory cytokines are critical for transendothelial migration (Persidsky *et al.*, 1997b). Pulliam *et al.* (1997) detected a high frequency of circulating activated monocytes expressing CD14/CD16 and CD14/CD69 in those with dementia. It remains plausible that differential activation of monocytes may determine whether sufficient HIV enters the CNS to trigger the pathophysiological processes which end in dementia.

HIV isolated from the CNS is most frequently macrophage-trophic, non-syncytial inducing, and is also associated with transmission of virus during early infection (Gartner *et al.*, 1986). Studies in SIV and with HIV *in vitro* have suggested that certain viruses are capable of infecting microvascular and endothelial cells (Mankowski *et al.*, 1994, 1997; Moses *et al.*, 1993).

The issue of whether the brain might serve as a significant reservoir for HIV remains undetermined. While HIV replication can occur in perivascular macrophages and microglia to high levels in some patients, in many the levels of HIV RNA and proviral DNA are relatively low at autopsy. Some perivascular macrophages return to the periphery after a sojourn within the brain. Theoretically, these could introduce CNS-derived strains of HIV into the

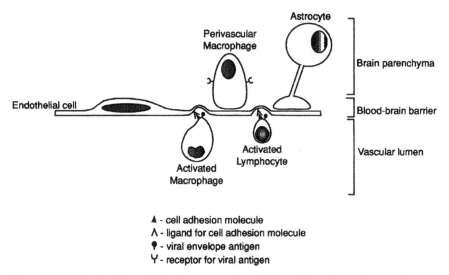

Figure 6.15   Mechanisms of viral entry – cell trafficking. An activated macrophage or lymphocyte infected with dual-tropic HIV may adhere to the endothelial cell and then pass directly through it bey the process of emperipolesis. The trafficking infected macrophage or lymphocyte would then transmit the virus to a perivascular macrophage. (From Zink, C., Carter, D., Flaherty, M., Mankowski, J. and Clements, J. (1998). The SIV/macaque model: Unravelling the mysteries of HIV encephalitis. In: Gendelman, H. E., Lipton, S. A., Epstein, L. and Swindells, S., (eds). *The Neurology of AIDS*, pp. 189–200. New York: Chapman and Hall).

systemic compartment. To date, however, there is no evidence that this occurs *in vivo*.

7 Specific neurovirulence of HIV

A concept has emerged in recent years, namely that certain strains of HIV-1 might have an increased propensity to invade (neurotropism) and cause damage in the nervous system (neurovirulence). This has significance because the development of HIV-D is not universal in advanced AIDS, suggesting that there may be viral determinants of heightened risk. Indeed distinct strains of HIV-1 isolated from both peripheral blood and the nervous system of the same individual can have different biological characteristics and cellular tropisms *in vitro* (Cheng-Mayer *et al.*, 1989; Chiodi *et al.*, 1989; Embretson *et al.*, 1993). Brain isolates tend to be more macrophage-tropic with specifically conserved regions in a portion of the envelope, the V3 domain (Chesebro *et al.*, 1992). *In vitro* neurotoxicity studies suggest that diversity in HIV envelope sequences may influence neuronal survival (Bratanich *et al.*, 1998). Extensive sequence heterogeneity has been demonstrated in brain-derived HIV genes that are critical for viral replication. This implies that *tat* and *env* genes may be important in the pathogenesis of HIV dementia and that *tat* sequence variation could account for the variation in the course and severity of dementia. Most of the mutations in the *tat* sequences from the HIV dementia group were located in the augmenting region of the first exon which influences viral replication. Parallel study models of SIV and FIV encephalitis have found that specific sequences in HIV *env* or *nef* confer neurovirulence (Power C, personal communication) (Flaherty *et al.*, 1997; Mankowski *et al.*, 1997). These observations suggest that infection with a 'neurotropic and neuroviru-lent' strain might lead to dementia. Alternatively, neurotropism may be less important than the evolution of neurovirulent HIV strains (Tersmette *et al.*, 1989; Richman, 1990). The clinical significance of these genotypic and phenotypic differences remains uncertain.

Pathogenetic mechanisms

The pathogenetic mechanisms involved in the production of HIV dementia remain obscure since in some patients with advanced dementia there may only be relatively mild neuropathological changes (de La Monte *et al.*, 1987; Price *et al.*, 1988) and only a small fraction of cells within inflammatory nodules or perivenular infiltrates contain viral antigens (Gabuzda *et al.*, 1986). (For recent reviews, see Epstein and Gendelman (1993) and Lipton (1994).) This dis-crepancy between the amounts of replicating HIV-1 and the severity of the dementia suggests that indirect mechanisms may be important in pathogenesis (Johnson *et al.*, 1988).

It appears likely that after the establishment of productive HIV infection in the CNS there is an activation of macrophages and microglia with the release of cytokines, metalloproteinases, and chemokines in the brain parenchyma. The cytokines may play a number of roles including the amplification of HIV replication, stimulation of astrocytosis, and, via autocrine feedback loops, lead to additional production of cytokines and arachidonic acid metabolites. Activated astrocytes may play a role in modulating and amplifying the release of neurotoxic substances. Chemokines may attract monocyte/macro-phages to the brain, while metalloproteinases break down the blood–brain barrier, both processes facilitating the ingress of HIV into the CNS.

As mentioned previously, direct neural cell infection does not occur, although there is a drop in neuronal density and dendritic 'pruning' (Ketzler *et al.*, 1990; Everall *et al.*, 1991; Wiley *et al.*, 1991). The putative mechanisms of these neuronal changes are not completely understood, and may be multi-factorial. Evidence suggests that both viral proteins and the products of macrophage activation might be neurotoxic. *In vitro*, different viral proteins including gp120 (the envelope glycoprotein of HIV-1), gp41, and *tat* (a regulatory protein) can lead to increases in intraneuronal free calcium, producing neuronal death (Dreyer *et al.*, 1990; Lipton, 1991; Magnuson *et al.*, 1995). This has not been demonstrated *in vivo*, however, increased parenchymal levels of these viral proteins might lead to neuronal damage in the same manner.

There is, however, abundant *in vivo* evidence of the importance of products of macrophage activation in the pathogenesis of HIV-D. Macrophages and microglia in the brain and spinal cord are intensely activated, and the relative levels of parenchymal activation correlate well with the severity of dementia (Glass *et al.*, 1995). CSF levels of immune activation markers also correlate with dementia (Brew *et al.*, 1990; McArthur *et al.*, 1992). The release of pro-inflammatory cytokines locally from infected or activated macrophages might impair cellular, neuronal or astrocytic function or modify neurotransmitter function (Navia *et al.*, 1986a; Johnson *et al.*, 1988). Alternatively, these soluble factors might cause alterations in the blood–brain barrier exposing the parenchyma to circulating toxins. *In vitro* studies have shown that HIV *tat* and TNF-α can induce neuronal apoptosis (Shi *et al.*, 1998). The potential for brain dysfunction to result from exposure to toxins has been demonstrated by the greatly elevated CSF levels of quinolinic acid (an excitatory neurotoxic metabolite of tryptophan) (Heyes *et al.*, 1990, 1991). Some of these mechanisms may act via glutamate overactivation of the NMDA (N-methyl-d-aspartate) receptor (Lipton, 1992), and the neurotoxic effects of nitric oxide (Adamson *et al.*, 1996), and this could be the final common pathway for several mechanisms of neuronal injury (Table 6.9). Several animal models have been developed to study these mechanisms *in vivo*. These include transgenic animals (Thomas *et al.*, 1994), SIV encephalitis (Zink *et al.*, 1998a, b) and SCID mice inoculated with HIV-infected macrophages (Persidsky *et al.*, 1997a). For example, transgenic mice expressing high levels of TNF-α in the CNS show widespread T lymphocytic infiltration which can be attenuated with antibodies to TNF-α (Probert *et al.*, 1995). The pattern of lymphocytic infiltration, however, obviously differs substantially from the widespread macrophage activation which occurs with HIV encephalitis. Furthermore, studies in knock-out mice in which TNF-α receptor expression is reduced have shown a heightened susceptibility to neuronal injury, even though microglial activation is attenuated (Bruce *et al.*, 1996).

Despite the potential importance of TNF-α and other pro-inflammatory cytokines, little progress has been made in clinical trials of TNF-α antagonists. In one early study of pentoxifylline, a phosphodiesterase-IV inhibitor which suppresses TNF-α gene expression by elevating intracellular levels of cyclic adenosine monophosphate (CAMP), little effect on neurological disease or plasma or CSF levels of TNF-α was noted (McArthur *et al.*, 1994). The agent, however, produced GI intolerance and pentoxifylline is only a relatively weak TNF-α antagonist. A novel antioxidant, CPI-1189, which may be a more potent TNF-α antagonist, is currently in trial in the USA.

Table 6.9   Potential steps in the pathogenesis of HIV dementia.

HIV infection of CNS macrophages (and ? evolution of neurovirulent strain)
Activation of macrophages
Expression of endothelial adhesion markers and chemoattractants
Facilitated CNS ingress of monocytes/macrophages
Damage to blood–brain barrier
Reduced inhibitory control of macrophage activation
Macrophage products/HIV proteins stimulate astrocyte proliferation and neuronal death

Studies of viral load in HIV-associated neurological disease

Higher levels of plasma HIV RNA are predictive of the development of dementia (Childs *et al.*, 1998). This suggests a strong relationship between the levels of active HIV replication in the systemic compartment and the subsequent seeding of the nervous system, ultimately triggering the pathophysiological events leading to neuronal dysfunction and dementia. Parallel observations have been made in SIV encephalitis, where animals with SIV encephalitis had higher plasma viral loads than those without (Westmoreland *et al.*, 1998).

Early studies of the relationship of HIV load to neurological disease suggested that neurological dysfunction is associated with increased CNS or CSF burden (Portegies *et al.*, 1989b; Buffet *et al.*, 1991; Goswami *et al.*, 1991; Steuler *et al.*, 1992; Bell *et al.*, 1993; Royal *et al.*, 1994). Several studies have now been completed using sensitive PCR techniques to examine CSF viral load in neurologically impaired persons. Initial results were discordant regarding the relationship between neurological disease and CSF HIV load (Chiodi *et al.*, 1992; Conrad *et al.*, 1995; Bossi *et al.*, 1997). More recently, however, studies using commercial assays have found a significant correlation between CSF HIV load and the severity of neurological disease (Sei *et al.*, 1995; Ellis *et al.*, 1997; Gisslen *et al.*, 1997; McArthur *et al.*, 1997).

One of the main questions in interpreting CSF HIV RNA levels is whether the CSF reflects brain tissue levels. Potential sources of CSF HIV RNA include the meninges, choroid plexus, parenchyma, and trafficking lymphocytes and monocytes. Presumably, the parenchymal levels are the most relevant for the study of neurological disease. From the studies to date, we do not have a clear answer to this. CSF HIV RNA might derive from different sources at different stages of HIV infection. Price and Staprans (1997) discuss this in a recent editorial, and use the phrases 'transitory' infection (trafficking cells) and 'autonomous' infection (parenchymal infection of macrophages and microglia). We have shown that while different brain regions have similar levels of HIV RNA, there is only a weak correspondence between brain and CSF HIV levels (McArthur *et al.*, 1997). Wiley *et al.* (1998) showed that CSF and parenchymal levels did not correlate when CSF levels were low (less than 10^5 copies/ml), but did correlate when CSF levels exceeded 10^6 copies/ml.

There is relatively little information about the effects of antiretroviral therapy on CSF constituents or HIV levels. CSF HIV RNA levels have not yet been validated as a measure of treatment effect, however, a recent study suggests that they may be a useful surrogate marker. LeTendre *et al.* (1998) assessed CSF HIV levels in 15 patients with minor cognitive/motor disorder (i.e. with definite neuropsychological deficits, but not frank dementia) who initiated HAART. Improvements in neuropsychological performance correlated with declines in CSF HIV RNA levels, and those who did *not* show CSF HIV RNA decreases did not have neuropsychological improvement. Recent studies in small series have begun to examine changes in CSF viral load after initiation of HAART, although none have focused on patients with HIV-D. The CSF penetrance of the protease inhibitors has conventionally been thought

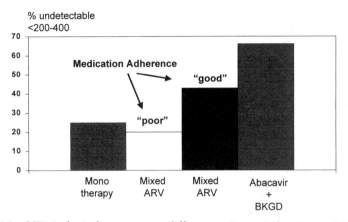

Figure 6.16   CSF virological responses to different antiretroviral regimens. Monotherapy indicates zidovudine; (Gisslen *et al.*, 1997) mixed ARV includes an observational study of different HAART regimens (McArthur *et al.*, 1998) where medication adherence was assessed; Abacavir + bkgd represents the relatively high levels of CSF virological suppression in a controlled clinical trial of abacavir + background HAART. (From McArthur, J. C., Sacktor, N. and Selnes, O. A. HIV-associated dementia. *Seminars in Neurology* (in press)).

to be poor, however, emerging studies have reported successful suppression of HIV in CSF with long-term use of protease inhibitors. Collier *et al.* (1997) reported nine individuals with CSF HIV levels determined before initiation of indinavir, and then after 8 weeks of therapy, significant reductions were observed. We examined plasma and CSF HIV RNA in 35 patients at variable times after the initiation of HAART. CSF HIV RNA levels were suppressed to undetectable levels in only 50% after 6 months of therapy. Self-reported adherence was a significant factor in the success of therapy, with 'poor' adherence associated with virological suppression in only 25% (Figure 6.16). Significantly better virological suppression was observed in a carefully monitored study using abacavir in combination with other ARTs (Lanier *et al.*, 1998).

Treatment of HIV dementia

Antiretroviral therapy: CNS penetration

There have been several important advances in the past few years which have lead to concrete improvements in the care and prognosis of HIV-infected individuals. The first is an understanding of the direct relationship between viral replication and immunological and disease progression, which reinforces the need to suppress viral replication at the earliest point to control the infection. This has lead to the so-called 'hit early, hit hard' philosophy arising out of the 1996 reports showing that HAART could suppress viral replication in patients who began therapy early in the course of their HIV disease. The second is the wider availability of multiple, potent antiretroviral regimes that can be combined in various ways to provide effective suppression of HIV. The third major change is the ability to monitor the response to therapy through regular measurement of plasma HIV RNA levels which, with CD4 counts, has become a routine part of clinical care. In addition, resistance to antiretrovirals can now be relatively easily measured with genotypic or phenotypic assays. In patients who fail to achieve HIV suppression with antiretroviral therapy it is often uncertain whether this reflects development of resistance, incomplete adherence, or inadequate delivery of antiretroviral agents to the target site. This is potentially of even greater importance for the treatment of CNS infection given the relatively limited penetrance of most of the available antiretroviral agents.

There are now 14 FDA-licensed antiretroviral agents in the USA, with several more in development with approval expected during 1999. The published pharmacokinetic data for CSF penetration for available agents is shown in Table 6.10 (Groothuis and Levy, 1997). Groothuis and Levy (1997) have summarized some of the issues in relating plasma, CSF and brain concentrations of antiretroviral agents. They stress that drug concentrations in the different compartments may be quite different, and that using CSF concentrations to estimate brain extracellular fluid levels may overestimate the latter. The estimation of brain tissue levels of drug needs to take into account not only the plasma concentration, but also the degree of protein binding, and lipophilicity. Additional factors which will tend to lower tissue levels include diffusion in brain tissue, and a lack of correction for drug which is within the intravascular space (Blasberg and Groothuis, 1986). The CSF:plasma ratios for available antiretrovirals are very variable, reflecting individual drug

Table 6.10   CSF:plasma-HIV RNA concentration ratios in humans (Brinkman et al., 1998; Clifford and Simpson, 1998; Howarth et al., 1998).

Compound	CSF-to-plasma ratio
Nucleoside reverse transcriptase inhibitors	
Zidovudine	0.3–1.35
Stavudine	0.16–0.97
Abacavir	0.3–0.42 (from Glaxo-Wellcome)
Didanosine	0.16–0.19
Lamivudine	0.11
Zalcitabine	0.09–0.37
Non-nucleoside reverse transcriptase inhibitors	
Nevirapine	0.45
Delavirdine	0.02
Efavirenz	0.01
Protease inhibitors	
Indinavir	0.02–0.06
Saquinavir	< 0.05
Nelfinavir	< 0.05
Ritonavir	< 0.05
Amprenavir	< 0.05

differences in lipid solubility, molecular size and the state of ionization. In fact, the relevance of this ratio to actual brain concentrations is uncertain, as relatively few data are available. As an example, the CSF : plasma ratios for several ARVs are shown in Table 6.10, however, many of these data are based on a few patient samples, and usually do not include patients with HIV dementia, where the blood–brain barrier may be more permeable (Hurwitz *et al.*, 1994). Other important factors include the active efflux of ARTs through transporters including p-glycoprotein (Kim *et al.*, 1998).

Despite the relatively low plasma : CSF ratios achieved with the potent protease inhibitors which suggests that CNS penetration would be poor, presumably CNS and CSF levels are adequate to suppress the trafficking of infected cells into the CNS and the minimal amount of protein binding in the CSF allows for adequate free levels of drug. There is now accumulating evidence that HAART regimens can improve neuropsychological performance and radiological abnormalities in HIV dementia (Sacktor *et al.*, 1999). Furthermore, virological suppression within the CSF can be obtained.

The effects of monotherapy on dementia

In the early years of the epidemic, from approximately 1987 (when zidovudine, the first licensed antiretroviral agent, was introduced) to around 1992 (when studies of dual therapy were published) antiretroviral therapy usually consisted of monotherapy. The more widespread and earlier use of AZT appeared to reduce the frequency/incidence of HIV dementia dramatically from 53% to 10% (Portegies *et al.*, 1989a). Early open label studies with zidovudine showed promising improvements in clinical functioning and neuropsychological per-formance (Yarchoan *et al.*, 1987). Tozzi *et al.* (1993) completed an open label study of AZT in HIV dementia and observed clinical improvements in two-thirds of patients.

Children treated with intravenous AZT showed improvement in neuropsy-chological performance and hypometabolism on PET scans (Pizzo *et al.*, 1988). Didanosine (ddl) was shown to improve IQ scores in children and plasma concentrations correlated with IQ improvement (Butler *et al.*, 1991). In one open-label study of zidovudine, after a few months of treatment, Tartaglione *et al.* (1991) noted neurological improvement in most patients with mild neurological abnormalities, but no relationship between treatment response and CSF AZT concentration, cumulative AZT dose, or HIV isolation from CSF. Arendt *et al.* (1998) presented data from an observational study in patients with dementia who were switched to stavudine. Many showed dramatic improvements in psychomotor speed function.

Surprisingly, only two placebo-controlled monotherapy antiretroviral trials for HIV dementia were completed, but these have provided important information on changes in neurological function with ART. First, evidence from the multi-centre licensing trial (Fischl *et al.*, 1987) of AZT in patients with AIDS or ARC suggested that this drug improved neuropsychological function (Schmitt *et al.*, 1988). This study was not specifically a trial of HIV dementia (in fact severely demented individuals were excluded), and it was several more years before a controlled trial of zidovudine in HIV dementia was completed. This study suggested that there was a dose effect, with more improvement with very high doses of AZT (2000 mg daily) (Sidtis *et al.*, 1993).

The effects of combination ART on dementia

There have been very few systematic studies of the effects of combination ART on neurocognitive deficits in HIV-D. In part, this reflects the difficulty and expense of performing controlled clinical trials in this disorder. It also reflects the dynamic nature of drug development in AIDS, where new agents may be introduced before dementia trials can be completed. Graham *et al.* (1996), using data from the Multicenter AIDS Cohort Study suggested that the use of combination ART (not including protease inhibitors) was associated with a reduced risk of developing HIV-D. The effects of adding a non-nucleoside RTI, nevirapine, to background ART were studied in a blinded clinical trial (ACTG193a) in very advanced HIV infection. Neuropsychological performance was improved in the nevirapine group (Price *et al.*, 1998). More recently, with the introduction of the potent protease inhibitors in 1996, several groups have completed open-label studies of combination regimens including protease inhibitors. In one study, 23 patients with HIV-associated cognitive impairment received neuropsychological testing before and after the initiation of combination regimens including protease inhibitors, and improvement was noted in 78% of the patients (Sacktor *et al.*, 1998a, b). Furthermore, the effect of combination antiretroviral therapy including protease inhibitors on neuropsychological testing performance was compared to combination antiretroviral therapy without protease inhibitors, monotherapy, and no treatment in subjects in the Multicenter AIDS Cohort Study (Sacktor *et al.*, 1998). Subjects using either combination ART with or without protease inhibitors had better neuropsychological testing performance than subjects using monotherapy or no treatment. In another cross-sectional study, Ferrando *et al.* (1998) found that combination therapy with protease inhibitors was associated with a lower prevalence of neuropsychological impairment in HIV positive homosexuals.

In 1998, a new reverse transcriptase inhibitor, abacavir, was tested in a placebo-controlled, double-blinded study in 99 patients with HIV dementia. The rationale for considering the use of abacavir included its penetration into cerebrospinal fluid (CSF), and its activity in macrophages, HIV's principal target cell within the brain (Brew *et al.*, 1998). Ninety-nine individuals with HIV dementia were randomized to add abacavir, 600 mg b.i.d., or placebo, onto stable background ART. The patients were heavily pretreated with ART, and in fact only 10% had wild type virus at entry. Perhaps surprisingly, very few subjects showed neurological deterioration during the 12 weeks of the study: only two in the placebo group, and none on abacavir. Overall, both groups showed improvements in neuropsychological performance on standardized tests, with a trend favouring abacavir. The more severely impaired group on abacavir showed a greater improvement than placebo recipients. The CSF virological response favoured abacavir with a 0.64 log drop during the study, while the placebo group showed a rise of 0.25 log. This was an important study partly because of the inherent difficulty of performing clinical trials in demented subjects, and partly because of the relatively limited treatment options available. The lack of any dramatic treatment effect emphasizes that a switch of one ART is unlikely to be an effective treatment for dementia, especially in heavily pretreated patients with multiple resistance mutations. The improvement in the background treatment group suggests that triple combination ART may produce neurological improvement which continues over several months. Thus, despite entering the study on 'stable' ART therapy, in fact, the placebo group overall were still improving. Abacavir did reduce CSF levels to a greater extent than background ART. There are multiple implications from this study including: single changes in ART are not likely to be very effective; the progression of dementia may be different in an era when combination therapies are used; and other types of outcome measures, in addition to neuropsychological testing may be needed to detect changes.

Suggestions for antiretroviral therapy in HIV-D

At this point, it is impossible to make definitive recommendations about the optimum antiretroviral therapy for HIV dementia. Stavudine and abacavir appear to be useful alternatives to include in a combination regimen for patients with dementia, based upon their pharmacokinetic properties, tolerability and b.i.d. dosing. New information is emerging that stavudine (d4T) may have a role in treating neurological disease, based upon favourable pharmacokinetic studies demonstrating that CSF levels are above the IC50 for the dose of 40 mg b.i.d. Improvements in neurological performance were observed by Arendt *et al.* (1998). The non-nucleoside reverse transcriptase inhibitor, nevirapine, achieves good CSF levels and may also be useful to include in ART regimens for patients with HIV-D.

The role of resistance testing may become important in selection of ART combinations for demented patients, most of whom are heavily pretreated and are likely to have multiple resistance mutations (as in the abacavir trial where 90% of subjects had resistance mutations at baseline). There does not appear to be any direct utility from examining resistance patterns in CSF. There is generally concordance between the CSF and plasma with respect to genotypic resistance mutations, although there may be occasional differences.

Adherence is clearly an important issue in maintaining virological suppression, particularly in patients with cognitive impairment. New techniques for improving adherence, including directly observed therapy, pill counts, intensive education, and electronic monitors, are being applied to this problem.

Adjunctive therapies for HIV dementia

The delineation of the pathophysiological steps contributing to HIV dementia has suggested that antiretroviral therapies alone may not be sufficient to prevent the self-sustaining macrophage activation, and the subsequent release of neurotoxic factors. This concept has led to the development of several

Table 6.11 Clinical Trials of Adjunctive Therapies for HIV Dementia.

Agent	Action	Conclusion	Reference
Nimodipine	Calcium channel	NP trend	Navia (Vinik et al., 1995)
Peptide T	Uncertain action	No effect	Heseltine (Heseltine et al., 1998)
OPC14117	Antioxidant	NP trend	Dana Consortium (The Dana Consortium on Therapy of HIV Dementia and Related Cognitive Disorders, 1997)
Thioctic acid vs selegiline	Antioxidant, neuroprotectant	Selegiline NP effect	Dana Consortium (The Dana Consortium on the Therapy of HIV Dementia and Related Cognitive Disorders, 1998)
Lexipafant	PAF antagonist	NP effect	Schiffito (in preparation)
Memantine	NMDA antagonist	Underway	B. Navia (personal communication)

adjunctive therapies aimed at interrupting or blocking these aberrant pathways (Table 6.11). These include inflammatory antagonists, such as Lexipafant, an antagonist of platelet activating factor, and neuroprotective agents, such as memantine, an open-channel NMDA antagonist. Other compounds have been tested in small phase I/II trials, in patients receiving stable ART, and have shown promising results. In one study of the licensed agent selegiline, significant improvements in memory were seen (The Dana Consortium on the Therapy of HIV Dementia and Related Cognitive Disorders, 1998). Larger scale studies are in the planning stages.

Symptomatic treatment is an important adjunct to antiviral treatment. Patients with HIV dementia are extremely susceptible to the adverse effects of psychoactive drugs, so hypnotics and anxiolytics should be avoided. Small doses of neuroleptics, such as risperidol may be needed in the agitated or combative patient. If marked inertia is present, activating selective serotonin reuptake inhibitors or methylphenidate (Ritalin) can be tried. In patients with progressive dementia, medico-legal issues should be discussed at any early stage before the dementia becomes too severe: establishing a power of attorney, completion of a living will, and arrangement for the dispersal of assets.

Future projections

HIV dementia is estimated to develop eventually in 15–20% of individuals with advanced HIV disease. With about one million individuals already infected in the USA alone, we can anticipate an annual incidence of 10 000 cases of HIV dementia, similar to the annual incidence of multiple sclerosis. HIV dementia has thus become one of the leading causes of dementia in young Americans. Our hope is that this new era of potent combination antiretroviral therapy will result in a reduction in HIV dementia. However, combination therapies are complex, have side-effects, and are expensive enough to be beyond the reach of 90% of HIV-infected individuals world-wide. New approaches to improving adherence with complex medication regimens are needed to maximize virological suppression.

Acknowledgement

The following support is acknowledged: NIH A135042, NS 26643, RR 00722, and Glaxo Wellcome Inc.

References

Adamson, D. C., Wildemann, B., Sasaki, M. *et al.* (1996). Immunologic nitric oxide synthase: Elevation in severe AIDS dementia and induction by HIV-1 coat protein, gp41. *Science*, **274**, 1917–1921.

Arendt, G., v.Giesen, H.-J. and Jablonowski, H. (1998). Stavudine stops neuro-AIDS in AZT-non-responders (abstract #32207). *12th World AIDS Conference, Geneva*, June 28–July 3.

Asare, E., Dunn, G., Glass, J. *et al.* (1996). Neuronal pattern correlates with the severity of human immunodeficiency virus-associated dementia complex. Usefulness of spatial pattern analysis in clincopathological studies. *Am. J. Pathol.*, **148**, 31–38.

Aylward, E. H., Henderer, J. D., McArthur, J. C. *et al.* (1993). Reduced basal ganglia volume in HIV-1-associated dementia: results from quantitative neuroimaging. *Neurology*, **43**, 2099–2104.

Bell, J. E., Busuttil, A., Ironside, J. W. *et al.* (1993). Human immunodeficiency virus and the brain: investigation of virus load and neuropathic changes in pre-AIDS subjects. *J. Infect. Dis.*, **168**, 818–824.

Belman, A. L., Diamond, G., Dickson, D. *et al.* (1988). Pediatric acquired immunodeficiency syndrome. Neurologic syndromes (published erratum appears in *Am. J. Dis. Child.*, 1988 May; **142**(5), 507). *Am. J. Dis. Child.*, **142**, 29–35.

Belman, A. L., Lantos, G., Horoupian, D. *et al.* (1986). AIDS: calcification of the basal ganglia in infants and children. *Neurology*, **36**, 1192–1199.

Berger, J. R., Anderson, A. H. and Avison, M. J. (1996). Blood brain barrier breakdown in AIDS dementia: An MRI study. *Neuroscience of HIV Infection: Basic and Clinical Frontiers Paris*, March 6–9.

Blasberg, R. G. and Groothuis, D. R. (1986). Chemotherapy of brain tumours: physiological and pharmacokinetic considerations. *Sem. Oncol.*, **13**, 70–83.

Bossi, P., Dupin, N., Coutellier, A. *et al.* (1997). Absence of any clinical interest of HIV-1 RNA in CSF for diagnosis of HIV encephalitis (abstract). *Interscience Conference of Antimicrobial Agents and Chemotherapy, Toronto*, Sept 27–Oct 1.

Bouwman, F. H., Skolasky, R., Hes, D. *et al.* (1998). Variable progression of HIV-associated dementia. *Neurology*, 50, 1814–1820.

Bratanich, A. C., Liu, C., McArthur, J. C. *et al.* (1998). Brain-derived HIV-1 tat sequences from AIDS patients with dementia show increased molecular heterogeneity. *J. Neurovirol.*, 4, 387–393.

Brew, B. J., Bhalla, R. B., Paul, M. *et al.* (1990). Cerebrospinal fluid neopterin in human immunodeficiency virus type-I infection. *Ann. Neurol.*, 28, 556–560.

Brew, B. J., Brown, S. J., Catalan, J. *et al.* (1998). Safety and efficacy of abacavir (ABC, 1592) in AIDS dementia complex (Study CNAB 3001) (abstract #32192). *12th World AIDS Conference, Geneva*, June 28–July 3.

Brinkman, K., Kroon, F., Hugen, P. W. H. and Burger, D. M. (1998). Therapeutic concentrations of indinavir in cerebrospinal fluid of HIV-1-infected patients (letter). *AIDS*, 12, 537.

Brodt, H. R., Kamps, B. S., Gute, P., Knupp, B., Staszewski, S. and Helm, E. B. (1997). Changing incidence of AIDS-defining illnesses in the era of antiretroviral combination therapy. *AIDS*, 11, 1731–1738.

Bruce, A. J., Boling, W., Kindy, M. S. *et al.* (1996). Altered neuronal and microglial responses to excitotoxic and ischemic brain injury in mice lacking TNF receptors. *Nature Med.*, 2, 788–794.

Budka, H. (1986). Multinucleated giant cells in brain: a hallmark of the acquired immune deficiency syndrome (AIDS). *Acta Neuropathol. (Berl.)*, 69, 253–258.

Budka, H., Wiley, C. A., Kleihues, P. *et al.* (1991). HIV-associated disease of the nervous system: review of nomenclature and proposal for neuropathology-based terminology. *Brain Pathol.*, 1, 143–152.

Buffet, R., Agut, H., Chieze, F. *et al.* (1991). Virological markers in the cerebrospinal fluid from HIV-1 infected individuals. *AIDS*, 5, 1419–1424.

Butler, K. M., Husson, R. N., Balis, R. M. *et al.* (1991). Dideoxyinosine in children with symptomatic human immunodeficiency virus infection. *N. Engl. J. Med.*, 324, 137–144.

Centers for Disease Control (1987). Revision of the CDC surveillance case definition for acquired immunodeficiency syndrome. *MMWR*, 36(suppl. 1S), 3S–15S.

Centers for Disease Control and Prevention (1995). *HIV/AIDS Surveillance Report*, 7(2), 1–39.

Centers for Disease Control and Prevention (1997). *HIV/AIDS Surveillance Report*, 9, 1–43.

Chaisson, R. E., Keruly, J. C. and Moore, R. D. (1995). Race, sex, drug use, and progression of human immunodeficiency virus disease. *N. Engl. J. Med.*, 333, 751–756.

Cheng-Mayer, C., Weiss, C., Seto, D. and Levy, J. A. (1989). Isolates of human immunodeficiency virus type 1 from the brain may constitute a special group of the AIDS virus. *Proc. Natl Acad. Sci. USA*, 86, 8575–8579.

Chesebro, B., Wehrly, K., Nishio, J. and Perryman, S. (1992). Macrophage-tropic human immunodeficiency virus isolates from different patients exhibit unusual V3 envelope sequence homogeneity in comparison with T-cell-tropic isolates: definition of critical amino acids involved in cell tropism. *J. Virol.*, **66**, 6547–6554.

Childs, E., Lyles, R., Selnes, O. A. *et al.* (1999). Plasma viral load and CD4 lymphocytes predict HIV-associated dementia and sensory neuropathy. *Neurology*, **52**, 607–613.

Chiodi, F., Keys, B., Albert, J. *et al.* (1992). Human immunodeficiency virus type 1 is present in the cerebrospinal fluid of a majority of infected individuals. *J. Clin. Microbiol.*, **30**, 1768–1771.

Chiodi, F., Valentin, A., Keys, B. *et al.* (1989). Biological characterization of paired human immunodeficiency virus type 1 isolates from blood and cerebrospinal fluid. *Virology*, **173**, 178–187.

Clifford, D. B. and Simpson, D. (1998). Targeting HIV therapy for the brain. *HIV Adv. Res. Ther.*, **8**, 10–17.

Coffin, J. (1996). HIV viral dynamics. *AIDS*, **10**(suppl. 3), S75–S84.

Collier, A., Marra, C. and Coombs, R. W. (1997). Cerebrospinal fluid (CSF) HIV RNA levels in patients on chronic indinavir therapy (abstract 22). *Abstracts of the infectious Disease Society of America, 35th annual meeting, San Francisco*, Sept. 13–16.

Conant, K., Garzinodemo, A., Nath, A. *et al.* (1998). Induction of monocyte chemoattractant protein-1 in HIV-1 tat-stimulated astrocytes and elevation in AIDS dementia. *Proc. Natl Acad. Sci. USA*, **95**, 3117–3121.

Connor, E. M., Sperling, R. S., Gelber, R. *et al.* (1994). Reduction of maternal-infant transmission of human immunodeficiency virus type 1 infection with zidovudine treatment. *N. Engl. J. Med.*, **331**, 1173–1180.

Conrad, A. J., Schmid, P., Syndulko, K. *et al.* (1995). Quantifying HIV-1 RNA using the polymerase chain reaction on cerebrospinal fluid and serum of seropositive individuals with and without neurologic abnormalities. *J. AIDS*, **10**, 425–435.

Dal Pan, G. J., McArthur, J. H., Aylward, E. *et al.* (1992). Patterns of cerebral atrophy in HIV-1 infected individuals: results of a quantitative MRI analysis. *Neurology*, **42**, 2125–2130.

De-The, G., Giordano, C., Gessain, A. *et al.* (1989). Human retroviruses HTLV-I, HIV-1, and HIV-2 and neurological diseases in some equatorial areas of Africa. *J. AIDS*, **2**, 550–556.

de la Monte, S. M., Ho, D. D., Schooley, R. T., Hirsch, M. S. and Richardson, E. P. JR (1987). Subacute encephalomyelitis of AIDS and its relation to HTLV-III infection. *Neurology*, **37**, 562–569.

Deeks, S., Grant, R., Horton, C., Simmonds, N., Follansbee, S. and Eastman, S. (1997). Virologic effect of ritonavir (RTV) plus saquinavir (SQV) in subjects who have failed indinavir (IDV) (Abstract I-205). *Interscience Conference on Antimicrobial Agents and Chemotherapy (ICAAC), Toronto*, Sept. 28–Oct. 1. 282.

Di Sclafani, V., Mackay, R. D., Meyerhoff, D. J., Norman, D., Weiner, M. W. and Fein, G. (1997). Brain atrophy in HIV infection is more strongly associated with CDC clinical stage than with cognitive impairment. *J. Int. Neuropsychol. Soc.*, **3**, 276–287.

Dreyer, E. B., Kaiser, P. K., Offermann, J. T. and Lipton, S. A. (1990). HIV-1 coat protein neurotoxicity prevented by calcium channel antagonists. *Science*, **248**, 364–367.

Ellis, R. J., Hsia, K., Spector, S. A. *et al.* (1997). Cerebrospinal fluid human immunodeficiency virus type 1 RNA levels are elevated in neurocognitively impaired individuals with acquired immunodeficiency syndrome. *Ann. Neurol.*, **42**, 679–688.

Elovaara, I., Iivanainen, M., Valle, S. L., Suni, J., Tervo, T. and Lahdevirta, J. (1987). CSF protein and cellular profiles in various stages of HIV infection related to neurological manifestations. *J. Neurol. Sci.*, **78**, 331–342.

Embretson, J., Zupancic, M., Beneke, J. *et al.* (1993). Analysis of human immunodeficiency virus-infected tissues by amplification and in situ hybridization reveals latent and permissive infections at single cell resolution. *Proc. Natl Acad. Sci. USA*, **90**, 357–361.

Epstein, L. G. and Gendelman, H. E. (1993). Human immunodeficiency virus type 1 infection of the nervous system: pathogenetic mechanisms. *Ann. Neurol.*, **33**, 429–436.

Epstein, L. G., Sharer, L. R., Joshi, V. V., Fojas, M. M., Koenigsberger, M. R. and Oleske, J. M. (1985). Progressive encephalopathy in children with acquired immune deficiency syndrome. *Ann. Neurol.*, **17**, 488–496.

Everall, I. P., Glass, J. D., McArthur, J., Spargo, E. and Lantos, P. (1994). Neuronal density in the superior frontal and temporal gyri does not correlate with the degree of human immunodeficiency virus-associated dementia. *Acta Neuropathol.*, **88**, 538–544.

Everall, I. P., Luthert, P. J. and Lantos, P. L. (1991). Neuronal loss in the frontal cortex in HIV infection. *Lancet*, **337**, 1119–1121.

Ferrando, S., Rabkin, J., van Gorp, W. and McElhiney, M. (1998). Protease inhibitors are associated with less neuropsychological impairment in HIV infection (abstract 186). *5th Conference on Retroviruses and Opportunistic Infections Chicago*, Feb. 1–5. 113.

Finzi, D., Hermankova, M., Pierson, T. *et al.* (1997). Identification of a reservoir for HIV-1 in patients on highly active antiretroviral therapy. *Science*, **278**, 1295–1300.

Fischl, M. A., Richman, D. D., Grieco, M. H. *et al.* (1987). The efficacy of azidothymidine (AZT) in the treatment of patients with AIDS and AIDS-related complex. *N. Engl. J. Med.*, **317**, 185–191.

Flaherty, M. T., Hauer, D. A., Mankowski, J. L., Zink, M. C. and Clements, J. E. (1997). Molecular and biological characterization of a neurovirulent molecular clone of simian immunodeficiency virus. *J. Virol.*, **71**, 5790–5798.

Fox, L., Alford, M., Achim, C., Mallory, M. and Masliah, E. (1997). Neurodegeneration of somatostatin-immunoreactive neurons in HIV encephalitis. *J. Neuropathol. Exp. Neurol.*, **56**, 360–368.

Fujimura, R. K., Goodkin, K., Petito, C. K. *et al.* (1997). HIV-1 proviral DNA load across neuroanatomic regions of individuals with evidence for HIV-1-associated dementia. *J. AIDS*, **16**, 146–152.

Gabuzda, D. H., Ho, D. D., de la Monte, S. M., Hirsch, M. S., Rota, T. R. and Sobel, R. A. (1986). Immunohistochemical identification of HTLV-III antigen in brains of patients with AIDS. *Ann. Neurol.*, **20**, 289–295.

Gartner, S., Markovits, P., Markovitz, D. M., Kaplan, M. H., Gallo, R. C. and Popovic, M. (1986). The role of mononuclear phagocytes in HTLV-III/LAV infection. *Science*, **233**, 215–219.

Gisslen, M., Norkrans, G., Svennerholm, B. and Hagberg, L. (1997). The effect of human immunodeficiency virus type 1 RNA levels in cerebrospinal fluid after initiation of zidovudine or didanosine. *J. Infect. Dis.*, **175**, 434–437.

Glass, J. D., Fedor, H., Wesselingh, S. L. and McArthur, J. C. (1995). Immunocytochemical quantitation of HIV in the brain: correlations with HIV-associated dementia. *Ann. Neurol.*, **38**, 755–762.

Glass, J. D., Wesselingh, S. L., Selnes, O. A. and McArthur, J. C. (1993). Clinical-neuropathologic correlation in HIV-associated dementia. *Neurology*, **43**, 2230–2237.

Goswami, K. K., Miller, R. F., Harrison, M. J., Hamel, D. J., Daniels, R. S. and Tedder, R. S. (1991). Expression of HIV-1 in the cerebrospinal fluid detected by the polymerase chain reaction and its correlation with central nervous system disease. *J. AIDS*, **5**, 797–803.

Graham, N. M. H., Hoover, D. R., Park, L. P. *et al.* (1996). Survival in HIV-infected patients who have received zidovudine. Comparison of combination therapy with sequential monotherapy and continued zidovudine monotherapy. *Ann. Intern. Med.*, **124**, 1031–1038.

Grant, I., Atkinson, J. H., Hesselink, J. R. *et al.* (1987). Evidence for early central nervous system involvement in the acquired immunodeficiency syndrome (AIDS) and other human immunodeficiency virus (HIV) infections. Studies with neuropsychologic testing and magnetic resonance imaging (published erratum appears in *Ann. Intern. Med.*, 1988 **108**(3), 496). *Ann. Intern. Med.*, **107**, 828–836.

Greene, W. C. (1991). The molecular biology of human immunodeficiency virus type 1 infection. *N. Engl. J. Med.*, **324**, 308–317.

Groothuis, D. R. and Levy, R. M. (1997). The entry of antiviral and antiretroviral drugs into the central nervous system. *J. Neurovirol.*, **3**, 387–400.

Gyorkey, F., Melnick, J. L. and Gyorkey, P. (1987). Human immunodeficiency virus in brain biopsies of patients with AIDS and progressive encephalopathy. *J. Infect. Dis.*, **155**, 870–876.

Handelsman, L., Aronson, M., Maurer, G. *et al.* (1992). Neuropsychological and neurological manifestations of HIV-1 dementia in drug users. *J. Neuropsychiatr. Clin. Neurosci.*, **4**, 21–28.

Harrison, M. J. G. and McArthur, J. C. (1995). *AIDS and Neurology*. Edinburgh: Churchill Livingstone.

Haverkos, H. W. and Quinn, T. C. (1995). The third wave: HIV infection among heterosexuals in the United States and Europe. *Int. J. STD AIDS*, **6**, 227–232.

Haworth, S. J., Christofalo, B., Anderson, R. D. and Dunkle, L. M. (1988). A single-dose study to assess the penetration of stavudine into human cerebrospinal fluid in adults. *J. AIDS*, **17**, 235–238.

He, J., Chen, Y., Farzan, M. *et al.* (1997). CCR3 and CCR5 are co-receptors for HIV-1 infection of microglia. *Nature*, **385**, 645–649.

Heseltine, P. N. R., Goodkin, K., Atkinson, J. H. *et al.* (1998). Randomized double-blind placebo-controlled trial of peptide T for HIV-associated cognitive impairment. *Arch. Neurol.*, **55**, 41–51.

Heyes, M. P., Brew, B. J., Martin, A. *et al.* (1991). Quinolinic acid in cerebrospinal fluid and serum in HIV-1 infection: relationship to clinical and neurologic status. *Ann. Neurol.*, **29**, 202–209.

Heyes, M. P., Mefford, I. N., Quearry, B. J., Dedhia, M. and Lackner, A. (1990). Increased ratio of quinolinic acid to kynurenic acid in cerebrospinal fluid of D retrovirus-infected Rhesus macaques: relationships to clinical and viral status. *Ann. Neurol.*, **27**, 666–675.

Ho, D. D., Neumann, A. U., Perelson, A. S., Chen, W., Leonard, J. M. and Markowitz, M. (1995). Rapid turnover of plasma virions and CD4 lymphocytes in HIV-1 infection. *Nature*, **373**, 123–126.

Holland, N. R., Power, C., Matthew, V. P., Glass, J. D., Forman, M. and McArthur, J. C. (1994). CMV encephalitis in acquired immunodeficiency syndrome (AIDS). *Neurology*, **44**, 507–514.

Hriso, E., Kuhn, T., Masdeu, J. C. and Grundman, M. (1991). Extrapyramidal symptoms due to dopamine-blocking agents in patients with AIDS encephalopathy. *Am. J. Psych.*, **148**, 1558–1561.

Hurwitz, A. A., Berman, J. W. and Lyman, W. D. (1994). The role of blood–brain barrier in HIV infection of the central nervous system. *Adv. Neuroimmunol.*, **4**, 249–256.

Janssen, R. S., Cornblath, D. R., Epstein, L. G. *et al.* (1991). Nomenclature and research case definitions for neurological manifestations of human immunodeficiency virus type-1 (HIV-1) infection. Report of a Working Group of the American Academy of Neurology AIDS Task Force. *Neurology*, **41**, 778–785.

Janssen, R. S., Nwanyanwu, O. C., Selik, R. M. and Stehr-Green, J. K. (1982). Epidemiology of human immunodeficiency virus encephalopathy in the United States. *Neurology*, **42**, 1472–1476.

Janssen, R. S., Saykin, A. J., Kaplan, J. E. *et al.* (1988). Neurological complications of human immunodeficiency virus infection in patients with lymphadenopathy syndrome. *Ann. Neurol.*, **23**, 49–55.

Johnson, R. T., McArthur, J. C. and Narayan, O. (1988). The neurobiology of human immunodeficiency virus infections. *FASEB. J.*, **2**, 2970–2981.

Kamin, S. S. and Petito, C. K. (1988). Vacuolar myelopathy in immuocompromised non-AIDS patients (abstract). *J. Neuropathol. Exp. Neurol.*, **47**, 385.

Ketzler, S., Weis, S., Haug, H. and Budka, H. (1990). Loss of neurons in the frontal cortex in AIDS brains. *Acta Neuropathol. (Berl.)*, **80**, 92–94.

Kim, R. B., Fromm, M. F., Wandel, C. *et al.* (1998). The drug transporter P-glycoprotein limits oral absorption and brain entry of HIV-1 protease inhibitors. *J. Clin. Invest.*, **101**, 289–294.

Koralnik, I. J., Beumanoir, A., Hausler, R. *et al.* (1990). A controlled study of early neurologic abnormalities in men with asymptomatic human immunodeficiency virus infection. *N. Engl. J. Med.*, **323**, 864–870.

Kure, K., Weidenheim, K. M., Lyman, W. D. and Dickson, D. W. (1990). Morphology and distribution of HIV-1 gp41-positive microglia in subacute AIDS encephalitis. Pattern of involvement resembling a multisystem degeneration. *Acta Neuropathol. (Berl.)*, **80**, 393–400.

LaFrance, N., Pearlson, G. D., Schaerf, F. W. *et al.* (1988). I-123 IMP-SPECT in HIV-related dementia. *Adv. Funct. Imag.*, **1**, 9–15.

Lanier, R., McArthur, J., Atkinson, J. H. *et al.* (1998). Viral resistance and viral load response to abacavir (ABC, 1592) in an AIDS dementia complex trial (CNAB 3001). (abstract #32293). *12th World AIDS Conference, Geneva*, June 28–July 3.

Le Tendre, S., Ellis, R., Heaton, R. K., Atkinson, J. H. and McCutchan, J. A. (1998). Change in CSF RNA level correlates with the effects of maximal antiretroviral therapy of HIV associated cognitive disorder. *12th World AIDS Conference, Geneva*, 32198.

Levy, J. A. (1989). Human immunodeficiency viruses and the pathogenesis of AIDS (Review). *J. Am. Med. Assoc.*, **261**, 2997–3006.

Levy, R. M., Bredesen, D. E. and Rosenblum, M. L. (1985). Neurological manifestations of the acquired immunodeficiency syndrome (AIDS): experience at UCSF and review of the literature. *J. Neurosurg.*, **62**, 475–495.

Levy, R. M., Rosenbloom, S. and Perrett, L. V. (1986). Neuroradiologic findings in AIDS: a review of 200 cases. *Am. J. Roentgenol.*, **147**, 977–983.

Lipton, S. A. (1991). HIV-related neurotoxicity. *Brain Pathol.*, **1**, 193–199.

Lipton, S. A. (1992). Models of neuronal injury in AIDS: another role for the NMDA receptor? *Trends Neurosci.*, **15**, 75–79.

Lipton, S. A. (1994). Neurobiology – HIV displays its coat of arms. *Nature*, **367**, 113–114.

Magnuson, D. S. K., Knudsen, B. E., Geiger, J. D., Brownstone, R. M. and Nath, A. (1995). Human immunodeficiency virus type 1 tat activates non-N-methyl-D-aspartate excitatory amino acid receptors and causes neurotoxicity. *Ann. Neurol.*, **37**, 373–380.

Mankowski, J. L., Flaherty, M. T., Spelman, J. P. *et al.* (1997). Pathogenesis of simian immunodeficiency virus encephalitis: viral determinants of neurovirulence. *J. Virol.*, **71**, 6055–6060.

Mankowski, J. L., Spelman, J. P., Ressetar, H. G. *et al.* (1994). Neurovirulent simian immunodeficiency virus replicates productively in endothelial cells of the central nervous system in vivo and in vitro. *J. Virol.*, **68**, 8202–8208.

Marder, K., Albert, S. M., McDermott, M. and The Dana Consortium on the Therapy of HIV Dementia and Related Disorders (1998). Prospective study of neuro-cognitive impairment in HIV (Dana Cohort): dementia and mortality outcomes (abstract). *J. Neurovirol.*, **4**, 358.

Masliah, E., Ge, N., Morey, M., Deteresa, R., Terry, R. D. and Wiley, C. A. (1992a). Cortical dendritic pathology in human immunodeficiency virus encephalitis. *Lab. Invest.*, **66**, 285–291.

Masliah, E., Achim, C. L., Ge, N., Deteresa, R., Terry, R. D. and Wiley, C. A. (1992b). Spectrum of human immunodeficiency virus-associated neocortical damage. *Ann. Neurol.*, **32**, 321–329.

Masliah, E., Ge, N., Achim, C. L., Hansen, L. A. and Wiley, C. A. (1992c). Selective neuronal vulnerability in HIV encephalitis. *J. Neuropathol. Exp. Neurol.*, **51**, 585–593.

Masliah, E., Ge, N., Achim, C. L. and Wiley, C. A. (1995). Differential vulnerability of calbindin-immunoreactive neurons in HIV encephalitis. *J. Neuropathol. Exp. Neurol.*, **54**, 350–357.

Mayeux, R., Stern, Y., Tang, M. X. *et al.* (1993). Mortality risks in gay men with human immunodeficiency virus infection and cognitive impairment. *Neurology*, **43**, 176–182.

McArthur, J. C. (1987). Neurologic manifestations of AIDS. *Medicine (Baltimore)*, **66**, 407–437.

McArthur, J. C. (1998), Understanding measurement of CSF HIV levels. *HIV Neurol. Newsletter*, **1**, 1–8.

McArthur, J. C., Cohen, B. A., Selnes, O. A. *et al.* (1989). Low prevalence of neurological and neuropsychological abnormalities in otherwise healthy HIV-1-infected individuals: results from the Multicenter AIDS Cohort Study. *Ann. Neurol.*, **26**, 601–611.

McArthur, J. C., Hoover, D. R., Bacellar, H. *et al.* (1993). Dementia in AIDS patients: incidence and risk factors. *Neurology*, **43**, 2245–2252.

McArthur, J. C., McClernon, D. R., Cronin, M. F. *et al.* (1997). Relationship between human immunodeficiency virus-associated dementia and viral load in cerebrospinal fluid and brain. *Ann. Neurol.*, **42**, 689–698.

McArthur, J. C., Nance-Sproson, T., Childs, E., Jackson, J. B., Lanier, E. R. and McClernon, D. (1998). Virologic response in cerebrospinal fluid after initiation of antiretroviral therapy. *Neuroscience of HIV Infection, Chicago*, June 3–6.

McArthur, J. C., Nance-Sproson, T. E., Griffin, D. E. *et al.* (1992). The diagnostic utility of elevation in cerebrospinal fluid b2 microglobulin in HIV-1 dementia. *Neurology*, **42**, 1707–1712.

McArthur, J. C., Selnes, O. A., Dal Gan, G. J. *et al.* (1994). Phase I/II trial of pentoxifylline in HIV-associated dementia and myelopathy. *Neuroscience of HIV Infection: Basic and Clinical Frontiers, Vancouver*, Aug. 2–5.

Mellors, J. W., Kingsley, L. A., Rinaldo, C. R. *et al.* (1995). Quantitation of HIV-1 RNA in plasma predicts outcome after seroconversion. *Ann. Intern. Med.*, **122**, 573–579.

Mellors, J. W., Munoz, A., Giorgi, J. V. *et al.* (1997). Plasma viral load and CD4+ lymphocytes as prognostic markers of HIV-1 infection. *Ann. Intern. Med.*, **126**, 946–954.

Melnick, S. L., Sherer, R., Louis, T. A. *et al.* (1994). Survival and disease progression according to gender of patients with HIV infection. The Terry Beirn Community Programs for Clinical Research on AIDS. *J. Am. Med. Assoc.*, **272**, 1915–1921.

Menon, D. K., Baudouin, C. J., Tomlinson, D. and Hoyle, C. (1990). Proton MR spectroscopy and imaging of the brain in AIDS: evidence of neuronal loss in regions that appear normal with imaging. *J. Comput. Assist. Tomogr.*, **14**, 882–885.

Merigan, T. C. and Schooley, R. T. (1995). Surrogate markers of HIV: strategies and issues for selection and use. *Acquired Immune Def. Synd. Hum. Retrovirol.*, **10**(suppl. 2), S1–S116.

Mertens, T. E. and Low-Beer, D. (1996). HIV and AIDS: where is the epidemic going? *Bull. WHO*, **74**, 121–129.

Michael, N. L., Vahey, M., Burke, D. S. and Redfield, R. R. (1992). Viral DNA and mRNA expression correlate with the stage of human immunodeficiency virus (HIV) type 1 infection in humans: evidence for viral replication in all stages of HIV disease. *J. Virol.*, **66**, 310–316.

Mijch, A. M., Clezy, K. and Furner, V. (1997). Women and HIV. In: *Managing HIV*, (G., Stewart, (ed.)) North Sydney: Australian Medical Publishing Company Limited. pp. 128–130.

Mintz, M., Epstein, L. G. and Koenigsberger, M. R. (1989). Neurological manifestations of acquired immunodeficiency syndrome in children. *Int. Pediatr.*, **4**, 161–171.

Moore, J. P. (1997). Coreceptors: implications for HIV pathogenesis and therapy. (Review.) *Science*, **276**, 51–52.

Moore, R., Keruly, J. C., Gallant, J. and Chaisson, R. E. (1998). Decline in mortality rates and opportunistic disease with combination antiretroviral therapy (abstract #22374). *12th World AIDS Conference, Geneva*, June 28–July 3.

Moore, R. D., Keruly, J. C. and Chaisson, R. E. (1997). Effectiveness of combination antiretroviral therapy in clinical practice (abstract). *Interscience Conference on Antimicrobial Agents and Chemotherapy (ICAAC), Toronto*, Sept. 28–Oct. 1.

Moses, A. V., Bloom, F. E., Pauza, C. D. and Nelson, J. A. (1993). Human immunodeficiency virus infection of human brain capillary endothelial cells occurs via a CD4 galactosylceramide-independent mechanism. *Proc. Natl Acad. Sci. USA*, **90**, 10474–10478.

Mucke, L. and Buttini, M. (1998). Molecular basis of HIV-associated neurologic disease. In: *Molecular Neurology*, (J. B. Martin, (ed.)). New York: Scientific American. pp. 135–154.

Navia, B., Lee, L., Ernst, T. *et al.* (1998). In vivo proton MRS studies of HIV brain injury and HIV dementia. *12th World AIDS Conference, Geneva*, June 28–July 3. Abstract #32204.

Navia, B. A., Cho, E. S., Petito, C. K. and Price, R. W. (1986a). The AIDS dementia complex: II. Neuropathology. *Ann. Neurol.*, **19**, 525–535.

Navia, B. A., Jordan, B. D. and Price, R. W. (1986b). The AIDS dementia complex: I. Clinical features. *Ann. Neurol.*, **19**, 517–524.

Navia, B. A. and Price, R. W. (1987). The acquired immunodeficiency syndrome dementia complex as the presenting or sole manifestation of human immuno-deficiency virus infection. *Arch. Neurol.*, **44**, 65–69.

Newman, S. P., Lunn, S. and Harrison, M. J. G. (1995). Do asymptomatic HIV-seropositive individuals show cognitive deficit? *AIDS*, **9**, 1211–1220.

Nuwer, M. R., Miller, E. N., Visscher, B. R. *et al.* (1992). Asymptomatic HIV infection does not cause EEG abnormalities: results from the Multicenter AIDS Cohort Study (MACS). *Neurology*, **42**, 1214–1219.

O'Brien, W. A., Hartigan, P. M., Martin, D. *et al.* (1996). Changes in plasma HIV-1 RNA and CD4+ lymphocyte counts and the risk of progression to AIDS. *N. Engl. J. Med.*, **334**, 426–431.

Pantaleo, G., Graziosi, C., Dernarest, J. F. *et al.* (1993). HIV infection is active and progressive in lymphoid tissue during the clinically latent stage of disease. *Nature*, **362**, 355–358.

Persidsky, Y., Buttini, M., Limoges, J., Bock, P. and Gendelman, H. E. (1997a). An analysis of HIV-1-associated inflammatory products in brain tissue of humans and SCID mice with HIV-1 encephalitis. *J. Neurovirol.*, **3**, 401–416.

Persidsky, Y., Stins, M., Way, D. *et al.* (1997b). A model for monocyte migration through the blood–brain barrier during HIV-1 encephalitis. *J. Immunol.*, **158**, 3499–3510.

Petito, C. K., Navia, B. A., Cho, E. S., Jordan, B. D., George, D. C. and Price, R. W. (1985). Vacuolar myelopathy pathologically resembling subacute combined degeneration in patients with the acquired immunodeficiency syndrome. *N. Engl. J. Med.*, **312**, 874–879.

Pialoux, G., Fournier, S., Moulignier, A., Poveda, J. D., Clavel, F. and Dupont, B. (1997). Central nervous system (CNS) as sanctuary of HIV-1 in a patient treated

Sei, S., Saito, K., Stewart, S. K. *et al.* (1995). Increased human immunodeficiency virus (HIV) type 1 DNA content and quinolinic acid concentration in brain tissues from patients with HIV encephalopathy. *J. Infect. Dis.*, **172**, 638–647.

Selnes, O. A., McArthur, J. C., Royal, W. *et al.* (1992). HIV-1 infection and intravenous drug use: longitudinal neuropsychological evaluation of asymptomatic subjects. *Neurology*, **42**, 1924–1930.

Selnes, O. A., Miller, E., McArthur, J. C. *et al.* (1990). HIV-1 infection: no evidence of cognitive decline during the asymptomatic stages. *Neurology*, **40**, 204–208.

Sharer, L. R., Cho, E. S. and Epstein, L. G. (1985). Multinucleated giant cells and HTLV-III in AIDS encephalopathy. *Hum. Pathol.*, **16**, 760.

Sharer, L. R. and Kapila, R. (1985). Neuropathologic observations in acquired immunodefficiency syndrome (AIDS). *Acta Neuropathol. (Berl.)*, **66**, 188–198.

Shi, B., De Girolami, U., He, J. *et al.* (1996). Apoptosis induced by HIV-1 infection of the central nervous system. *J. Clin. Invest.*, **98**, 1979–1990.

Shi, B., Raina, J., Lorenzo, A., Busciglio, J. and Gabuzda, D. (1998). Neuronal apoptosis induced by HIV-1 Tat protein and TNF-alpha: potentiation of neurotoxicity mediated by oxidative stress and implications for HIV-1 dementia. *J. Neurovirol.*, **4**, 281–290.

Sidtis, J. J., Gatsonis, C., Price, R. W. *et al.* (1993). Zidovudine treatment of the AIDS dementia complex: results of a placebo-controlled trial. *Ann. Neurol.*, **33**, 343–349.

Silberstein, C. H., McKegney, F. P., O'Dowd, M. A. *et al.* (1987). A prospective longitudinal study of neuropsychological and psychosocial factors in asymptomatic individuals at risk of HTLV-III/LAV infection in a methadone program: preliminary findings. *Int. J. Neurosci.*, **32**, 669–676.

Snider, W. D., Simpson, D. M., Nielsen, S., Gold, J. W., Metroka, C. E. and Posner, J. B. (1983). Neurological complications of acquired immune deficiency syndrome: analysis of 50 patients. *Ann. Neurol.*, **14**, 403–418.

So, Y. T., Engstrom, J. W. and Olney, R. K. (1990). The spectrum of electrodiagnostic abnormalities in patients with human immunodeficiency virus infection. *Muscle Nerve*, **13**, 855 (Abstract).

Sorell, T. and Kesson, A. (1995). The HIV-infected woman. In: *Management of the HIV Infected Patient*, (S. M. Crowe, J. Hoy and J. Mills, (eds)). Cambridge: Cambridge University Press.

Steuler, H., Munzinger, S., Wildemann, B. and Storch-Hagenlocher, B. (1992). Quantitation of HIV-1 proviral DNA in cells from cerebrospinal fluid. *J. AIDS*, **5**, 405–408.

Stoler, M. H., Eskin, T. A., Benn, S., Angerer, R. C. and Angerer, L. M. (1986). Human T-cell lymphotropic virus type III infection of the central nervous system. A preliminary in situ analysis. *J. Am. Med. Assoc.*, **256**, 2360–2364.

Takahashi, K., Wesselingh, S. L., Griffin, D. E., McArthur, J. C., Johnson, R. T. and Glass, J. D. (1996) Localization of HIV-1 in human brain using polymerase chain reaction/in situ hybridization and immunocytochemistry. *Ann. Neurol.*, **39**, 705–711.

Tartaglione, T. A., Collier, A. C., Coombs, R. W. *et al.* (1991). Acquired immunodeficiency syndrome: cerebrospinal fluid findings in patients before and during long-term oral zidovudine therapy. *Arch. Neurol.*, **48**, 695–699.

Tersmette, M., Gruters, R. A., de Wolf, F. *et al.* (1989). Evidence for a role of virulent human immunodeficiency syndrome: studies of sequential HIV isolates. *J. Virol.*, **63**, 2118–2125.

The Dana Consortium on Therapy for HIV Dementia and Related Cognitive Disorders (1996). Clinical confirmation of the American Academy of Neurology algorithm for HIV-1 associated cognitive/motor disorder. *Neurology*, **47**, 1247-1253.

The Dana Consortium on Therapy of HIV Dementia and Related Cognitive Disorders (1997). Safety and efficacy of the antioxidant OPC-14117 in HIV associated cognitive impairment. *Neurology*, **49**, 142–146.

The Dana Consortium on the Therapy of HIV Dementia and Related Cognitive Disorders (1998). A randomized, double-blind, placebo-controlled trial of deprenyl and thioctic acid in human immunodeficiency virus-associated cognitive impairment. *Neurology*, **50**, 645–651.

Thomas, F. P., Chalk, C., Lalonde, R., Robitaille, Y. and Jolicouer, P. (1994). Expression of human immunodeficiency virus type 1 in the nervous system of transgenic mice leads to neurological disease. *J. Virol.*, **68**, 7099–7107.

Tozzi, V., Narciso, P., Galgani, S. *et al.* (1993). Effects of zidovudine in 30 patients with mild to end-stage AIDS dementia complex. *AIDS*, **7**, 683–692.

Tyor, W. R., Griffin, J. W., Wesselingh, S., McArthur, J. C. and Griffin, D. E. (1995). A unifying hypothesis for the pathogenesis of HIV-associated dementia complex, vacuolar myelopathy, and sensory neuropathy. *J. AIDS*, **9**, 379–388.

Vinik, A. I., Suwanwalaikorn, S., Stansberry, K. B., Holland, M. T., McNitt, P. M. and Colen, L. E. (1995). Quantitative measurement of cutaneous perception in diabetic neuropathy. *Muscle Nerve*, **18**, 574–584.

Weis, S., Haug, H. and Budka, H. (1993). Neuronal damage in the cerebral cortex of AIDS brains: a morphometric study. *Acta Neuropathol.*, **85**, 185–189.

Westmoreland, S. V., Halpern, E. and Lackner, A. A. (1998). Simian immunodeficiency virus encephalitis in rhesus macaques is associated with rapid disease progression. *J. Neurovirol.*, **4**, 260–268.

Wiley, C. A. and Achim, C. (1994). Human immunodeficiency virus encephalitis is the pathological correlate of dementia in aquired immunodeficiency syndrome. *Ann. Neurol.*, **26**, 673–676.

Wiley, C. A., Masliah, E. and Achim, C. L. (1994). Measurement of CNS HIV burden and its association with neurologic disease. *Adv. Neuroimmunol.*, **4**, 319–325.

Wiley, C. A., Masliah, E., Morey, M. *et al.* (1991). Noncortical damage during HIV infection. *Ann. Neurol.*, **29**, 651–657.

Wiley, C. A., Schrier, R. D., Nelson, J. A., Lampert, P. W. and Oldstone, M. B. (1986). Cellular localization of human immunodeficiency virus infection within the brains of acquired immune deficiency syndrome patients. *Proc. Natl Acad. Sci. USA*, **83**, 7089–7093.

Wiley, C. A., Soontornniyomkij, V., Radhakrishnan, L. *et al.* (1998). Distribution of brain HIV load in AIDS. *Brain Pathol.*, **8**, 277–284.

Wong, J. K., Hezareh, M., Gunthard, H. F. *et al.* (1997). Recovery of replication-competent HIV despite prolonged suppression of plasma viremia. *Science*, **278**, 1291–1295.

Yarchoan, R., Berg, G., Brouwers, P. *et al.* (1987). Response of human-immuno-deficiency-virus-associated neurological disease to 3′-azido-3′-deoxythymidine. *Lancet*, **1**, 132–135.

Zhang, H., Dornadula, G., Beumont, M. *et al.* (1988). Human immunodeficiency virus type 1 in the semen of men receiving highly active antiretroviral therapy. *N. Engl. J. Med.*, **339**, 1803–1809.

Zink, C., Carter, D., Flaherty, M., Mankowski, J. and Clements, J. (1988a). The SIV/macaque model: unraveling the mysteries of HIV encephalitis. In: *The Neurology of AIDS* (H. E. Gendelman, S. A. Lipton, L. Epstein and S. Swindells (eds)). New York: Chapman & Hall. pp. 189–200.

Zink, M. C., Spelman, J. P., Robinson, R. B. and Clements, J. E. (1998b). SIV infection of macaques – modeling the progression to AIDS dementia. *J. Neurovirol.*, **4**, 249–259.

This chapter has been modified from:

McArthur, J. C. *HIV-associated dementia. Seminars In Neurology* (in press).

McArthur, J. C. *AIDS 1999 and Advances in Therapy. AIDS and the Nervous System Course.* American Academy of Neurology, Minneapolis, MN, April 23, 1999.

McArthur, J. C. and Grant, I. HIV neurocognitive disorders. In: Geneelman H. E., Lipton, S. A., Epstein, L., Swindells, S. (eds). *The Neurology of AIDS.* Chapman & Hall, New York, 1998, pp. 499–523.

7

Human prion diseases

Rajith de Silva and Robert G. Will

Introduction

The human prion diseases are a group of rare neurodegenerative disorders, which are characterized by spongiform change in the central nervous system and natural or experimental transmissibility. The commonest of these, sporadic Creutzfeldt-Jakob disease (CJD), occurs throughout the world with an incidence of 0.5 to 1.0 case/million/year. Up to 15% of cases are familial, with an autosomal dominant mode of inheritance. Inherited forms of prion disease include Gerstmann-Sträussler syndrome (GSS) and fatal familial insomnia (FFI). A small, but increasing, number of cases of iatrogenic human prion disease have been identified world-wide. The observation that a single group of disorders can straddle a spectrum of mechanisms by which human disease is thought to arise (from inherited to infectious) has been a source of fascination to scientists, and recent theories on the pathogenesis of spongiform encephalopathy attempt to explain this apparent conundrum.

Although H. G. Creutzfeldt (Creutzfeldt, 1920) and A. Jakob (Jakob, 1921, 1923), are credited with the first descriptions of CJD, by current criteria probably only two of the original six cases, both described by Jakob, are examples of human spongiform encephalopathy (Masters and Gajdusek, 1982). Perhaps the most accurate early clinical descriptions of the entity that we recognize as CJD were given by Nevin and colleagues (Jones and Nevin, 1954; Nevin et al., 1960), in which they described a neurodegenerative process of subacute onset and rapid progression culminating invariably in death. They drew attention to the combination of pyramidal and cerebellar disturbance, the presence of involuntary movements especially myoclonus, the occurrence of visual failure, paratonic rigidity and speech disturbance, and the recurrence of primitive reflexes. They also described the characteristic electroencephalogram (EEG) findings, but felt that these were unlikely to be specific for the diagnosis. Crucially they gave details of the neuropathological appearances, but erroneously concluded that the spongiform change was due to microvascular dysfunction. Other notable early descriptions include cases of CJD characterized by occipital blindness (Heidenhain, 1929; Meyer et al., 1954), and an unusual form of the illness dominated in the early stages by progressive cerebellar ataxia (Brownell and Oppenheimer, 1965).

Kuru is a progressive and eventually fatal neurodegenerative disorder characterized by cerebellar dysfunction and personality change. It predominantly affects the Fore-speaking people of the highlands of Papua New Guinea, and reached epidemic proportions up to the mid-1950s probably as a consequence of endocannibalistic rituals. After it was confirmed to be a transmissable disease (Gajdusek *et al.*, 1966), CJD, which shares some clinical and histopathological similarities with kuru, was demonstrated to be experimentally transmissible (Gibbs, 1968). This observation led to a series of epidemiological surveys world-wide to investigate the possibility that sporadic CJD arose from case-to-case or zoonotic transmission (Galvez *et al.*, 1980; Tsuji and Kuroiwa, 1983; Brown *et al.*, 1987; Harries-Jones, *et al.*, 1988). While no such evidence emerged, a large amount of data on the clinical and epidemiological features of CJD were collected. These studies may be criticized for relying on the criteria suggested by Masters *et al.* for 'establishing' the diagnosis (Table 7.1) (Masters *et al.*, 1979), but the validity of these criteria has been supported by more recent work in which only neuropathologically confirmed or experimentally transmitted cases have been studied (Brown *et al.*, 1986; Brown, 1994). Taken together, these epidemiological surveys provide a comprehensive, and remarkably consistent, picture of the characteristics of sporadic CJD.

Spongiform encephalopathies affect a number of mammalian species in addition to humans (Table 7.2), and the sheep disorder scrapie was recognized first in 1755 in Britain (Brown and Bradley, 1998). The number of species affected has increased recently, following the emergence of bovine spongiform encephalopathy (BSE). Transmission experiments give convincing evidence that these 'new' forms of spongiform encephalopathy, such as feline spongiform encephalopathy and spongiform encephalopathy of captive exotic ungulates, are related to BSE (Bruce *et al.*, 1997). In 1996 Will *et al.* described a 'new variant' of CJD in the UK (Will *et al.*, 1996), which appears on the basis of transmission studies (Bruce *et al.*, 1997), immunblotting experiments (Collinge *et al.*, 1996) and epidemiological grounds (Will, 1999) to be associated with BSE also.

In this chapter, the clinical characteristics of all forms of human spongiform encephalopathy are described. The salient neurophysiological, imaging and laboratory findings are presented. The differential diagnosis is discussed, and criteria for the positive clinical diagnosis during life explored. Practical issues concerning the 'management' of CJD are finally discussed. We start, however,

Table 7.1 The Masters' criteria for the diagnosis of CJD.

Definite CJD	Pathologically confirmed CJD
Probable CJD	Rapidly progressive dementia
	+ Periodic sharp wave complexes in all leads throughout electroen-cephalogram recording
	+ At least two of the following clinical features: myoclonus; cerebellar or pyramidal or extrapyramidal signs; cortical blindness; akinetic mutism; early neurogenic muscle atrophy
Possible CJD	Rapidly progressive dementia
	+ At least three of the above clinical features

Adapted from Masters, 1979

Table 7.2   The spongiform encephalopathies

Disorder	Species
Sporadic Creutzfeldt-Jakob disease	Human
Inherited Creutzfeldt-Jakob disease (includes Gerstmann-Sträussler syndrome and fatal familial insomnia)	Human
Iatrogenic Creutzfeldt-Jakob disease	Human
Kuru	Human
New variant Creutzfeldt-Jakob disease*	Human
Scrapie	Sheep/goat/moufflon
Transmissible mink encephalopathy	Mink
Chronic wasting disease	Deer/elk
Bovine spongiform encephalopathy*	Cattle
Feline spongiform encephalopathy*	Cat/cheetah/puma/ocelot
Spongiform encephalopathy of captive exotic ungulates*	Kudu/nyala/oryx/gemsbok/eland

* These disorders are associated with the same agent of infectivity

with an exploration of the theories regarding the causative 'agent' of CJD and the other spongiform encephalopathies.

Pathogenesis

The suggestion that the agent of scrapie infectivity was devoid of nucleic acid was first made by Tikvah Alper and colleagues as far back as 1967 (Alper *et al.*, 1967). This hypothesis was based on the observation that scrapie infectivity was resistant to irradiation, including ultraviolet at 254 nm. Stanley Prusiner resurrected the concept in the early 1980s, and argued that the agent was composed mainly, if not wholly, of protein; hence the term prion, or proteinaceous infectious particle (Prusiner, 1982). Prusiner's suggestion was met with considerable scepticism, but over the next 20 years he performed a series of experiments to support the prion theory. He demonstrated that scrapie infectivity copurified with a protein of 27–30 kDa molecular weight and that this infectivity was not dependent on polynucleotides (Bolton *et al.*, 1982; Prusiner, 1982). Transgenic mice carrying a mutation in the gene (*PRNP*) encoding prion protein (PrP) developed spontaneous neurodegeneration (Hsiao *et al.*, 1990), and transmission of brain tissue from these animals into Syrian hamsters and homotypic transgenic mice was successful. In other laboratories, it was shown that PrP null mice were resistant to the intracerebral inoculation of scrapie (Büeler *et al.*, 1993), and that the conversion of a protease-sensitive prion protein (PrP^c) to a protease-resistant and probably 'infective' form (PrP^{Sc}) could be achieved in a cell-free system (Kocisko *et al.*, 1995). Taken together the results of these experiments provide strong evidence in favour of Prusiner's hypothesis, and his contribution was recognized by the Nobel Prize for Medicine in 1997.

The theory at present holds that PrP^c is a nascent and non-infectious cell surface protein that has the capacity to interact with the physiochemically altered and infectious PrP^{Sc}. As well as causing neurotoxicity, PrP^{Sc} converts more PrP^c to PrP^{Sc}. The ease with which transmissibility occurs according to this model would be dependent on the homotypic similarities between interacting prion proteins. It is suggested that this accounts for the low rate of successful transmission of inherited cases of CJD to experimental animals: PrP molecules derived from mutated alleles may have difficulty interacting with the 'normal' PrP of the inoculated animal. Sporadic CJD is thought to arise from the chance conformational change of PrP^c to PrP^{Sc}, a process which then proceeds autocatalytically.

The theory is less successful in accounting for the strain variability that is, for example, observed with scrapie. This is intuitively attributed to the agent containing nucleic acids and modifications to the PrP structure are not thought to be capable of mediating this variability. In amendments to the theory it is argued that an essential but small nucleic acid component is protected by its close and integral association with PrP (the 'virino' model) (Kimberlin, 1990), or that the agent has the capacity to recruit cellular nucleic acid from the cell which it is infecting for replication (the 'coprion' or 'unified' theory) (Weissmann, 1991). Others, including Prusiner, argue that the variability of the agent resides in glycoprotein modifications of the basic prion molecule, or in conformational differences in the β-pleated quaternary structure of PrP^{Sc}.

Evidence to support the prion hypothesis has emerged from the study of the inherited form of CJD. More than 20 separate mutations of the open reading frame (ORF) of the gene encoding PrP in man (*PRNP*) have been linked with cases of inherited CJD. These mutations have not been identified in normal controls, and to date there have been no reported cases of inherited CJD world-wide not associated with a *PRNP* ORF mutation. A site of common polymorphism at codon 129 of the *PRNP* ORF (which encodes methionine or valine) appears to confer increased susceptibility to the development of sporadic, iatrogenic and, possibly, new variant CJD. In the case of sporadic CJD, around 80% of subjects in Caucasian series are homozygous for methionine at this site (as compared with 37% of the normal population) (Laplanche *et al.*, 1994; Windl *et al.*, 1996). In one large pedigree with inherited CJD, the age at death was influenced by the codon 129 polymorphic status, carriers who were heterozygous having an older age of death compared with those who were homozygous (Poulter *et al.*, 1992). These observations are consistent with the prion theory: PrP molecules that are derived from *PRNP* genes that are homozygous at codon 129 may have an enhanced capacity for polymerization, whereas this process may be less efficient when PrP molecules are derived from *PRNP* genes that are heterozygous at this site. In the latter case, patients may not only be afforded a degree of protection from disease development, but once established (as in the inherited CJD pedigree) the disease may progress less rapidly and there may be an older age at death.

The normal function of PrP is unknown. Early studies appeared to show that PrP null mice developed normally and that they had normal gross behavioural characteristics (Büeler *et al.*, 1993). This was surprising, given the high conservation of PrP among mammalian species and its wide expression in early embryogenesis. However, more recent experiments have demonstrated abnormal sleep patterns, altered electrophysiological characteristics and accelerated cerebellar Purkinje cell loss in these animals. All of these observations have possible clinical correlates in CJD.

Clinical presentations

The analysis of symptoms and signs at the start of and during the course of sporadic CJD from large published surveys reveals that at the debut of their illnesses, 30–40% of patients had cognitive impairment alone, 30–40% had neurological disease in isolation (most with cerebellar ataxia) and 20–30% had mixed features. Furthermore, dementia was almost always present during the course of illness. Myoclonus (which was rarely present at disease onset) was frequently noted during the course of disease, features of cerebellar, visual, pyramidal and extra-pyramidal dysfunction were noted regularly but were not universal, and features of lower motor neuron dysfunction and convulsions were rare presenting features and were unusual even during the course of illness. As the disease progresses, evidence of multifocal central nervous system dysfunction emerges, with the reappearance of primitive reflexes and the development of akinetic mutism. Terminally, patients are rigid, mute and unresponsive, and may have abnormal patterns of respiration. The mean age of onset of sporadic CJD is around 65 years and the mean disease duration is around 4 months.

As mentioned earlier, atypical presentations of CJD have long been recognized. In the Heidenhain variant, the early course is dominated by cortical visual disturbance (homonymous hemianopia and occipital blindness). As the disease progresses, the phenotype increasingly resembles sporadic CJD. In some pathological studies, the cerebral spongiform change has been especially marked in the occipital lobes (Meyer et al., 1954). This and other 'focal' presentations of CJD probably account for no more than 10% of cases, but it is worth bearing in mind that cases may present with features as diverse as dysphasia, dyspraxia, hemiparesis, oculomotor disturbance and parkinsonism. The form of CJD characterized by progressive cerebellar ataxia (in which cognitive impairment is a late development, appearing weeks or months after the presentation with ataxia) is highly unusual accounting for less than 5% of sporadic cases. A recent study has drawn attention to the acute presentation of CJD resembling stroke (McNaughton and Will, 1997), and there are well described (and pathologically confirmed) cases of CJD found in association with other neurodegenerative processes especially dementia of Alzheimer-type where the course can be protracted and 'bi-phasic' (Muramoto et al., 1992).

Early descriptions of cases of CJD of long duration (greater than 2 years) were confounded by the inclusion of familial cases, which have a longer course. In P. Brown and colleagues' paper on CJD of longer than 2 years, the cases represented 9% of those with histopathologically verified CJD (Brown et al., 1984). Also that year, Will and Matthews gave clinical descriptions of their 'intermediate' cases, representing 6% of their series (Will and Matthews,

1984). They identified three distinct types of disease progression: a form characterized by slow but inexorable progression, a form in which slow neurodegeneration is followed by a rapid terminal phase; and a form in which rapid early decline is followed by a protracted terminal state (two of their 12 cases had family histories of neurodegeneration and may have had familial CJD). In Brown's later series, sporadic cases were defined by the absence of known *PRNP* ORF mutations or family histories of CJD, which will have excluded the vast majority of familial cases (Brown *et al.*, 1994). The proportion of cases with disease durations longer than 2 years was 4%, the longest duration was 4.5 years and there were three patients each in the slow, slow-fast and fast-slow categories. Parchi and colleagues have identified a small number of sporadic CJD cases which are methionine homozygous at codon 129 of the *PRNP* ORF and have long disease durations, with a distinctive protease-resistant PrP profile on Western blotting (Parchi *et al.*, 1996). These authors argued that differences in the structure of PrP governed disease duration, but host factors including *PRNP* genotype and age must also influence the disease phenotype. The codon 129 polymorphic status does not appear to influence disease duration in sporadic CJD significantly, but in one series heterozygous patients had a mean disease duration of 8.8 months compared with disease durations of 3.0 and 6.0 months in methionine and valine homozygous patients respectively (Laplanche *et al.*, 1994).

Signs of lower motor neuron dysfunction are encountered in CJD, but they are uncommon, rarely appear at the start of the illness and never occur in the absence of more widespread cortical and cerebellar disease. In a seminal paper, Salazar and colleagues argued that cases of so called 'amyotrophic CJD' were distinct from cases of CJD and '... do not represent transmissible disease caused by unconventional viruses as presently understood' (Salazar *et al.*, 1983). They based this conclusion on negative transmission studies and on the atypical neuropathological appearances of these cases. The most consistent feature of the latter examinations was neuronal loss and gliosis of the frontotemporal cortex, now recognized as being the pathological hallmark of the dementia that can accompany motor neuron disease. (There may also be secondary spongiform change in these regions, a possible explanation for the confusion.) The general consensus is that 'amyotrophic CJD' is a misnomer, and that the majority of these cases are patients with motor neuron disease and dementia. In the Salazar series, only two out of 33 cases with dementia and early lower motor neuron signs transmitted. Both cases had typical CJD brain pathology, and were probably cases of CJD that had developed by chance in individuals with chronic neuropathy.

The clinical spectrum associated with familial CJD is wide. In general, the disorders linked with the *PRNP* ORF missense mutations at codons 200 (Pro-Leu), 210 (Val-Ile) and 178 (Asp-Asn, in association with valine at codon 129), and extra base pair insertions in the octapeptide repeat region resemble sporadic CJD. GSS is a form of familial CJD characterized by slowly progressive (relative to sporadic CJD) cerebellar incoordination, pyramidal signs and dementia. The pathological appearances are dominated by multi-centric argyrophilic plaques (staining positively with anti-PrP antibody)

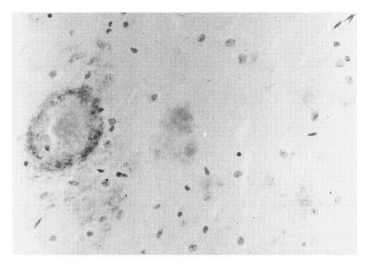

Figure 7.1 A typical amyloid deposit in the cerebellar molecular layer in GSS comprises a rounded amyloid core (left), with multiple smaller deposits in the adjacent neuropil (right), forming a multicentric plaque. Haematoxylin and eosis, × 270

throughout the brain and minimal spongiform change (Figure 7.1). This form of familial CJD is classically associated with the missense mutation at codon 102 (Pro-Leu) (Hsiao *et al.*, 1989). Mutations at codons 117 (Ala-Val), 198 (Phe-Ser) and 217 (Gln-Arg) are also associated with this clinical phenotype, but in the case of the latter two the pathological appearances include neurofibrillary tangles, the Indiana variant (Dlouhy *et al.*, 1992). The mutation at codon 117 (Ala-Val) has also been described in association with the 'telencephalic' form of familial CJD, in which dementia is accompanied by pyramidal and extra-pyramidal features, and variable cerebellar signs (Hsiao *et al.*, 1991). There is considerable phenotypic variability within large pedigrees with GSS, but to date it has proved difficult to account for this on the basis of the codon 129 polymorphic status or other sites of genotypic variability (Barbanti *et al.*, 1996).

FFI is now recognized as a relatively common form of familial prion disease. It is characterized clinically by disturbances of the wake-sleep cycle, dysautonomia, myoclonus, ataxia, dysarthria, spasticity and cognitive impairment. Neuropathological examination reveals marked thalamic and inferior olivary atrophy with variable degrees of cortical spongiform change. The disease has been linked with the codon 178 (Asp-Asn) mutation of the *PRNP* ORF, in association with methionine at codon 129 of the mutated allele (Goldfarb *et al.*, 1992). (As noted earlier, when the latter site encodes valine the same mutation results in inherited CJD.) Recent data suggest that methionine homozygous subjects have a shorter duration of disease than heterozygotes (Montagna *et al.*, 1998).

In summary, familial forms of the illness can manifest highly unusual clinical features for CJD including insomnia, dysautonomia and (in the case of the codon 105 (Pro-Leu) mutation) progressive spastic paraparesis. There is considerable overlap between the clinical features associated with each mutation, and 'typical' phenotypes cannot always be attributed accurately to specific mutations. For example, the clinical and neuropathological features of FFI have been described in a subject bearing the codon 200 (Glu-Lys) mutation (Chapman *et al.*, 1996). In general, familial cases of CJD tend to present about a decade earlier than sporadic cases (around 55 years) and have a disease duration that is twice as long (around 8 months) (de Silva, 1998).

The clinical presentation of forms of iatrogenic CJD may be influenced by the route through which the agent of infectivity gains entry. Cases in which 'peripheral' (outside the central nervous system or eye) inoculation has taken place are characterized by progressive cerebellar ataxia and minimal early cognitive impairment. This is the characteristic presentation of CJD in recipients of contaminated human pituitary-derived hormones. Despite increasing neurological disability, these patients may retain awareness and the ability to communicate until late in the clinical course. With disease progression, more 'typical' features of CJD emerge, including rigidity, myoclonus, startle responses and akinetic mutism. In contrast, those patients who have had the CJD agent inoculated centrally (for example, recipients of infected human dura mater grafts) have disease phenotypes consistent with sporadic CJD (Brown *et al.*, 1992).

The description by Will and colleagues in 1996 of a form of CJD with a unique and previously unrecognized pathological phenotype has extended the spectrum of human spongiform encephalopathy (Will *et al.*, 1996). Clinically, these cases are characterized by a younger age of onset and a longer duration of disease than sporadic CJD. The first 14 cases of new variant CJD (nvCJD) had a mean age of onset of 29 years (range 16 to 48) and a median disease duration of 14 months (range 9 to 35) (Zeidler *et al.*, 1997). All these patients had early psychiatric symptoms (most often depression) and around half had persistent and often painful sensory symptoms early in the illness. As the disease evolved, neurological signs including ataxia and involuntary movements were seen, and terminally most patients had akinetic mutism. The analysis of clinical signs noted during the course of nvCJD revealed that while some features associated with CJD such as spasticity, myoclonus and recurrent primitive reflexes were common, others (especially cortical blindness) were not (Zeidler *et al.*, 1997). None of the nvCJD cases reported to date have been shown to have a *PRNP* mutation and all have been methionine homozygous with respect to the common polymorphism at codon 129. The unifying pathological feature in all cases has been the presence of unusual PrP plaques (termed 'florid' plaques) with dense anti-PrP staining characteristics throughout the brain (Figure 7.2).

The clinical presentations of sporadic, familial, iatrogenic and new variant CJD while sharing similarities, are associated with distinctive features. These need to be considered in the context of the other available clinical data such as age of onset, past operative and drug therapy, family history, *PRNP* genome analysis and (eventually) disease duration. Clearly laboratory data and the likely differential diagnosis will also influence the interpretation of clinical

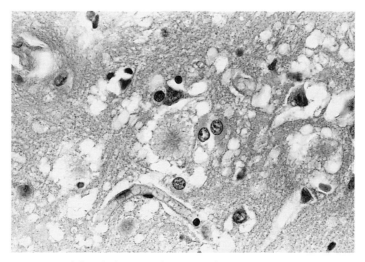

Figure 7.2   A typical florid plaque in the occipital cortex in nvCJD comprises a central amyloid core with radiating fibris, surrounded by a rim of spongiform change (centre). Similar smaller lesions are present on both sides. Haematoxylin and eosin, × 300

features, and the decision as to whether a patient has CJD or not; these issues are discussed next.

Laboratory findings

Abnormal liver 'function' tests are a relatively common observation during the course of illness. In the series by Will and Matthews (1984), 32 out of 80 cases had mild elevations of hepatic enzymes but overt liver failure never occurred. Where enzyme levels have been measured serially, the elevations have been noted to be transient (Tanaka *et al.*, 1993). The cerebrospinal fluid (CSF) protein content can also be raised, usually less than 1 g/l, and is not associated with a cellular response.

The EEG recording remains one of the most useful diagnostic tests in CJD. Contrary to the opinion of Nevin *et al.* (1960), in the appropriate clinical setting the finding of periodic sharp wave complexes in all leads throughout the recording is virtually diagnostic of CJD (in other words, this finding has high specificity for the diagnosis). A proportion of cases, however, never manifests this feature, thereby reducing its sensitivity. The proportion of cases with 'typical' EEG abnormalities is difficult to estimate accurately from the large epidemiological series, as its inclusion in the Masters' criteria will have led to the over-ascertainment of cases with this characteristic and, given the subjective nature of EEG interpretation, there will have been some variation in the types of abnormalities considered 'typical'. Knight has probably provided the most comprehensive data on EEG findings in CJD, based on the prospective surveillance of CJD in the UK between 1980 and 1984. In 60 pathologically confirmed, sporadic CJD cases, data were available in 57: 74% of cases had 'highly suggestive' or 'typical' appearances (Knight, personal communication). In the current UK prospective surveillance study, between 1990 and 1998, two cases with 'typical' EEGs have turned out to have Alzheimer-type dementia (Will, personal communication).

Conventional neuroimaging studies are usually normal in CJD. Computerized tomography may reveal cerebral atrophy, especially in long duration cases, but it must be borne in mind that there will be a tendency to overemphasize any degree of atrophy in view of the clinical history of progressive dementia. High T2 signal emanating from the basal ganglia on cranial magnetic resonance imaging has been described (Finkenstaedt et al., 1996), but at the present time there is inadequate systematic data on how consistent a finding this is. In nvCJD, high T2 signal emanating from the pulvinar region of the thalamus may be a relatively specific finding (Sellar et al., 1997).

Recent studies have attempted to identify markers of CJD infection in the CSF. These include neuron-specific enolase, S100 protein and τ protein, all of which may be relatively non-specific markers of neuronal damage and astrocytic change. Western blot analysis for the 14-3-3 protein on CSF optimally stored after collection has yielded a sensitivity and positive predictive value in excess of 90% in sporadic CJD (Zerr et al., 1998). False positive results do occur, especially in encephalitic subjects. In familial CJD and nvCJD its sensitivity is lower.

Efforts to identify ante-mortem diagnostic tests for nvCJD (where typical EEG appearances are never encountered) have generated some novel approaches. Following the discovery that a tonsil-specific isoform of PrP[Sc] existed in nvCJD, a small number of nvCJD cases have been studied: in all nine subjects this isoform was demonstrable by Western blotting or immunocyto-chemistry in tonsil, spleen and lymph node tissue (Hill et al., 1999). Interestingly, it was absent in all the cases of sporadic, familial and iatrogenic CJD that were studied.

The authors of the latter paper have suggested that tonsil biopsy obviates the need for brain biopsy in order to establish a diagnosis of nvCJD. It could be argued that in nvCJD and all other forms of CJD, brain biopsy is indicated clinically only if a potentially treatable condition is suspected (such as central nervous system vasculitis or Whipple's disease). The main limitations to brain biopsy are the potential risks to health care workers and the need to destroy all biopsy equipment if the diagnosis of spongiform encephalopathy is confirmed. In the case of tonsil biopsy, these risks and expenses are not diminished and will not aid diagnosis (unless it confirms nvCJD, the diagnosis considered most likely on clinical grounds).

Differential diagnosis, and criteria for diagnosis

The differential diagnosis in cases with suspected CJD is wide. During the prospective surveillance of CJD in the UK between 1990 and 1994, a proportion of cases suspected clinically of having CJD turned out to have an alternative neurodegenerative process pathologically (Table 7.3). There were

Table 7.3   Cases referred to the UK surveillance unit as suspect CJD whose final neuropathological diagnosis was not CJD, 1990–1994.

Alzheimer-type dementia (ATD)	17
ATD + multi-infarct disease (MID)	5
MID	3
Dementia of Lewy body-type (DLBT)	1
ATD + DLBT	1
Motor neuron disease	1
Cerebrovascular disease	1
Pick's disease	1
Progressive supranuclear palsy	1
Multiple system atrophy	1
Corticobasal degeneration	1
Viral encephalomyelitis	1
Metastatic carcinoma	1
Hypoxia	1
Epilepsy	1
No abnormality found	1

examples of a range of neurodegenerative processes affecting the central nervous system, but the majority (almost 60%) had Alzheimer-type dementia either in isolation or in combination with another form of dementia. Cases of non-CJD, with a median disease length of 16 months, had a significantly longer disease duration than patients with sporadic CJD. This was a useful indicator of whether a suspect case had CJD or not.

As clinical data during the course of illness were collected systematically on the non-CJD group, as well as on patients with confirmed CJD, it was possible to estimate the relative sensitivities and specificities of the various clinical features (Table 7.4). In addition to demonstrating that the various components of Masters criteria, such as elements of cognitive impairment, cerebellar

Table 7.4   Sensitivity and specificity of clinical characteristics for the diagnosis of CJD.

Clinical feature	Sensitivity	Specificity
Personality change	0.5	0.6
Abnormal behaviour	0.6	0.5
Memory impairment	0.6	0.4
Disorientation	0.8	0.2
Expressive dysphasia	0.4	0.7
Dyspraxia	0.6	0.5
Pyramidal dysfunction	0.6	0.4
Parkinsonism	0.3	0.7
Myoclonus	0.8	0.4
Cortical blindness	0.5	0.8
Cerebellar incoordination	0.8	0.6
Muscle wasting	0.2	0.8
Primitive reflexes	0.6	0.6
Paratonic rigidity	0.4	0.7
Akinetic mutism	0.7	0.8

dysfunction, cortical blindness, myoclonus and akinetic mutism, had reasonable diagnostic value, other less well-recognized features, including paratonic rigidity, recurrent primitive reflexes, dyspraxia and expressive dysphasia, emerged as useful signs. Of the original criteria, 'early neurogenic muscle wasting' stands alone in having a low sensitivity for the diagnosis of CJD (of 0.2). This observation echoes our previous statement that 'amyotrophic CJD' is unlikely to represent true CJD, and is likely to be motor neuron disease with dementia.

Prognosis and management

It is difficult not to be nihilistic in discussing the 'treatment' of CJD. Despite the advances that have been made in understanding the pathogenesis of the spongiform encephalopathies, to this day it remains a relentlessly progressive and untreatable disorder which culminates inevitably in death. Nevertheless, the provision of accurate information about the diagnosis and expected outcome is important when speaking with the relatives of affected patients, and it can be helpful to explain that many patients are unlikely to be aware of their suffering in the terminal stages. The expected rapidity of decline should be stressed. The devastating effect of seeing a relative in an akinetic mute and rigid state with frequent myoclonic jerks, cannot be overemphasized, and it may be important to discuss end of life decisions with the patient's family. Myoclonus may respond to clonazepam and valproate, and are worth trying.

Amantadine and amphotericin have both been discarded as potential agents with efficacy against the agent of CJD. Current research efforts are directed towards interfering with prion replication and accumulation, but therapeutic trials are some way off. Sulphated glycosaminoglycans appear to have some effect on these processes (Priola and Caughey, 1994).

Prevention is another important consideration. Iatrogenic CJD can be prevented or reduced by banning or minimizing the use of human-derived tissues (particularly those derived from the central nervous system and eyes) as medicinal products and during operations. Recent work appears to implicate cellular blood components, plasma and plasma fractions as potential, albeit minimal, sources of infectivity (Brown, 1998; Brown et al., 1998). In the UK, in view of the potential risk of nvCJD transmission, blood supplies derived from donors are leucodepleted and all plasma products are obtained from abroad (Warden, 1998).

The risks to health care workers of acquiring CJD by occupational contact, and the transmission of CJD from patient to patient during hospital procedures are probably minimal. Nevertheless, guidelines have been published on the safe handling of potentially infected tissue (Advisory Committee on Dangerous Pathogens, 1994) and on carrying out electrophysiological procedures (Evans et al., 1993). Recent guidelines issued by the Department of Health in the UK, attempt to stratify the risks associated with all surgical procedures depending on how secure the diagnosis of CJD is, whether the patient is considered to be in an 'at risk' category (for example, individuals who have received human pituitary-derived growth hormone therapy) and the type of procedure involved (those involving the central nervous system or eyes are considered as more likely to be associated with the potential for transmission) (Department of Health, 1998).

References

Advisory Committee on Dangerous Pathogens (1994). *Precautions for Work with Human and Animal Spongiform Encephalopathies.* HMSO, pp. 1–35.

Alper,T., Cramp, W. A., Haig, D. A. and Clarke, M. C. (1967). Does the agent of scrapie replicate without nucleic acid. *Nature*, **214**, 764–766.

Barbanti, P., Fabbrini, G., Salvatore, M. *et al.* (1996). Polymorphism at codon 129 or codon 219 of *PRNP* and clinical heterogeneity in a previously unreported family with Gerstmann-Straussler-Scheinker disease (PrP-P102L mutation). *Neurology*, **47**, 734–741.

Bolton, D. C., McKinley, M. P. and Prusiner, S. B. (1982). Identification of a protein that purifies with the scrapie prion. *Science*, **218**, 1309–1311.

Brown, P., Rodgers-Johnson, P., Cathala, F. *et al.* (1984). Creutzfeldt-Jakob disease of long duration: clinicopathological characteristics, transmissibility, and differential diagnosis. *Ann. Neurol.*, **16**, 295–304.

Brown, P., Cathala, F., Castaigne, P. and Gajdusek, D. C. (1986). Creutzfeldt-Jakob disease: clinical analysis of a consecutive series of 230 neuropathologically verified cases. *Ann. Neurol.*, **20**, 597–602.

Brown, P., Preece, M. A., and Will, R. G. (1992). 'Friendly fire' in medicine: hormones, homografts, and Creutzfeldt-Jakob disease. *Lancet*, **340**, 24–27.

Brown, P., Gibbs, C. J. JR, Rodgers-Johnson, P. *et al.* (1994). Human spongiform encephalopathy: the National Institutes of Health series of 300 cases of experimentally transmitted disease. *Ann. Neurol.*, **35**, 513–529.

Brown, P. (1998). Commentary: donor pool size and the risk of blood-borne Creutzfeldt-Jakob disease. *Transfusion*, **38**, 312–315.

Brown, P. and Bradley, R. (1998). 1755 and all that: a historical primer of transmissible spongiform encephalopathy. *Br. Med. J.*, **317**, 1688–1692.

Brown, P., Rohwer, R., Dunstan, B. C. *et al.* (1998). The distribution of infectivity in blood components and plasma derivatives in experimental models of transmissible spongiform encephalopathy. *Transfusion*, **38**, 810–816.

Brownell, B. and Oppenheimer, D. R. (1965). An ataxic form of subacute presenile polioencephalopathy (Creutzfeldt-Jakob disease). *J. Neurol. Neurosurg. Psych.*, **28**, 350–361.

Bruce, M. E., Will, R. G., Ironside, J. W. *et al.* (1997). Transmissions to mice indicate that 'new variant' CJD is caused by the BSE agent. *Nature*, **389**, 498–501.

Büeler, H., Aguzzi, A., Sailer, A. *et al.* (1993) Mice devoid of PrP are resistant to scrapie. *Cell*, **73**, 1339–1347.

Chapman, J., Arlazoroff, A., Goldfarb, L. G. *et al.* (1996). Fatal familial insomnia in a case of familial Creutzfeldt-Jakob disease with the codon 200(Lys) mutation. *Neurology*, **46**, 758–761.

Collinge, J., Sidle, K. C. L., Meads, J. *et al.* (1996). Molecular analysis of prion strain variation and the aetiology of 'new variant' CJD. *Nature*, **383**, 685–690.

Creutzfeldt, H. G. (1920). Uber eine eigenartige herdformige Erkrankung des Zentralnervensystems. *Z. ges. Neurol. Psychiat.*, **57**, 1.

de Silva, R. (1998). A correlative study of the clinical, pathological and molecular biological features of Creutzfeldt-Jakob disease. *Thesis for MD*, University of Edinburgh.

Department of Health (1998). *Advisory Committee on Dangerous Pathogens (ACDP)/ Spongiform Encephalopathy Advisory Committee (SEAC) guidance – 'Transmissible Spongiform Encephalopathy Agents: Safe working and the Prevention of Infection'.* London.

Dlouhy, S. R., Hsiao, K., Farlow, M. R. *et al.* (1992). Linkage of the Indiana kindred of Gerstmann-Straussler-Scheinker disease to the prion protein gene. *Nature Genet.*, **1**, 64–67.

Evans, B. M., Kriss, A., Jeffries, D., Boland, M., Carter, P. and Fowler, C. (1993). British Society for Clinical Neurophysiology Guidelines for preventing transmission of infective agents and toxic substances by clinical neurophysiological procedures: an update. *J. Electrophysiological Technology*, **19**, 129–135.

Finkenstaedt, M., Szudra, A., Zerr, I. *et al.* (1996). MR imaging of Creutzfeldt-Jakob disease. *Radiology*, **199**, 793–798.

Gajdusek, D. C., Gibbs, C. J. JR. and Alpers, M. (1966). Experimental transmission of a kuru-like syndrome in chimpanzees. *Nature*, **209**, 794–796.

Galvez, S., Masters, C., and Gajdusek, D. C. (1980). Descriptive epidemiology of Creutzfeldt-Jakob disease in Chile. *Arch. Neurol.*, **37**, 11–14.

Gibbs, C. J., Gajdusek, D. C., Asher, D. M. *et al.* (1968). Creutzfeldt-Jacob disease (spongiform encephalopathy) transmission to the chimpanzee. *Science*, **161**, 388–389.

Goldfarb, L. G., Petersen, R. B., Tabaton, M. *et al.* (1992). Fatal familial insomnia and familial CJD: disease phenotype determined by a DNA polymorphism. *Science*, **258**, 806–808.

Harries-Jones, R., Knight, R., Will, R. G. *et al.* (1988). Creutzfeldt-Jakob disease in England and Wales, 1980–1984: a case-control study of potential risk factors. *J. Neurol. Neurosurg. Psych.*, **51**, 1113–1119.

Heidenhain, A. (1929). Klinische und Anatomische Untersuchungen uber eine eigenartige Erkrankung des Zentralnervensystems in Praesenium. *Z. ges. Neurol. Psychiat.*, **118**, 49–114.

Hill, A. F., Butterworth, R. J., Joiner, S. *et al.* (1999). Investigation of variant Creutzfeldt-Jakob disease and other human prion diseases with tonsil biopsy samples. *Lancet*, **353**, 183–184.

Hsiao, K., Baker, H. F., Crow, T. J. *et al.* (1989). Linkage of a prion protein missense variant to Gerstmann-Straussler syndrome. *Nature*, **338**, 342–345.

Hsiao, K. K., Scott, M., Foster, D. *et al.* (1990). Spontaneous neurodegeneration in transgenic mice with mutant prion protein. *Science*, **250**, 1587–1590.

Hsiao, K. K., Cass, C., Schellenberg, G. D. *et al.* (1991). A prion protein variant in a family with the telencephalic form of Gerstmann-Straussler-Scheinker syndrome. *Neurology*, **41**, 681–684.

Jakob, A. (1921). Uber eine der multiplen sklerose klinisch nahenstehende erkrankung des zentralnervensystems (spastiche pseudosklerose) mit bemerkswertem anatomishen befunde. *Med. Klin.*, **13**, 372–376.

Jakob, A. (1923). Spastische Pseudosklerose. *Die Extrapyramidalen Erkrankungen*. Berlin: Julius Springer. pp. 215–245.

Jones, D. P. and Nevin, S. (1954). Rapidly progressive cerebral degeneration (subacute vascular encephalopathy) with mental disorder, focal disturbance, and myoclonic epilepsy. *J. Neurol. Neurosurg. Psych.*, **17**, 148–159.

Kimberlin, R. H. (1990). Scrapie and possible relationships with viroids. *Sem. Virol.*, **1**, 153–162.

Kocisko, D. A., Come, J. H., Priola, S. A. *et al.* (1995) Cell-free formation of protease-resistant prion protein. *Nature*, **370**, 471–474.

Laplanche, J.-L., Delasnerie-Laupretre, N., Brandel, J. P. *et al.* (1994). Molecular genetics of prion diseases in France. *Neurology*, **44**, 2347–2351.

Masters, C. L., Harris, J. O., Gajdusek, D. C. *et al.* (1979). Creutzfeldt-Jakob disease: patterns of worldwide occurrence and the significance of familial and sporadic clustering. *Ann. Neurol.*, **5**, 177–188.

Masters, C. L. and Gajdusek, D. C. (1982). The spectrum of Creutzfeldt-Jakob disease and virus induced subacute spongiform encephalopathies. In: *Recent Advances in Neuropathology* II (W. Thomas Smith and J. B. Cavanagh, eds). Edinburgh: Churchill Livingstone. pp. 139–163

McNaughton, H. K. and Will, R. G. (1997). Creutzfeldt-Jakob disease presenting acutely as stroke: an analysis of 30 cases. *Neurol. Infect. Epidemiol.*, **2**, 19–24.

Meyer, A., Leigh, D. and Bagg, C. E. (1954). A rare presenile dementia associated with cortical blindness (Heidenhain's syndrome). *J. Neurol. Neurosurg. Psych.*, **17**, 129–133.

Montagna, P., Cortelli, P., Avoni, P. *et al.* (1998). Clinical features of fatal familial insomnia: phenotypic variability in relation to a polymorphism at codon129 of the prion protein gene. *Brain Pathol.*, **8**, 515–520.

Muramoto, T., Kitamoto, T., Koga, H., and Tateishi, J. (1992). The coexistence of Alzheimer's disease and Creutzfeldt-Jakob disease in a patient with dementia of long duration. *Acta Neuropathol.*, **84**, 686–689.

Nevin, S., McMenemey, W. H., Behrman, S., and Jones, D. P. (1960). Subacute spongiform encephalopathy – a subacute form of encephalopathy attributable to vascular dysfunction (spongiform cerebral atrophy). *Brain*, **83**, 519–563.

Parchi, P., Castellani, R., Capellari, S. *et al.* (1996). Molecular basis of phenotypic variability in sporadic Creutzfeldt-Jakob disease. *Ann. Neurol.*, **39**, 767–778.

Poulter, M., Baker, H. F., Frith, C. D. *et al.* (1992). Inherited prion disease with 144 base pair gene insertions. 1. Genealogical and molecular studies. *Brain*, **115**, 675–685.

Priola, S. A. and Caughey, B. (1994). Inhibition of scrapie-associated PrP accumulation. *Mol. Neurobiol.*, **8**, 113–120.

Prusiner, S. B. (1982). Novel proteinaceous infectious particles cause scrapie. *Science*, **216**, 136–144.

Salazar, A. M., Masters, C. L., Gajdusek, D. C. and Gibbs, C. J. JR (1983). Syndromes of amyotrophic lateral sclerosis and dementia: relation to transmissible Creutzfeldt-Jakob disease. *Ann. Neurol.*, **14**, 17–26.

Sellar, R. J., Will, R. G., and Zeidler, M. (1997). MR imaging of new variant Creutzfeldt-Jakob disease: the pulvinar sign. *Neuroradiology*, **39**, S53.

Tanaka, M., Tanaka, K. and Tadashi, M. (1993). Lymphocytes in Creutzfeldt-Jakob disease. *Neurology*, **43**, 2155–2156.

Tsuji, S. and Kuroiwa, Y. (1983). Creutzfeldt-Jakob disease in Japan. *Neurology*, **33**, 1503–1506.

Warden, J. (1998). Blood supplies to be treated to reduce CJD risk. *Br. Med. J.*, **317**, 232.

Weissmann, C. (1991) A 'unified theory' of prion propagation. *Nature*, **352**, 679–683.

Will, R. G. and Matthews, W. B. (1984). A retrospective study of Creutzfeldt-Jakob disease in England and Wales 1970–79 I: Clinical features. *J. Neurol. Neurosurg. Psych.*, **47**, 134–140.

Will, R. G., Ironside, J. W., Zeidler, M. *et al.* (1996). A new variant of Creutzfeldt-Jakob disease in the UK. *Lancet*, **347**, 921–925.

Will, R. G. (1999). New variant Creutzfeldt-Jakob disease. *Biomed. Pharmacother.*, **53**, 9–13.

Windl, O., Dempster, M., Estibeiro, J. P. *et al.* (1996). Genetic basis of Creutzfeldt-Jakob disease in the United Kingdom: a systematic analysis of predisposing mutations and allelic variation in the *PRNP* gene. *Hum. Genet.*, **98**, 259–264.

Zeidler, M., Stewart, G. E., Barraclough, C. R. *et al.* (1998). Detection of 14-3-3 protein in the cerebrospinal fluid supports the diagnosis of Creutzfeldt-Jakob disease. *Ann. Neurol.*, **43**, 32–40.

Zerr, I., Bodemer, M., Gefeller, O. *et al.* (1998). Detection of 14-3-33 protein in the cerebrospinal fluid supports the diagnosis of Creutzfeldt-Jacob disease. *Ann. Neurol.*, **43**, 32–40.

8
Japanese encephalitis

V. Ravi, Anita Desai, S. K. Shankar and M. Gourie-Devi

Introduction

An acute encephalitic illness occurred for the first time in horses and human beings in Japan as early as 1871. However, it was not until 1924 that this illness was designated Japanese B encephalitis to differentiate it from Von Economo's disease or encephalitis lethargica which at that time was referred to as Japanese A encephalitis. The letter B was subsequently dropped from the terminology following changes in taxonomy (Bu'lock, 1986). Since its original description in Japan in the early part of this century, Japanese encephalitis (JE) has spread extensively to several countries in Asia.

Japanese encephalitis virus (JEV)

JEV is an RNA virus and a member of the family of Flaviviridae. Initially it was classified as a member of the group B arboviruses and later as a member of the family of Togaviridiae. Recent advances in the molecular biology and immunology have however resulted in its classification as a member of Flaviviridae. In this family it is closely related to other members of the subgroup, e.g. Murray Valley encephalitis (MVE), West Nile (WN) and St Louis encephalitis (SLE) viruses (Monath and Tsai, 1997). It is a spherical virus with an icosahedral symmetry measuring approximately 40–60 nm in diameter, which includes an outer bilayered lipid envelope derived from the host. Lipases, organic solvents, and detergents disrupt the virus envelope and inactivate JEV.

Embedded in the lipid envelope are two structural proteins of the virus – the envelope (E) protein which projects from the surface giving the virus a spiky appearance and the matrix (M) protein which is situated closely by its side. A third structural protein, the capsid (C) protein, surrounds the single-stranded RNA of the virus. The E protein is glycosylated and has a molecular weight of 50–53 kDa (Shapiro *et al.*, 1971). All of the biological properties of the virus such as haemagglutination (HA), neutralization (Nt) and attachment to host cells are associated with the E protein (Takagami *et al.*, 1982). Virus-specific as well as cross-reactive neutralizing epitopes for JE have been identified on this protein. The M and C proteins are not glycosylated and measure 8 and 14 kDa respectively. Besides these three structural proteins JEV has five non-structural proteins designated NS1 to NS5. NS1 is a glycoprotein whose function is as yet unclear although it induces a protective immune response in mice. Recent studies have shown that NS3 serves as a virus specific protease and enables the cleavage of a single large polyprotein produced upon translation of the viral genome. In addition it also has helicase and RNA triphosphatase activity. NS2a, NS2b, NS4a and NS4b are poorly conserved membrane associated proteins whose function is currently unclear. It has been suggested that NS5 may be involved in the methylation of the 5' cap of the nucleic acid.

The genome of JEV is a single-stranded infectious RNA of positive polarity measuring approximately 11 kilobases in length, the most notable feature being the presence of a single open reading frame (ORF) of approximately 10 kb. The structural genes encoding the C protein, the M (pre-M and M) protein and the E protein occupy 25% of the genome at the 5' end. The rest of the ORF ($\sim 75\%$) encodes NS proteins in the following order; NS1, NS2a, NS2b, NS3, NS4a, NS4b and NS5. The 5' end is comprised of a short non-coding region while the 3' end is a looped structure that is usually devoid of poly A tracts (Chambers et al., 1990; Rice, 1996).

Attempts have been made to type and group JEV isolates from different regions by determining the reactivity of the virus with anti-JEV envelope protein monoclonal antibodies (Kobayashi et al., 1984; Kedarnath et al., 1986). However, no distinct geographic or chronologic antigenic types have been identified. On the contrary, genetic analysis carried out by sequencing JEV isolates obtained from various regions has been more rewarding (Chen et al., 1992; Ni and Barrett, 1995; Sumiyoshi et al., 1995). Based on genomic analysis four distinct groups have emerged: group I – isolates from North Thailand and Cambodia; group II – isolates from South Thailand, Malaysia and Indonesia; group III – isolates from Japan, China, India, Nepal and Sri Lanka; and group IV – a recently identified genotype recognized in Indonesia.

Epidemiology

JE is a major public health problem in several parts of Asia particularly China, India, Nepal, Sri Lanka, Vietnam, Cambodia and Thailand. Close to 3 billion people are now living in JE-endemic regions, where more than 70 million children are born each year (WHO, 1998). Consequently it is recognized as the commonest cause of mosquito-borne encephalitis world-wide (Johnson, 1987). The annual incidence of clinical infection in these endemic areas ranges from 10 to 100 per 100 000 population. The World Health Organization (WHO) estimates that over 50 000 cases and 10 000 deaths occur in these countries every year (WHO, 1998). JE is also reported from other Asian countries such as Indonesia, Malaysia, Myanmar, Philippines, Republic of Korea and Japan albeit to a lesser extent. Most of these countries have a similar environmental, ecological and agricultural background that favours JEV transmission. JE is predominantly reported from rural areas, especially among the lower socio-economic group.

Although sweeping epidemics of JE have occurred in rural areas of India, it has been noted that only a few cases are seen in villages. This is because of the high ratio of asymptomatic to symptomatic infections reported in JE. Estimates ranging from 1000 : 1 in Japan to 200 : 1 to 6300 : 1 in other parts of Asia have been reported (Gajanana *et al.*, 1995; Monath and Tsai, 1997). Exposure to JEV occurs in childhood and antibody prevalence rates approaching 80–90% by early adulthood have been recorded.

JE exhibits a seasonal pattern with incidence of disease peaking during or shortly after the rainy season. However, variations within the same region are known. For instance, epidemics occur during or soon after rainy seasons in the northern regions of Vietnam and Thailand, while the disease has been reported throughout the year in the southern parts of these countries (Umenai *et al.*, 1985).

The epidemiology of JE has undergone a remarkable change in recent years and it is emerging in many new geographic regions of Asia. Until recently Indonesia was the southern limit for JE while the Eastern States of India were the western limit. In the past 5 years it has emerged in some countries beyond these limits which had hitherto not reported the disease (Figure 8.1). Consequently, the geographic 'boundaries' have now extended to Pakistan in the West (Igarashi *et al.*, 1994) and Australia in the South (Hanna *et al.*, 1996). Furthermore, in countries where JE has been endemic for several decades the virus has been gradually spreading to newer areas, e.g. Goa (Mohan Rao *et al.*, 1983), Haryana (Prasad *et al.*, 1993) and Kerala (Dhanda *et al.*, 1997) which are in the Western half of India and where cases of JE have not been recorded

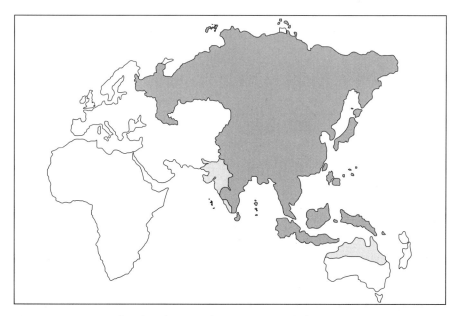

Figure 8.1 Geographic distribution of Japanese encephalitis (JE) cases. Countries in South Asia (dark grey) have been endemic for several years, however, very recently it has emerged in newer geographical areas in Asia and Australia (light grey).

earlier. This is presumably due to the changing ecological pattern brought about by a shift towards paddy cultivation in these regions.

Japanese encephalitis is a zoonosis transmitted by the bite of an infected mosquito wherein human beings act as a dead end host. The virus is maintained in nature among water birds of the Ardeidae family, chiefly pond herons and cattle egrets. Pigs play a vital role in the natural cycle of this disease. They serve as excellent amplifiers. They do not suffer from any major illness, although they circulate virus to high titres in their blood. Whenever climatic conditions favour the prevalence of a high mosquito density (especially following the monsoon season) infection spills over to human beings. Man-to-man transmission has never been recorded probably because viraemia is very transient and of a low order in humans. Virus infection rates in mosquito vectors ranges from 1 to 3% (WHO, 1998). The low incidence of JE in some parts of India has been attributed to a zooprophylactic role of cattle, which also serve as dead end hosts by diverting mosquitoes from biting pigs (Rodrigues, 1984). Elegant studies carried out in Japan and other countries including India (Scherer *et al.*, 1959; Dandawate *et al.*, 1969) have shown that Culicine mosquitoes of the *Culex vishnui* complex (*C. tritaenorhyncus*, *C. pseudo-vishnui* and *C. vishnui*) are the chief vectors involved in transmission, although some species of Anopheline mosquitoes (*A. barbirostrus* and *A. hyrcanus*) and *Mansoni* have also been incriminated in some instances. Transovarial transmission has been noted among field collected larvae and this observation offers an explanation for the 'overwintering' of the virus in the interepidemic period (Rosen *et al.*, 1978). Paddy fields serve as an excellent breeding ground for these species of mosquitoes and therefore JE is more often reported in areas where paddy cultivation is in vogue. Thus the most conducive combination of ecological factors contributing to the JE outbreak include a large number of domestic pigs living adjacent to human dwellings, and prolific mosquito breeding sites such as inundated paddy fields frequented often by migratory water birds such as pond herons and cattle egrets.

Pathogenesis and pathology

Various groups have studied the molecular determinants of JEV virulence. Attenuation of neurovirulence by limited or prolonged passage in cell cultures has been achieved. The high frequency of amino acid changes in the E protein of these attenuated viruses suggests that this protein is endowed with neurovirulence and/or neuroinvasiveness determinants (McMinn, 1997). Sequencing the E genes of attenuated neutralization escape variants selected with anti-E protein monoclonal antibodies has yielded valuable information (Cecilia and Gould, 1991). The escape variant displayed diminished neuroinvasiveness in mice, low haemagglutination activity and a single alteration in the amino acid residue of the E protein at position 720 (I → S). Similarly, it has also been suggested that mutations in the E protein of the virus may affect the virus–receptor interactions following conformational changes in the receptor binding domain of this protein (Cao *et al.*, 1995).

The course and outcome of the disease is influenced by the dose, the route of inoculation, the species, the age of the host, immune sensitization by earlier infection by the same group of cross–reacting viruses in the endemic areas and the virulence of the infecting virus. Among the host factors that affect the outcome, the immune status, reticuloendothelial clearance mechanism, nutritional status and probably genetic factors play a role. The immature brain is generally more susceptible to the infection and evolves into fatal encephalitis (Ogata *et al.*, 1991), thus explaining the greater incidence of mortality and morbidity among children. The neuronal permissiveness to flavivirus replication decreases with age and the slower replication probably allows host immune intervention and clearance before clinical signs manifest. However, a study from South India revealed persistence of viral antigen in CSF, along with high titres of IgM and neutralizing antibodies, indicating that this humoral response may not be capable of offering protection in the presence of an overwhelming antigen load (Desai *et al.*, 1995a). Immunochemical localization of antigen in the neurons beyond the tenth day of illness (Desai *et al.*, 1995a), and at 151 days after the onset of illness (Kimoto *et al.*, 1968), implies that the virus can persist in tissues for longer periods (Ravi *et al.*, 1993), contrary to earlier suggestions (Johnson *et al.*, 1985). This contention is further supported by the detection of many antigen bearing yet cytologically well preserved neurons with no associated microglial reaction and neuronophagia at different sites of the brain, in some cases.

The pathological lesions in the brain of fatal cases of JE are polymorphic and diffuse involving various parts of the nervous system. The brains show severe degree of vascular congestion and cerebral oedema, leading to uncal and cerebellar tonsillar herniation. This has been a consistent feature, except in cases treated earlier with vigorous antioedema measures. The more significant and fairly characteristic change on closer gross examination of the brain is the presence of small, circular necrolytic zones seen in the superficial cortical and deep grey matter (Figure 8.2).

Histologically, the leptomeninges have a variable degree of mononuclear cell infiltrate, extending to the deep parenchyma, along the perivascular space. In nearly one-quarter of cases the inflammatory reaction is severe, admixed with polymorphs. During the first 3 days, the brain shows intense vascular congestion and oedema, with sparse inflammation. Diffuse microglial proliferation and formation of gliomesenchymal nodules in the brain, the hallmark of JE, is similar to other viral encephalitides and these lesions are consistently seen from the third day of illness. Focal aggregates of microglial cells and lymphocytes around degenerating neuronal perikarya form these nodules. The gliomesenchymal nodules are seen consistently in the inferior olivary complex of medulla oblongata (Figure 8.3), pars compacta of substantia nigra, thalamus, molecular layer of the cerebellar folia, cerebral cortex and less frequently in pontine nuclei, reticular nuclei of the brainstem, cerebellar nuclei and spinal grey matter. Though many of the glial nodules are found around neurons undergoing neuronophagia, many antigen-bearing neurons are relatively well preserved, the microglial cells forming satellites. The neurons of the substantia nigra in many cases reveal depletion of melanin pigment of

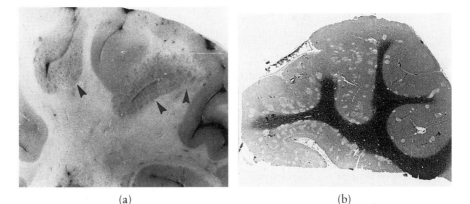

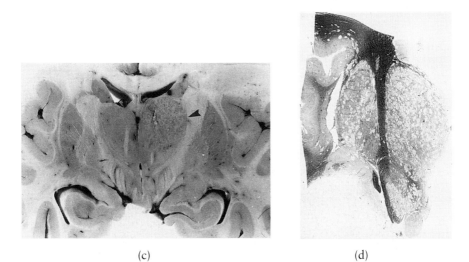

Figure 8.2 (a) Close up view of parietal cortex showing multiple necrolytic lesions involving grey matter (arrowheads). (b) Whole mount picture showing the necrolytic lesions in the grey matter. (LFB × 5). (c) Coronal slice of the brain from a case of JE showing necrolytic lesions involving the thalamus unilaterally (30-year-old male from endemic area with 4 days illness – arrow head). (d) Whole mount preparation showing florid necrolytic lesions involving thalamus and putamen, globus pallidus and adjacent internal capsule (3-year-old female child from an endemic area, 9 days illness).

variable degree. In an occasional case the microglial response can be seen in the superficial white matter.

The second most characteristic microscopic finding of JE is the focal, discrete or confluent, small, round to oval areas of cystic necrosis. These 'necrolytic' areas are seen in abundance in the cerebral grey matter, thalamic nuclei, midbrain, pons (Figures 8.2 and 8.4), corpus striatum and less frequently in medulla oblongata. These lesions are well circumscribed, pale, rarefied zones in the neuropil, usually around a capillary. During the early stages of evolution, they contain abundant microglia, polymorphs (Figure 8.5a) and

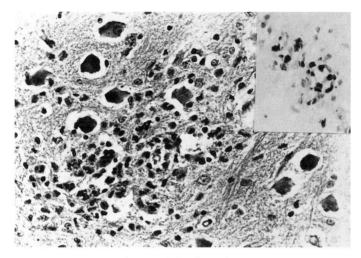

Figure 8.3   Large aggregates of microglial cells with neuronophagia in inferior olivary nucleus (HE × 320). Inset: Immunohistochemical localization of JEV antigen in microglia (immunoperoxidase × 280).

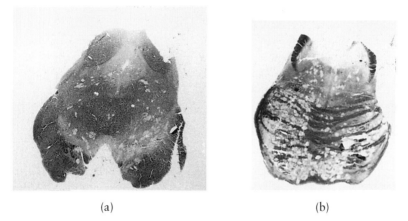

(a)   (b)

Figure 8.4   (a) Necrolytic lesions involving substantia nigra and peri-aqueductal grey matter (LFB × 2). (b) Florid necrolytic lesions involving the pontine nuclei and tegmentum (3-year-old female child, from endemic area, with 9 days of illness) (LFB × 3).

neutral fat-containing macrophages. Later these zones look pale, relatively accellular with loss of axons and myelin (Figure 8.5b and c). These lesions do not contain myelin breakdown products. Astroglial reaction is conspicuously absent. No intracytoplasmic or intranuclear inclusions are observed in any of the cells. Though the pathological changes are essentially in the grey matter, a few areas of white matter destruction involving the internal capsule, transverse pontine fibres, cerebellar peduncle and occasionally medial funicules are also seen. In nearly 2–4% of JE cases, large haemorrhagic areas are found bilaterally in the thalamus, pons and cerebellum (Figure 8.6) that resemble

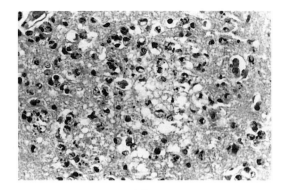

(a)

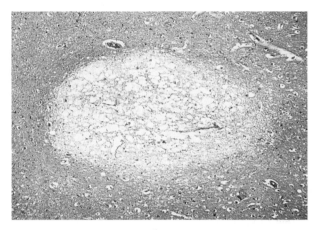

(b)

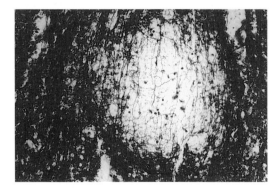

(c)

Figure 8.5   (a) Early necrolytic lesion showing rarefaction of neuropil and acute inflammatory cell infiltrate (fourth day of illness (HE × 400). (b) Late necrolytic lesion is
relatively acellular, and pale, well circumscribed and spongy (10th day of illness
(HE × 60). (c) Late necrolytic lesion in the superficial white matter showing marked
axonal loss (10th day of illness) (Bielschowsky's silver × 240).

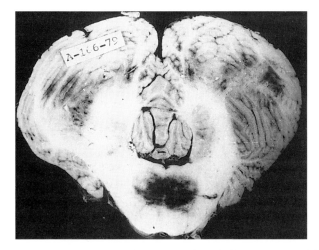

Figure 8.6   Haemorrhagic lesions in the pons and cerebellum (20-year-old female from endemic area, 5 days of illness. Similar haemorrhagic lesions were also seen in the thalamus, bilaterally, leading to diagnosis of deep venous system thrombosis).

lesions found in cases of deep venous system thrombosis. However, the pathogenesis of these lesions is not clear. The vascular system does not reveal any structural alteration. Intraneuronal or neuropil calcification that was reported earlier by Zimmerman (1946) has not been noted in the cases reported from India (Shankar *et al.*, 1983). Ishii *et al.* (1977) studied serologically confirmed cases of JE and reported the persistence of rarefied necrolytic lesions in thalamus, hippocampus and brainstem and focal calcified neurons even after 12 to 67 years of initial illness. These appear to represent residual neuropathological stigmata of an earlier encephalitic process.

The aforementioned pathological lesions were also observed in a virologically confirmed case of West Nile encephalitis from South India. The characteristic microglial nodule formation and necrolytic lesions in various regions of the brain seen in cases of JE can also be found in some cases of tick-borne encephalitis as well, thereby making differentiation difficult on morphological grounds alone.

The histological changes in the spinal grey matter such as the significant microglial response and formation of nodular aggregates by microglia especially around the neurons (see Figure 8.6) and perivascular mononulear cuffing are similar to that noted in poliomyelitis and tick-borne encephalitis (Jervis and Higgins, 1952). However, the astroglial reaction in JE is negligible in comparison to poliomyelitis. The relatively acellular necrolytic lesions noted in the cortex in JE are not found in the spinal cord in either of the two conditions. The feature discriminating JE and tick-borne encephalitis from poliomyelitis is that in poliomyelitis, the inferior olivary nucleus and thalamus are marginally and only occasionally involved (Kornyey, 1978).

By immunochemical staining, JE viral antigen can be localized in the neurons of the affected areas. The neurons in the hippocampus, the adjoining temporal cortex and thalamus, pars compacta in substantia nigra, the neurons of inferior olivary nucleus, hypoglossal and vagal nuclei usually show a high density of viral antigen in the soma during the acute phase, while microglia are devoid of antigen (Johnson et al., 1985; Desai et al., 1995a). In the hippocampus, the large pyramidal neurons of Ammon's horn and in the subiculum and entorrhinal cortex, the superficial layer of the cortex contain the viral antigen, while in the temporal isocortex, the antigen positive neurons are usually found in layers 4–6. In the cerebellum, Purkinje cells, the stellate cells in the molecular layer and granular layer, are positive for viral antigen in a few cases. During the first 3–4 days, the viral antigen can be found in morphologically normal neurons with no microglial reaction. Over the next few days, the antigen-bearing neurons have around them microglial satellites that are devoid of antigen. In the later stages, with active neuronophagia, the viral antigen is largely confined to macrophages in microglial shrubs (see Figure 8.3, inset) and perivascular zones. Very rarely the antigen can be found in an occasional astrocyte, ependymal cell or capillary endothelial cell, but not in oligodendroglial cells (Johnson et al., 1985; Desai et al., 1995a).

Very few studies have been undertaken using biopsied or autopsied human material to determine the ultrastructural alterations taking place within the infected cells. Oyanagi et al. (1969) described the ultrastructural features in the brain and spinal cord of mice infected with JEV. Seventy two hours post inoculation, when the mice began to show encephalitic symptoms, the majority of the cortical neurons and spinal anterior horn cells were found to contain viral particles in smooth endoplasmic reticulum and a few in granular endoplasmic reticulum. By 96 h, the neurons revealed large vacuoles and vesicles containing scattered viral particles. The satellite and Purkinje cells revealed viral particles at a later time than cortical and spinal neurons, while none could be found in glial cells.

The controversy regarding the evolution of the localized, relatively acellular rarefaction necrosis in the grey matter is not resolved. Wake (quoted by Miyake) considered direct toxic action of the virus as the cause of cerebral necrosis with rarefaction, while Miyake (1964) suggested vascular spasm secondary to circulatory disturbances as the cause. Histology of the necrolytic lesions during the early stages revealed an acute polymorph reaction and a mild macrophage response, leading to breakdown of myelin and axons, finally resulting in acellular rarefied lesions (see Figure 8.5), suggesting an active role for the inflammatory cells in the process. Antigen-bearing microglia are sparse in these areas both during the early and healing phase. Khanna et al. (1994) described a JEV stimulated splenic macrophage derived neutrophilic chemotactic factor (MDF) in mice, which enhanced vascular permeability and neutrophil emigration. This response was found to be sensitive to and abrogated by pretreatment of the animal with H_1 and H_2 histamine receptor blockers. This MDF could be actively modulating the evolution of necrotic lesions. The inflammatory cells in the brain parenchymal lesions and perivascular space were mostly T-helper cells and a few T-suppressor cells and a large number of macrophages. Antibody-forming B cells comprised 10% of the cells in the perivascular space, but these were not found outside the perivascular regions (Johnson *et al.*, 1985). The cells in CSF from patients with JE also showed a high ratio of T-helper/T-suppressor cells and a variable number of B cells and macrophages, both in fatal and non-fatal cases. Thus, the fatality due to encephalitis does not appear to be related to failure of the antibody-synthesizing B cells or clearance of the virus by T cells and macrophages.

A temporal relationship to the evolution of various lesions in JE is noted in the cases studied from South India (Shankar *et al.*, 1983). In fulminant cases, where death occurred in less than 3 days, the cellular response was poor, but the vascular congestion and oedema were prominent. The cellular reaction, especially the microglial and polymorph response, was intense from the fourth day onwards, manifesting as microglial nodules with neuronophagia and heralding necrolytic lesions. By the tenth day the cellular response is observed to wane and relatively acellular necrolytic lesions predominate, these features being more obvious after 15 days of illness.

The spectrum of pathological features described in JE is not specific and diagnostic, as these are common to different types of arbovirus and tick-borne viral encephalitis. The early and frequent brainstem infection, the preponderance of the viral antigen in the rostral neurons, the perivascular lymphocytic cuffing, and the presence of viral antigen in the vascular endothelial cells all suggest invasion of the nervous system by the virus via the haematogenous route. The presence of the viral antigen in the long dendritic arborization and in the axons, suggests transcellular spread of virus to distant, but functionally related neurons. This is further supported by our experimental studies where following intramuscular inoculation of the virus, the viral antigen could be traced in the corresponding segment of dorsal root ganglion and the spinal motor neurons (unpublished observation). The intraneuronal antigen localization and the absence of neuropil immunostaining at different times suggest that extracellular spread of JE virus to distant areas may not occur. The astroglia and vascular endothelial cells appear occasionally to ingest the virus by phagocytosis and thus have a limited role in the spread of the virus, but may have an accessory function of antigen presentation, similar to microglia.

The involvement of critical neuronal targets in the brainstem and the resultant secondary effect rather than failure of viral specific immunity appear to determine the mortality and clinical outcome. The infection and destruction of the reticular and other neurons in brainstem and thalamus account for the deep coma and respiratory failure. Involvement of the spinal motor neurons, with florid microglial reaction and neuronophagia during the acute phase of illness can lead to acute flaccid paralysis in children that has clinical and pathological features similar to poliomyelitis thus leading to diagnostic dilemma (Solomon *et al.*, 1998). The involvement of the striatum and pars compacta of the substantia nigra is consistent with the frequent tremors noted during the acute phase and parkinsonian features as the long-term sequelae (Gourie-Devi, 1984; Misra and Kalita, 1997a). The topographic distribution of antigen-bearing neurons in the hippocampus and temporal cortex are found to have a curious correspondence to the zones affected in neurodegenerative diseases like Alzheimer's disease, in which cholinergic neuronal deficit is implicated in the pathogenesis. In endemic areas, arboviral

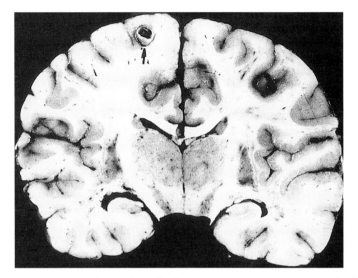

Figure 8.7   Association of JE and cerebral cysticercosis (arrow). Note multiple necrolytic lesions in the thalamic nuclei.

infection may contribute to the post-infectious cognitive deficits, leading to dementia as a long-term sequela.

Cysticercosis–JE: with the first report by Hsu (1940) of co-occurrence of cerebral cysticercosis and JE and the elegant experimental studies describing the synergistic role of *Toxocara canis* in the evolution of JEV infection, the modulating role of the parasite on the progression, course and outcome of the viral encephalitis has been recognized (Pavri *et al.*, 1975). During epidemics in South India, serological and autopsy studies have revealed coexistence of cerebral cysticercosis and JE (Figure 8.7), in nearly one third of cases, with high mortality and morbidity (Shankar *et al.*, 1983; Desai *et al.*, 1997). With the coexistence of cysticercosis, the numerical density and diffusion of the topographic distribution of the pathological lesions is enhanced (Liu *et al.*, 1957). Interestingly, the necrolytic lesions were found to be numerous and more florid on the ipsilateral side bearing the parasitic cyst. A short peptide capable of opening the blood–brain barrier, identified in the cysticercal cyst fluid (Shankar *et al.*, 1994) could be modulating the diffusion of the viral particles in the brain, entering through the haematogenous route.

Immune response

Natural immunization is considered the most important factor restricting this disease (Huang, 1982). In epidemic regions the incidence of the disease has been shown to decrease with increase in immune groups (Chakravarty *et al.*, 1975). Studies carried out in adult mice have shown that a prior inapparent infection protects against lethal challenge with virulent virus suggesting that a similar mechanism may be operative in humans. Information on humoral and cell-mediated immunity in JE has been largely obtained from experimental studies in mice. Passive transfer of antibodies seemed to afford protection against primary infection in mice. Similarly, administration of monoclonal antibodies on the fifth day post infection protected 82% of mice (Kimura-Kuroda and Yasui, 1988). These observations have been validated in several human studies. The presence of intrathecal anti-JEV antibodies on the day of admission into the hospital has been associated with a favourable outcome suggesting an important role for antibody-mediated virus neutralization (Burke et al., 1985a; Ravi et al., 1989a; Desai et al., 1994a). Although antibody dependent enhancement (ADE) of JEV has been observed using monoclonal antibodies in an in vitro system, its role in vivo with respect to immunopathology is unclear. Observations from the author's laboratory, however, suggest that two important factors probably contribute to immunopathological damage in the brain. First, the presence of intrathecal antibodies to neural antigens such as neurofilament proteins and/or myelin basic protein in 49% of JE cases has been associated with a fatal outcome (Desai et al., 1994b). Secondly, JEV specific immune complexes present in the CSF of 17% of cases have also been associated with a fatal outcome (Desai et al., 1995b). Cell-mediated immunity studies have been carried out extensively in experimental animals such as mice. Adoptive transfer of spleen cells, especially cytotoxic T cells obtained from immunized mice, have protected recipient mice against lethal intracerebral challenge (Muralikrishna et al., 1994). However, this protection was restricted to adult mice and was not observed in younger mice (Muralikrishna et al., 1996a). Recent studies in mice seem to suggest that the non-structural proteins of JEV are also capable of inducing cytotoxic T lymphocyte (CTL) responses (Muralikrishna et al., 1996b). The generation of virus specific suppressor T cells has also been demonstrated in mice (Mathur et al., 1986). Limited studies carried out in humans have shown that immune T cells derived from the peripheral venous blood proliferate in response to JEV or its infected cell lysates. These proliferative responses did not show any association with the clinical outcome in JE patients (Desai et al., 1995c). High levels of TNFα in the CSF has also been correlated with a fatal outcome in JE patients (Ravi et al., 1997).

Clinical features

Only one in several hundred JEV infections manifests as clinical illness. In most of the epidemics and in sporadic cases children are most frequently affected (Figure 8.8), although regional variations are not unusual within the same country. For instance, in South India children under 15 years constitute 80% of cases, while in Eastern and North-eastern India the proportion was less than 50% (Gourie-Devi and Deshpande, 1982; Chatterjee and Banerjee, 1975). The clinical course of the disease can be conveniently divided into three phases, the prodromal, acute encephalitic and convalescent stages. The prodromal stage is characterized by the occurrence of fever, headache, nausea and vomiting, chills

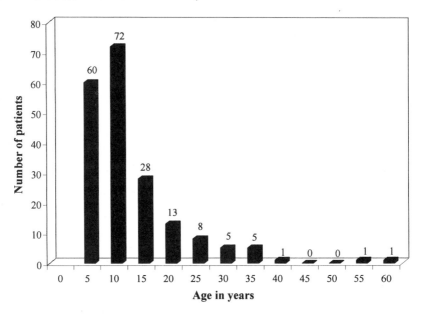

Figure 8.8   The age distribution in laboratory confirmed Japanese encephalitis cases ($n = 194$) in Karnataka, South India.

and anorexia. Diarrhoea may be a prominent feature in children. The onset of this prodromal stage may be abrupt (1–6 h), acute (6–24 h) or more commonly subacute (2–5 days). In more than 75% of the patients the onset is subacute (Gourie-Devi, 1984). Although spontaneous recovery is known from this stage, the disease usually progresses to the acute encephalitic stage. As the symptoms are non-specific during the prodromal stage, the diagnosis can only be suspected on epidemiological evidence and confirmed by appropriate serological and virological tests.

During the encephalitic phase on the background of symptoms noted in the prodromal phase, convulsions, alteration of sensorium, behavioural changes, motor paralysis and involuntary movements supervene. Although the main symptoms suggest encephalitis in more than one-third of the patients frank signs of meningitis are also seen. Alteration in sensorium ranging from mild mental clouding to drowsiness to stupor and coma is a common feature. Two-thirds of the patients develop seizures that may be generalized or focal motor in type which occur more frequently in children than adults. Status epilepticus as the presenting symptom on a background of fever is not an uncommon feature. Isolated case reports of diencephalic epilepsy during the acute phase are of interest in view of the pathological lesions observed in the thalamus (Misra *et al.*, 1980; Shankar *et al.*, 1983). Focal neurological deficit, particularly hemiplegia, is seen during the course of illness in nearly half of the patients and in less than 10% of cases as the presenting feature. Behavioural abnormalities in the form of confusion, disorientation, restlessness, talking irrelevantly, and delirium are seen in a small proportion of cases. Onset of illness with behaviour change may lead to errors in diagnosis.

Table 8.1 Clinical features noted in Japanese encephalitis patients during the 1979–1980 epidemic, Karnataka, South India (*n* = **133**)*.

Symptoms/signs	Number of patients	(%)
Fever	126	(94.7)
Headache	83	(62.4)
Altered sensorium	114	(85.7)
Convulsions	90	(67.7)
Behaviour disturbances	13	(9.8)
Motor paralysis	66	(53.1)
Meningitis	45	(35.2)
Speech disorder	19	(14.8)
Movement disorders	14	(10.5)
Gaze paralysis	8	(6.0)
Cranial nerve disorder (II and VI nerves)	3	(2.3)
Papilloedema	2	(1.6)
Incoordination	2	(1.6)

* From Gourie-Devi, 1984, with permission.

A variety of movement disorders have been reported including head nodding, coarse tremors, choreoathetosis, dystonia and features suggestive of parkinsonism (mask-like face, rigidity and oculogyric crisis) especially during the late stage of the encephalitic phase or 2–3 weeks following the acute stage of the disease. Incoordination due to cerebellar involvement, and hypotonic hyporeflexic paralysis of limbs suggestive of lower motor neuron involvement are rare features and sensory deficits are exceptional (Misra *et al.*, 1980; Gourie-Devi, 1984). Although symptoms of increased intracranial tension are obvious, frank papilloedema is a rare occurrence.

Cranial nerves including optic, oculomotor and facial are rarely affected. Sinus tachycardia, gallop rhythm, tachypnoea have been noted in critically ill patients. Isolated cases with respiratory paralysis as the presenting symptom have been observed. Although no clinical manifestations of hepatic involvement are evident biochemical abnormalities have been reported. The acute encephalitic phase usually lasts for a week, but when complications supervene it may be prolonged for a few weeks. Other most common complications are bacterial infections especially pneumonia and stasis ulcers.

Most of the deaths in JE occur within the first 7 days after the onset of symptoms. Among patients who survive the illness steady improvement to full recovery or stabilization of the neurological deficit is seen. The duration of this convalescent phase is however prolonged and may vary from a few weeks to a few months.

JE acquired during the first and second trimesters of pregnancy has led to fetal death and abortion with recovery of virus from the products of conception (Chaturvedi *et al.*, 1980). Recently, a number of variations have been noted in the clinical manifestations of JE. These include a subacute form of the disease in which the clinical course is rather prolonged. Recurrence of symptoms has been reported in some children, more than a year after the acute encephalitic phase with recovery of latent virus from the peripheral blood mononuclear cells (Sharma *et al.*, 1991). Persistence of IgM antibodies and viral antigen has been noted in the CSF for prolonged periods in about 5% of children and virus could be isolated in one of these patients at 90 and 110 days after the onset of symptoms (Ravi *et al.*, 1993). The precise clinical significance of these laboratory observations is at present unclear. Other flavivirus infections have been associated with chronic progressive central nervous system infection, suggesting a similar mechanism may be operative in JE as well (Monath and Tsai, 1997). JE occasionally may present as Guillian–Barré syndrome, especially in adults from endemic areas (Ravi *et al.*, 1994).

Muscle wasting has also been noted in JEV infection and this has been attributed to the involvement of anterior horn cells (Misra and Kalita, 1997b). Very recently JEV has been reported to cause a poliomyelitis-like illness in 12 (55%) of the 22 Vietnamese children (Solomon *et al.*, 1998). Compared with JEV-negative patients, the onset of weakness in JEV infected children was more rapid, tended to be asymmetrical but was less likely to involve the arms. Nerve conduction and electromyographic studies indicated damage to the anterior horn cells.

Diagnosis

The diagnosis of JE is based on the clinical features suggestive of acute encephalitis which include fever, headache, vomiting, convulsions and focal neurological deficits of a few days' duration. JEV can also be suspected on epidemiological grounds. Polymorphonuclear leucocytosis in the peripheral blood, elevated ESR and mild biochemical abnormality of liver function tests are typical. A constant finding is the pleocytosis in CSF with predominance of lymphocytes, though a significant number of polymorphs may also be seen. Generally the average cell count is about 150–200 but rarely more than 1000 cells/μl may also be observed (Gourie-Devi, 1984). It is noteworthy that, in a significant number of patients, the CSF cell count may be normal. In cases with an elevated CSF cell count, if a repeat CSF analysis is performed within the next 24 h to 6 days, and shows a return to normal without specific antibacterial treatment, viral encephalitis is the likely diagnosis. The CSF protein shows mild to moderate elevation in two-thirds of patients with values ranging from 50 to 150 mg/dl. However, higher levels up to 300 mg/dl may be encountered.

The electroencephalogram (EEG) is consistently abnormal in the acute encephalitic stage and shows diffuse slowing of background activity in all patients and asymmetry between the two hemispheres in some patients. Though clinical seizures are a common feature, spikes or seizure discharges are rarely seen. In general EEG changes reflect the severity of CNS damage but do not provide an accurate guideline to the final outcome (Gouri-Devi and Deshpande, 1982). Recent imaging techniques, computerized tomography and magnetic resonance imaging have provided valuable insights into the topographic distribution of lesions. The most frequent abnormalities are diffuse white matter hypodensities suggestive of cerebral oedema and low density areas in the cerebral cortex in the frontal, parietal, and temporal areas. Bilateral low density areas and abnormal signal intensities in the thalamus and basal ganglia including putamen have been considered to be characteristic features of JE (Shoji *et al.*, 1989, 1990; Misra *et al.*, 1994).

Differential diagnosis

The clinical features of acute encephalitis, seen during an epidemic, especially in children, hailing from endemic areas, strongly suggests a diagnosis of JE. However, there is a risk of overdiagnosis since a number of other clinical conditions such as cerebral malaria, Reye's syndrome, acute pyogenic meningitis and tuberculous meningitis may present with similar clinical features. Differentiating JE from acute tuberculous meningitis, particularly in children, is fraught with difficulties since in both the diseases lymphocytic predominance is noted in CSF, and positive culture for *Mycobacterium tuberculosis* is observed in less than 15% of cases in India (Gouri-Devi *et al.*, 1989). The cell count in viral encephalitis shows a rapid decrease while in tuberculous meningitis without specific treatment either there is no change or there is a further increase in cell count. Other disorders that overlap in their clinical presentation with JE are febrile convulsions in children and encephalitis caused by other viral agents like West Nile virus (George *et al.*, 1987).

Laboratory diagnosis

CSF, plasma and brain tissue (post-mortem) collected early in the illness are suitable specimens for virus isolation, while CSF and paired serum samples are necessary for antibody estimation. JEV has been isolated from CSF and brain tissue more often during the early part of the illness and very rarely from the plasma and peripheral blood mononuclear cells. Inoculation of CSF/brain specimen intracerebrally into suckling mice and observing them for signs of sickness is the commonly adopted procedure. However, this procedure is time consuming. Inoculation of mosquito cell cultures especially *Aedes albopictus* C6/36 and *Aedes pseudoscutellaris* cell lines, is a sensitive and rapid method for isolation of JEV from clinical specimens (Leake *et al.*, 1986; Ravi *et al.*, 1989a). However, antibody detection is the most widely used method for diagnosis (Table 8.2). Conventional antibody detection methods such as haemagglutination inhibition (HI), complement fixation (CFT) and neutralization tests (Nt) have paved the way for more rapid and sensitive assays such as the IgM capture ELISA (MAC-ELISA). This test has a sensitivity approaching 100% when CSF and serum samples collected after the first week of illness are tested (Burke *et al.*, 1985b). Samples obtained prior to this time point may be negative for IgM antibodies in about 50% cases. Immunofluorescent localization of viral antigen in the cells of the CSF (Mathur *et al.*, 1990; Desai *et al.*, 1994c), and detection of soluble antigens in the CSF by reverse passive haemagglutina-

Table 8.2 Laboratory procedures in use for the diagnosis of Japanese encephalitis.

Procedures used (Reference)	Specimen used	Testing time (days)	Comments on the test
Antibody detection			
HI & CFT (Clarke and Cassals, 1956)	Paired serum sample	10–15	Cumbersome. Cross reactions with other flaviviruses. Not widely used at present.
MAC-ELISA (Burke *et al.*, 1985)	Single CSF sample	1–2	Most sensitive and widely used test. Invariably positive after 7 days, may give negative results in 50% of patients during the first week.
Neutralization test (Desai *et al.*, 1994)	Paired sera and CSF	10–15	Very Specific test. Cumbersome and cannot be used as routine test.
Antigen detection			
RPHA (Ravi *et al.*, 1989b)	Single CSF sample	1–2	Useful in the first week of illness especially in antibody negative cases.
IFA (Mathur *et al.*, 1990)	Cells smears from a single CSF sample	1–2	
Virus isolation			
Suckling mouse brain inoculation (Clarke and Cassals, 1956)	CSF/serum sample, preferably acute phase sample	10–20	Gold standard – the best method to confirm diagnosis. Not feasible in routine labs.
Mosquito cell line inoculation (Leake *et al.*, 1986)	CSF/serum sample	3–7	
Immune complexes (Desai *et al.*, 1995b)	Single CSF sample	1–2	Specific but not sensitive. Useful lab indicator of final outcome.

HI = haemagglutination inhibition; CFT = complement fixation test; MAC-ELISA = IgM antibody capture ELISA; RPHA = reverse passive haemagglutination assay.

tion (Ravi *et al.*, 1989b) are useful, rapid methods for confirming the diagnosis during the first week of illness (Table 8.2). Using a combination of various methods such as virus isolation, antigen and antibody detection, diagnosis could be confirmed in 80% of clinically suspected cases (Ravi *et al.*, 1989a). Molecular methods such as PCR have not been evaluated extensively and their utility as a routine diagnostic test is therefore unclear at this stage.

Treatment

No specific antiviral therapy is available. In an open labelled clinical trial of recombinant interferon (IFN) $\propto$ in 14 patients in Thailand, 13 survived (Harinasuta *et al.*, 1985). However, more detailed, double-blind controlled studies are essential before any conclusions can be drawn. General measures such as maintenance of fluid and electrolyte balance and good nursing care are of paramount importance. Since cerebral oedema is a prominent feature in many JE patients and perhaps the most important cause of death, energetic management of raised intracranial pressure by intravenous infusion of high doses of mannitol and parenteral steroids are recommended. However, in a recent study which evaluated high dose of dexamethasone in a randomized double-blind method, no significant difference in the final outcome was noted (Hoke *et al.*, 1992). Oral glycerol is advocated when anti-oedema measures are required over a long period of time and frusemide can be given if there is additional evidence of pulmonary oedema. Recurrent convulsions and status epilepticus are treated by the standard regimens. Superadded pulmonary infection, a common occurrence particularly when adequate nursing care is not available, has to be treated with appropriate antibiotics.

Outcome

The case fatality rates in Southern and East Asian countries varies from 10 to 40% (Umenai *et al.*, 1985). In India it has been observed that approximately one-third of the patients die during the acute stage of the illness (Gourie-Devi and Deshpande, 1982; Rodrigues, 1984). Cerebral oedema, neuronal damage and acute pulmonary oedema are responsible for early deaths and broncho-pneumonia for late deaths. Poor prognostic indicators are the duration of the acute encephalitic stage, severity and duration of unconsciousness, recurrent uncontrolled seizures and status epilepticus, marked increase of cells in CSF and severe degree of slowing observed in the EEG. Among those who survive the illness, more than half are left with residual neurological or developmental deficits and only one-third of the patients fully recover from the illness. Mental deficiency, behavioural abnormalities, motor paralysis, speech and movement disorders are among the commonly encountered sequelae while convulsions and cranial nerve palsies are rare (Gourie-Devi, 1984). In a 5-year follow up of these patients from South India it was observed that neurological deficits persisted in as many as 42 (75%) of the 56 patients who had deficits at the time of discharge from hospital. The majority of them were children and many had more than one type of deficit. Mental retardation and learning disability were the major problems leading to poor scholastic performance. Similar observations have also been reported from Thailand (Plubrukarn *et al.*, 1991). Movement disorders, chiefly of the parkinsonian variety, are also seen in some children (Gouri-Devi, 1984; Misra and Kalita, 1997a). Thus the recognition of these mental and motor sequelae suggest that there is a larger public health impact of JE than is generally appreciated.

Prevention

A multitude of approaches is needed for the effective control of JE. They include vector control, environmental control and vaccination of pigs and human beings. Vector control can be achieved through thermal fogging with insecticides such as pyrethrum or malathion but it is not feasible to cover extensive rural areas. A more sustainable approach is to use personal protection methods such as mosquito repellents and bed nets especially those impregnated with pyrethroid insecticides (Luo *et al.*, 1994).

Although vector control and changes in agricultural practices do contribute to the reduction of transmission, vaccination of affected populations with effective and affordable vaccines appears to be the most logical control measure. The impact of large scale vaccination is clearly documented in the literature (Hoke *et al.*, 1988). Three types of vaccines are currently in large scale production and use (WHO, 1998) namely: (i) mouse brain derived inactivated vaccine; (ii) cell culture derived inactivated vaccine; and (iii) cell culture derived live attenuated vaccine. Among these, the mouse brain derived inactivated vaccine is the most widely used in several Asian countries except China where an inactivated cell culture vaccine (Chinese SA-14-2 strain) is used. A crude version of the mouse brain derived vaccine was first produced as early as the 1930s, although purification (to reduce myelin basic protein content) and large scale production was not achieved until 1969 (WHO, 1998). Two prototype strains are used in the preparation, the original Nakayama strain and the Beijing strain. This vaccine is given subcutaneously in doses of 1 ml for older children and adults and 0.5 ml for children between 1 and 3 years of age. The primary schedule comprises of two doses of vaccine spaced 1–2 weeks apart. This may be followed by a booster one year later and subsequently every 3–4 years in endemic areas. Seroconversion (a Nt antibody titre of >10) is reported to occur in 80–85% of the vaccinees after the two dose primary schedule and in a majority of them Nt antibody titres declined below the protective levels by 6–12 months. In general the mouse brain derived vaccine is considered to be relatively safe. Local reactions such as tenderness, erythema and oedema with mild systemic symptoms such as headache, myalgia and fever are known to occur in about 10–20% of vaccinees (WHO, 1998). However, in recent years there have been several vaccine related adverse reactions reported in literature. These have ranged from allergic mucocutaneous reactions (1–17 per 10 000) to serious neurological complications (1 per 64 000) in European recipients (Andersen and Ronne, 1991; Othaki *et al.*, 1995; Plesner and Renne, 1997; Plesner *et al.*, 1998), although it is much less in Asians, at 1–2 per million vaccinees (Hsu *et al.*, 1971; Hoke *et al.*, 1988). The attenuated cell culture vaccine which is widely used in China on the other hand is reported to be devoid of such serious complications while offering the same degree of protection as the mouse brain derived vaccine. A number of new approaches towards the development of effective vaccines are being pursued currently. They include poxvirus based recombinant vaccines (Konishi *et al.*, 1997a), DNA vaccines (Lin *et al.*, 1998; Konishi *et al.*, 1998), chimearic vaccines (Pugachev *et al.*, 1995), and subunit vaccines (Konishi *et al.*, 1997b) and oral immunization using conventional immunogens (Ramakrishna *et al.*, 1999). However, all these approaches are in the experimental stages and will need further evaluation.

References

Andersen, M. M. and Ronne, T. (1991). Side effects with Japanese encephalitis vaccine. *Lancet*, **337**, 1044.

Bu'lock, F. A. (1986). Japanese B encephalitis virus in India – a growing problem *Q. J. Med.*, **60**, 825–836.

Burke, D. S., Nisslak, A., Ussery, M. A. *et al.* (1985a). Kinetics of IgM and IgG response to Japanese encephalitis virus in human serum and CSF. *J. Infect. Dis.*, **155**, 797–799.

Burke, D. S., Lorsuomrudee, W., Leake, C. J. *et al.* (1985b). Fatal outcome in Japanese encephalitis. *Am. J. Trop. Med. Hyg.*, **34**, 1203–1210.

Cao, J. X., Ni, H., Willis, M. R. *et al.* (1995). Passage of Japanese encephalitis virus in HeLa cells results in attenuation of virulence in mice. *J. Gen. Virol.*, **76**, 2757–2764.

Cecilia, D. and Gould, E. A. (1991). Nucleotide changes responsible for loss of neuroinvasiveness in Japanese encephalitis virus neutralization-resistant mutants. *Virology*, **181**, 70–77.

Chakravarty, S. K., Sarkar, J. K., Chakravarty, M. S. *et al.* (1975). The first epidemic of Japanese encephalitis in India – virological studies. *Ind. J. Med. Res.*, **63**, 77–82.

Chambers, T. J., Hahn, C. S., Galler, R. and Rice, C. M. (1990). Flavivirus genome organization, expression and replication. *Ann. Rev. Microbiol.*, **44**, 649–688.

Chatterjee, A. K. and Banerjee, K. (1975). Epidemiological studies on the encephalitis epidemic in Bankura. *Ind. J. Med. Res.*, **63**, 1164–1177.

Chaturvedi, U. C., Mathur, A., Chandra, A. *et al.* (1980). Transplacental infection with Japanese encephalitis virus. *J. Infect. Dis.*, **141**, 712–715.

Chen, W. R., Rico-Hess, R. and Test, R. B. (1992). A new genotype of Japanese encephalitis virus from Indonesia. *Am. J. Trop. Med. Hyg.*, **47**, 61–68.

Clarke, D. H. and Casals, J. (1958). Technique for haemagglutination of arboviruses. *Am. J. Trop. Med. Hyg.*, **7**, 561–573.

Dandawate, C. N., Rajagopalan, P. K., Pavri, K. M. and Work, T. H. (1969). Virus isolations from mosquitoes collected in North Arcot district, Madras State, and Chittoor district, Andhra Pradesh, November 1955 and October 1957. *Ind. J. Med. Res.*, **57**, 1420–1424.

Desai, A., Ravi, V., Chandramuki, A. *et al.* (1994a). Detection of neutralizing antibodies to Japanese encephalitis virus in the cerebrospinal fluid using a rapid micro-neutralization test. *Serodiag. Immunother. Infect. Dis.*, **6**, 130–134.

Desai, A., Ravi, V., Guru, S. C. *et al.* (1994b). Detection of autoantibodies to neural antigens in the CSF of Japanese encephalitis patients and correlation of findings with outcome. *J. Neurol. Sci.*, **122**, 109–116.

Desai, A., Ravi, V., Chandramuki, A. and Gourie-Devi, M. (1994c). Detection of Japanese encephalitis virus antigen in the CSF using monoclonal antibodies. *Clin. Diag. Virol.*, **2**, 191–199.

Desai, A., Shankar, S. K., Ravi, V. *et al.* (1995a). Japanese encephalitis virus antigen in the human brain and its topographic distribution, *Acta Neuropathol.*, **89**, 368–373.

Desai, A., Ravi, V., Chandramuki, A. and Gourie-Devi, M. (1995b). Proliferative response of human peripheral blood mononuclear cells to Japanese encephalitis virus. *Microbiol. Immunol.*, **39**, 269–273.

Desai, A., Ravi, V., Chandramuki, A. and Gourie-Devi, M. (1995c). Detection of immune complexes in the CSF of Japanese encephalitis patients: correlation of findings with outcome. *Intervirology*, **37**, 352–355.

Desai, A., Shankar, S. K., Jayakumar, P. N. *et al.* (1997). Coexistence of cerebral cysticercosis and Japanese encephalitis – a prognostic modulator. *Epidemiol. Infect.*, **118**, 165–171.

Dhanda, V., Thenmozhi, V., Kumar, N. P. *et al.* (1997). Virus isolation from wild caught mosquitoes during JE outbreak in Kerala in 1996. *Ind. J. Med. Res.*, **106**, 4–6.

Gajanana, A., Thenmozhi, V., Samuel, P. P. and Reuben, R. (1995). A community-based study of subclinical flavivirus infections in children in an area of Tamil Nadu, India, where Japanese encephalitis is endemic. *Bull. World Hlth. Org.*, **73**, 237–244.

George, S., Prasad, S. R., Rao, J. R. *et al.* (1987). Isolation of Japanese encephalitis and West Nile viruses from fatal cases of encephalitis in Kolar districts of Karnataka. *Ind. J. Med. Res.*, **86**, 131–134.

Gourie-Devi, M. (1984). Clinical aspects and experiences in the management of Japanese encephalitis patients. In: *Proceedings of the National Conference on Japanese Encephalitis*. New Delhi: Indian Council of Medical Research. pp. 25–29.

Gourie-Devi, M. and Deshpande, D. H. (1982). Japanese encephalitis. In: *Pediatric Problems*, (L. S. Prasad, L. L. Kukzkeyi, eds). New Delhi: S. Chand and Co. pp. 340–356.

Gourie-Devi, M. Satishchandra, P., Gokul, B. N. *et al.* (1989). Short course treatment in culture positive tuberculous meningitis. *Neurol. Ind.*, **37**, 581–587.

Hanna, J. N., Ritchie, S. A., Phillips, D. A. *et al.* (1996). An outbreak of Japanese encephalitis in Torres Strait, Australia, 1995. *Med. J. Aust.*, **165**, 256–260.

Harinasuta, C., Nimmanitya, S. and Titsyakorn, U. (1985). The effect of Interferon Alpha on cases of Japanese encephalitis in Thailand. *Southeast Asian J. Trop. Med. Publ. Hlth.*, **16**, 332–336.

Hoke, C. H., Nisalak, A., Nadhirat, S. *et al.* (1988). Protection against Japanese encephalitis by inactivated vaccines. *N. Engl. J. Med.*, **319**, 608–614.

Hoke, C. H. JR., Vaughn, D. W., Nisalak, A. *et al.* (1992). Effects of high dose dexamethasone on the outcome of acute Japanese encephalitis. *J. Infect. Dis.*, **165**, 131–136.

Hsu, Y. K. (1940). Cerebral cysticercosis and acute poliomyeloencephalitis. *Chinese Med. J.*, **57**, 318–319.

Hsu, T. C., Chow, L. P., Wei, H. Y. *et al.* (1971). A completed trial for an evaluation of the effectiveness of mouse brain Japanese encephalitis vaccine. In: *Immunization for Japanese Encephalitis* (W. H. Hammon, M. Kitaoka, and K. H. Downs, eds). Williams and Wilkins, pp. 258–265.

Huang, C. H. (1982). Studies of Japanese encephalitis in China. *Adv. Virus Res.*, **27**, 71–101.

Igarashi, A., Tanaka, M., Morita, K. *et al.* (1994). Detection of West Nile and Japanese encephalitis viral genome sequences in cerebrospinal fluid from acute encephalitis cases in Karachi, Pakistan. *Microbiol. Immunol.*, **38**, 827–830.

Ishii, T., Matsushita, M. and Hamada, S. (1977). Characteristic residual neuropathological features of Japanese B-encephalitis. *Acta Neuropathol.*, **38**, 181–186.

Jervis, G. and Higgins, G. (1953). Russian Spring-Summer encephalitis. *J. Neuropathol. Exp. Neurol.*, **12**, 1–10.

Johnson, R. T. (1987). The pathogenesis of acute viral encephalitis and post infectious encephalomyelitis. *J. Infect. Dis.*, **155**, 359–364.

Johnson, R. T., Burke, D. S., Elwell, M. *et al.* (1985). Japanese encephalitis: immunocytochemical studies of viral antigen and inflammatory cells in fatal cases. *Ann. Neurol.*, **18**, 567–573.

Kedarnath, N., Cecilia, D., Sathe, P. S. *et al.* (1986). Monoclonal antibodies against Japanese encephalitis virus. *Ind. J. Med. Res.*, **84**, 125–133.

Khanna, N., Mathur, A., Chaturvedi, U. C. *et al.* (1994). Regulation of vascular permeability by macrophage-derived chemotactic factor produced in Japanese encephalitis. *Immunol. Cell Biol.*, **72**, 200–204.

Kimoto, T., Yamada, T., Uebe, N. *et al.* (1968). Laboratory diagnosis of Japanese encephalitis: comparison of the fluorescent antibody technique with virus isolation and serological tests. *Biken J.*, **11**, 157–168.

Kimura Kuroda, J. and Yasui, K. (1988). Protection of mice against Japanese encephalitis virus by passive administration with monoclonal antibodies. *J. Immunol.*, **141**, 3606–3610.

Kobayashi, Y., Hasegawa, H., Omaya, T. *et al.* (1984). Antigenic analysis of Japanese encephalitis virus using monoclonal antibodies. *Infect. Immun.*, **44**, 117–123.

Konishi, E., Kurane, I., Mason, P. W. *et al.* (1997a). Poxvirus based Japanese encephalitis virus vaccine candidates induce JE virus-specific CD8 + cytotoxic T lymphocytes in mice. *Virology*, **227**, 353–360.

Konishi, E., Win, K. S., Kurane, I. *et al.* (1997b). Particulate vaccine candidate for Japanese encephalitis induces long-lasting virus specific memory T lymphocytes in mice. *Vaccine*, **15**, 281–286.

Konishi, E., Yamaoka, M., Win, K. S. *et al.* (1998). Induction of protective immunity against Japanese encephalitis in mice by immunization with a plasmid encoding Japanese encephalitis virus premembrane and envelope genes. *J. Virol.*, **72**, 4925–4930.

Kornyey, S. (1978). Contribution to the histology of tick-borne encephalitis. *Acta Neuropathol.*, **43**, 179–183.

Leake, C. J., Burke, D. S., Nisalak, A. *et al.* (1986). Isolation of Japanese encephalitis virus from clinical specimens using a continuous mosquito cell line. *Am. J. Trop. Med. Hyg.*, **35**, 1045–1050.

Lin, Y. L., Chen, L. K., Liao, C. L. *et al.* (1998). DNA immunization with Japanese encephalitis virus nonstructural proteins NS1 elicits protective immunity in mice. *J. Virol.*, **72**, 191–200.

Liu, Y. F., Teng, C. I. and Liu, K. (1957). Cerebral cysticercosis as a factor aggravating Japanese B-encephalitis. *Chinese Med. J.*, **75**, 101–107.

Luo, D., Zhang, K., Song, J. *et al.* (1994). The protective effect of bed nets impregnated with pyrethroid insecticide and vaccination against Japanese encephalitis. *Trans. Roy. Soc. Trop. Med. Hyg.*, **88**, 632–634.

Mathur, A., Rawat. S., Chaturvedi, U. C. *et al.* (1986). Macrophage transmission of suppressor signal for delayed hypersensitivity and humoral response in Japanese encephalitis virus infected mice. *Br. J. Exp. Pathol.*, **67**, 171–179.

Mathur, A., Kumar, R., Sharma, S. *et al.* (1990). Rapid diagnosis of Japanese encephalitis by immunofluorescent examination of cerebrospinal fluid. *Ind. J. Med. Res.*, **91**, 1–4.

McMinn, P. C. (1997). The molecular basis of virulence of the encephalitogenic flaviviruses. *J. Gen. Virol.*, **78**, 2711–2722.

Misra, U. K., Nag, D., Shukla, R. and Kar, A. M. (1980). Diencephalic epilepsy and parkinsonism as sequelae of Japanese encephalitis. *Neurol. Ind.*, **28**, 252.

Misra, U. K., Kalita, J., Jain, S. K. and Mathur, A. (1994). Radiological and neuro-physiological changes in Japanese encephalitis. *J. Neurol. Neurosurg. Psych.*, **57**, 1484–1487.

Mishra, U. K. and Kalita, J. (1997a). Movement disorders in Japanese encephalitis. *J. Neurol.*, **234**, 299.

Misra, U. K. and Kalita, J. (1997b). Anterior horn cells are also involved in Japanese encephalitis. *Acta Neurol. Scand.*, **96**, 114.

Miyake, M. (1964). The pathology of Japanese encephalitis: a review. *Bull. World Hlth. Org.*, **30**, 153–160.

Mohan Rao, C. V. R., Prasad, S. R., Rodrigues, J. J. *et al.* (1983). The first laboratory proven outbreak of Japanese encephalitis in Goa. *Ind. J. Med. Res.*, **78**, 745–750.

Monath, T. P. and Tsai, T. F. (1997). Flaviviruses. In: *Clinical Virology*, (D. D. Richman, R. J. Whitley and F. G. Hayden, eds). Edinburgh: Churchill Livingstone. pp. 1133–1185.

Muralikrishna, K., Ravi, V. and Manjunath, R. (1994). Cytotoxic T lymphocytes against Japanese encephalitis virus: effector cell phenotype, target specificity and in vitro clearance. *J. Gen. Virol.*, **75**, 799–807.

Muralikrishna, K., Ravi, V. and Munjunath, R. (1996a). Protection of adult but not newborn mice against intracerebral challenge with Japanese encephalitis virus by adoptively transferred virus specific T lymphocytes: requirement of L3T4 + cells. *J. Gen. Virol.*, **77**, 705–714.

Muralikrishna, K., Ramireddy, B., Ravi, V. and Manjunath, R. (1996b). Recognition of non-structural protein peptides by cytoxic T lymphocytes raised against Japanese encephalitis virus. *Microbiol. Immunol.*, **39**, 1021–1024.

Ni, H. and Barrett, A. D. T. (1995). Nucleotide and deduced amino acid sequence of structural protein genes of Japanese encephalitis viruses from different geographical locations. *J. Gen. Virol.*, **76**, 401–408.

Ogata, A., Nagashira, K., Hall, W. W. *et al.* (1991). Japanese encephalitis virus neurotropism is dependent on degree of neuronal maturity. *J. Virol.*, **65**, 880–886.

Othaki, E., Matsuishe, T., Hiranu, Y. and Maekawa, K. (1995). Acute disseminated encephalomyelitis after treatment with Japanese B encephalitis vaccine (Nakayama Yolken and Beijing strains). *J. Neurol. Neurosurg. Psych.*, **59**, 316–317.

Oyanagi, S., Ikuta, F. and Ross, E. R. (1969). Electron microscopic observations in mice infected with Japanese encephalitis. *Acta Neuropathol. (Ber.)*, **13**, 169–181.

Pavri, K. M., Ghalasasi, G. R., Dastur, D. K. *et al.* (1975). Dual infections in mice: visceral larva migraines and sublethal infection with Japanese encephalitis. *Trans. Roy. Soc. Trop. Med. Hyg.*, **69**, 99–110.

Plesner, A. and Renne, T. (1997). Allergic mucocutaneous reactions to Japanese encephalitis vaccine. *Vaccine*, **15**, 1239–1243.

Plesner, A., Arlien-Sorberg, P. and Herning, M. (1998). Neurological complications to vaccination against Japanese encephalitis. *Eur. J. Neurol.*, **5**, 479–485.

Plubrukarn, R., Thaeramanoparb, S. and Nimmanitya, S. (1991). Clinical sequelae after Japanese encephalitis: a five year follow up study. *Bull. Dep. Med. Serv.*, **16**, 125–132.

Prasad, S. R., Kumar, V., Marwah, R. K. *et al.* (1993). An epidemic of encephalitis in Haryana: serological evidence for Japanese encephalitis in a few patients. *Ind. Paediatr.*, **30**, 905–910.

Pugachev, K. V., Mason, P. W., Shope, R. E. and Frey, T. K. (1995). Double-subgenomic Sindbis virus recombinants expressing immunogenic proteins of Japanese encephalitis virus induce significant protection in mice against lethal JEV infection. *Virology*, **212**, 587–594.

Ramakrishna, C., Desai, A., Shankar, S. K. *et al.* (1999). Oral immunization of mice with live Japanese encephalitis virus induces a protective immune response. *Vaccine*, **17**, 3102–3108.

Ravi, V., Vanajakshi, S., Gowda, A. and Chandramuki, A. (1989a). Laboratory diagnosis of Japanese encephalitis using monoclonal antibodies and correlation of findings with outcome. *J. Med. Virol.*, **29**, 221–223.

Ravi, V., Premkumar, S., Chandramuki, A. and Kimura-Kuroda, J. (1989b). A reverse passive haemagglutination test for the detection of Japanese encephalitis virus antigens in the cerebrospinal fluid. *J. Virol. Meth.*, **23**, 291–298.

Ravi, V., Desai, A., Shenoy, P. K. *et al.* (1993). Persistence of Japanese encephalitis virus in the human nervous system. *J. Med. Virol.*, **40**, 326–329.

Ravi, V., Taly, A. B., Shankar, S. K. *et al.* (1994). Association of Japanese encephalitis virus infection with Guillian-Barré syndrome in endemic areas in South India. *Acta Neurol. Scand.*, **90**, 67–72.

Ravi, V., Parida, S., Desai, A. *et al.* (1997). Correlation of TNF levels in the serum and CSF of Japanese encephalitis patients. *J. Med. Virol.*, **51**, 132–136.

Rice, C. M. (1996). Flavivirdae: the viruses and their replication. In: *Fields Virology*, 3rd edn, (B. N. Fields, D. M. Knipe and P. M. Howley, eds). Philadelphia: Lippincot-Raven. pp. 931–959.

Rodrigues, F. M. (1984). Epidemiology of Japanese encephalitis in India: a brief overview. In: *Proceedings of the National Conference on Japanese Encephalitis*. New Delhi: Indian Council of Medical Research. pp. 1–9.

Rosen, L., Tesh, R. B., Lien, J. C. *et al.* (1978). Transovarial transmission of Japanese encephalitis virus by mosquitoes. *Science*, **199**, 909–911.

Scherer, W. F., Buescher, E. L. and Mclure, H. E. (1959). Ecolgical studies of Japanese encephalitis virus in Japan. V. Avian factors. *Am. J. Trop. Med. Hyg.*, **8**, 689–694.

Shankar, S. K., Vasudeva Rao, T., Mruthyunjayanna, B. P. *et al.* (1983). Autopsy study of brains during an epidemic of Japanese encephalitis in Karnataka. *Ind. J. Med. Res.*, **78**, 431–440.

Shankar, S. K., Suryanarayana, V., Vasantha, S. *et al.* (1994). Biology of neurocysti-cercosis – parasite related factors modulating host response. *Med. J. Armed Forces Ind.*, **50**, 79–88.

Shapiro, D., Brandt, W. E., Cardiff, R. D. *et al.* (1971). The proteins of Japanese encephalitis Virus. *Virology*, **44**, 108–124.

Sharma, S., Mathur, A., Prakash, V. *et al.* (1991). Japanese encephalitis virus latency in the peripheral blood lymphocytes and recurrence of infection in children. *Clin. Exp. Immunol.*, **85**, 85–89.

Shoji, H., Hiraki, V., Kuwasaki, N. *et al.* (1989). Japanese encephalitis in the Kurumke region of Japan – CT and MRI findings. *J. Neurol.*, **236**, 255–259.

Shoji, H., Murakami, T., Murai, I. *et al.* (1990). A follow up study by CT and MRI in 3 cases of Japanese encephalitis. *Neuroradiology*, **32**, 215–219.

Solomon, T., Kneen, R., Dung, N. M. *et al.* (1998). Poliomyelitis-like illness due to Japanese encephalitis virus. *Lancet*, **351**, 1094–1097.

Sumiyoshi, H., Tignor, G. H. and Shope, R. E. (1995). Characterization of a highly attenuated Japanese encephalitis virus generated from a molecular cloned cDNA. *J. Infect. Dis.*, **171**, 1144–1151.

Takagami, T., Miyamoto, H., Nakamura, H. *et al.* (1982). Biological activities of structural proteins of Japanese encephalitis virus. *Acta Virol.*, **26**, 312–320.

Umenai, T., Krzysko, R., Bektimirov, T. A. and Assad, F. A. (1985). Japanese encephalitis: current worldwide status. *Bull World Hlth Org.*, **63**, 625–631.

WHO (1998). Japanese encephalitis vaccine – WHO position paper. *Wkly Epidemiol. Rec.*, **73**, 337–344.

Zimmerman, H. M. (1946). The pathology of Japanese B encephalitis. *Am. J. Pathol.*, **22**, 965–991.

9

Vaccines to prevent bacterial meningitis

J. Simon Kroll and Jennifer M. MacLennan

Introduction

At least a million cases of bacterial meningitis occur each year resulting in a massive burden of acute and chronic ill health on individuals and their families and on society. Infection appears to strike capriciously and may progress rapidly, carrying off individuals who were in robust good health only days before. It naturally generates considerable public anxiety and media attention, especially when clusters of cases occur.

Before the antibiotic era, death was almost inevitable. Even now, with highly effective drugs, the case fatality rate in most countries remains around 10%, and a similar proportion of individuals are left with significant neurological problems. The development of vaccines effective against meningitis pathogens is correspondingly seen widely to be a matter of importance and urgency.

While bacterial meningitis can occur in individuals of any age, it is predominantly a disease of young children. The organisms generally responsible are among those commonly found colonizing mucosal surfaces, particularly of the upper respiratory tract (URT). In the neonatal period, heavy contamination of the oropharynx with bacterial flora of the maternal lower gastrointestinal and genital tract transiently – over the first 3 months – increases the risk of invasive infection and meningitis caused by *Streptococcus agalactiae* (Group B streptococcus), *Escherichia coli* and other enterobacteriaceae, and *Listeria monocytogenes*. As small compensation, during the first months of life infants are relatively protected against invasive infection by the more usual colonists of the URT, thanks to the presence of antibody acquired by transfer across the placenta during the last trimester of pregnancy. However, as the concentration of this maternally-derived antibody declines, infants become increasingly susceptible to meningitis due to *Haemophilus influenzae*, *Streptococcus pneumoniae* (pneumococcus) and *Neisseria meningitidis* (meningococcus) – the major meningitis pathogens.

Meningitis is a seasonal infection, rates peaking in the winter months (Figure 9.1). The age-specific attack rate for disease caused by all these organisms is greatest during the second half of the first year of life. After 2 years of age, the risk of meningitis due to *H. influenzae* and pneumococcus declines, but older

Quarterly notifications

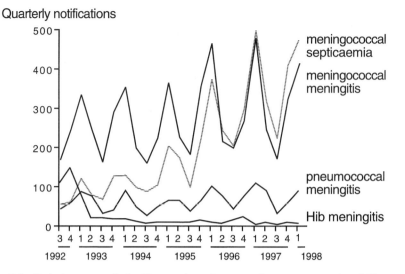

Figure 9.1 Relative quarterly incidence of meningococcal, pneumococcal and *Haemophilus influenzae* type b (Hib) meningitis (and meningococcal septicaemia): 1992–1998. The striking increase in meningococcal septicaemia notification coincides with heightened clinical awareness and improved non-culture diagnostic techniques. Adapted from Communicable Disease Report 9 (Suppl. 3) 1999. S3, by permission of PHLS CDSC.

children remain at significant risk of meningococcal disease. In industrialized countries, a secondary peak in age-specific incidence occurs in late adolescence, while in the developing world major outbreaks of meningococcal disease occur periodically in older children and young adults. Beyond adolescence, unusual host susceptibility becomes a more and more prominent association with meningitis caused by any of these pathogens, cases increasingly occurring in patients with conditions that compromise host defences.

Pathogenesis

Understanding the interaction between the major meningitis pathogens and their human hosts at different stages of colonization and infection has led to successful vaccination strategies in some cases – best illustrated in the case of *H. influenzae* type b (Hib) – but has also thrown into prominence the considerable difficulties to be faced in developing protective vaccines in others – exemplified by serogroup B meningococcus.

As common commensals of the human URT, the major meningitis pathogens pass from one individual to another by the airborne route in droplets of respiratory secretions. Nearly all such acquisitions are either entirely harmless to the new host – resulting merely in transient, symptomless, carriage of bacteria on the mucosal surface – or positively advantageous, stimulating an immune response that protects against subsequent infection. Life-threatening invasive disease such as meningitis is very rare and from the bacterial perspective represents an ecological dead-end, terminating as it does opportunities for bacterial survival or spread. The paradox that these otherwise quite innocuous organisms exhibit such considerable virulence once in the human bloodstream may be explained by the inherently opposing nature of attributes which best allow bacteria on the one hand to survive in the harsh environment of a rapidly desiccating respiratory droplet passing from host to host, and on the other efficiently to colonize the mucosal surface.

A thick hydrated layer of polysaccharide on the bacterial surface facilitates transmission, allowing organisms to resist desiccation between hosts. By covering adhesive structures on the bacterial outer membrane beneath, important for anchoring organisms to host cells, capsule may also promote detachment from one epithelial surface in anticipation of departure, but the price to pay is a reduction in the efficiency with which organisms can then colonize a new host. In Hib and meningococcus, where the events of colonization and invasion have been extensively studied at the molecular and cellular level, this dilemma is resolved by a combination of phenotypic and phase variation. On arriving at the URT mucosal surface, thickly encapsulated Hib organisms adhere relatively weakly to non-ciliated epithelial cells initially via long pili that extend through the polysaccharide layer. In the new environment, in response to changes in the concentrations of nutrients, ions, temperature and pH, an altered pattern of gene expression leads to a considerable reduction in polysaccharide synthesis, with thinning of the capsule to expose other, shorter, adhesive structures which bind the bacteria more firmly to the mucosa (St-Geme and Cutter, 1996) (Figure 9.2).

Capsulate meningococci not only down-regulate capsule synthesis, but even extinguish it altogether by genetic rearrangement leading to inactivation of critical capsulation genes either by the insertion element *IS*1301, or through a mechanism of slipped-strand mispairing (Hammerschmidt *et al.*, 1996a, b). Changes in gene expression of these kinds take an appreciable time to become manifest at the phenotypic level, and both Hib and meningococcus have evolved contingency strategies to ensure that at any time a proportion of the bacterial population is generously capsulated and able to survive if ejected into the harsh outside world. Extinction of capsulation in meningococcus is

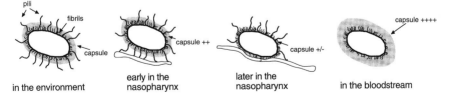

Figure 9.2 Hib colonization and invasion. Organisms in the environment between hosts have a substantial capsule. Early on in epithelial colonization, bacteria are attached by relatively scanty, long pili. Later, capsule is down-regulated and bacteria become more tightly attached by fibrils. Organisms that reach the bloodstream are non-piliated and thickly capsulate through operation of a contingency mechanism at the capsulation locus (see text), evading opsonophagocytic host defences.

reversible, precise excision of the transposable element or DNA strand slippage restoring the capsulate phenotype in a stochastic process that ensures that a small proportion of the bacterial population is capsulate and 'ready to go' at any time. A different strategy is found in the case of Hib. The capsulation locus *cap* is maintained in a quasi-stable direct repeat configuration that can be amplified to high copy-number (Kroll *et al.*, 1991). At any time a small proportion of the bacterial population will have an amplified *cap* locus and consequently a thicker capsule (Corn *et al.*, 1993), more readily detached from the mucosal surface and better able to survive between hosts.

Below the polysaccharide capsule layer, and relatively better exposed to the host as capsule is thinned or removed altogether, protein structures on the surface of Hib and meningococcus mediate interaction with a variety of host cells, allowing these organisms efficiently to spread and colonize different niches in their human hosts. Exposed as they are to components of the host immune system, some of these proteins are extremely antigenically diverse, to reduce the chance that prior exposure of the host to a colonizing strain of the same species will have led to cross-reactive immunity.

While organisms remain on the mucosal surface, no significant host pathology ensues. Problems follow if by chance organisms invade, a process which may perhaps be more likely if concurrent viral infection, cigarette smoking, or drying of the mucosa in desert air, reduces the integrity of the nasopharyngeal mucosa. Operation of these same colonization/dissemination-promoting mechanisms can then occasionally lead to disaster. If organisms penetrate the mucosal surface, by migration through intercellular clefts in the case of Hib or in endocytic vacuoles in the case of meningococcus (Stephens and Farley, 1991) then the stochastic processes maintaining a small population of heavily capsulate organisms will furnish a founder bacterial population well equipped to resist the action of humoral and cell-mediated host defences (Figure 9.2). While polysaccharide capsule is a relatively inert substance that plays a negligible role in inducing a host inflammatory response, it can protect bacteria against opsonization by the alternative pathway of complement, inhibiting phagocytosis by neutrophils, macrophages and reticuloendothelial cells. Antibody is crucial for protection against capsulate bacteria, but at birth human infants cannot mount an effective immune response to polysaccharide antigens. This capability does not develop until towards the end of the second year of life, so that once in the bloodstream, encapsulated organisms are singularly invulnerable to infant hosts. Further, some bacterial capsular polysaccharides are chemically similar or identical to host cell molecules, so failing to elicit a protective antibody response at any age. If, in addition, antibody-accessible structures on the subcapsular bacterial surface are highly antigenically variable so that the likelihood is low of a host having preformed bactericidal antibody, specific immune responses may be virtually powerless to protect the host. If such organisms reach the bloodstream, in the worst circumstances they can multiply almost unchecked, rapidly spreading to sites such as the CSF space to cause meningitis.

In this chapter we focus on vaccines to prevent disease due to Hib, pneumococcus and meningococcus. The problems these pathogens present illustrate the general principles used for the development of effective vaccines, and the considerable challenges that remain.

Haemophilus influenzae

Epidemiology

H. influenzae is a Gram-negative coccobacillus whose only natural host is man. About 4% of *H. influenzae* isolates are capsulate (Moxon, 1986) and these strains are subdivided into six serotypes based on the nature of the capsular polysaccharide. Serotype b organisms (Hib), with a capsule composed of polyribosyl-ribitol phosphate (PRP), are responsible for the great majority of cases of childhood meningitis, as well as other serious invasive infections such as pneumonia, septic arthritis and epiglottitis, and also cause most occult *Haemophilus* bacteraemia. Other capsular serotypes (a–f) much less commonly cause serious disease, but unencapsulated (non-typable) organisms are important causes of respiratory illness and otitis media and may cause invasive disease in newborn infants. Hib disease is almost exclusively restricted to children under the age of 5 years (Booy *et al.*, 1993), and susceptibility to disease is inversely correlated with the natural development of anti-PRP serum antibody titres, induced by asymptomatic carriage of Hib in the nasopharynx or of bacteria expressing cross-reacting antigens in the gastrointestinal tract (Bradshaw *et al.*, 1971; Handzel *et al.*, 1975; Robbins *et al.*, 1975; Schneerson and Robbins, 1975).

The population at risk

The window of susceptibility to invasive Hib infection in early childhood is the consequence of the universal incapacity of the infant immune system (until the age of about 2 years) to respond with protective antibody to exposure to capsule polysaccharide antigens. Beyond that age, individuals with quantitative or qualitative antibody deficiencies remain prone to invasive infection (reviewed by Rijkers *et al.*, 1993). Within the age range that infants are normally susceptible, some populations show a particularly high incidence of Hib disease. Thus while in the pre-Hib vaccine era in the USA, as in many European countries, the incidence of invasive infection in under 5s varied between 40–100/100 000, peaking at 6–11 months (Broome, 1987), in native American populations such as Navajo and Apache Indians or the Alaskan Inuit, rates of >400/100 000 were recorded (Losonsky *et al.*, 1984; Ward *et al.*, 1981, 1986). Both genetic (Petersen *et al.*, 1985, 1987) and environmental factors (extremely high Hib carriage and transmission rates in crowded dwellings) are thought to have contributed to this population's very high infection risk, which was characterized also by peaking of infection at a particularly young age (4–7 months).

Vaccines to prevent Hib disease

The first vaccine introduced to prevent Hib disease consisted of purified PRP. As a pure polysaccharide, PRP does not recruit T-lymphocyte help in the course of stimulating an immune response, and is therefore only poorly immunogenic in infants in whom the T-independent pathway to immunity is undeveloped. Although it induced reasonable antibody concentrations in those older than 2 years, PRP vaccine could not protect the younger children in whom more than half of the disease occurred, and suffered the additional drawback of failing to generate immunological memory (Makela, 1984). The challenge remained to produce a vaccine inducing a protective antibody response in the young children most at risk from Hib disease. This was triumphantly met by conversion of the polysaccharide from a T-independent to a T-dependent antigen by chemical linkage, conjugation, to one of a range of proteins. In currently licensed vaccines, PRP has been conjugated variously to tetanus toxoid (PRP-T), to diphtheria toxoid (PRP-D), to a recombinant modified diphtheria toxin CRM_{197} (HbOC), or to a meningococcal outer membrane protein complex (PRP-OMP). The effect of this modification is fundamentally to alter the pattern of immune response to the antigen. After internalization, processing of the protein portion by antigen presenting cells leads to recruitment of T-lymphocyte help and the production of the appropriate cytokine milieu to result in production of high affinity anti-polysaccharide antibody and to the establishment of a pool of memory B lymphocytes which confer immunological memory (the ability to respond rapidly when subsequently exposed to the organism) (Siber, 1994).

Hib conjugate vaccines have by now been introduced into routine infant immunisation schedules in many countries with spectacular success. Courses of three doses of vaccine given at 2, 3 and 4 months of age (in the UK) (2, 4 and 6 months in the USA) have been found to be highly effective. Vaccination has been shown to be effective even when commenced in infants as young as 6 weeks of age (Heath, 1998). The PRP-OMP formulation can induce protective levels of antibody and immunological memory even after only two doses and has therefore been used as the vaccine of preference in native American and Australian aboriginal populations considered at particular risk of early-onset infection (Hanna and Will, 1991; Santosham et al., 1991). Wherever vaccine has been introduced, whether in the developed or the developing world, rates of Hib disease have plummeted. The pattern seen in the UK is typical. The sawtooth pattern of seasonal peaks and troughs in the incidence of Hib meningitis was abolished in late 1992 when infant vaccination was introduced into the infant schedule, and disease has remained at a minimal level ever since (Figure 9.3).

In many areas, rates of Hib disease have dropped much more rapidly than expected, even in unvaccinated children. This has been explained by the finding that vaccination can bring about a degree of herd immunity through greatly reducing or even virtually eliminating carriage throughout the population (Barbour et al., 1995). This effect on carriage may be a significant part of vaccine protective efficacy in the immunized as well. In an Inuit population

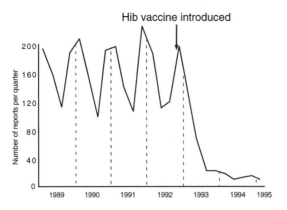

Figure 9.3   Quarterly incidence of Hib meningitis in England and Wales (1989–1995). The high rate of infection, with obvious winter peaks and summer troughs, was obliterated from late 1992, with introduction of Hib conjugate vaccine. Similar patterns have been seen in many other countries. (Data from PHLS CDSC)

where Hib carriage before introduction of vaccination was extremely high, introduction of PRP-OMP vaccine did not eliminate carriage, although the rate of cases of invasive disease declined sharply. When a change in the vaccination regimen led to exchange of the PRP-OMP vaccine for the different formulation HbOC, which is less protective after the first and second doses, persisting Hib carriage led to a resurgence of cases of meningitis (Galil *et al.*, 1999).

Some remaining Hib vaccine issues

As the first of the polysaccharide conjugates to be introduced into schedules of infant vaccination, after extensive safety testing that was of necessity conducted over a limited time span, Hib vaccines represent the proving ground for the technology, and a very wide range of questions continue to be asked about their long term efficacy and safety in different vaccine formulations and when given in combination with other vaccines. Long-term studies over many years will be needed to resolve some questions. For example, the question of whether Hib vaccination might induce type I diabetes mellitus has only recently been answered, reassuringly in the negative (Karvonen *et al.*, 1999).

Among many important issues, the following practical ones stand out.

The vaccines can in general be used interchangeably to immunize infants. Switching from one vaccine to another during the primary vaccination course is not recommended but limited data suggest that this still leads to robust immunity; and regardless of the product used in the primary series, any conjugate can be given to elicit a booster response in the second year of life (Anderson *et al.*, 1995; Goldblatt *et al.*, 1998a). The question, however, of whether such a booster is needed remains controversial. Data from US infants have shown a rapid decline in antibody concentrations to approximately 20% of the peak concentration by 1 year of age, in some cases to levels below those regarded as conferring protection. On this basis an additional booster dose has been recommended for US children between 12 and 15 months of age, and this recommendation is followed in many countries. The importance accorded to serum antibody concentration acknowledges the evidence, from *passive* immunisation studies, that a particular concentration of anti-PRP antibody (>0.15 mg/ml) is correlated with present protection (Makela *et al.*, 1977). The *active* immunity following successful vaccination can reasonably be expected to afford much greater protection. Reduced exposure to Hib in the circumstances of reduced Hib carriage following community-wide vaccination makes it scarcely surprising that antibody concentration may fall to low levels in a vaccinated individual, but the important thing is whether there is robust immunological memory, manifest as rapid synthesis of high-affinity antibody if invasive infection threatens (Granoff *et al.*, 1993). Measurement of antibody concentration after a booster dose of Hib vaccine shows that there is indeed rapid and substantial rise in high-affinity antibody (Goldblatt *et al.*, 1998b), the result of the continued presence of adequate numbers of circulating memory T lymphocytes, and in the UK the present recommendation remains not to give any further dose of Hib vaccine after the primary three-dose schedule. This policy has so far been satisfactory, with no evidence of substantial decline in protection in the first 4 years of life (Booy *et al.*, 1997) but remains under review. It diverges from the policy in most of the rest of the world, where generally the American practice is followed of giving a booster in the second year of life. Clearly the necessity – and if so, the cost – of a booster dose of Hib vaccine is a very important issue when it comes to making recommendations for delivering vaccine to infants in the resource-poor nations of the developing world.

The reformulation of Hib conjugates in multivalent vaccines has prompted continuing re-evaluation of their efficacy. Various mixtures of the different Hib vaccines with other infant vaccines have been assessed for compatibility and efficacy of the individual components. In the UK HibTITER (Wyeth Laboratories' preparation of PRP-CRM$_{197}$ conjugate) is licensed for administration in the same syringe as Trivax-AD (Evans Medical's preparation of adsorbed diphtheria/tetanus/pertussis (DTP) vaccine).

There is a drive in some countries to replace the traditional whole-cell pertussis vaccine in the infant schedule with a less reactogenic acellular preparation. This has raised the question of whether there will be any impact on other vaccines administered concurrently. In the case of Hib conjugates, Eskola and colleagues (1996) have shown that the anti-PRP antibody concentration achieved after vaccination is substantially lower if acellular pertussis is mixed with the conjugate than if whole cell pertussis vaccine in conventional DTP is used. The key question is whether this translates into reduced efficacy. This has been investigated by Bell and colleagues (1998), with results which seem broadly reassuring. Although post-vaccination serum concentrations of anti-PRP antibody were lower than those achieved when the Hib conjugate was given with whole cell pertussis vaccine, there appeared to be satisfactory priming for a memory response.

In summary, no major reversals have (yet) emerged in the crusade to prevent Hib meningitis by vaccination. Post-marketing surveillance continues to provide the opportunity to assess many important practical issues of protein-polysaccharide conjugate vaccine immunogenicity and effectiveness which will be invaluable in formulating policy for the introduction of other meningitis vaccines.

Is *Haemophilus* meningitis finished?

The great success of Hib vaccines in virtually eradicating Hib meningitis in many countries, coupled with the substantially reduced levels of Hib carriage generally found in vaccinated populations, has raised the theoretical possibility that Hib strains, and with them, invasive *Haemophilus* disease, could one day be eliminated. Disappointingly, current insights into the molecular genetic basis for *Haemophilus* virulence suggest that this will not be possible, and indeed that other strains of *Haemophilus* might come to replace serotype b strains as meningitis pathogens.

The continued success of Hib PRP-conjugate vaccines is predicated on the assumption that the enhanced virulence of serotype b strains is a consequence of their expression of serotype b polysaccharide capsule. An alternative possibility, however, is that there is linkage but not congruence between genes for serotype b capsulation and genes encoding some other trait responsible for virulence. The overwhelming predominance of serotype b strains among invasive isolates might then reflect either very close physical genetic linkage of such traits or a highly clonal bacterial population in which perhaps a whole range of traits are fortuitously in linkage disequilibrium with serotype b capsulation genes. In fact both possibilities must be admitted. Musser and colleagues (1990) have demonstrated striking clonality in the capsulate *Haemophilus* population, so that serotype b strains differ in many respects other than capsule from non-b strains. Also, studies of the genetic basis for *Haemophilus* capsulation have revealed a potential virulence-modifying locus adjacent to genes necessary for synthesis of serotype b polysaccharide. In serotype b strains, but not in other capsular serotypes, the capsulation locus *cap* consists of a large duplicated segment of DNA that crucially is stabilized by a small deletion mutation at one end (Hoiseth *et al*, 1986; Kroll *et al.*, 1988, 1991). This arrangement allows ready multimerization of the *cap* locus, and has apparently conferred such biological advantage that virtually all serotype b isolates, from cases of invasive disease all over the world, are descended from one original mutant strain (Kroll *et al*, 1993). The effect of this mutation has been to convert *cap* into a contingency locus as described above, allowing hypercapsulate strains quickly to proliferate if the bacteria invade the bloodstream. While the mutation conferring this amplification phenotype lies very close on the chromosome to serotype b-specific genes, it is physically separable from them. Capsule serotype-specific genes are clustered in a cassette of DNA (Kroll *et al.*, 1989) which, through a process of transformation and recombination, can come to be replaced by other serotype-specific genes, leading to generation of non-b serotype strains which retain the amplification phenotype. Where this has happened naturally, non-serotype b strains of increased virulence have come to clinical prominence, causing meningitis (Kroll *et al.*, 1994).

The prospect of universal Hib vaccination

The impact of Hib vaccination on *Haemophilus* meningitis rates has been dramatic wherever it has been introduced (Pan American Health Organisation, 1996; Peltola *et al.*, 1999). However there are many nations, both in the industrialized and developing world, which have yet to introduce it. In some cases there is a perception that Hib disease is a comparatively rare problem that does not merit such an expensive step. While Hib meningitis does indeed seem to be an unusual childhood infection in some societies, for example in various oriental populations (Sung *et al.*, 1997), in other countries an explicit surveillance exercise has overturned misperceptions about its rarity (Almuneef *et al.*, 1998). In many more countries of the developing world the real problem is cost. The Hib conjugate vaccines are much more expensive than the established childhood vaccines to prevent DTP, polio and measles, and universal implementation would place a huge strain on national resources (Miller, 1998). At a heavily discounted price of around US$1–3 for a three-dose schedule (compared to about £30 for a three dose course in the UK), a cost benefit analysis showed clear economic advantage in Chile to universal implementation (Levine *et al.*, 1993), but in the poorest countries this would still be a prohibitive cost. Reduced-dose vaccination schedules that do not compromise efficacy (Lagos *et al.*, 1998) can bring the cost down significantly, and a philanthropic donation on an heroic scale from such as the recently launched Bill and Melinda Gates Children's Vaccine Program may provide the resources to vaccinate the world's children.

Streptococcus pneumoniae

More than 90 different serotypes of *Streptococcus pneumoniae* (pneumococcus) can be distinguished on the basis of their capsular polysaccharides. The different capsules confer a varying degree of resistance to host defences aimed at limiting pneumococcal survival on mucosal surfaces and in the bloodstream, with the result that, like *H. influenzae*, the pneumococcus is an important cause of infection in young children all over the world. In the UK it is a leading cause of community-acquired pneumonia and otitis media, and an important cause of meningitis both in children and the elderly.

Epidemiology

Pneumococci are extremely common colonists of the nasopharynx. During the first 2 years of life virtually all children carry the organism at some time (Gray *et al.*, 1980) but the diversity of strains means that regardless of what protection such carriage may confer, there continues to be a significant risk to individuals of all ages of meeting a serotype for the first time that has the capacity to cause invasive infection. Life-threatening pneumococcal disease may follow symptomatic URT infection, commonly otitis media, or follow occult pneumococcal bacteraemia originating from asymptomatic URT mucosal colonization. Epidemiological associations of pneumococcal meningitis in childhood include the child having older siblings (Takala *et al.*, 1995) and being in day care (Levine *et al.*, 1999) circumstances which plausibly increase the risk of exposure to previously unencountered strains.

The population at risk

Some individuals are particularly susceptible to invasive pneumococcal disease. The spleen provides a key defence against progression of pneumococcal bacteraemia, and where this organ has been removed (after trauma or in the management of lymphoma) or has ceased to function normally (as in sickle cell anaemia and other haemoglobinopathies after early childhood), fulminant pneumococcal infection may occur. Antibody deficiency (quantitative deficiency, as in hypogammaglobulinaemia or IgG_2 subclass deficiency, or as increasingly recognized, qualitative inadequacy of antibody affinity) is also associated with an increased risk of severe pneumococcal infection. In conditions such as these, or where there is a physical connection, congenital or acquired, between the subarachnoid space and the URT mucosal surface, recurrent attacks of pneumococcal meningitis are well recognized.

Vaccines to prevent pneumococcal disease

Although the morbidity and mortality of pneumococcal meningitis is generally higher than Hib or meningococcal meningitis, its comparative rarity means that the search for effective pneumococcal vaccines has primarily been driven by the enormous burden of mucosal and respiratory disease. These have substantial impact in older children and adults, and as such individuals may be protected by pure polysaccharide vaccines, considerable efforts have for some time gone into developing such a formulation. Results of trials indicating high efficacy of 6- and 12-valent polysaccharide vaccines in young South African gold miners, who had a high rate of pneumococcal pneumonia, were reported in the mid-1970s (Smit *et al.*, 1977). Subsequent developments culminated in formulation of a 23-component pneumococcal polysaccharide vaccine, representing serotypes responsible for 85– >90% of invasive pneumococcal infection in diverse populations (Smart *et al.*, 1987; Jorgenson *et al.*, 1991; Gratten *et al.*, 1996; Laurichesse *et al.*, 1998). The vaccine is currently licensed and recommended for use in adults and children older than 2 years of age who are considered to be at high risk of pneumococcal disease: for example those with immunodeficiency, but also those with disorders such as congestive cardiac failure, chronic obstructive airways disease, chronic liver disease or diabetes mellitus. In the USA it has been recommended for everyone aged over 65 years.

Since a substantial burden of pneumococcal disease falls on children under 2 years of age in whom a pure polysaccharide vaccine is ineffective, efforts are now being focused, as they have been with Hib PRP, on developing poly-saccharide conjugate vaccines which should be effective at all ages. However, a substantial logistical problem is created by the great diversity of pneumococcal serotypes that may cause serious disease (in contrast to the single serotype b responsible for nearly all *Haemophilus* meningitis). The expense of conjugate vaccines increases in proportion to the number of components they contain, and it is necessary to establish, through well-conducted surveys, both which serotypes to include, and the point at which inclusion of further serotypes is no longer economically viable. Nine pneumococcal serotypes (14, 6B, 19F, 18C, 9V, 23F, 7F, 1 and 5) have recently been found responsible for between 70% (developing world) and 90% (developed world) of cases of pneumococcal pneumonia in children, although the prevalence of disease due to each serotype varies substantially between different geographical areas. A nonavalent conjugate vaccine with these constituents might be a reasonable compromise for a universally applicable pneumococcal vaccine (Sniadack *et al.*, 1995). Alternatively, country- or region-specific vaccines may be developed.

Various conjugate vaccines containing between 4 and 11 different serotypes are being assessed in clinical trials. A number of efficacy studies are underway, and the first trial of a heptavalent vaccine in the USA involving 30 000 infants has just been completed (Black *et al.*, 1998) revealing 100% efficacy in preventing invasive disease caused by the serotypes contained in the vaccine. While this is very exciting, a number of considerations have to be borne in mind if/when these vaccines come to be used routinely over the coming years.

Many different serotypes can cause disease, and as vaccination has been found to lead to reduction in the nasopharyngeal carriage of vaccine serotypes (Dagan *et al.*, 1996, 1997) the result may be a corresponding increase in carriage of non-vaccine strains (Obaro *et al.*, 1996). This population shift may occur not only as the result of displacement by existing serotypes of pneumococci, but through genetic exchange. This process, in which genes, including those responsible for capsular type, may be transferred from one strain to another, occurs naturally between pneumococci to give rise to novel chimeras (Nesin *et al.*, 1998). There must therefore be a reasonable concern that with time, immune selective pressure may simply result in an increase in disease caused by serotypes not contained in the vaccine. Surveillance on a trans-national scale of pneumococcal serotypes responsible for invasive disease will be very important once the vaccines are routinely introduced. This is a considerable departure from normal Public Health policy which will require international cooperation.

Neisseria meningitidis

Epidemiology

Of the 13 meningococcal serogroups, differentiated by their capsular poly-saccharides, five (A, B, C, W135 and Y) are responsible for nearly all disease, and the focus of attention as potentially vaccine-preventable infections. Three

(A, B and C) cause >90% of cases worldwide (Harrison, 1995; Kaczmarski, 1997). However, the prevalence of individual serogroups causing disease varies significantly from country to country. In the developed world serogroup B and C strains greatly predominate (Ramsay et al., 1998), but the proportion of cases due to each serotype varies in a cyclical manner. In England and Wales serogroups B and C account for more than 95% of cases of invasive infection, but in the period 1984–1994, serogroup C was responsible for anything from 25% to 39% of cases annually. In 1995 there was apparently a large increase in the number of cases (1890 laboratory confirmed cases), 43% more than in 1994 (Kaczmarski, 1997), and serogroup C was responsible for the main increase. This may to some extent be explained by better case ascertainment due to an increase in public awareness of meningococcal disease, and the introduction of sensitive non-culture diagnostic tools. In any event, further rises in notifications of meningococcal disease have been reported year on year since then, reaching a 50-year high of 2659 in 1997 (Communicable Disease Report, 1999). This has coincided with the emergence of a new serogroup C clone, known as ET-37, that has been responsible for multiple small outbreaks, and a similar general trend has been widely reported elsewhere (Sacchi et al., 1992; Harrison, 1995; Jackson et al., 1995; Krizova et al., 1995; Whalen et al., 1995, Fogarty, 1998, Mateo et al., 1998). Although other serogroups are generally much less common as causes of meningococcal disease in the developed world, local variation means that some are becoming sufficiently prominent to cause real concern. Since 1989, the USA has seen a dramatic increase in cases due to serogroup Y. (Morbidity and Mortality Weekly Report, 1996; Racoosin et al., 1998).

In complete contrast to the situation in the developed world, in the 'meningitis belt' of sub-Saharan Africa – a broad band extending from The Gambia in the west into Uganda and Ethiopia in the east – serogroup A strains are the predominant cause of meningococcal disease. Serogroup C is in addition responsible for up to 20% of cases (Greenwood, 1987). Endemic rates of meningococcal disease are typically five to ten times higher than in countries of the developed world (Campagne et al., 1999) but this statistic is often forgotten, dwarfed by the enormous serogroup A epidemics that occur every 8–14 years during the dry season (Greenwood et al., 1979) (Figure 9.4). During an epidemic, up to 1% of the population may fall ill, and more than 200 000 cases and 25 000 deaths have been recorded in a single year (Robbins et al., 1997).

Development of natural immunity

Immunity to meningococcal infection caused by serogroup A and C strains correlates with the presence of bactericidal anti-capsular antibody in the serum (Goldschneider et al., 1969; Artenstein et al., 1971a). The situation with serogroup B disease is more obscure, and the bacterial component(s) that elicit protective immunity are yet to be identified. Natural immunity is thought to develop through intermittent carriage of different strains of pathogenic and non-pathogenic Neisseria such as N. lactamica, and through exposure to other

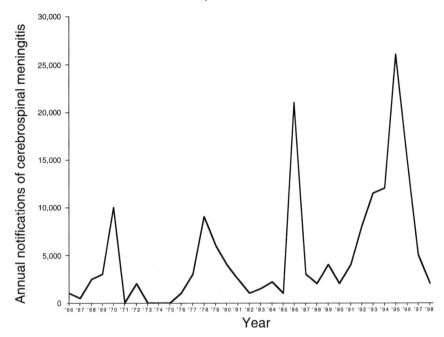

Figure 9.4   Annual notifications of meningitis in Niger, 1966–1998. 8–10 year peaks of serogroup A meningococcal disease dwarf the incidence of meningococcal disease in the developed world (compare Figure 9.1). (World Health Organisation unpublished data.)

organisms bearing cross-reacting surface structures – in the case of serogroup A meningococcus, for example, the capsular polysaccharides of *E. coli* K51 and K93 (Goldschneider *et al.*, 1969; Artenstein *et al.*, 1971b; Robbins *et al.*, 1972; Peller *et al.*, 1973; Gold *et al.*, 1978; Guirguis *et al.*, 1985; Jones *et al.*, 1998).

The population at risk

Most cases of meningococcal disease occur in previously healthy individuals with no apparent risk factors predisposing them to infection. An association has long been recognized between genetically-determined deficiency in components of the terminal attack complex of complement and susceptibility to neisserial infection, but while such defects may greatly increase an individual's risk, they account for only a tiny proportion of the human burden of disease. A search for potentially modifiable factors operating in populations at risk has identified exposure to cigarette smoke as an independent risk factor for infection (Fischer *et al.*, 1997), but while careful avoidance might reduce individual risk, only vaccination can give reliable protection. Vaccines consisting of purified capsular polysaccharide from serogroups A, C, W135 and Y are available and offer useful, although short-lived, protection against infection in older children and adults. Development of protein-polysaccharide vaccines analogous to Hib vaccines, to protect infants against serogroups A and C infection, are well advanced. However, serogroup B meningococcus poses unique problems as its polysaccharide is non-immunogenic, and will be considered separately.

Vaccines to prevent meningococcal serogroups A and C disease

Meningococcal polysaccharide vaccines

Vaccines consisting of purified polysaccharides of serogroups A and C, or serogroups A, C, W135 and Y, have been available for about 25 years. They have been used successfully to control epidemics, particularly in the meningitis belt of sub-Saharan Africa, (Wahdan et al., 1973; 1977; Erwa et al., 1973; Peltola et al., 1977; Ettori et al., 1977; Greenwood and Wali, 1980; Mohammed and Zaruba, 1981; Binkin and Band, 1982; Reingold et al., 1985; Greenwood et al., 1986; Cochi et al., 1987; Moore et al., 1992; Lennon et al., 1992; Pinner et al., 1992; Whitney et al., 1996) and are routinely offered to groups at high risk of disease such as Haj pilgrims and military recruits (Artenstein et al., 1970; Gold and Artenstein, 1972; Stroffolini, 1990; Biselli et al., 1993; Al-Gahtani et al., 1995).

It has been suggested that serogroup A polysaccharide vaccine might offer some short-term protection to infants from about 6 months, which could be useful in an epidemic situation (Gold et al., 1977). There might even be a little protection in these circumstances to be gained from a serogroup C polysaccharide vaccine (Mitchell et al., 1996). However, in general purified meningococcal polysaccharides share with Hib PRP all the limitations as vaccine antigens previously discussed (Gold and Lipow, 1976; Gotschlich et al., 1978). There is the added problem that, as meningococcal disease risk extends far beyond infancy, the limited duration of immunity that they provide means that for continued protection, boosters would probably be needed every 3 years or so. While these vaccines have good (80–100%) short-term efficacy in older children and adults, from about 3 years after vaccination an unacceptable rate of breakthrough infection has been seen, particularly in younger recipients (Taunay et al., 1978; Reingold et al., 1985; Lennon et al., 1992). This is consistent with immunogenicity data which shows an age-related antibody response to vaccination, and age-related persistence of antibody. (Lepow et al., 1977; Gold et al., 1979).

Although they clearly have great value in epidemic control, there have been concerns about repeated vaccination with meningococcal polysaccharides, relating to the possibility that second and subsequent doses may be less and less effective in providing protection (inducing tolerance) (Gold et al., 1977; Leach et al., 1997). For this reason, as well as because of their inadequacy in infants, there is great pressure to develop conjugate vaccines for use at all ages.

Meningococcal serogroup A and C conjugate vaccines

Meningococcal conjugate vaccines using the same technology as the very successful Hib conjugate vaccines are in the final phases of clinical trials prior to licensure (Table 9.1). Carrier proteins used in clinical trials of

Table 9.1   Meningococcal conjugate vaccines currently under development.

Manufacturer	Carrier protein	Polysaccharide component
Chiron	CRM_{197}	C
Lederle	CRM_{197}	C
NAVA	Tetanus toxoid	C
Pasteur Mérieux*	Diphtheria toxoid	A/C

* Development of this vaccine is being discontinued in favour of an A/C/W135/Y quadrivalent conjugate vaccine.

meningococcal conjugate vaccines have included diphtheria toxoid, CRM_{197}, and tetanus toxoid.

Group C conjugate vaccines are expected imminently to be licensed and introduced routinely in the UK (Miller et al., 1998). Development of quadrivalent meningococcal conjugate vaccines containing serogroups A/C/W135/Y for use world-wide are likely to follow shortly. In the run-up to the introduction of group C conjugates, large scale safety trials have been undertaken in the USA, and further safety data will be available from trials in the UK in the near future. In all published studies, the safety profile has been excellent. Local and systemic reactions have been, if anything, less with the conjugate vaccines than with pure polysaccharide (Twumasi et al., 1995; Lieberman et al., 1996; Maclennan et al., 1997). Of course pre-licensure clinical trials cannot exclude rare, serious, side-effects and, as with the Hib and other new vaccines, post-licensure safety data will have to be collected for a very extended period (discussed at http://www.niaid.nih.gov/publications/Vaccine/safervacc. htm).

Meningococcal conjugates appear to be highly immunogenic at all ages (Costantino et al., 1992; Anderson et al., 1994; Twumasi et al., 1995; Fairley et al., 1996; Lieberman et al., 1996; Leach et al., 1997; Maclennan et al., 1997, 1998a; Campagne et al., 1997; Borrow et al., 1998; Choo et al., 1998; MacDonald et al., 1998; Plotkin, 1998; Richmond et al., 1998a, b). Bactericidal antibody titres are significantly higher in groups receiving C conjugate vaccine than polysaccharide vaccine (Lieberman et al., 1996) and, in addition, immunological memory is induced that lasts for at least 5 years after even apparently a single dose of conjugate in infancy (Maclennan et al., 1998a). Induction of memory has however not yet been proven conclusively for meningococcal group A conjugate vaccines (Plotkin, 1998). Notwithstanding concerns expressed about a possible tolerizing effect, prior vaccination with group C meningococcal polysaccharide does not appear to prevent the induction of immunological memory by a subsequent dose of meningococcal conjugate vaccine (Maclennan et al., 1998b).

No meningococcal conjugate vaccine has been evaluated in a large efficacy trial, but it is unlikely that this will be required by licensing authorities in the case of serogroup C vaccines (Carl Frasch, personal communication). Convincing data from efficacy studies of the closely similar Hib and pneumococcal conjugate vaccines make it reasonable to anticipate similar high efficacy for the meningococcal conjugates in preventing cognate infection, although the impact on the total burden of meningococcal disease is impossible to predict. There are no data on the effect of vaccination with meningococcal conjugates on meningococcal carriage. Based on experience using Hib and pneumococcal conjugate vaccines, it is reasonable to expect that the meningococcal vaccines will reduce carriage of the cognate strains and so provide a degree of herd immunity, with an even more significant effect on the incidence of meningococcal disease with vaccine-serogroup strains.

Challenges facing meningococcal polysaccharide conjugate vaccines

The immediate challenge is the large-scale pharmaceutical production and successful widespread introduction of these vaccines, especially of serogroup A vaccines that have the potential to make such a difference in the developing world. While there are technological challenges to be met – the serogroup A conjugates appear to be less stable than others – the real challenge will be to overcome financial obstacles to allow the vaccines to be used widely where they are most urgently needed. This is currently being addressed by a World Health Organization working group.

A second challenge is the need for meningococcal vaccines, in contrast to Hib vaccines, to provide extended protection against disease which may strike in an unvaccinated population over an extended age range. While almost all Hib disease occurs in children less than 5 years of age, high rates of meningococcal disease continue for at least a further 15 years. Different patterns are also seen in nasopharyngeal carriage of these organisms. Carriage of Hib is highest in children 3–4 years of age (Coen *et al.*, 1998), while meningococcal carriage is highest in teenagers and young adults (Caugant *et al.*, 1994). It remains to be seen whether vaccination in infancy alone will provide protection for this period of time. The question of whether booster vaccinations are required and the timing of such boosters can only be answered by extended careful surveillance.

A third challenge is to avoid displacement of the meningococcal disease problem into non-vaccine serogroups. As with pneumococcus but in contrast to the situation with Hib, more than one serogroup regularly causes clinical disease. Could the clinical problem shift on introduction of a C-conjugate vaccine, more to B, or to Y, W135 or even A? Currently we see little serogroup Y disease in the UK, but neither did the USA before 1989, and their disease rate due to this serogroup is now over 30% even without selective pressure from vaccination (Morbidity and Mortality Weekly Report, 1996). An Italian study of meningococcal nasopharyngeal colonization of army recruits gives pause for thought. Before meningococcal (A + C) polysaccharide vaccination, the meningococcal carriage rate was 32% with 9% serogroup C and 17% serogroup Y. Three weeks later overall carriage had risen to 52%, with no serogroup C or A but 40% serogroup Y (Stroffolini *et al.*, 1996). In Saudi Arabia, where widespread vaccination in the region around Mecca with A/C polysaccharide has been undertaken for the last 15 years, about 25% of disease is now reported to be from serogroup W135 (WHO, 1998). So there is legitimate concern that selective pressure from serogroup C conjugate vaccination alone could alter meningococcal disease patterns rather than simply reduce the numbers of infections. While one mechanism by which this shift in the pattern of meningococcal disease might be brought about is opportunistic filling by existing strains of the colonizing niche vacated by serogroup C, as with pneumococcus, another is through genetic exchange. This occurs readily *in vitro* between meningococci, and allelic exchange of the polysialyltransferase gene has been demonstrated to have been responsible for capsular switching from B to C during a mixed outbreak of serogroups B and C strains in Oregon, USA (Swartley *et al.*, 1997). Do current widely prevalent serogroup C strains have attributes which, if transferred to a different serogroup, might cause a major problem? This has already been raised as a concern in Canada where mass vaccination with serogroup C polysaccharide during an outbreak was followed by a number of cases of group B disease with the same distinctive subtype (Kertesz *et al.*, 1998). There is currently no answer to this question since we do not know what the critical determinants of meningococcal virulence are, and this is an important area for research.

Vaccines to prevent serogroup B meningococcal disease

In contrast to the polysaccharides contained in the quadrivalent meningococcal vaccine, native group B meningococcal polysaccharide (GBMP) – a long-chain homopolymer of alpha-2,8-linked N-acetylneuraminic acid (polysialic acid) – is very poorly immunogenic in humans (Wyle *et al.*, 1972; Mandrell and Zollinger, 1982). This is probably because it is recognized as a self-antigen through the presence of polysialic acid in various mammalian tissues, in particular as a constituent of neural cell adhesion molecule (N-CAM). This membrane glycoprotein is highly sialylated in the embryonic and neonatal human brain (Finne *et al.*, 1983; Troy, 1992) and although the polysialic acid chain length decreases after birth, the longer, embryonic, form has been detected in some adult tissues such as NK cells, regenerating muscle and some tumour cell types. In this form it can bind anti-GBMP antibodies, which has caused considerable concern over the theoretical possibility that, were immune tolerance to be circumvented, autoreactive antibodies might be elicited with the potential to damage the host. Rejection of GBMP as a vaccine candidate, however, poses very substantial problems. Various subcapsular surface structures, such as outer membrane proteins or lipopolysaccharide, are immunogenic and elicit protective antibody (reflected in serum bactericidal activity (SBA) and/or enhanced opsonophagocytosis after experimental vaccination or natural infection) (Lehmann *et al.*, 1999), but they frequently show a high degree of antigenic variation. The major porin protein PorA (also referred to as P1, the serosubtyping antigen) is a case in point. This meningococcal surface protein elicits bactericidal antibody of high-affinity through the immunodominance of two prominent surface-exposed peptide loops, but the protein sequence in these domains is hypervariable. There are hundreds of serosubtypes, differing at the genetic level by insertions, deletions or single base changes of DNA in the segments of the gene corresponding to these antibody binding domains. Many serogroup B strains of different P1-serosubtypes circulate simultaneously in the population, and over time the spectrum of serosubtypes changes. As antibody that kills one P1-serosubtype may fail altogether to kill another (McGuinness et al., 1991), a vaccine based on a currently prevalent PorA protein can only be anticipated to have a limited efficacy reflected both in the proportion of infections it can be expected to prevent and the time over which it will be useful.

Possible ways out of this dilemma are to identify an invariant meningococcal antigen that is capable of eliciting protective immunity, or to formulate a multivalent vaccine based on variant antigens that can cover a range of prevalent strains. Both approaches are being energetically followed, but an effective vaccine to protect against serogroup B meningococcal disease remains frustratingly elusive.

Several investigators have argued that as GBMP is a critical determinant of meningococcal virulence, and as invariant subcapsular meningococcal antigens have proved so hard to identify, the best approach may be to develop a vaccine based on the polysaccharide despite the theoretical concerns this approach raises. Chemical modification of a high molecular weight fraction of polysialic acid, replacing the N-acetyl with N-propionyl groups, and conjugation to tetanus toxoid, has produced a vaccine antigen that apparently mimics a unique bactericidal capsular epitope and elicits monoclonal antibodies that can passively protect mice infected experimentally with serogroup B meningococci (Pon et al., 1997). Jennings and colleagues (1989) have hypothesized that this protective epitope is a complex conformational one, formed on the meningococcal surface by interaction of native GBMP with some other bacterial molecule and by inference not present in human tissues. They speculate that this has successfully been mimicked by their vaccine antigen through conformational changes wrought by chemical modification. It remains essential to establish beyond doubt that the vaccine cannot elicit auto-antibodies in humans. The vaccine is approaching clinical trials.

Several non-capsular meningococcal antigens are under evaluation for their ability to evoke protective immunity. Brodeur and colleagues have identified a low molecular weight outer membrane protein NspA of unknown function, apparently invariant and conserved over an extensive range of meningococcal strains, which elicits mouse-protective monoclonal antibodies (Martin et al., 1997). Natural human antibody to this protein is detectable after infection, though at low levels (Farrant et al., 1998). Clinical trials of an NspA vaccine are anticipated shortly. The transferrin binding proteins TbpA and TbpB are outer membrane proteins expressed by meningococci under conditions of iron limitation, as occur during natural infection. They are variable between strains, though much less so than PorA, and elicit protective antibody against the homologous meningococcal strain when injected into rodents (Danve et al., 1993). A mixture of different TbpBs has been proposed for a human vaccine (Lissolo et al., 1995) and is undergoing clinical trials, although recent immunogenicity data have been rather disappointing (Danve et al., 1998).

A radically different approach has been pioneered by scientists at the Norwegian National Institute of Public Health (NIPH) and at the Finlay

Institute, Havana, Cuba (FI) in response to increasing rates of serogroup B disease in their respective countries in the 1970s. Meningococci shed blebs of outer membrane during growth, and these blebs, outer membrane vesicles (OMVs), can be harvested and formulated as a vaccine. OMVs contain PorA in its native conformation – felt to be a major component of their antigenicity – but similarly all other outer membrane antigens, each speculatively best placed to elicit a natural protective immune response. OMV vaccine prepared from the Norwegian epidemic strain showed 57% efficacy in a randomized trial in Norwegian school-children (Bjune et al., 1991) and this rather disappointing result, coupled with a decline in disease rate, led to the decision to develop the vaccine further rather than press forward with full-scale implementation. OMV vaccine prepared from the (different) Cuban epidemic strain had 80% protective efficacy in adolescents (Sierra et al., 1991; Peltola, 1998) and was introduced into the Cuban national vaccination programme. It is the only serogroup B meningococcal vaccine in current routine use anywhere in the world. These two vaccines and analogues prepared from strains of different P1 serosubtypes have subsequently been submitted to very extensive clinical trials. In response to meningococcal outbreaks in various South American countries, more than 40 million doses of the FI vaccine have been given, with a broadly consistent pattern of responsiveness observed in each case. Judging by the rate of cases reported in vaccinees compared to non-vaccinees, the vaccine appeared more effective in older children than in those under 4 years old, in whom unfortunately the burden of disease is greatest but in whom at best only a low level of protection was seen (de Moraes et al., 1992; Boslego et al., 1995). However, the difficult circumstances in which these enormous efficacy trials had to be carried out has not entirely resolved the question of whether the vaccine is of population-wide value. For example, the disappointing apparent lack of efficacy in infants could conceivably still reflect a positive effect of the vaccine. It might for example be that vaccine converted a proportion of fulminant cases of meningococcal septicaemia – so rapidly fatal that they never reached medical attention – to less severe cases which were recognized and reported. A prospective randomised double-blind controlled trial comparing immunogenicity of FI and NIPH vaccines based on different group B meningococcal serosubtypes has recently been reported from Santiago, Chile (Tappero et al., 1999) with interesting results. On the basis of changes in SBA titres, neither vaccine conferred reliable cross-protection at all ages against either the other vaccine strain or the then current Chilean epidemic strain, although there was more cross-protection in older recipients. With other evidence, this emphasizes the importance of PorA as an important component of the vaccine. However, after three doses there was a substantial increase in SBA against the homologous vaccine strain, regardless of the age of the vaccinee. Infants under 1 year old showed a comparable response rate to adults, 67% in each group developing a post-third dose SBA $>1:8$ compared to a pre-trial $<1:2$. This very encouraging result suggests that a three-dose schedule of OMV vaccine prepared from an epidemic strain can usefully protect even very young infants against infection.

The appreciation that PorA makes a major contribution to immunogenicity of OMV vaccines has led to the development of second-generation OMV vaccines, prepared from genetically modified meningococci carrying multiple *porA* genes. A hexavalent vaccine containing P1 serosubtype antigens found in the majority of case isolates in many countries has been developed (Peeters *et al.*, 1996; Van d *et al.*, 1996) and is being evaluated in clinical trials in UK infants (Cartwright *et al.*, 1999). At this stage these vaccines hold out the greatest promise for the prevention of serogroup B meningococcal disease.

Conclusion

This is a time of rapid development in the implementation of vaccines to prevent meningitis. Vaccines against Hib infection have been a remarkable success. Pneumococcal conjugate vaccines have already been demonstrated to be effective against invasive disease in clinical trials, and a cocktail of conjugates that will cover the main pneumococcal meningitis isolates should not be far off. It is reasonable to expect meningococcal conjugate vaccines imminently to be introduced that will be highly successful in preventing disease caused by serogroups A and C. Group B meningococcal disease remains the greatest challenge and it could well be 5–10 years before an effective vaccine has been identified and carried through all the hurdles to licensure. Nevertheless, the virtual eradication of bacterial meningitis is no longer an idle dream – major progress should be seen over the next decade.

References

Al-Gahtani, Y. M., El Bushra, H. E., Al-Qarawi, S. M. *et al.* (1995). Epidemiological investigation of an outbreak of meningococcal meningitis in Makkah (Mecca), Saudi Arabia,1992. *Epidemiol. Infect.*, **115**, 399–409.

Almuneef, M., Memish, Z., Khan, Y., Kagallwala, A. and Alshaalan, M. (1998). Childhood bacterial meningitis in Saudi Arabia. *J. Infect.*, **36**, 157–160.

Anderson, E. L., Bowers, T., Mink, C. M. *et al.* (1994). Safety and immunogenicity of meningococcal A and C polysaccharide conjugate vaccine in adults. *Infect. Immun.*, **62**, 3391–3395.

Anderson, E. L., Decker, M. D., Englund, J. A. *et al.* (1995). Interchangeability of conjugated *Haemophilus influenzae* type b vaccines in infants. *J. Am. Med. Assoc.*, **273**, 849–853.

Artenstein, M. S., Gold, R., Zimmerly, J. G., Wyle, F. A., Schneider, H. and Harkins, C. (1970). Prevention of meningococcal disease by group C polysaccharide vaccine. *N. Engl. J. Med.*, **282**, 417–420.

Artenstein, M. S., Brandt, B. L., Tramont, E. C., Branche, W. C. JR, Fleet, H. D. and Cohen, R. L. (1971a). Serologic studies of meningococcal infection and polysaccharide vaccination. *J. Infect. Dis.*, **124**, 277–288.

Artenstein, M. S., Schneider, H. and Tingley, M. D. (1971b). Meningococcal infections. 1. Prevalence of serogroups causing disease in US Army personnel in 1964–70. *Bull. World Hlth Org.*, **45**, 275–278.

Barbour, M. L., Mayon, W. R., Coles C, Crook, D. W. and Moxon, E. R. (1995). The impact of conjugate vaccine on carriage of *Haemophilus influenzae* type b. *J. Infect. Dis.*, **71**, 93–98.

Bell, F., Heath, P., Shackley, F. *et al.* (1998). Effect of combination with an acellular pertussis, diphtheria, tetanus vaccine on antibody response to Hib vaccine (PRP-T). *Vaccine*, **16**, 637–642.

Binkin, N. and Band, J. (1982). Epidemic of meningococcal meningitis in Bamako, Mali: epidemiological features and analysis of vaccine efficacy. *Lancet*, **2**, 315–318.

Biselli, R., Fattorossi, A., Matricardi, P. M., Nisini, R., Stroffolini, T. and D'Amelio, R. (1998). Dramatic reduction of meningococcal meningitis among military recruits in Italy after introduction of specific vaccination. *Vaccine*, **11**, 578–581.

Bjune, G., Hoiby, E. A., Gronnesby, J. K. *et al.* (1991). Effect of outer membrane vesicle vaccine against group B meningococcal disease in Norway. *Lancet*, **338**, 1093–1096.

Black, S., Shinefield, H., Ray, P. *et al.* (1998). Efficacy of heptavalent conjugate pneumococcal vaccine (Wyeth Lederle) in 37 000 infants and children: results of the Northern California Kaiser Permanente Trial. (Abstract). *Pneumococcal Vaccines for the World 1998 Conference*, Washington, DC, 18.

Borrow, R., Richmond, P., Fox, A. J. *et al.* (1998). Induction of immunological memory in UK infants by a meningococcal A/C conjugate vaccine. *Abstracts of the 11th International Pathogenic Neisseria Conference*, Nice 1998, 157.

Boslego, J., Garcia, J., Cruz, C. *et al.* (1995). Efficacy, safety, and immunogenicity of a meningococcal group B (15:P1.3) outer membrane protein vaccine in Iquique, Chile. Chilean National Committee for Meningococcal Disease. *Vaccine*, **13**, 821–829.

Booy, R., Hodgson, S. A., Slack, M. P., Anderson, E. C., Mayon, W. R. and Moxon E. R. (1993). Invasive *Haemophilus influenzae* type b disease in the Oxford region (1985–91). *Arch Dis. Child*, **69**, 225–228.

Booy, R., Heath, P. T., Slack, M. P., Begg, N. and Moxon, E. R. (1997). Vaccine failures after primary immunisation with *Haemophilus influenzae* type-b conjugate vaccine without booster (published erratum appears in *Lancet* 1997, **349**, 1630). *Lancet*, **349**, 1197–1202.

Bradshaw, M. W., Schneerson, R., Parke, J. C. J. and Robbins, J. B. (1971). Bacterial antigens cross-reactive with the capsular polysaccharide of *Haemophilus influenzae* type b. *Lancet*, **1**, 1095–1096.

Broome, C. V. (1987). Epidemiology of *Haemophilus influenzae* type b infections in the United States. *Pediatr. Infect. Dis. J.*, **6**, 779–782.

Campagne, G., Garber, A. and Fabre, P. (1997). Safety and immunogenicity of three doses of a N. *meningiitidis* A/C diphtheria conjugate vaccine in infants in Niger (Abstract G-1). *Abstracts of the 37th Interscience Conference on Antimicrobial Agents and Chemotherapy*, Toronto, Canada 1997, 192.

Campagne, G., Schuchat, A., Djibo, S., Ousseini, A., Cisse, L. and Chippaux, J. P. (1999). Epidemiology of bacterial meningitis in Niamay, Niger, 1981–1996. *Bull. World Hlth Org.*, **77**, 499–508.

Cartwright, K., Morris, R., Rumke, H. C. *et al.* (1999). Immunogenicity and reactogenicity in UK infants of a novel meningococcal vesicle vaccine containing multiple class 1 (PorA) outer membrane proteins. *Vaccine*, **17**, 2612–2619.

Caugant, D. A., Hoiby, E. A., Magnus, P. *et al.* (1994). Asymptomatic carriage of *Neisseria meningitidis* in a randomly sampled population. *J. Clin. Microbiol.*, **32**, 323–330.

Choo, S., Everard, J., Goilav, C., Hatzmann, E., Zuckerman, J. and Finn, A. (1998). Immunogenicity and reactogenicity of a serogroup C meningococcal conjugate vaccine compared with a serogroup A & C meningococcal polysaccharide vaccine in adolescents. *Abstracts of the 11th International Pathogenic Neisseria Conference*, Nice 1998, 164.

Cochi, S. L., Markowitz, L. E., Joshi, D. D. *et al.* (1987). Control of epidemic group A meningococcal meningitis in Nepal. *Int. J. Epidemiol.*, **16**, 91–97.

Coen, P. G., Heath, P. T., Barbour, M. L. and Garnett, G. P. (1998). Mathematical models of *Haemophilus influenzae* type b. *Epidemiol. Infect.*, **120**, 281–295.

Communicable Disease Report (1999). Infectious disease in England and Wales: October to December 1998. *Commun. Dis. Rep. CDR.* Suppl. **9**, S5.

Corn, P. G., Anders, J., Takala, A. K., Kayhty, H. and Hoiseth, S. K. (1993). Genes involved in *Haemophilus influenzae* type b capsule expression are frequently amplified. *J. Infect. Dis.*, **167**, 356–364.

Costantino, P., Viti, S., Podda, A., Velmonte, M. A., Nencioni, L. and Rappuoli, R. (1992). Development and phase 1 clinical testing of a conjugate vaccine against meningococcus A and C. *Vaccine*, **10**, 691–698.

Dagan, R., Melamed, R., Muallem, M. *et al.* (1996). Reduction of nasopharyngeal carriage of pneumococci during the second year of life by a heptavalent conjugate pneumococcal vaccine. *J. Infect. Dis.*, **174**, 1271–1278.

Dagan, R., Muallem, M., Melamed, R., Leroy, O. and Yagupsky, P. (1997). Reduction of pneumococcal nasopharyngeal carriage in early infancy after immunization with tetravalent pneumococcal vaccines conjugated to either tetanus toxoid or diphtheria toxoid. *Pediatr. Infect. Dis. J.*, **16**, 1060–1064.

Danve, B., Lissolo, L., Mignon, M. *et al.* (1993). Transferrin-binding proteins isolated from *Neisseria meningitidis* elicit protective and bactericidal antibodies in laboratory animals. *Vaccine*, **11**, 1214–1220.

Danve, B., Lissolo, L., Guinet, F. *et al.* (1998). Safety and immunogenicity of a *Neisseria meningitidis* group B transferrin binding protein vaccine in adults. *Abstracts of the 11th International Pathogenic Neisseria Conference*, Nice 1998, 53.

de-Moraes, J. C., Perkins, B. A., Camargo, M. C. *et al.* (1992). Protective efficacy of a serogroup B meningococcal vaccine in Sao Paulo, Brazil (published erratum appears in *Lancet*, 1992 **340**, 1554). *Lancet*, **340**, 1074–1078.

Erwa, H. H., Haseeb, M. A., Idris, A. A., Lapeyssonnie, L., Sanborn, W. R. and Sippel, J. E. (1973). A serogroup A meningococcal polysaccharide vaccine: studies in the Sudan to combat cerebrospinal meningitis caused by *Neisseria meningitidis* group A. *Bull.World Hlth Org.*, 49, 301–305.

Eskola, J., Olander, R. M., Hovi, T., Litmanen, L., Peltola, S. and Kayhty, H. (1996). Randomised trial of the effect of co-administration with acellular pertussis DTP vaccine on immunogenicity of *Haemophilus influenzae* type b conjugate vaccine. *Lancet*, 348, 1688–1692.

Ettori, D., Saliou, P., Renaudet, J. and Stoeckel, P. (1977). Le vaccin antimeningococcique polysaccharidique du type A:premiers essais controles en Afriques de l'ouest. *Med. Trop.*, 37, 225–230.

Fairley, C. K., Begg, N., Borrow, R., Fox, A. J., Jones, D. M. and Cartwright, K. (1996). Conjugate meningococcal serogroup A and C vaccine: reactogenicity and immunogenicity in United Kingdom infants. *J. Infect. Dis.*, 174, 1360–1363.

Farrant, J. L., Kroll, J. S., Brodeur, B. R. and Martin, D. (1998). Detection of anti-NspA antibodies in sera from patients convalescent after meningococcal infection. *Abstracts of the 11th International Pathogenic Neisseria Conference*, Nice 1998, 208.

Finne, J., Leinonen, M. and Makela, P. H. (1983). Antigenic similarities between brain components and bacteria causing meningitis. Implications for vaccine development and pathogenesis. *Lancet*, 2, 355–357.

Fischer, M., Hedberg, K., Cardosi, P. *et al.* (1997). Tobacco smoke as a risk factor for meningococcal disease. *Pediatr. Infect. Dis. J.*, 16, 979–983.

Fogarty, J. (1998). Trends in serogroup C meningococcal disease in the Republic of Ireland. *Eurosurveillance*, 2, 75–76.

Galil, K., Singleton, R., Levine, O. S. *et al.* (1999). Reemergence of invasive *Haemophilus influenzae* type b disease in a well-vaccinated population in remote Alaska. *J. Infect. Dis.*, 179, 101–106.

Gold, R. and Artenstein, M. S. (1971). Meningococcal infections. 2. Field trial of group C meningococcal polysaccharide vaccine in 1969–70. *Bull. World Hlth Org.*, 45, 279–282.

Gold, R. and Lepow, M. L. (1976). Present status of polysaccharide vaccines in the prevention of meningococcal disease. *Adv. Pediatr.*, 23, 71–93.

Gold, R., Lepow, M. L., Goldschneider, I. and Gotschlich, E. C. (1977). Immune response of human infants to polysaccharide vaccines of group A and C *Neisseria meningitidis*. *J. Infect. Dis.*, 136 (suppl), S31–S35.

Gold, R., Goldschneider, I., Lepow, M. L., Draper, T. F. and Randolph, M. (1978). Carriage of *Neisseria meningitidis* and *Neisseria lactamica* in infants and children. *J. Infect. Dis.*, 137, 112–121.

Gold, R., Lepow, M. L., Goldschneider, I., Draper, T. F. and Gotschlich, E. C. (1979). Kinetics of antibody production to group A and group C meningococcal polysaccharide vaccines administered during the first six years of life: prospects for routine immunization of infants and children. *J. Infect. Dis.*, 140, 690–697.

Goldblatt, D., Miller, E., McCloskey, N. and Cartwright, K. (1998a). Immunological response to conjugate vaccines in infants: follow up study. **316**, 1570–1571.

Goldblatt, D., Vaz, A. R. and Miller, E. (1998b). Antibody avidity as a surrogate marker of successful priming by *Haemophilus influenzae* type b conjugate vaccines following infant immunization. *J. Infect. Dis.*, **177**, 1112–1115.

Goldschneider, I., Gotschlich, E. C. and Artenstein, M. S. (1969). Human immunity to the meningococcus. II. Development of natural immunity. *J. Exp. Med.*, **129**, 1327–1348.

Gotschlich, E. C., Austrian, R., Cvjetanovic, B. and Robbins, J. B. (1978). Prospects for the prevention of bacterial meningitis with polysaccharide vaccines. *Bull. World Hlth Org.*, **56**, 509–518.

Granoff, D. M., Holmes, S. J., Osterholm, M. T. *et al.* (1993). Induction of immunologic memory in infants primed with *Haemophilus influenzae* type b conjugate vaccines. *J. Infect. Dis.*, **168**, 663–671.

Gratten, M., Torzillo, P., Morey, F. *et al.* (1996). Distribution of capsular types and antibiotic susceptibility of invasive *Streptococcus pneumoniae* isolated from aborigines in central Australia. *J. Clin. Microbiol.*, **34**, 338–341.

Gray, B. M., Converse, G. M. and Dillon-H. C. J. (1980). Epidemiologic studies of *Streptococcus pneumoniae* in infants: acquisition, carriage, and infection during the first 24 months of life. *J. Infect. Dis.*, **142**, 923–33.

Greenwood, B. M. (1987). The epidemiology of acute bacterial meningitis in tropical Africa. In: *Bacterial Meningitis*. London: Academic Press, pp. 61–84.

Greenwood, B. M. and Wali, S. S. (1980). Control of meningococcal infection in the African meningitis belt by selective vaccination. *Lancet*, **1**, 729–732.

Greenwood, B. M., Bradley, A. K., Cleland, P. G. *et al.* (1979). An epidemic of meningococcal infection at Zaria, Northern Nigeria. 1. General epidemiological features. *Trans. R. Soc. Trop. Med. Hyg.*, **73**, 557–562.

Greenwood, B. M., Smith, A. W., Hassan King, M. *et al.* (1986). The efficacy of meningococcal polysaccharide vaccine in preventing group A meningococcal disease in The Gambia, West Africa. *Trans. R. Soc. Trop. Med. Hyg.*, **80**, 1006–1007.

Guirguis, N., Schneerson, R., Bax, A. *et al.*, (1985). *Escherichia coli* K51 and K93 capsular polysaccharides are crossreactive with the group A capsular polysaccharide of *Neisseria meningitidis*. Immunochemical, biological, and epidemiological studies. *J. Exp. Med.*, **162**, 1837–1851.

Hammerschmidt, S., Hilse, R., van-Putten, J. P., Gerardy, S. R., Unkmeir, A. and Frosch, M. (1996a). Modulation of cell surface sialic acid expression in *Neisseria meningitidis* via a transposable genetic element. *EMBO J.*, **15**, 192–198.

Hammerschmidt, S., Muller, A., Sillmann, H. *et al.* (1996b). Capsule phase variation in *Neisseria meningitidis* serogroup B by slipped-strand mispairing in the polysialyltransferase gene (siaD): correlation with bacterial invasion and the outbreak of meningococcal disease. *Mol. Microbiol.*, **20**, 6, 1211–1220.

Handzel, Z. T., Argaman, M., Parke,-J. C. J., Schneerson, R. and Robbins, J. B. (1975). Heteroimmunization to the capsular polysaccharide of *Haemophilus influenzae* type b induced by enteric cross-reacting bacteria. *Infect. Immun.*, **11**, 1045–1052.

Hanna, J. N. and Wild, B. E. (1991). Bacterial meningitis in children under five years of age in Western Australia. *Med. J. Aust.*, **155**, 160–164.

Harrison, L. H. (1995). The worldwide prevention of meningococcal infection. Still an elusive goal. *J. Am. Med. Assoc.*, **273**, 419–421.

Heath, P. T. (1998). *Haemophilus influenzae* type b conjugate vaccines: a review of efficacy data. *Pediatr. Infect. Dis. J.*, **17**, S117–S122.

Hoiseth, S. K., Moxon, F. R. and Silver, R. P. (1986). Genes involved in *Haemophilus influenzae* type b capsule expression are part of an 18-kilobase tandem duplication. *Proc. Natl Acad. Sci. USA*, **83**, 1106–1110.

Jackson, L. A., Schuchat, A., Reeves, M. W. and Wenger, J. D. (1995). Serogroup C meningococcal outbreaks in the United States. An emerging threat. *J. Am. Med. Assoc.*, **273**, 383–389.

Jennings, H. J., Gamian, A., Michon, F. and Ashton, F. E. (1989). Unique intermolecular bactericidal epitope involving the homosialopolysaccharide capsule on the cell surface of group B *Neisseria meningitidis* and *Escherichia coli* K1. *J. Immunol.*, **142**, 3585–3591.

Jones, G. R., Christodoulides, M., Brooks, J. L., Miller, A. R., Cartwright, K. A. and Heckels, J. E. (1998). Dynamics of carriage of *Neisseria meningitidis* in a group of military recruits: subtype stability and specificity of the immune response following colonization. *J. Infect. Dis.*, **178**, 451–459.

Jorgenson, J. H., Howell, A. W., Maher, L. A. and Facklam, R. R. (1991). Serotypes of respiratory isolates of *Streptococcus pneumoniae* compared with the capsular types included in the current pneumococcal vaccine. *J. Infect. Dis.*, **163**, 644–646.

Kaczmarski, E. B. (1997). Meningococcal disease in England and Wales: 1995. *Commun. Dis. Rep. CDR Rev.*, **7**, R55–59.

Karvonen, M., Cepaitis, Z. and Tuomilehto, J. (1999). Association between type 1 diabetes and *Haemophilus influenzae* type b vaccination: birth cohort study. *Br. Med. J.*, **318**, 1169–1172.

Kertesz, D. A., Coulthart, M. B., Ryan, J. A., Johnson, W. M. and Ashton, F. E. (1998). Serogroup B, electrophoretic type 15 *Neisseria meningitidis* in Canada. *J. Infect. Dis.*, **177**, 1754–1757.

Krizova, P., Vlckova, J. and Bobak, M. (1995). [Evaluation of the effectiveness of targeted vaccination with the meningococcal polysaccharide A and C vaccine in one location in the Czech Republic]. *Epidemiol. Mikrobiol. Imunol.*, **44**, 9–14.

Kroll, J. S., Hopkins, I. and Moxon, E. R. (1988). Capsule loss in *H. influenzae* type b occurs by recombination-mediated disruption of a gene essential for polysaccharide export. *Cell*, **53**, 347–356.

Kroll, J. S., Zamze, S., Loynds, B. and Moxon, E. R. (1989). Common organization of chromosomal loci for production of different capsular polysaccharides in *Haemophilus influenzae. J. Bacteriol.*, **171**, 3343–3347.

Kroll, J. S., Loynds, B. M. and Moxon, E. R. (1991). The *Haemophilus influenzae* capsulation gene cluster: a compound transposon. *Mol.Microbiol.*, **5**, 1549–1560.

Kroll, J. S., Moxon, E. R. and Loynds, B. M. (1993). An ancestral mutation enhancing the fitness and increasing the virulence of *Haemophilus influenzae* type b. *J. Infect. Dis.*, **168**, 172–176.

Kroll, J. S., Moxon, E. R. and Loynds, B. M. (1994). Natural genetic transfer of a putative virulence-enhancing mutation to *Haemophilus influenzae* type a. *J. Infect. Dis.*, **169**, 676–679.

Lagos, R., Valenzuela, M. T., Levine, O. S. *et al.*, (1998). Economisation of vaccination against *Haemophilus influenzae* type b: a randomised trial of immunogenicity of fractional-dose and two-dose regimens. *Lancet*, **351**, 1472–1476.

Laurichesse, H., Grimaud, O., Waight, P., Johnson, A. P., George, R. C. and Miller, E. (1998). Pneumococcal bacteraemia and meningitis in England and Wales, 1993 to 1995. *Commun. Dis. Public Hlth*, **1**, 22–27.

Leach, A., Twumasi, P. A., Kumah, S. *et al.* (1997). Induction of immunologic memory in Gambian children by vaccination in infancy with a group A plus group C meningococcal polysaccharide-protein conjugate vaccine. *J. Infect. Dis.*, **175**, 200–204.

Lehmann, A. K., Halstensen, A., Aaberge, I. S. *et al.* (1999). Human opsonins induced during meningococcal disease recognize outer membrane proteins PorA and PorB. *Infect. Immun.*, **67**, 2552–2560.

Lennon, D., Gellin, B., Hood, D., Voss, L., Heffernan, H. and Thakur, S. (1992). Successful intervention in a group A meningococcal outbreak in Auckland, New Zealand. *Pediatr. Infect. Dis. J.*, **11**, 617–623.

Lepow, M. L., Goldschneider, I., Gold, R., Randolph, M. and Gotschlich, E. C. (1977). Persistence of antibody following immunization of children with groups A and C meningococcal polysaccharide vaccines. *Pediatrics*, **60**, 673–680.

Levine, O. S., Ortiz, E., Contreras, R. *et al.* (1993). Cost-benefit analysis for the use of *Haemophilus influenzae* type b conjugate vaccine in Santiago, Chile. *Am. J. Epidemiol.*, **137**, 1221–1228.

Levine, O. S., Farley, M., Harrison, L. H., Lefkowitz, L., McGeer, A. and Schwartz, B. (1999). Risk factors for invasive pneumococcal disease in children: a population-based case-control study in North America. *Pediatrics*, **103**, E28.

Lieberman, J. M., Chiu, S. S., Wong, V. K. *et al.* (1996). Safety and immunogenicity of a serogroups A/C *Neisseria meningitidis* oligosaccharide-protein conjugate vaccine in young children. A randomized controlled trial. *J. Am. Med. Assoc.*, **275**, 1499–1503.

Lissolo, L., Maitre, W. G., Dumas, P., Mignon, M., Danve, B. and Quentin, M. M. (1995). Evaluation of transferrin-binding protein 2 within the transferrin-binding protein complex as a potential antigen for future meningococcal vaccines. *Infect. Immun.*, **63**, 884–890.

Losonsky, G. A., Santosham, M., Sehgal, V. M., Zwahlen, A. and Moxon, E. R. (1984). *Haemophilus influenzae* disease in the White Mountain Apaches: molecular epidemiology of a high risk population. *Pediatr. Infect. Dis.*, **3**, 539–547.

MacDonald, N. E., Halperin, S., Law, B., Forrest, B. D., Danzig, L. E. and Granoff, D. M. (1998). Induction of imunologic memory by conjugated vs plain meningococcal C polysaccharide vaccine in toddlers: a randomized controlled trial. *J. Am. Med. Assoc.*, **280**, 1685–1689.

McGuinness, B. T., Clarke, I. N., Lambden, P. R. *et al.* (1991). Point mutation in meningococcal por A gene associated with increased endemic disease. *Lancet*, **337**, 514–517.

Maclennan, J. M., Shackley, F. and Heath, P. T. (1997). Induction of immunological memory by a *Neisseria meningitidis* group C conjugate vaccine (Abstract O19). *Abstracts of the 15th Annual Meeting of the European Society of Paediatric Infectious Diseases*, Paris, France 1997, 10.

Maclennan, J. M., Deeks, J. J., Obaro, S. *et al.* (1998a). Meningococcal serogroup C conjugate vaccination in infancy induces persistent immunological memory. *Abstracts of the 11th International Pathogenic Neisseria Conference*, Nice 1998, 151.

Maclennan, J. M., Deeks, J. J., Obaro, S. *et al.* (1998b). Reduced response to revaccination with meningococcal A/C polysaccharide. *Abstracts of the 16th Annual Meeting of the European Society for Paediatric Infectious Diseases*, Bled 1998, 36.

Makela, P. H. (1984). Capsular polysaccharide vaccines today. *Infection*, **12** (suppl. 1), 7.

Makela, P. H., Peltola, H., Kayhty, H. *et al.* (1977). Polysaccharide vaccines of group A *Neisseria meningitidis* and *Haemophilus influenzae* type b: a field trial in Finland. *J. Infect. Dis.*, **136** (suppl.), S43–50.

Mandrell, R. E. and Zollinger, W. D. (1982). Measurement of antibodies to meningococcal group B polysaccharide: low avidity binding and equilibrium binding constants. *J. Immunol.*, **129**, 2172–2178.

Martin, D., Cadieux, N., Hamel, J. and Brodeur, B. R. (1997). Highly conserved *Neisseria meningitidis* surface protein confers protection against experimental infection. *J. Exp. Med.*, **185**, 1173–1183.

Mateo, S., Cano, R. and Garcia, C. (1998). Changing epidemiology of meningococcal disease in Spain, 1989–1997. *Eurosurveillance*, **2**, 71–74.

Miller, M. A. (1998). An assessment of the value of *Haemophilus influenzae* type b conjugate vaccine in Asia. *Pediatr. Infect. Dis. J.*, **17**, (suppl.), S152–S159.

Miller, E., Richmond, P., Borrow, R. *et al.* (1998). UK strategy for introduction of meningococcal C conjugate vaccines. (Abstract) *Abstracts of the 11th International Pathogenic Neisseria Conference*, Nice 1998, 57.

Mitchell, L. A., Ochnio, J. J., Glover, C., Lee, A. Y., Ho, M. K. and Bell, A. (1996). Analysis of meningococcal serogroup C-specific antibody levels in British Columbian children and adolescents. *J. Infect. Dis.*, **173**, 1009–1013.

Mohammed, I. and Zaruba, K. (1981). Control of epidemic meningococcal meningitis by mass vaccination. *Lancet*, **2**, 80–82.

Moore, P. S., Hierholzer, J., DeWitt, W. *et al.* (1990). Respiratory viruses and mycoplasma as cofactors for epidemic group A meningococcal meningitis. *J. Am. Med. Assoc.*, **264**, 1271–1275.

Morbidity and Mortality Weekly Report (1996). Serogroup Y meningococcal disease – Illinois, Connecticut, and selected areas, United States, 1989–1996. **45**, 1010–1013.

Moxon, E. R. (1986). The carrier state: *Haemophilus influenzae. J. Antimicrob. Chemother.*, **18** (suppl. A), 17–24.

Musser, J. M., Kroll, J. S., Granoff, D. M. *et al.* (1990). Global genetic structure and molecular epidemiology of encapsulated *Haemophilus influenzae. Rev. Infect. Dis.*, **12**, 75–111.

Nesin, M., Ramirez, M. and Tomasz, A. (1998). Capsular transformation of a multidrug-resistant *Streptococcus pneumoniae* in vivo. *J. Infect. Dis.*, **177**, 707–713.

Obaro, S. K., Adegbola, R. A., Banya, W. A. and Greenwood, B. M. (1996). Carriage of pneumococci after pneumococcal vaccination. *Lancet*, **348**, 271–272.

Pan America Health Organisation. (1996) Impact of Uruguay's introduction of the *Haemophilus influenzae* type b (Hib) vaccine. *EPI newsletter* **18**, 6.

Peeters, C. C., Rumke, H. C., Sundermann, L. C. *et al.* (1996). Phase I clinical trial with a hexavalent PorA containing meningococcal outer membrane vesicle vaccine. *Vaccine*, **14**, 1009–1015.

Peltola, H. (1998). Meningococcal vaccines. Current status and future possibilities. *Drugs*, **55**, 347–366.

Peltola, H., Makela, H., Kayhty, H. *et al.* (1977). Clinical efficacy of meningococcus group A capsular polysaccharide vaccine in children three months to five years of age. *N. Engl. J. Med.*, **297**, 686–691.

Peltola, H., Aavitsland, P., Hansen, K. G., Jonsdottir, K. E., Nokleby, H. and Romanus V. (1999). Perspective: a five-country analysis of the impact of four different *Haemophilus influenzae* type b conjugates and vaccination strategies in Scandinavia. *J. Infect. Dis.*, **179**, 223–229.

Petersen, G. M., Silimperi, D. R., Scott, E. M., Hall, D. B., Rotter, J. I. and Ward, J. I. (1985). Uridine monophosphate kinase 3: a genetic marker for susceptibility to *Haemophilus influenzae* type b disease. *Lancet*, **2**, 417–419.

Petersen, G. M., Silimperi, D. R., Rotter, J. I. *et al.* (1987). Genetic factors in *Haemophilus influenzae* type b disease susceptibility and antibody acquisition. *J. Pediatr.*, **110**, 228–233.

Pinner, R. W. Onyango, F., Perkins, B. A. *et al.* (1992). Epidemic meningococcal disease in Nairobi, Kenya, 1989. The Kenya/Centers for Disease Control (CDC) Meningitis Study Group. *J. Infect. Dis.*, **166**, 359–364.

Plotkin, S. (1998). Diphtheria toxoid conjugated vaccines against meningococcal group A and C infections. *Abstracts of the 16th Annual Meeting of the European Society for Paediatric Infectious Diseases*, Bled 1998, 11.

Pon, R. A., Lussier, M., Yang, Q. L. and Jennings, H. J. (1997). N-Propionylated group B meningococcal polysaccharide mimics a unique bactericidal capsular epitope in group B *Neisseria meningitidis. J. Exp. Med.*, **185**, 1929–1938.

Racoosin, J. A., Whitney, C. G., Conover, C. S. and Diaz, P. S. (1998). Serogroup Y meningococcal disease in Chicago, 1991–1997. *J. Am. Med. Assoc.*, **280**, 2094–2098.

Ramsay, M., Collins, M., Rush, M. and Kaczmarski, E. (1998). The epidemiology of meningococcal disease in England and Wales, 1996 and 1997. *Eurosurveillance*, **2**, 74–75.

Reingold, A. L., Broome, C. V., Hightower, A. W. *et al.* (1985). Age-specific differences in duration of clinical protection after vaccination with meningococcal polysaccharide vaccine. *Lancet*, **2**, 114–118.

Reller, L. B., MacGregor, R. R. and Beaty, H. N. (1973). Bactericidal antibody after colonization with *Neisseria meningitidis. J. Infect. Dis.*, **127**, 56–62.

Richmond, P., Cartwright, K., Borrow, R. *et al.* (1998a). An investigation of the immunogenicity and reactogenicity of three meningococcal serogroup C conjugate vaccines administered as a single dose in UK toddlers. *Abstracts of the 11th International Pathogenic Neisseria Conference*, Nice 1998, 153.

Richmond, P., Miller, E., Borrow, R. *et al.* (1998b). Reactogenicity, immunogenicity and priming of two different strengths of a meningococcal serogroup C conjugate vaccine in UK infants. *Abstracts of the 11th International Pathogenic Neisseria Conference*, Nice 1998, 156.

Rijkers, G. T., Sanders, L. A. and Zegers, B. J. (1993). Anti-capsular polysaccharide antibody deficiency states. *Immunodeficiency*, **5**, 1–21.

Robbins, J. B., Myerowitz, L., Whisnant, J. K. *et al.* (1972). Enteric bacteria cross-reactive with *Neisseria meningitidis* groups A and C and *Diplococcus pneumoniae* types I and 3. *Infect. Immun.*, **6**, 651–656.

Robbins, J. B., Schneerson, R., Glode, M. P. *et al.* (1975). Cross-reactive antigens and immunity to diseases caused by encapsulated bacteria. *J. Allergy Clin. Immunol.*, **56**, 141–51.

Robbins, J. B., Towne, D. W., Gotschlich, E. C. and Schneerson, R. (1997). 'Love's labours lost': failure to implement mass vaccination against group A meningococcal meningitis in sub-Saharan Africa. *Lancet*, **350**, 880–882.

Sacchi, C. T., Zanella, R. C., Caugant, D. A. *et al.* (1992). Emergence of a new clone of serogroup C *Neisseria meningitidis* in Sao Paulo, Brazil. *J. Clin. Microbiol.* **30**, 1282–1286.

Santosham, M., Wolff, M., Reid, R. *et al.* (1991). The efficacy in Navajo infants of a conjugate vaccine consisting of *Haemophilus influenzae* type b polysaccharide and *Neisseria meningitidis* outer-membrane protein complex. *N. Engl. J. Med.*, **324**, 1767–72.

Schneerson, R. and Robbins, J. B. (1975). Induction of serum *Haemophilus influenzae* type b capsular antibodies in adult volunteers fed cross-reacting *Escherichia coli* 075:K100:H5. *N. Engl. J. Med.*, **292**, 1093–1096.

Shapiro, E. D., Capobianco, L. A., Berg, A. T. and Zitt, M. Q. (1989). The immunogenicity of *Haemophilus influenzae* type B polysaccharide-*Neisseria meningitidis* group B outer membrane protein complex vaccine in infants and young children. *J. Infect. Dis.*, **160**, 1064–1067.

Siber, G. R. (1994). Pneumococcal disease: prospects for a new generation of vaccines. *Science*, **265**, 1385–1387.

Sierra, G. V., Campa, H. C., Varcacel, N. M. *et al.* (1991). Vaccine against group B *Neisseria meningitidis*: protection trial and mass vaccination results in Cuba. *NIPH Ann.*, **14**, 195–207.

Smart, L. E., Dougall, A. J. and Girdwood, R. W. (1987). New 23-valent pneumococcal vaccine in relation to pneumococcal serotypes in systemic and non-systemic disease. *J. Infect.*, **14**, 209–215.

Smit, P., Oberholzer, D., Hayden, S. S., Koornhof, H. J. and Hilleman, M. R. (1977). Protective efficacy of pneumococcal polysaccharide vaccines. *J. Am. Med. Assoc.*, **238**, 2613–2616.

Sniadack, D. H., Schwartz, B., Lipman, H. *et al.* (1995). Potential interventions for the prevention of childhood pneumonia: geographic and temporal differences in serotype and serogroup distribution of sterile site pneumococcal isolates from children – implications for vaccine strategies. *Pediatr. Infect. Dis. J.*, **14**, 503–510.

St-Geme, J. W. and Cutter, D. (1996). Influence of pili, fibrils, and capsule on in vitro adherence by *Haemophilus influenzae* type b. *Mol. Microbiol.*, **21**, 21–31.

Stephens, D. S. and Farley, M. M. (1991). Pathogenic events during infection of the human nasopharynx with *Neisseria meningitidis* and *Haemophilus influenzae*. *Rev. Infect. Dis.*, **13**, 22–33.

Stroffolini, T. (1990). Vaccination campaign against meningococcal disease in army recruits in Italy. *Epidemiol. Infect.*, **105**, 579–583.

Stroffolini, T., Angelini, L., Galanti, I., Occhionero, M., Congiu, M. E. and Mastrantonio, P. (1990). The effect of meningococcal group A and C polysaccharide vaccine on nasopharyngeal carrier state. *Microbiologica*, **13**, 225–229.

Swartley, J. S., Marfin, A. A., Edupuganti, S. *et al.* (1997). Capsule switching of *Neisseria meningitidis*. *Proc. Natl Acad. Sci. USA*, **94**, 271–276.

Sung, R. Y., Senok, A. C., Ho, A., Oppenheimer, S. J. and Davies, D. P. (1997) Meningitis in Hong Kong children, with special reference to the infrequency of Haemophilus and meningococcal infection. *J. Paediatr. Child Hlth.*, **33**, 296–299.

Takala, A. K., Jero, J., Kela, E., Ronnberg, P. R., Koskenniemi, E. and Eskola, J. (1995). Risk factors for primary invasive pneumococcal disease among children in Finland. *J. Am. Med. Assoc.*, **273**, 859–864.

Tappero, J. W. *et al.* (1999). Immunogenicity of two serogroup B outer-membrane protein meningococcal vaccines. *J. Am. Med. Assoc.*, **281**, 1520–1527.

Taunay, A. E., Feldman, R. A., Bastos, C. O., Galvao, P. A. A., Morais, J. S. and Castro, I. O. (1978). Assessment of the protection conferred by anti-group C meningococcal polysaccharide vaccine to 6 to 36 month-old children. *Rev. Inst. Adolfo Lutz.*, **38**, 77–82.

Troy, F. A. (1992). Polysialylation: from bacteria to brains. *Glycobiology*, **2**, 5–23.

Twumasi, P. A., JR, Kumah, S., Leach, A. *et al.* (1995). A trial of a group A plus group C meningococcal polysaccharide-protein conjugate vaccine in African infants. *J. Infect. Dis.*, **171**, 632–638.

Van d, V., van-der-Ley, P., van-der-Biezen, J. *et al.* (1996). Specificity of human bactericidal antibodies against PorA P1.7,16 induced with a hexavalent meningococcal outer membrane vesicle vaccine. *Infect. Immun.*, **64**, 2745–2751.

Wahdan, M. H., Rizk, F., el-Akkad, A. M. *et al.* (1973). A controlled field trial of a serogroup A meningococcal polysaccharide vaccine. *Bull. World Hlth Org.*, **48**, 667–673.

Wahdan, M. H., Sallam, S. A., Hassan, M. N. *et al.* (1977). A second controlled field trial of a serogroup A meningococcal polysaccharide vaccine in Alexandria. *Bull. World Hlth Org.*, **55**, 645–651.

Ward, J. I., Margolis, H. S., Lum, M. K., Fraser, D. W., Bender, T. R. and Anderson, P. (1981). *Haemophilus influenzae* disease in Alaskan Eskimos: characteristics of a population with an unusual incidence of invasive disease. *Lancet*, **1**, 1281–1285.

Ward, J. I., Lum, M. K., Hall, D. B., Silimperi, D. R. and Bender, T. R. (1986). Invasive *Haemophilus influenzae* type b disease in Alaska: background epidemiology for a vaccine efficacy trial. *J. Infect. Dis.*, **153**, 17–26.

Whalen, C. M., Hockin, J. C., Ryan, A. and Ashton, F. (1995). The changing epidemiology of invasive meningococcal disease in Canada, 1985 through 1992. Emergence of a virulent clone of *Neisseria meningitidis*. *J. Am. Med. Assoc.*, **273**, 390–394.

Whitney, C. G., Dondoc, N., Enktuja, B. *et al.* (1996). Control of epidemic serogroup A meningococcal disease, Mongolia (poster 20.011). (Abstract). *7th International Congress for Infectious Diseases, Hong Kong, 1996*.

WHO (1998). *Report of the Third International Coordinating Group (ICG) Meeting on Vaccine Provision for Epidemic Meningitis Control*. Geneva: World Health Organization. p. 6.

Wyle, F. A., Artenstein, M. S., Brandt, B. L. *et al.* (1972). Immunologic response of man to group B meningococcal polysaccharide vaccines. *J. Infect. Dis.*, **126**, 514–521.

10

Neurological complications of varicella-zoster virus

Donald H. Gilden, James J. LaGuardia, Ravi Mahalingam, Tiffany M. White and Randall J. Cohrs

Naturally occurring varicella: epidemiology and clinical features

Primary varicella-zoster virus (VZV) infection produces varicella (chickenpox), a highly contagious, but typically mild disease of childhood. By adult life, nearly everyone in North America is seropositive. An estimated four million cases occur annually in the USA, 90% of which are in individuals 1–14 years of age (Preblud, 1986). In northern regions, only 2% of varicella occurs after age 20. This differs from countries in tropical climates, where a higher incidence of varicella is seen in adults (Nassar and Touma, 1986; Longfield *et al.*, 1990).

In temperate climates, chickenpox peaks in the spring, with another, smaller peak in winter (Preblud and D'Angelo, 1979; Preblud *et al.*, 1984). Disease is presumably transmitted by direct contact or aerosols containing virus (Leclair *et al.*, 1980; Gustafson *et al.*, 1982; Josephson and Gombert, 1988). Infection is probably respiratory, followed by viral replication, most likely in the pharynx and regional lymph nodes (Tomlinson, 1939; Fenner, 1948; Grose, 1981). The incubation period in healthy children is 9–21 days (Fenner, 1948; Grose, 1981; Preblud *et al.*, 1984). Viraemia in immunocompetent varicella patients has been demonstrated 1–11 days before rash (Asano *et al.*, 1985; Källander *et al.*, 1989), predominantly in lymphocytes (Ozaki *et al.*, 1986; Vonsover *et al.*, 1987; Koropchak *et al.*, 1989). Immunological evidence indicates that subclinical reinfection with VZV is fairly common (Baba *et al.*, 1986; Wharton, 1996). Fever, myalgia and arthralgias precede or coincide with rash.

The exanthem of chickenpox consists of macules and papules that develop into vesicles surrounded by an erythematous halo. Vesicles, which reflect degenerative changes of the corium and dermis, develop quickly and are characterized by multinucleated giant cells and intranuclear Cowdry type A inclusions (Tyzzer, 1906), a hallmark of herpesvirus family infection. Vesicles contain abundant infectious virus which can be isolated in cell culture (Weller *et al.*, 1958). Rash usually begins on the trunk, spreads to the face, limbs, and often to the buccal and pharyngeal mucosa. Compared with healthy skin, areas that are sunburned or subject to irritation (e.g. from nappies (diapers)) often exhibit a more dense rash. Eventually, vesicles burst and their fluid hardens, a process referred to as crusting. New vesicles form within the first 4 days after outbreak, while crusting starts after 2–3 days; thus, both crusting and fresh vesicles may be seen at the same time. Patients are considered infectious from 2 days before rash until all vesicles have crusted, typically 6 days after the onset of rash. Immunization of children 12–18 months old with a live attenuated varicella vaccine (Oka strain) may eventually shift the average age of infection to older susceptible individuals (Halloran, 1996).

Classification

In the second century AD, Claudius Galen first described vesicular skin lesions which he named herpes because the lesions crept or crawled over the skin. Nearly 1800 years later, the cause was shown to be a member of the family of herpesviruses. Herpesviruses infect mammals, birds, reptiles, amphibians and fish, and are classified by shared characteristics of *in vitro* cytopathology, the duration of replicative cycle, and their ability to become latent.

Standard virology

VZV is exclusively a human pathogen. It is readily propagated in multiple human and primate cell lines (Weller *et al.*, 1958; Gilden *et al.*, 1978, 1982), and is maintained *in vitro* by cocultivation of infected cells with uninfected cells. Figure 10.1 shows the typical VZV-induced multinucleated cytopathic

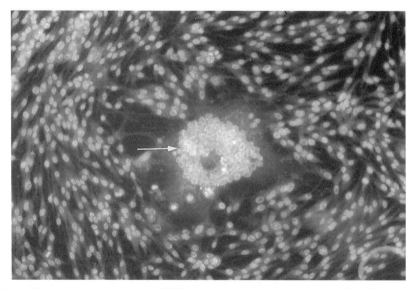

Figure 10.1   Arrow points to a VZV-induced multinucleated giant cell × 400.

effect in human melanoma cells stained 4 days after infection. Virtually every region of the virus genome is transcribed during productive infection (Reinhold *et al.*, 1988). Thus, the low virus yield associated with VZV grown in culture has been attributed to errors either in virion assembly or maturation.

Molecular virology

The entire 125 884 bp VZV genome has been sequenced and shown to have a high degree of homology to herpes simplex virus (HSV)-1, the prototype human alphaherpesvirus (Davison and Scott, 1986; McGeoch *et al.*, 1985, 1986, 1988; Perry and McGeoch, 1988). The VZV genome comprises a unique long (U_L) segment of 104 836 bp and a unique short (U_S) segment of 5232 bp. Each unique segment of VZV DNA is bound by inverted repeats (88 bp inverted repeats around the U_L and 7320 bp inverted repeats around the U_S). Figure 10.2 shows the location, relative size and direction of transcription of the 71 predicted open reading frames (ORFs) potentially encoding proteins ranging from eight to 300 kDa in size (Davison and Scott, 1986). Although transcripts mapping to most VZV ORFs have been identified in VZV-infected cells in culture, fewer than 20 VZV genes have been analysed in detail (Ostrove *et al.*, 1985; Maguire and Hyman, 1986; Reinhold *et al.*, 1988; Cohen and Straus, 1996). In the VZV genome, the 71 ORFs are separated by an average of 211 bp, indicating that the promoters are closely associated with the genes they regulate. During virus DNA replication, in approximately 50% of virus DNA molecules, the U_S and its attendant repeats (IR_S and TR_S) invert with respect to U_L (Straus *et al.*, 1982; Kinchington *et al.*, 1985; Hayakawa and Hyman, 1987; Davison, 1991). The biological significance of VZV genome isomerization has yet to be determined; however, the presence of inverted repeats results in duplication of genes contained within them. Thus VZV genes 62 and 63 are present in two copies per genome.

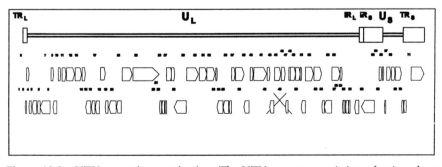

Figure 10.2   VZV genomic organization. The VZV genome consisting of unique long (U_L) and short segments (U_S) bound by internal repeats (IR) and terminal repeats (TR) contains 71 tightly packed open reading frames (ORFs), numbered consecutively from the left. The relative size, location and direction of transcription of the predicted ORFs are indicated (Davison and Scott, 1986).

Zoster (shingles) epidemiology

Herpes zoster is a common disorder. More than 300 000 cases are estimated to occur annually in the USA. Except in immunocompromised individuals (especially AIDS patients), zoster is a disease of the elderly. The incidence among people over age 50 is double that of people under 50 (Harnisch, 1984), which ultimately translates into an 8–10-fold increased frequency in people over age 60 compared with those under 60. As the ageing population increases (by the year 2000, an estimated 20–25% of Americans will be older than 65), the incidence of zoster-associated morbidity and mortality is also expected to increase. Varicella in infancy may predispose to zoster earlier in life (Guess *et al.*, 1985). The incidence of recurrent zoster is less than 5% (Hope-Simpson, 1965). Although varicella outbreaks occur most often in the spring, zoster may develop at any time of the year. The risk of zoster in vaccinated individuals compared with those who developed naturally occurring chickenpox will not be known for decades. Meanwhile, some investigators have predicted an increased incidence of zoster with widespread use of the live attenuated varicella vaccine (Garnett and Grenfell, 1992; Wharton, 1996).

Pathology and pathogenesis

Despite the ubiquitous nature and frequency of VZV infection, the pathogenesis of zoster remains largely unknown. Our present understanding of virus spread, localization and replication is based on *in vitro* studies of infected human or primate cells in tissue culture, correlation of the presence of VZV in human tissues with pathological changes in different clinical situations, and attempts to produce disease experimentally.

Pathological changes in ganglia corresponding to the segmental distribution of rash were first noted by von Barensprung (1863), and more extensively detailed by Head and Campbell (1900) and Denny-Brown *et al.* (1944). The older literature accurately reflects the true pathology of zoster, since the lesions described were those of localized zoster in immunocompetent individuals, except perhaps for occasional zoster that developed in syphilis patients treated with arsenic. The cardinal pathological features were inflammation and haemorrhagic necrosis, often associated with neuritis, localized leptomeningitis, unilateral segmental poliomyelitis, and degeneration of related motor and sensory roots. Demyelination was also seen in areas of mononuclear cell infiltration and microglial proliferation.

Later, intranuclear inclusions (Cheatham *et al.*, 1956; Ghatak and Zimmerman, 1973), viral antigen and herpesvirus particles (Esiri and Tomlinson, 1972; Nagashima *et al.*, 1975) were detected in ganglia, and VZV was isolated from ganglia (Bastian *et al.*, 1974). However, those studies were performed on ganglia from patients with underlying malignancies or other disorders of immune function who developed disseminated zoster just before death. There is a single report in which VZV antigen was detected and virus isolated from ganglia of a fatal case of bacterial pneumonitis on which acute thoracic zoster was superimposed (Shibuta *et al.*, 1974).

Zoster is presumed to reflect reactivation and retrograde transport of virus from ganglia to skin in a host partially immune to VZV. Viraemia has also been demonstrated in otherwise immunocompetent zoster patients (Gilden *et al.*, 1987a). Although the significance of viraemia in zoster patients remains to be determined, VZV DNA has been detected by *in situ* hybridization (ISH) in blood mononuclear cells (MNCs) of four uncomplicated zoster patients for 3–7 weeks after rash (Gilden *et al.*, 1988a), coinciding with the period during which these patients experienced pain.

In immunocompromised patients with localized and disseminated zoster, VZV can be isolated from blood (Gold, 1966; Feldman and Epp, 1976; Feldman *et al.*, 1977; Gershon *et al.*, 1978; Myers, 1979), suggesting a role for haematogenous spread in the pathogenesis of zoster in such individuals. VZV in blood is cell-associated (Myers, 1979) and has been detected by electron microscopy in monocytes (Twomey *et al.*, 1974). A loss of cell-mediated immunity to VZV may be responsible for an increased risk of zoster in immunocompromised patients (Wharton, 1996).

The detection of VZV in macrophages (Arbeit *et al.*, 1982), in B cells (Leventon-Kriss *et al.*, 1979; Cauda *et al.*, 1986), and in T cells (Gilden *et al.*, 1987a), particularly in activated T lymphocytes (Koropchak *et al.*, 1989), provides indirect evidence that blood MNCs represent a site for VZV persistence. Nucleic acid hybridization studies revealed that VZV DNA did not replicate in human MNCs (Gilden *et al.*, 1987a), a finding confirmed by Koropchak *et al.* (1989).

Zoster (shingles, ganglionitis)

Herpes zoster is characterized by pain and a vesicular eruption on an erythematous base in one to three dermatomes. All levels of the neuraxis may be involved in zoster. Thoracic zoster is most common, followed by lesions on the face, most often in the ophthalmic division of the trigeminal nerve. The latter is frequently accompanied by zoster keratitis, a potential cause of blindness if not recognized and treated promptly. All patients with ophthalmic distribution zoster should have an immediate slitlamp examination by an ophthalmologist. Maxillary and mandibular trigeminal distribution zoster with osteonecrosis and spontaneous tooth exfoliation has also been described in adults (Manz *et al.*, 1986) and children (Garty *et al.*, 1985). The seventh cranial nerve is also commonly involved. Weakness of all facial muscles of one side develops in conjunction with rash in the ear (zoster oticus) or on the ipsilateral anterior two-thirds of the tongue or hard palate. Unless searched for in patients with facial weakness, vesicles in either site are easily overlooked. The combination of zoster oticus and peripheral facial weakness constitutes the Ramsay Hunt syndrome, and the prognosis for recovery from facial weakness or paralysis is not as favourable as in idiopathic Bell's palsy. Zoster may be accompanied by ophthalmoplegia, most commonly affecting the third cranial nerve (Thomas and Howard, 1972), optic neuritis (Miller *et al.*, 1986), or both (Carroll and Mastaglia, 1979), and less often lower cranial nerve palsies

(Crabtree, 1968; Steffen and Selby, 1972). Zoster-associated cranial neuropathy often occurs weeks after acute VZV infection. One explanation for late-onset zoster cranial neuropathy is that virus spreads slowly along trigeminal and other ganglionic afferent fibres to small vessels supplying cranial nerves. This appears to happen in granulomatous arteritis (described below) preceded weeks earlier by trigeminal distribution zoster. All cranial nerves receive their blood supply from the carotid circulation (Lapresle and Lasjaunias, 1986). It is likely, but not yet proven, that the vasa vasorum of cranial nerves may also receive trigeminal afferents, as has been shown for larger extracranial and intracranial blood vessels (Mayberg et al., 1984).

Postherpetic neuralgia

Most neurological complications of zoster manifest as postherpetic neuralgia (PHN), operationally defined as pain persisting more than 4–6 weeks after rash. Age is the most important factor in predicting the development of PHN (Brown, 1976; Ragozzino et al., 1982). The risk of PHN in zoster patients over age 50 ranges from 43 to 47.5%. The incidence of PHN also appears to be slightly greater in women (Hope-Simpson, 1975) and after trigeminal distribution zoster (DeMoragas and Kierland, 1957; Rogers and Tindall, 1971; Hope-Simpson, 1975).

The mechanism of PHN is unknown. The detection of VZV-specific proteins in MNCs of patients with PHN (Vafai et al., 1988b) suggested that persistence of VZV may result in PHN. Later, VZV DNA was shown to persist in blood MNCs of PHN patients (Mahalingam et al., 1995) compared with zoster patients without PHN, thus providing further presumptive (albeit indirect) evidence that the abundance of VZV in ganglia of PHN patients may be greater than during latency. It is possible that MNCs trafficking through such ganglia encounter and engulf virus whose DNA can then be amplified by PCR. Ganglia need to be analysed at autopsy from individuals who suffered from PHN at the time of death. If a greater virus burden could be demonstrated in these ganglia than has been found during latency (Mahalingam et al., 1993), this would provide a rationale for aggressive treatment of PHN patients with antivirals. Meanwhile, the existence of ganglionitis without rash is further supported by the presence of radicular pain up to 100 days preceding zoster (Gilden et al., 1991), so-called preherpetic neuralgia. Further, a recent report described four patients with acute trigeminal distribution zoster who, after years free from pain, developed severe trigeminal 'PHN' (Schott, 1998).

Zoster paresis

Zoster in cervical, thoracic and lumbosacral dermatome distributions may be associated with muscle weakness developing 1–5 weeks after rash. Cervical distribution zoster has been associated with arm weakness, and rarely, diaphragmatic paralysis (Brostoff, 1966; Stowasser et al., 1990). The small incidence of thoracic zoster paresis probably reflects difficulty in diagnosing intercostal muscle weakness at the bedside. Lower in the neuraxis, lumbosacral distribution zoster may be associated with leg weakness as well as impairment of bladder and bowel function. Urinary retention, haemorrhagic cystitis and massive bladder haemorrhage have all been described with sacral distribution zoster (Izumi and Edwards, 1973; Jellinek and Tulloch, 1976). The incidence of zoster paresis has been estimated from as low as 0.5% to as high as 31%. Approximately 11% of patients with segmental zoster paresis have malignant disease (Thomas and Howard, 1972).

VZV encephalitis-arteritis

What has previously been called VZV encephalitis is for the most part a VZV vasculopathy which affects small or large vessels of the CNS, and often, both. Small vessel artery encephalitis and large vessel artery disease (granulomatous arteritis) are discussed below.

Zoster small-vessel encephalitis

Zoster small-vessel encephalitis is the most common form of CNS involvement. Disease usually develops on a background of cancer, immunosuppression (Horton et al., 1981) or AIDS. Neurological disease is subacute and death is common. Zoster encephalitis presents with headache, fever, vomiting, mental changes, seizures and focal deficit (Gilden et al., 2000). Brain MRI reveals large and small ischaemic or haemorrhagic infarcts, often both, of cortex and subcortical grey and white matter (Figure 10.3). Deep-seated white matter lesions often predominate, and are ischaemic or demyelinative, depending on the size of blood vessels involved and the amount of additional demyelination. The demyelinative lesions are smaller and less coalescent than those seen in progressive multifocal leucoencephalopathy. The CSF shows a mild pleocytosis (predominantly mononuclear), normal or mild elevation of protein, and a normal glucose, findings that do not differ significantly from zoster without encephalitis. Two reports describe hypoglycorrhachia in zoster meningoencephalitis (Reimer and Reller, 1981; Wolf, 1974). In suspected cases of zoster small-vessel encephalitis, the CSF should be studied for both VZV DNA and antibody to VZV. The presence of either, or both, in CSF, in the typical clinical setting described above, is strong presumptive evidence of VZV small-vessel encephalitis (Gilden et al., 1998). Zoster small-vessel encephalitis should be treated with acyclovir, 15–30 mg/kg/day for 10 days. Longer treatment may be necessary in severely immunocompromised patients.

Zoster large-vessel encephalitis (granulomatous arteritis)

Zoster large-vessel encephalitis (granulomatous arteritis) is characterized by acute focal deficit that develops weeks to months after contralateral trigeminal

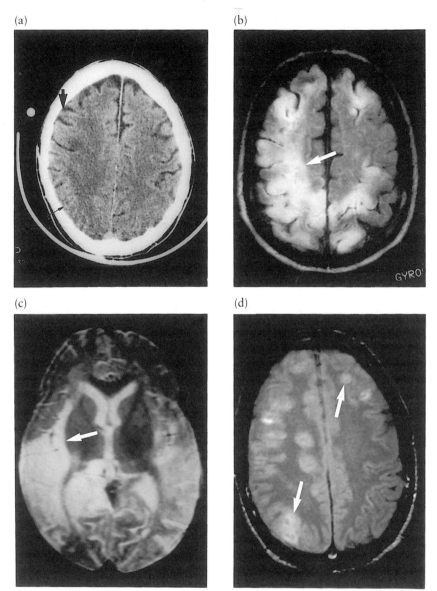

Figure 10.3 (a) CT changes that occur in most viral encephalitides. Brain computed tomography scan demonstrates relative effacement of sulci posteriorly in both hemispheres (thin arrow), compared with normal sulcal spaces anteriorly (thick arrow). (b) MRI changes that occur in most viral encephalitides. T2-weighted inversion recovery (fluid-attenuated inversion recovery (FLAIR)) MRI brain scan of the same patient demonstrates areas of increased signal in both hemispheres, greater on the right and even more so posteriorly (arrow), reflecting increased water content in mildly swollen brain. (c) Herpes simplex virus encephalitis. T2-weighted MRI brain scan demonstrates bilateral involvement of temporal lobes. The exaggerated signal does not extend beyond the insular cortex (arrow). (d) Varicella-zoster virus encephalitis. Proton-density brain MRI scan shows multiple areas of infarction in both hemispheres (arrows).

distribution zoster. Stroke results from a necrotizing arteritis, primarily of large cerebral arteries. In a comprehensive review by Hilt *et al.* (1983), most patients with zoster large-vessel encephalitis were over age 60, and there was no sex predilection. The mean onset of neurological disease was 7 weeks, and the longest interval was 6 months after zoster. Transient ischaemic attacks and mental symptoms were common. Twenty-five per cent of patients died. The majority of patients had CSF pleocytosis, usually fewer than 100 cells (predominantly mononuclear), oligoclonal bands, and increased CSF IgG. Besides contralateral hemiplegia, ipsilateral central retinal artery occlusion (Hall *et al.*, 1983) and posterior circulation involvement have been described. Angiographic examination reveals focal constriction and segmental narrowing primarily in middle cerebral, internal carotid and anterior cerebral arteries. Microscopic examination revealed a necrotizing arteritis, primarily involving the intima and adventitia, inflammation with multinucleated giant cells, VZV antigen, Cowdry A inclusions and herpes virus particles. Most zoster-associated granulomatous angiitis infarcts are pale (Kuroiwa and Furukawa, 1981), but haemorrhagic infarction also occurs (Eible, 1983). Afferent trigeminal ganglionic fibres to both intracranial and extracranial blood vessels (Mayberg *et al.*, 1984) provide an anatomic pathway for the spread of virus. How much disease is exclusively viral, a viral-induced immunopathology, or both, is unknown. Based on the collective pathological changes, granulomatous arteritis patients should receive intravenous acyclovir (10–15 mg/kg three times daily for 7–10 days) to kill persistent virus, and a short course of steroids (prednisone 60–80 mg daily for 3–5 days) can be added for their anti-inflammatory effect.

VZV myelitis

Myelitis, a rare complication of acute varicella or zoster, usually develops 1–2 weeks after rash. Clinical features are those of paraparesis with a sensory level and sphincter impairment. The CSF is either normal or may show a mild pleocytosis with a normal or mild elevation of protein. Although recovery is variable, most patients improve significantly, but some experience persistent lower extremity stiffness and weakness. This form of VZV-associated transverse myelitis has been presumed to be post-infectious, but requires pathological, virological and immunological verification.

In immunocompromised individuals, the development of myelopathy is often more insidious, progressive, and sometimes fatal. Spinal cord MRI scanning shows longitudinal serpiginous enhancing lesions (Gilden *et al.*, 1994a). Autopsy studies have demonstrated frank invasion of the spinal cord by VZV. A fatal case of ascending VZV myelitis was described after steroid treatment for thoracic zoster (Hogan and Krigman, 1973). The severity of the myelitis could have been influenced by steroid therapy, a notion supported by the development of zoster meningoencephalitis that occurred in a diabetic who had been treated for months with low-dose steroids (Tako and Rado, 1965). As in VZV encephalitis, an early search for VZV DNA or antibody to VZV in CSF is essential to make the diagnosis, particularly since aggressive treatment with acyclovir, even in AIDS patients, may produce a gratifying response (de Silva *et al.*, 1996).

Finally, although VZV myelopathy is usually diagnosed by the close temporal relationship between rash and the onset of myelopathy, the spectrum of VZV myelopathy is wide. Disease may be acute, remitting-exacerbating, or chronic; when myelopathy recurs, rash usually does not (Gilden *et al.*, 1994a).

Neuropathy

Postinfectious polyneuritis or the Guillain-Barré syndrome (GBS) is an uncommon, but well-documented neurological complication of both varicella and zoster. No neurological features distinguish polyneuritis after varicella or zoster from that seen in other clinical settings. The average interval between rash and neurological disease was 12 days (Underwood, 1935). Bilateral facial paralysis was present less often in VZV-associated GBS than in GBS unassociated with varicella (Underwood, 1935; Miller *et al.*, 1956). GBS after chickenpox is rare, as evidenced by its occurrence in only eight of 2534 cases of chickenpox (Bullowa and Wishik, 1935), and by the total absence of associated chickenpox in 50 extensively studied cases of GBS (Haymaker and Kernohan, 1949).

GBS after zoster is equally rare. Only 16 cases have been described since the initial report by Wohlwill (1924) and the first compilation of cases by Dayan *et al.* (1972). Polyneuritis usually occurs many days to a few weeks after rash, and in some instances 2 months later. The clinical course is usually acute, but occasionally subacute or indolent, especially in the cases that developed 1–2 months after rash. Neuropathological examination of teased nerve fibres revealed acute demyelination and remyelination. In addition, fibrinoid necrosis of blood vessels and infarction were seen in severely affected spinal ganglia, suggestive of an Arthus-type immunopathology (Dayan *et al.*, 1972).

Reye's syndrome

Reye's syndrome is a rapidly progressive, often fatal, non-inflammatory disorder of children and adolescents. The two most affected organs are the brain (which swells) and the liver (which becomes infiltrated by fat). Disease is associated with infection by the influenza viruses or VZV. Typically, an initial, apparently mild upper respiratory infection, or an episode of classic chickenpox is followed by an asymptomatic few days, after which patients develop intractable vomiting, seizures, lethargy, coma, and often death (Hurwitz *et al.*, 1982). Therapeutic amounts of salicylates increase the risk of developing Reye's syndrome (Remington *et al.*, 1986). Characteristic laboratory abnormalities include elevated serum transaminase and ammonia levels, as well as hypoglycaemia in approximately 40% of patients. A brain MRI may reveal sulcal effacement, loss of grey–white matter junctions, and small ventricles, all consistent with brain swelling. The exact metabolic abnormality in Reye's syndrome has not been determined. Patients require intensive care treatment to reverse rapidly developing cerebral oedema by hyperventilation and intravenous mannitol. Steroids have not been shown to be effective, probably because brain oedema is cytotoxic.

Zoster sine herpete

The concept of zoster sine herpete (shingles without rash) is nearly 100 years old. The first proposed case was that of a 38-year-old man who developed acute thoracic-distribution pain and hyperaesthesia, a dilated pupil, a CSF pleocytosis (predominantly mononuclear), and a negative serological test for syphilis (Widal, 1907). He was presumed to have zoster sine herpete even though serological tests for VZV were not done. Similarly, two patients who experienced segmental pain, hyperaesthesias and focal weakness were presumed to have zoster sine herpete despite lack of serological confirmation (Weber, 1916). The notion of zoster sine herpete received further credence when Lewis (1958) described numerous zoster patients who, days later, also developed pain without rash in a different dermatome distribution, often on the opposite side.

The first serological evidence of zoster sine herpete occurred in a physician who developed acute trigeminal distribution pain associated with a fourfold rise in complement-fixing antibody to VZV, but not to HSV (Easton, 1970). Virological confirmation of zoster sine herpete did not come until the analysis of two men with thoracic-distribution radicular pain that had lasted for months to years revealed amplifiable VZV DNA, but not HSV DNA, in their CSF and blood MNCs (Gilden et al., 1994b). After diagnosis, both men were treated successfully with intravenous acyclovir. A third virologically confirmed case of thoracic-distribution zoster sine herpete persisting for years included the demonstration of frequent fibrillation potentials restricted to chronically painful thoracic root segments (Amlie-Lefond et al., 1996). Unlike the gratifying response of the first two patients treated with antivirals, the third patient did not improve after treatment with intravenous acyclovir and oral famciclovir.

Although the nosological entity of zoster sine herpete as a clinical variant has now been established, its prevalence will not be known until more patients with prolonged radicular pain have been studied virologically. Analysis should include both PCR to amplify VZV DNA in CSF and in blood MNCs, as well as a search for antibody to VZV in CSF. Antibody to VZV in CSF, even in the absence of amplifiable VZV DNA, has been useful to support the diagnosis of encephalitis and myelitis produced by VZV without rash (Gilden et al., 1998). Analysis of serum anti-VZV antibody is of no value in the workup of patients with prolonged pain, because anti-VZV antibodies persist in nearly all adults throughout life, and the presence of antibodies in serum to different

VZV glycoproteins and non-glycosylated proteins is variable (Vafai *et al.*, 1988a).

Other non-zosteriform VZV infection of the nervous system without rash

Zoster sine herpete (reviewed above) is essentially a disorder of the peripheral nervous system (ganglioradiculopathy) produced by VZV without rash. VZV also produces disease of the CNS without rash. While cases are rare, at the University of Colorado Health Sciences Center, we have encountered more cases of VZV infection of the CNS (encephalitis and myelitis) without rash than we have of VZV infection of the peripheral nervous system (ganglioneuropathy) without rash.

In pathologically verified cases of VZV encephalitis without rash, the typical clinical picture has been an immunocompromised individual (usually AIDS) who develops CNS disease at the time of acute zoster, or may have a history of zoster weeks to months earlier, or even recurrent zoster. CNS disease in such patients develops more often in the absence of acute zoster than at the time of acute zoster (Amlie-Lefond *et al.*, 1995). Encephalitis is usually of the 'small vessel' type described above (see VZV encephalitis), and disease is usually protracted. Diagnosis may be difficult unless the clinician is alert to the history of recurrent zoster followed by the typical clinical features and multifocal lesions seen by brain MRI in 'small vessel' encephalitis. Many patients die of chronic progressive VZV encephalitis without ever having developed rash (Amlie-Lefond *et al.*, 1995; Gilden *et al.*, 1996). The most extreme example of VZV infection of the nervous system we have encountered was a 77-year-old man with T-cell lymphoma who developed a fatal meningoradiculitis and died 3 weeks after the onset of neurological disease (Dueland *et al.*, 1991). He did not develop zoster before or during neurological disease. At autopsy, haemorrhagic, inflammatory lesions with Cowdry A inclusions were found in meninges and nerve roots extending from cranial nerve roots to the cauda equina. The same lesions were present, although to a lesser extent, in the brain as well. We saw VZV antigen and nucleic acid, but not HSV or CMV antigen or nucleic acid, in infected tissue at all levels of the neuraxis. Thus, VZV may be included in the differential diagnosis of acute encephalomyeloradiculopathy, particularly since antiviral treatment is available.

Acute VZV myelopathy may also occur in the absence of rash. Heller *et al.* (1990) initially described a 31-year-old immunocompetent man who developed transverse myelitis with partial recovery. Disease was attributed to VZV based on the development of antibody in CSF. Later, we also encountered two patients with VZV myelopathy in the absence of rash (Gilden *et al.*, 1994b). The first patient developed zoster followed by myelopathy 5 months later, at which time amplifiable VZV DNA was detected in CSF. The second equally fascinating patient developed myelopathy at the time of acute zoster. The myelopathy resolved, but recurred 6 months later. Five months after the recurrence of myelopathy, the patient's CSF contained both amplifiable VZV

DNA as well as antibody to VZV. Overall, the spectrum of VZV myelopathy can be broad, ranging from acute to chronic and rarely recurrent myelopathy.

Further VZV involvement of the CNS without rash was verified by the intrathecal synthesis of antibodies to VZV in two patients with aseptic meningitis (Martinez-Martin *et al.*, 1985), later in four additional patients with aseptic meningitis (Echevarria *et al.*, 1987), and in one patient with acute meningoencephalitis (Vartdal *et al.*, 1982). We recently encountered an adult man who was taking low-dose methotrexate and developed acute encephalitis (fever, aphasia and a profound CSF mononuclear pleocytosis). His CSF contained amplifiable VZV and Epstein-Barr virus DNA. Zosteriform rash never developed, and he recovered completely after treatment with intravenous acyclovir.

There have been two instances of polyneuritis cranialis produced by VZV. The first occurred in a 70-year-old man who seroconverted to VZV during acute disease (Mayo and Booss, 1989). Another report described a 43-year-old man with acute polyneuritis cranialis who developed antibody in CSF to VZV, but not to other human herpesviruses, or to multiple ubiquitous paramyxoviruses or togaviruses (Osaki *et al.*, 1995). Both men were apparently immunocompetent. Finally, cases of acute unilateral facial (Bell's) palsy that developed in the absence of zosteriform rash have been attributed to VZV infection (so-called geniculate zoster sine herpete) based on 'a positive serum complement fixation test' (Aitken and Brain, 1933). Unfortunately, the serum was not tested for seroconversion to other human herpesviruses.

Latent VZV infection

Analysis of latent VZV is fraught with obstacles. VZV is exclusively a human pathogen and no rodent model exists in which to study virus latency and reactivation. VZV is latent only in ganglia (Gilden *et al.*, 1983, 1987b; Mahalingam *et al.*, 1990), a tissue not accessible in living individuals. Thus, analysis of latent VZV has been restricted to human ganglia obtained at autopsy.

Latent VZV DNA

During latency, 6–31 copies of the VZV genome per 10^5 cells are present in ganglia at all levels of the neuraxis (Mahalingam *et al.*, 1990, 1993). Our analysis of serial sections from trigeminal or thoracic ganglia revealed that VZV DNA is widely distributed throughout the entire latently infected human ganglion. Exploiting the fact that the U_L segment of the VZV genome rarely inverts with respect to the U_S segment (Straus *et al.*, 1982; Kinchington *et al.*, 1985; Hayakawa and Hyman, 1987; Davison, 1991), we selected PCR primers that amplified across the termini of the VZV genome and showed that in latently infected human ganglia, the ends of the VZV DNA molecule are covalently connected (Clarke *et al.*, 1995). The simplest interpretation of these PCR results is that during latency, the VZV genome assumes a circular, episomal state, similar to that identified in ganglia latently infected with HSV-1 (Rock and Fraser, 1983, 1985; Efstathiou *et al.*, 1986).

Site of VZV latency

Using *in situ* hybridization (ISH), VZV nucleic acids were detected exclusively in ganglionic neurons (Hyman *et al.*, 1983; Gilden *et al.*, 1987b) and later in non-neuronal satellite cells (Croen *et al.*, 1988; Meier *et al.*, 1993), or in both (Lungu *et al.*, 1995). Combined PCR and ISH revealed the presence of VZV DNA exclusively in neurons (Dueland *et al.*, 1995). Recently, a well-designed and carefully controlled study was conducted in which various groups investigating VZV latency submitted latently infected human ganglia to a single laboratory for analysis. The results showed that latent VZV DNA was found almost exclusively in neurons (Kennedy *et al.*, 1998). Thus, VZV latency in neurons appears to be the same as for other alpha-herpesviruses (Stevens *et al.*, 1987; Kutish *et al.*, 1990; Mitchell *et al.*, 1990; Priola *et al.*, 1990; Croen *et al.*, 1991; Bratanich *et al.*, 1992).

Latently transcribed VZV genes

While alpha-herpesviruses share similar biological features during latency (cell type harbouring latent virus and configuration of latent virus DNA), the transcriptional pattern of latent virus DNA differs. A single HSV-1 transcriptional unit has been detected consistently in human ganglia and in animal models. However, during VZV latency in human ganglia, no fewer than four VZV transcripts have been detected. The transcripts correspond to VZV genes 21, 29, 62 and 63. In addition, using rabbit antisera raised against VZV gene 63 protein (Debrus *et al.*, 1995), it was detected only in neurons of latently infected human ganglia (Mahalingam *et al.*, 1996).

VZV diagnosis: amplifiable VZV DNA by PCR and antibody to VZV

Rapid clinical diagnosis of VZV infection and any attendant systemic or neurological complications is essential since antiviral treatment exists. Standard diagnostic methods include histological analysis, attempts to isolate virus from infected tissue, serological assays that measure the humoral or cell-mediated immune response to VZV, and PCR analysis of VZV DNA.

Giemsa-stained smears of varicella vesicle scrapings have been used for histopathological diagnosis of VZV infection to detect multinucleated giant cells and Cowdry A intranuclear inclusions characteristic of any herpesvirus (Taylor-Robinson and Caunt, 1972). Inclusions have also been detected in smears of oral mucosa (Williams and Capers, 1959; Cooke, 1960, 1963). Occasionally, VZV can be isolated by cocultivation of infected pharyngeal tissue (Ozaki *et al.*, 1989) or blood MNCs (Gold, 1966) with indicator cells.

Various serological assays (FAMA, complement-fixation, haemagglutination, neutralization) have been used to diagnose VZV infection. The detection of VZV IgG is usually retrospective (Schmidt and Arvin, 1986). In contrast to serum, however, the detection of antibody to VZV in CSF, with or without the presence of amplifiable VZV DNA, is useful in the diagnosis of VZV encephalitis, myelitis and zoster sine herpete (Gilden *et al.*, 1994a, 1998). VZV IgG has been detected in CSF of four neonates with convulsions, indicating that intrauterine VZV infection can be acquired without skin lesions in the mother (Mustonen *et al.*, 1998). The sensitivity and specificity of different commercially available VZV IgG detection kits have been shown to be comparable (Gleaves *et al.*, 1996; Doern *et al.*, 1997).

In situ hybridization (ISH) has also been used to detect VZV DNA in the brains of patients with VZV encephalitis (Ryder *et al.*, 1986; Gilden *et al.*, 1988b), in VZV meningoradiculitis (Dueland *et al.*, 1991), in blood MNCs of patients with varicella and zoster (Gilden *et al.*, 1988a; Koropchak *et al.*, 1989), and in normal human ganglia (Hyman *et al.*, 1983; Gilden *et al.*, 1983, 1987b; Croen *et al.*, 1988; Meier *et al.*, 1993, Kennedy *et al.*, 1998). Although ISH can identify cells infected with VZV, its sensitivity compared with Southern blot hybridization is unknown.

Polymerase chain reaction (PCR) technology has provided a means to examine VZV at the molecular level with a specificity and precision not previously attainable. PCR has detected VZV DNA in throat swab samples (Koropchak *et al.*, 1991; Ozaki *et al.*, 1991), in blood MNCs (Koropchak *et al.*, 1991; Devlin *et al.*, 1992) and in vesicles from patients with chickenpox (Kido *et al.*, 1991). VZV DNA was detected in all throat swab samples within the first 3 days after the onset of chickenpox (Ozaki *et al.*, 1991). Further, in patients with acute peripheral facial palsy, the detection of VZV DNA by PCR in oropharyngeal swabs was more useful than currently available serological assays for the early diagnosis of zoster sine herpete (Furuta *et al.*, 1997).

PCR has also detected VZV DNA in blood MNCs of elderly patients with postherpetic neuralgia (Mahalingam *et al.*, 1995), in all of seven (100%) zoster patients with various neurological features (Puchhammer-Stockl *et al.*, 1991), in CSF from six of 84 (7%) of HIV-infected patients presenting with neurological symptoms, and in CSF of three of five (60%) children with post-varicella cerebellitis. The latter finding is particularly important, because it suggests that cerebellar ataxia days to weeks after chickenpox, thought to be immune-mediated, is more likely due to frank virus infection.

Recently, PCR has been used to detect VZV DNA in vitreous biopsy specimens from patients with viral retinitis (Knox *et al.*, 1998). VZV DNA has also been detected in cornea of seven of 14 (50%) patients after herpes zoster ophthalmicus (Mietz *et al.*, 1997). Also, PCR has shown that VZV is the most likely pathogen of atypical necrotizing herpetic retinopathies (Garweg and Bohnke, 1997).

PCR differentiates infection by herpes simplex and VZV (Rubben *et al.*, 1997; Beards *et al.*, 1998). Recently, VZV DNA was detected in synovial fluid of one patient with monoarthritis when blood MNCs were PCR-negative (Stebbings *et al.*, 1998) suggesting a direct role of VZV in causing the disease.

PCR has confirmed the presence of latent VZV DNA in human trigeminal and thoracic ganglia (Mahalingam *et al.*, 1990) and quantitative PCR showed that 6–31 copies of latent VZV DNA are present in 10^5 cells (Mahalingam *et al.*, 1993).

Overall, the combination of PCR and the detection of antibody to VZV in CSF is extremely useful, not only to evaluate disorders caused by VZV, but also to diagnose subclinical reactivation of the virus.

Simian varicella virus

Simian varicella virus (SVV) is an alpha-herpesvirus which causes a severe, disseminated, varicella-like disease in non-human primates (Soike *et al.*, 1984; Padovan and Cantrell, 1986). Outbreaks occur in epidemics and were first reported in the 1960s and 1970s at five different primate centres in the USA and the UK. Virus isolated from infected monkeys during each outbreak was shown to be closely related to the human VZV (Soike *et al.*, 1984). These initial findings provided a basis for further characterization of SVV and the use of SVV infection of non-human primates as an animal model for human VZV infections.

The clinical and virological features of SVV and VZV infections are summarized and compared in Table 10.1. Like VZV, SVV is an enveloped, double-stranded DNA virus with a linear genome 125 kilobase pairs (kb) in

Table 10.1 Clinical and virological features of VZV infection in humans and SVV infection in primates.

Features	VZV	SVV
Primary infection		
incubation period	7–21 days	7–9 days
rash	Vesicular	Vesicular
dissemination	Rare	Frequent
mortality	Rare	Frequent
Latency		
site	Ganglia	Ganglia
viral burden	6–31 genomes/10^5 cells	Unknown
transcription	Genes 21, 29, 62, 63	Gene 21
translation	Gene 63	Unknown
Reactivation	Frequent	Unknown
Viral immunology	Cross-reactivity to SVV	Cross-reactivity to VZV
Cell culture characteristics	Cell-associated	Cell-associated
	low titre	low titre
	multinucleated	multinucleated
Genomic characteristics		
structure	Double-stranded linear	Double-stranded linear
size	124 kb	124 kb
molecular weight	80×10^6 daltons	80×10^6 daltons
density (G + C)	46.0%	40.8%

length (Davison and Scott, 1986; Gray et al., 1992; Clarke et al., 1992). The genomes of SVV and VZV share 70–75% DNA homology (Gray and Oakes, 1984) and are collinear (Pumphrey and Gray, 1992; White et al., 1997). The genomic structures of SVV and VZV are similar. Both genomes include a 110 kb U_L sequence covalently linked to a 5.1 kb U_S sequence bracketed by 7.3 kb inverted repeat sequences (Straus et al., 1981; Ecker and Hyman, 1982; Davison and Scott, 1986; Gray et al., 1992). The U_L sequence of VZV is also bracketed by 88 kb inverted repeat sequences, but inverted repeats bracketing the SVV U_L have not been found. Like other herpesviruses, the U_S region of SVV can invert, allowing the genome to exist in two isoforms (Clarke et al., 1992; Gray et al., 1992). SVV DNA has a molecular weight of 80×10^6 (Davison and Scott, 1986), and a density of 1.700 ± 0.002 g/ml, corresponding to a $G + C$ ratio of 40.8%. Like VZV DNA, SVV DNA is infectious (Clarke et al., 1992). Also, SVV produces a cytopathic effect in tissue culture, character- ized by syncytia formation leading to cell lysis, low virus titre and cell- associated virus (Soike, 1992; Soike et al., 1984).

Clinical (Myers and Connelly, 1992; Padovan and Cantrell, 1986) and pathological (Wenner et al., 1977; Padovan and Cantrell, 1986; Dueland et al., 1992) changes produced by acute SVV infection of non-human primates are similar to human varicella. Simian varicella is characterized by an incubation period of one or more weeks followed by fever and a papulovesi- cular rash of skin and mucous membranes. Occasionally, rash becomes haemorrhagic, a poor prognostic sign (Soike, 1992). SVV infection frequently disseminates and has a high mortality (Soike et al., 1984). Although VZV reactivation in humans (zoster) is generally localized to one to three derma- tomes, SVV reactivation often appears as a whole-body rash. During reactiva- tion, SVV can be isolated from skin vesicles, but not from blood (Soike et al., 1984).

During primary infection, SVV-specific antigen and nucleic acid can be detected in liver, lung, spleen, adrenal gland, kidney, lymph node, bone marrow and ganglia at all levels of the neuraxis (Wenner et al., 1977; Roberts et al., 1984; Padovan and Cantrell, 1986; Dueland et al., 1992). Infected lesions are characterized by acute haemorrhagic necrosis, inflamma- tion and cells containing eosinophilic intranuclear inclusion bodies.

SVV and VZV encode antigenically related polypeptides, and SVV-specific antibodies cross-react with human VZV in serum neutralization and comple- ment fixation tests (Felsenfeld and Schmidt, 1975, 1977, 1979; Soike et al., 1987, Fletcher and Gray, 1992). Although VZV does not cause disease in non- human primates, it has been used to immunize and protect monkeys from SVV infection (Felsenfeld and Schmidt, 1979).

Like VZV, SVV becomes latent in dorsal root ganglia at multiple levels of the neuraxis (Mahalingam et al., 1990, 1991), and the entire genome appears to be present (Mahalingam et al., 1992). Furthermore, a region of SVV homologous to VZV gene 21 (one of four VZV genes known to be transcribed in latently infected human ganglia) has been found in latently infected monkey ganglia (Clarke et al., 1996). Already, 53 distinct SVV RNA species on the SVV genome have been mapped (Gray et al., 1993). We have recently constructed a recombinant SVV containing the green fluorescent protein gene under the control of a rous sarcoma virus (RSV) transcriptional promoter (Mahalingam *et al.*, 1998). We use the construct to study the cell type that is latently infected and to analyse further varicella transcription during latency. Thus, SVV provides an extremely useful animal model in which varicella pathogenesis and latency can be studied during life, an approach impossible in humans.

References

Aitken, R. S. and Brain, R. T. (1933). Facial palsy and infection with zoster virus. *Lancet* 1, 19–22.

Amlie-Lefond, C., Kleinschmidt-DeMasters, B. K., Mahalingam, R. *et al.* (1995). The vasculopathy of varicella zoster virus encephalitis. *Ann. Neurol.* 37, 784–790.

Amlie-Lefond, C., Mackin, G. A., Ferguson, M., *et al.* (1996). Another case of virologically confirmed zoster sine herpete, with electrophysiologic correlation. *J. Neuro. Virol.*, 2, 136–138.

Arbeit, R. D., Zaia, J. A., Valerio, M. A. and Levin, M. J. (1982). Infection of human peripheral blood mononuclear cells by varicella-zoster virus. *Intervirology*, 18, 56–65.

Asano, Y., Itakura, N., Hiroishi, Y., *et al.* (1985). Viremia is present in incubation period in nonimmunocompromised children with varicella. *J. Pediatr.*, 106, 69–71.

Baba, K., Yabuuchi, H. and Takahaski, M. (1986). Increased incidence of herpes zoster in normal children infected with varicella zoster virus during infancy: community-based follow-up study. *J. Pediatr.*, 108, 372–377.

Bastian, F. O., Rabson, A. S., Yee, C. L. and Tralka, T. S. (1974). Herpesvirus varicellae: isolated from human dorsal root ganglia. *Arch. Pathol.*, 97, 331–332.

Beards, G., Graham, C. and Pillay, D. (1998). Investigation of vesicular rashes for HSV and VZV by PCR. *J. Med. Virol.*, 54, 155–157.

Bratanich, A. C., Hanson, N. D. and Jones, C. J. (1992). The latency-related gene of bovine herpesvirus 1 inhibits the activity of immediate-early transcription unit 1. *Virology*, 191, 881–988.

Brostoff, J. (1966). Diaphragmatic paralysis after herpes zoster. *Br. Med. J.*, 2, 1571–1572.

Brown, G. R. (1976). Herpes zoster: correlation of age, sex, distribution, neuralgia and associated disorders. *South. Med. J.*, 69, 576–578.

Bullowa, J.G.M. and Wishik, S.M. (1935). Complications of varicella. I. Their occurrence among 2534 patients. *Am. J. Dis. Child.*, 49, 923–926.

Carroll, W.M. and Mastaglia, F.L. (1979). Optic neuropathy and ophthalmoplegia in herpes zoster oticus. *Neurology*, 29, 726–729.

Cauda, R., Chatterjee, S., Tiden, A. B. *et al.* (1986). Replication of varicella zoster virus in Raji cells. *Virus Res.*, 4, 337–342.

Cheatham, W. J., Weller, T. H., Dolan, T. F. and Dower, J. C. (1956). Varicella: Report on two fatal cases with necropsy, virus isolation, and serologic studies. *Am. J. Pathol.*, **32**, 1015–1035.

Clarke, P., Rabkin, S. D., Inman, M. V. *et al.* (1992). Molecular analysis of simian varicella virus DNA. *Virology*, **190**, 597–605.

Clarke, P., Beer, T., Cohrs, R. and Gilden, D. H. (1995). Configuration of latent varicella-zoster virus DNA. *J. Virol.*, **69**, 8151–8154.

Clarke, P., Matlock, W. L., Beer, T. and Gilden, D. H. (1996). A simian varicella virus (SVV) homolog to VZV gene 21 is expressed in monkey ganglia latently infected with SVV. *J. Virol.*, **70**, 5711–5715.

Cohen, J. J. and Straus, S. E. (1996). Varicella-zoster virus and its replication. In: *Fields Virology*, 3rd edn. (B. N. Fields, D. M. Knipe and P. M. Howley, eds). Philadelphia: Lippicott-Raven. pp. 2525–2547.

Cooke, B. E. D. (1960). Epithelial smears in diagnosis of herpes simplex and herpes zoster affecting the oral mucosa. *Brit. Dent. J.*, **109**, 83–96.

Cooke, B. E. D. (1963). Exfoliative cytology in evaluating oral lesions. *J. Dent. Res.*, **42**, 343–347.

Crabtree, J.A. (1968). Herpes zoster oticus. *Laryngoscope*, **78**, 1853–1879.

Croen, K. D., Ostrove, J. M., Dragovic, L. J. and Straus, S. E. (1988). Patterns of gene expression and sites of latency in human nerve ganglia are different for varicella-zoster and herpes simplex viruses. *Proc. Natl Acad. Sci. USA*, **85**, 9773–9777.

Croen, K. D., Dragovic, L., Ostrove, J. M. and Straus, S. E. (1991). Characterization of herpes simplex virus type 2 latency associated transcription in human sacral ganglia and in cell culture. *J. Infect. Dis.*, **163**, 23–28.

Davison, A. J. (1991). Varicella-zoster virus: the fourteenth Fleming Lecture. *J. Gen. Virol.*, **72**, 475–486.

Davison, A. J. and Scott, J. E. (1986). The complete DNA sequence of varicella-zoster virus. *J. Gen. Virol.*, **67**, 1759–1816.

Dayan, A. D., Ogul, E. and Graveson, G. S. (1972). Polyneuritis and herpes zoster. *J. Neurol. Neurosurg. Psych.*, **35**, 170–175.

de Silva, S. M., Mark, A. S., Gilden, D. H. *et al.* (1996). Zoster myelitis: improvement with antiviral therapy in two cases. *Neurology*, **47**, 929–931.

Debrus, S., Sadzot-Delvaux, C., Nikkels, A.F. *et al.* (1995). Varicella-zoster virus gene 63 encodes an immediate-early protein that is abundantly expressed during latency. *J. Virol.*, **69**, 3240–3245.

DeMoragas, J.M. and Kierland, R.R. (1957). The outcome of patients with herpes zoster. *Arch. Dermatol.*, **75**, 193–196.

Denny-Brown, D., Adams, R. D. and Fitzgerald, P. J. (1944). Pathologic features of herpes zoster: A note on 'geniculate herpes'. *Arch. Neurol. Psych.*, **51**, 216–231.

Devlin, M. E., Gilden, D. H., Mahalingam, R. *et al.* (1992). Peripheral blood mono-nuclear cells of the elderly contain varicella-zoster virus DNA. *J. Infect. Dis.*, **165**, 619–622.

Doern, G. V., Robbie, L. and St Armand, R. (1997). Comparison of the Vidas and Bio-Whittaker enzyme immunoassays for detecting IgG reactive with varicella-zoster virus and mumps virus. *Diagn. Microbiol. Infect. Dis.*, **28**, 31–34.

Dueland, A. N., Devlin, M., Martin, J. R. *et al.* (1991). Fatal varicella zoster virus meningoradiculitis without skin involvement. *Ann. Neurol.*, **29**, 569–572.

Dueland, A. N., Martin, J. R., Devlin, M. E. *et al.* (1992). Acute simian varicella infection: clinical, laboratory, pathologic, and virologic features. *Lab. Invest.*, **66**, 762–773.

Dueland, A. N., Ranneberg-Nilsen, T. and Degre, M. (1995). Detection of latent varicella zoster virus DNA and human gene sequences in human trigeminal ganglia by in situ amplification combined with in situ hybridization. *Virology*, **140**, 2055–2066.

Easton, H. G. (1970). Zoster sine herpete causing acute trigeminal neuralgia. *Lancet*, **2**, 1065–1066.

Echevarria, J. M., Martinez-Martin, P., Tellez, A. *et al.* (1987). Aseptic meningitis due to varicella-zoster virus: antibody levels and local synthesis of specific IgG, IgM and IgA. *J. Infect. Dis.*, **155**, 959–967.

Ecker, J. R. and Hyman, R. W. (1982). Varicella zoster virus DNA exists as two isomers. *Proc. Natl Acad. Sci. USA*, **79**, 156–160.

Efstathiou, S., Minson, A. C., Field, H. J. *et al.* (1986). Detection of herpes simplex virus-specific sequences in latently infected mice and in humans. *J. Virol.*, **57**, 446–455.

Eible, R. J. (1983). Intracerebral hemorrhage with herpes zoster ophthalmicus. *Ann. Neurol.*, **14**, 591–592.

Esiri, M. M. and Tomlinson, A. H. (1972). Herpes zoster: demonstration of virus in trigeminal nerve and ganglion by immunofluorescence and electron microscopy. *J. Neurol. Sci.*, **15**, 35–48.

Feldman, S. and Epp, E. (1976). Isolation of varicella-zoster virus from blood. *J. Pediatr.*, **88**, 265–267.

Feldman, S., Chaudary, S., Ossi, M. and Epp, E. (1977). A viremic phase for herpes zoster in children with cancer. *J. Pediatr.*, **91**, 597–600.

Felsenfeld, A. D. and Schmidt, N. J. (1975). Immunological relationship between delta herpesviruses of Patas monkeys and varicella zoster virus of humans. *Infect. Immun.*, **12**, 261–266.

Felsenfeld, A. D. and Schmidt, N. J. (1977). Antigenic relationships between several simian varicella-like viruses and varicella-zoster virus. *Infect. Immun.*, **15**, 807–812.

Felsenfeld, A.D. and Schmidt, N.J. (1979). Varicella-zoster virus immunizes Patas monkeys against simian varicella-like disease. *J. Gen. Virol.*, **42**, 171–178.

Fenner, F. (1948). The pathogenesis of the acute exanthems: an interpretation based on experimental investigations with mousepox (infectious ectromelia of mice). *Lancet*, ii, 915–920.

Fletcher, T. M., III. and Gray, W. L. (1992). Simian varicella virus: characterization of virion and infected cell polypeptides and the antigenic crossreactivity with varicella zoster virus. *J. Gen. Virol.*, **73**, 1209–1215.

Furuta, Y., Fukuda, S., Suzuki, S. *et al.* (1997). Detection of varicella-zoster virus DNA in patients with acute peripheral facial palsy by the polymerase chain reaction, and its use for early diagnosis of zoster sine herpete. *J. Med. Virol.*, **52**, 316–319.

Garnett, G. P. and Grenfell, B. T. (1992). The epidemiology of varicella-zoster virus infections: the influence of varicella on the prevalence of herpes zoster. *Epidemiol. Infect.*, **108**, 513–528.

Garty, B.-Z., Dinari, G., Sarnat, H. *et al.* (1985). Tooth exfoliation and osteonecrosis of the maxilla after trigeminal herpes zoster. *J. Pediatr.*, **106**, 71–73.

Garweg, J. and Bohnke, M. (1997). Varicella-zoster virus is strongly associated with atypical necrotising herpetic retinopathies. *Clin. Infect. Dis.*, **24**, 603–608.

Gershon, A. A., Steinberg, S. and Silber, R. (1978). Varicella-zoster viremia. *J. Pediatr.*, **92**, 1033–1034.

Ghatak, N. R. and Zimmerman, H. M. (1973). Spinal ganglion in herpes zoster. *Arch. Pathol.*, **95**, 411–415.

Gilden, D. H., Wroblewska, Z., Kindt, V. *et al.* (1978). Varicella-zoster virus infection of human brain cells and ganglion cells in tissue culture. *Arch. Virol.*, **56**, 105–117.

Gilden, D. H., Shtram, Y. Friedmann, A. *et al.* (1982). Extraction of cell-associated varicella-zoster virus DNA with triton X-100-NaC1. *J. Virol. Meth.*, **4**, 263–275.

Gilden, D. H., Vafai, A., Shtram, Y. *et al.* (1983). Varicella-zoster virus DNA in human sensory ganglia. *Nature*, **306**, 478–480.

Gilden, D. H., Hayward, A. R., Krupp, J. *et al.* (1987a). Varicella-zoster virus infection of human mononuclear cells. *Virus Res.*, **7**, 117–129.

Gilden, D. H., Rozemann, Y., Murray, R. *et al.* (1987b). Detection of varicella-zoster virus nucleic acid in neurons of normal human thoracic ganglia. *Ann. Neurol.*, **22**, 377–380.

Gilden, D. H., Devlin, M. E., Wellish, M. *et al.* (1988a). Persistence of varicella-zoster virus DNA in blood mononuclear cells of patients with varicella or zoster. *Virus Genes*, **2**, 299–305.

Gilden, D. H., Murray, R. S., Wellish, M. *et al.* (1988b). Chronic progressive varicella-zoster virus encephalitis in an AIDS patient. *Neurology*, **38**, 1150–1153.

Gilden, D. H., Dueland, A. N., Cohrs, R. *et al.* (1991). Preherpetic neuralgia. *Neurology*, **41**, 1215–1218.

Gilden, D. H., Beinlich, B. R., Rubinstein, E. M. *et al.* (1994a). VZV myelitis: an expanding spectrum. *Neurology*, **44**, 1818–1823.

Gilden, D. H., Wright, R. R., Schneck, S. A. *et al.* (1994b). Zoster sine herpete, a clinical variant. *Ann. Neurol.*, **35**, 530–533.

Gilden, D. H., Kleinschmidt-DeMasters, B. K., Wellish, M. *et al.* (1996). Varicella zoster virus, a cause of waxing and waning vasculitis. NEJM case 5-1995 revisited. *Neurology*, **47**, 1441–1446.

Gilden, D. H., Bennett, J. L., Kleinschmidt-DeMasters, B.K. *et al.* (1998). The value of cerebrospinal fluid antiviral antibody in the diagnosis of neurologic disease produced by varicella zoster virus. *J. Neurol. Sci.*, **159**, 140–144.

Gilden, D. H., Kleinschmidt-DeMasters, B. K., LaGuardia, J. J. *et al.* (2000). Neurologic complications of the reactivation of varicella-zoster virus. *N. Engl. J. Med.*, **342**, 635–645.

Gleaves, C. A., Schwarz, K. A. and Campbell, M. B. (1996). Determination of varicella-zoster virus (VZV) immune status with the VIDAS immunoglobulin G automated immunoassay and the VZV Scan latex agglutination assay. *Clin. Diagn. Lab. Immunol.*, **3**, 365–367.

Gold, E. (1966). Serologic and virus-isolation studies of patients with varicella or herpes-zoster infection. *N. Engl. J. Med.*, **274**, 181–185.

Gray, W. L. and Oakes, J. E. (1984). Simian varicella virus DNA shares homology with human varicella-zoster virus DNA. *Virology*, **136**, 241–246.

Gray, W. L., Pumphrey, C. Y., Ruyechen, W. T. and Fletcher, T. M. (1992). The simian varicella virus and varicella zoster virus geomes are similar in size and structure. *Virology*, **186**, 562–572.

Gray, W. L., Gusick, N., Fletcher, T. M. and Pumphrey, C. Y. (1993). Characterization and mapping of simian varicella virus transcripts. *J. Gen. Virol.*, **74**, 1639–1643.

Grose, C. (1981). Variation on a theme by Fenner: The pathogenesis of chickenpox. *Pediatrics*, **68**, 735–737.

Guess, H. A., Broughton, D. D., Melton, L. J. and Kurland, L. T. (1985). Epidemiology of herpes zoster in children and adolescents: A population-based study. *Pediatrics*, **76**, 512–517.

Gustafson, T. L., Lavely, G. B., Brawner, E. R. JR *et al.* (1982). An outbreak of airborne nosocomial varicella. *Pediatrics*, **70**, 550–556.

Hall, S., Carlin, L., Roach, S. E. *et al.* (1983). Herpes zoster and central retinal artery occlusion. *Ann. Neurol.*, **13**, 217–218.

Halloran, M. E. (1996). Epidemiologic effects of varicella vacinnation. *Infect. Dis. Clin. North Am.*, **10**, 631–655.

Harnisch, J. P. (1984). Zoster in the elderly: clinical, immunologic and therapeutic considerations. *J. Am. Geriatr. Soc.*, **32**, 789–793.

Hayakawa, Y. and Hyman, R. W. (1987). Isomerization of the U_L region of varicella-zoster virus DNA. *Virus Res.*, **8**, 25–31.

Haymaker, W. and Kernohan, J. W. (1949). The Landry-Guillain-Barré syndrome. *Medicine*, **28**, 59–141.

Head, H. and Campbell, A. W. (1900). The pathology of herpes zoster and its bearing on sensory localization. *Brain*, **23**, 353–523.

Heller, H. M., Carnevale, N. T. and Steigbigel, R. T. (1990). Varicella zoster virus transverse myelitis without cutaneous rash. *Am. J. Med.*, **88**, 550–551.

Hilt, D. C., Buchholz, D., Krumholz, A. *et al.* (1983). Herpes zoster ophthalmicus and delayed contralateral hemiparesis caused by cerebral angiitis: diagnosis and management approaches. *Ann. Neurol.*, **14**, 543–553.

Hogan, E. L. and Krigman, M. R. (1973). Herpes zoster myelitis: Evidence for viral invasion of spinal cord. *Arch. Neurol.*, **29**, 309–313.

Hope-Simpson, R. E. (1965). The nature of herpes zoster: a long-term study and a new hypothesis. *Proc. R. Soc. Med.*, **58**, 9–20.

Hope-Simpson, R. E. (1975). Postherpetic neuralgia. *J. Roy. Coll. Gen. Pract.*, **25**, 571–575.

Horton, B., Price, R. W. and Jimenez, D. (1981). Multifocal varicella-zoster virus leukoencephalitis temporally remote from herpes zoster. *Ann. Neurol.*, **9**, 251–266.

Hurwitz, E. S., Nelson, D. B., Davis, C. *et al.* (1982). National surveillance for Reye syndrome: a five-year review. *Pediatrics*, **70**, 895–900.

Hyman, R. W., Ecker, J. R. and Tenser, R. B. (1983). Varicella-zoster virus RNA in human trigeminal ganglia. *Lancet*, **2**, 814–816.

Izumi, A. I. and Edwards, J. (1973). Herpes zoster and neurogenic bladder dysfunction. *J. Am. Med. Assoc.*, **224**, 1748–1749.

Jellinek, E. H. and Tulloch, W. S. (1976). Herpes zoster with dysfunction of bladder and anus. *Lancet*, **2**, 1219–1222.

Josephson, A. and Gombert, M. E. (1988). Airborne transmission of nosocomial varicella from localized zoster. *J. Infect. Dis.*, **158**, 238–241.

Källander, C. F., Gronowitz, J. S. and Olding-Stenkvist, E. (1989). Varicella zoster virus deoxythymidine kinase is present in serum before the onset of varicella. *Scand. J. Infect. Dis.*, **21**, 255–257.

Kennedy, P. G. E., Grinfeld, E. and Gow, J. W. (1998). Latent varicella-zoster virus is located predominantly in neurons in human trigeminal ganglia. *Proc. Natl Acad. Sci. USA*, **95**, 4658–4662.

Kido, S., Ozaki, T., Asada, H. *et al.* (1991). Detection of varicella-zoster virus (VZV) DNA in clinical samples from patients with VZV by the polymerase chain reaction. *J. Clin. Microbiol.*, **29**, 76–79.

Kinchington, P. R. Reinhold, W. C., Casey T. A. *et al.* (1985). Inversion and circularization of the varicella-zoster virus genome. *J. Virol.*, **56**, 194–200.

Knox, C. M., Chandler, D., Short, G. A. and Margolis, T. P. (1998). Polymerase chain reaction-based assays of vitreous samples for the diagnosis of viral retinitis. Use in diagnostic dilemmas. *Ophthalmology*, **105**, 37–44.

Koropchak, C. M., Solem, S. D., Diaz, P. S. and Arvin, A. M. (1989). Investigation of varicella-zoster virus infection of lymphocytes by in situ hybridization. *J. Virol.*, **63**, 2392–2395.

Koropchak, C. M., Graham, G., Palmer, J. *et al.* (1991). Investigation of varicella-zoster virus infection by polymerase chain reaction in the immunocompetent host with acute varicella. *J. Infect. Dis.*, **163**, 1016–1022.

Kuroiwa, Y. and Furukawa, T. (1981). Hemispheric infarction after herpes zoster ophthalmicus: computed tomography and angiography. *Neurology*, **31**, 1030–1032.

Kutish, G., Mainprize, T. and Rock, D. (1990). Characterization of the latency-related transcriptionally active region of bovine herpesvirus 1 genome. *J. Virol.*, **64**, 5730–5737.

Lapresle, J. and Lasjuanias, P. (1986). Cranial nerve ischemic arterial syndromes. *Brain*, **109**, 207–215.

Leclair, J. M., Zaia, J. A., Levin, M.J. *et al.* (1980). Airborne transmission of chickenpox in a hospital. *N. Engl. J. Med.*, **302**, 450–453.

Leventon-Kriss, S., Gotlieb-Stematsky, T., Vonsover, A. *et al.* (1979). Infection and persistence of varicella-zoster virus in lymphoblastoid raji cell line. *Med. Microbiol. Immunol.*, **167**, 275–283.

Lewis, G. W. (1958). Zoster sine herpete. *Br. Med. J.*, **2**, 418–421.

Longfield, J. N., Winn, R. E., Gibson, R. L. *et al.* (1990). Varicella outbreaks in army recruits from Puerto Rico. *Arch. Intern. Med.*, **150**, 970–973.

Lungu, O., Annunziato, P.W., Gershon, A. *et al.* (1995). Reactivated and latent varicella-zoster virus in human dorsal root ganglia. *Proc. Natl Acad. Sci. USA*, **92**, 10980–10984.

Maguire, H. F. and Hyman, R. W. (1986). Polyadenylated, cytoplasmic transcripts of varicella-zoster virus. *Intervirology*, **26**, 181–191.

Mahalingam, R., Wellish, M., Wolf, W. *et al.* (1990). Latent varicella-zoster viral DNA in human trigeminal and thoracic ganglia. *N. Engl. J. Med.*, **323**, 627–631.

Mahalingam, R., Smith, D., Wellish, M. *et al.* (1991). Simian varicella virus DNA in dorsal root ganglia. *Proc. Natl Acad. Sci. USA*, **88**, 2750–2752.

Mahalingam, R., Clarke, P., Wellish, M. *et al.* (1992). Prevalence and distribution of latent simian varicella virus DNA in monkey ganglia. *Virology*, **188**, 193–197.

Mahalingam, R., Wellish, M., Lederer, D. *et al.* (1993). Quantitation of latent varicella-zoster virus DNA in human trigeminal ganglia by polymerase chain reaction. *J. Virol.*, **67**, 2381–2384.

Mahalingam, R., Wellish, M., Brucklier, J. and Gilden, D. H. (1995). Persistence of varicella-zoster virus DNA in elderly patients with postherpetic neuralgia. *J. NeuroVirol.*, **1**, 130–133.

Mahalingam, R., Wellish, M., Cohrs, R. *et al.* (1996). Expression of protein encoded by varicella-zoster virus open reading frame 63 in latently infected human ganglionic neurons. *Proc. Natl Acad. Sci. USA*, **93**, 2122–2124.

Mahalingam, R., Wellish, M., White, T. *et al.* (1998). Infectious simian varicella virus expressing the green fluorescent protein. *J. Neurovirol.*, **4**, 438–444.

Manz, H. J., Canter, H. G. and Melton, J. (1986). Trigeminal herpes zoster causing mandibular osteonecrosis and spontaneous tooth exfoliation. *South. Med. J.*, **79**, 1026–1028.

Martinez-Martin, P., Garcia-Saiz, A., Rapun, J. L. and Echevarria, J. M. (1985). Intrathecal synthesis of IgG antibodies to varicella-zoster virus in two cases of acute aseptic meningitis syndrome with no cutaneous lesions. *J. Med. Virol.*, **16**, 201–209.

Mayberg, M. R., Zervas, N. T. and Moskowitz, M. A. (1984). Trigeminal projections to supratentorial pial and dural blood vessels in cats demonstrated by horseradish peroxidase histochemistry. *J. Comp. Neurol.*, **223**, 46–56.

Mayo, D. R. and Booss, J. (1989). Varicella zoster-associated neurologic disease without skin lesions. *Arch. Neurol.*, **46**, 313–315.

McGeoch, D. J., Dolan, A., Donald, S. and Rixon, F. J. (1985). Sequence determination and genetic content of the short unique region in the genome of herpes simplex virus type 1. *J. Mol. Biol.*, **181**, 1–13.

McGeoch, D. J., Dolan, A., Donald, S. and Brauer, D. H. K. (1986). Complete DNA sequence of the short repeat region in the genome of herpes simplex virus type 1. *Nucl. Acid Res.*, **14**, 1727–1745.

McGeoch, D. J., Dalrymple, M. A., Davion, A. J. *et al.* (1988). The complete DNA sequence of the long unique region in the genome of herpes simplex virus type 1. *J. Gen. Virol.*, **69**, 1531–1574.

Meier, J. L., Holman, R. P., Croen, K. D. *et al.* (1993). Varicella-zoster virus transcription in human trigeminal ganglia. *Virology*, **193**, 193–200.

Mietz, H., Eis-Hubinger, A. M., Sundmacher, R. and Font, R. L. (1997). Detection of varicella-zoster virus DNA in keratectomy specimens by use of the polymerase chain reaction. *Arch. Ophthalmol.*, **115**, 590–594.

Miller, D. H., Kay, R., Schon, F. *et al.* (1986). Optic neuritis following chickenpox in adults. *J. Neurol.*, **233**, 182–184.

Miller, H. G., Stanton, J. B. and Gibbons, J. (1956). Para-infectious encephalomyelitis and related syndromes: a critical review of the neurological complications of certain specific fevers. *Q. J. Med.*, **25**, 427–505.

Mitchell, W. J. Lirette, R. P. and Fraser, N. W. (1990). Mapping of low abundance latency-associated RNA in the trigeminal ganglia of mice latently infected with herpes simplex virus type 1. *J. Gen. Virol.*, **71**, 125–132.

Mustonen, K., Mustakangas, P., Smeds, M. *et al.* (1998). Antibodies to varicella zoster virus in the cerebrospinal fluid of neonates with seizures. *Arch. Dis. Child. Fetal Neonatal Ed.*, **78**, F57–F61.

Myers, M. G. (1979). Viremia caused by varicella-zoster virus: Association with malignant progressive varicella. *J. Infect. Dis.*, **140**, 229–233.

Myers, M. G. and Connelly, B. L. (1992). Animal models of varicella. *J. Infect. Dis.*, **166**, 548–550.

Nagashima, K., Nakazawa, M. and Endo, H. (1975). Pathology of the human spinal ganglia in varicella-zoster virus infection. *Acta Neuropathol.*, **33**, 105–117.

Nassar, N. T. and Touma, H. C. (1986). Susceptibility of Filipino nurses to the varicella-zoster virus. *Infect. Control*, 7, 71–72.

Osaki, Y., Matsubayashi, K., Okumiya, K. *et al.* (1995). Polyneuritis cranialis due to varicella-zoster virus in the absence of rash. *Neurology*, 45, 2293.

Ostrove, J. M., Reinhold, W., Fan, C. M. *et al.* (1985). Transcription mapping of the varicella-zoster virus genome. *J. Virol.*, 56, 600–606.

Ozaki, T., Ichikawa, T., Matsui, Y. *et al.* (1986). Lymphocyte-associated viremia in varicella. *J. Med. Virol.*, 19, 249–253.

Ozaki, T., Matsui, Y., Asano, Y. *et al.* (1989). Study of virus isolation from pharyngeal swabs in children with varicella. *Am. J. Dis. Child.*, 143, 1448–1450.

Ozaki, T., Miwata, H., Matsui, Y. *et al.* (1991). Varicella zoster virus DNA in throat swabs. *Arch. Dis. Child.*, 66, 333–334.

Padovan, D. and Cantrell, C. A. (1986). Varicella-like herpesvirus infections of non-human primates. *Lab. Anim. Sci.*, 36, 7–13.

Perry, L. J. and McGeoch, D. J. (1988). The DNA sequences of the long report region and adjoining parts of the long unique region in the genome of herpes simplex virus type 1. *J. Gen. Virol.*, 69, 2831–2846.

Preblud, S. R. (1986). Varicella: complications and costs. *Pediatrics*, 78, 728–735.

Preblud, S. R. and D'Angelo, L. J. (1979). From the Center for Disease Control: Chickenpox in the United States. *J. Infect. Dis.*, 140, 257–260.

Preblud, S. R., Orenstein, W. A. and Bart, K. J. (1984). Varicella: clinical manifestations, epidemiology and health impact in children. *Pediatr. Infect. Dis.*, 3, 505–509.

Priola, S. A., Gustafson, D. P., Wagner, E. K. and Stevens, J. G. (1990). A major portion of the latent pseudorabies virus genome is transcribed in trigeminal ganglia of pigs. *J. Virol.*, 64, 4755–4760.

Puchhammer-Stockl, E., Popow-Kraupp, T., Heinz, F. X. *et al.* (1991). Detection of varicella-zoster virus DNA by polymerase chain reaction in the cerebrospinal fluid of patients suffering from neurological complications associated with chickenpox or herpes zoster. *J. Clin. Microbiol.*, 29, 1513–1516.

Pumphrey, C. Y. and Gray, W. L. (1992). The genomes of simian varicella and varicella zoster virus are collinear. *Virus Res.*, 26, 255–266.

Ragozzino, M. W., Melton, L. J. III, Kurland, L. T. *et al.* (1982). Population-based study of herpes zoster and its sequelae. *Medicine*, 61, 310–316.

Reimer, L. G. and Reller, L. B. (1981). CSF in herpes zoster meningo-encephalitis. *Arch. Neurol.*, 38, 668.

Reinhold, W. C., Straus, S. E. and Ostrove, J. M. (1988). Directionality and further mapping of varicella zoster virus transcripts. *Virus Res.*, 9, 249–261.

Remington, P. L., Rowley, D., McGee, H. *et al.* (1986). Decreasing trends in Reye syndrome and aspirin use in Michigan, 1979 to 1984. *Pediatrics*, 77, 93–98.

Roberts, E. D., Baskin, G. B., Soike, K. and Gibson, S. V. (1984). Pathologic changes of experimental simian varicella (Delta herpesvirus) infection in African green monkeys (*Cercopithecus aethiops*). *Am. J. Vet. Res.*, **45**, 523–530.

Rock, D. L. and Fraser, N. W. (1983). Detection of HSV-1 genome in central nervous system of latently infected mice. *Nature (Lond.)*, **302**, 523–525.

Rock, D. L. and Fraser, N. W. (1985). Latent herpes simplex virus type 1 DNA contains two copies of the virion DNA joint region. *J. Virol.*, **55**, 849–852.

Rogers, R. S. and Tindall, J. P. (1971). Geriatric herpes zoster. *J. Am. Geriatr. Soc.*, **19**, 495–503.

Rubben, A., Baron, J. M. and Grussendorf-Conen, E. I. (1997). Routine detection of herpes simplex virus and varicella-zoster virus by polymerase chain reaction reveals that initial herpes zoster is frequently misdiagnosed as herpes simplex. *Br. J. Dermatol.*, **137**, 259–261.

Ryder, J. W., Croen, K., Kleinschmidt-DeMasters, B. K. *et al.* (1986). Progressive encephalitis three months after resolution of cutaneous zoster in a patient with AIDS. *Ann. Neurol.*, **19**, 182–188.

Schmidt, N. Y. and Arvin, A. M. (1986). Sensitivity of different assay systems for immunoglobulin in responses to varicella zoster virus in reactivated infections (zoster). *J. Clin. Microbiol.*, **19**, 310–316.

Schott, G. D. (1998). Triggering of delayed-onset postherpetic neuralgia. *Lancet*, **351**, 419–420.

Shibuta, H., Ishikawa, T., Hondo, R. *et al.* (1974). Varicella virus isolation from spinal ganglion. *Arch. Virusforsch*, **45**, 382–385.

Soike, K. F. (1992). Simian varicella virus infection in African and Asian monkeys. The potential for development of antivirals for animal diseases. *Ann. N. Y. Acad. Sci.*, **653**, 323–333.

Soike, K. F., Rangan, S. R. S. and Gerone, P. J. (1984). Viral disease models in primates. *Adv. Vet. Sci. Comp. Med.*, **28**, 151–199.

Soike, K. F., Keller, P. M. and Ellis, R. W. (1987). Immunization of monkeys with varicella zoster virus glycoprotein antigens and their response to challenge with simian varicella virus. *J. Med. Virol.*, **22**, 307–313.

Stebbings, S., Highton, J., Croxson, M.C. *et al.* (1998). Chickenpox monoarthritis: demonstration of varicella-zoster in joint fluid by polymerase chain reaction. *Br. J. Rheumatol.*, **37**, 311–313.

Steffen, R. and Selby, G. (1972). 'Atypical' Ramsay Hunt syndrome. *Med. J. Aust.*, **1**, 227–230.

Stevens, J. G., Wagner, E. K., Devi-Rao, G. B. *et al.* (1987). RNA complementary to a herpesvirus α gene mRNA is prominent in latently infected neurons. *Science*, **235**, 1056–1059.

Stowasser, M., Cameron, J. and Oliver, W. A. (1990). Diaphragmatic paralysis following cervical herpes zoster. *Med. J. Aust.*, **153**, 555–556.

Straus, S. E., Aulakh, H. S., Ruychan, W. T. *et al.* (1981). Structure of varicella virus DNA. *J. Virol.*, **40**, 516–525.

Straus, S. E., Owens, J., Ruyechan, W. T. *et al.* (1982). Molecular cloning and physical mapping of varicella-zoster virus DNA. *Proc. Natl Acad. Sci. USA*, **79**, 993–997.

Tako, J. and Rado, J. P. (1965). Zoster meningoencephalitis in a steroid-treated patient. *Arch. Neurol.*, **12**, 610–612.

Taylor-Robinson, D. and Caunt, A. E. (1972). Varicella virus. In: *Virology Monographs* (S. Gard, C. Hallauer and K.F. Meyer, eds). New York: Springer-Verlag. pp. 13–17.

Thomas, E. J. and Howard, F. M. (1972). Segmental zoster paresis – a disease profile. *Neurology*, **22**, 459–466.

Tomlinson, T. H. (1939). Giant cell formation in the tonsils in the prodromal stage of chickenpox. *Am. J. Path.*, **15**, 523–526.

Twomey, J. J., Gyorkey, F. and Norris, S. M. (1974). The monocyte disorder with herpes zoster. *J. Lab. Clin. Med.*, **83**, 768–777.

Tyzzer, E.E. (1906). The histology of the skin lesions in varicella. *Philippine J. Sci.*, **1**, 349–372.

Underwood, E.A. (1935). The neurological complications of varicella: a clinical and epidemiological study. *Br. J. Child. Dis.*, **32**, 83–107.

Vafai, A., Mahalingam, R., Zerbe, G. *et al.* (1988a). Detection of antibodies to varicella-zoster virus proteins in sera from the elderly. *Gerontology*, **34**, 242–249.

Vafai, A., Murray, R. S., Wellish, M. *et al.* (1988b). Expression of varicella-zoster virus and herpes simplex virus in normal human trigeminal ganglia. *Proc. Natl Acad. Sci. USA*, **85**, 2362–2366.

Vartdal, F., Vandvik, B. and Norby, E. (1982). Intrathecal synthesis of virus-specific oligoclonal IgG, IgA and IgM antibodies in a case of varicella-zoster meningoencephalitis. *J. Neurol. Sci.*, **57**, 121–132.

von Barensprung, F.G.F. (1863). Beiträge zur Kenntnis des Zoster. *Ann. Chir. Krankenh*, **11**, 96–104.

Vonsover, A., Leventon-Kriss, S., Langer, A. *et al.* (1987). Detection of varicella-zoster virus in lymphocytes by DNA hybridization. *J. Med. Virol.*, **21**, 57–66.

Weber, F.P. (1916). Herpes zoster: its occasional association with a generalized eruption and its occasional connection with muscular paralysis – also an analysis of the literature of the subject. *Int. Clin.*, **3**, 185–202.

Weller, T. H., Witton, H. M and Bell, E. J. (1958). The etiologic agents of varicella and herpes zoster. Isolation, propagation, and cultural characteristics in vitro. *J. Exp. Med.*, **108**, 843–868.

Wenner, H. A., Abel, D., Barrick, S. and Seshummurty, P. (1977). Clinical and pathogenetic studies of Medical Lake macaque virus infection in cynomolgus monkeys (simian varicella). *J. Infect. Dis.*, **135**, 611–622.

Wharton, M. (1996). The epidemiology of varicella-zoster virus infections. *Infect. Dis. Clin. North Am.*, **10**, 571–581.

White, T. M., Mahalingam, R., Kolhatkar, G. and Gilden, D. H. (1997). Identification of simian varicella virus homologues of varicella zoster virus genes. *Virus Genes*, **15**, 265–269.

Widal (1907). *J. Med. Chiropractic Pract.*, **78**, 12.

Williams, B. and Capers, T.H. (1959). The demonstration of intranuclear inclusion bodies in sputum from a patient with varicella pneumonia. *Am. J. Med.*, **27**, 836–839.

Wohlwill, F. (1924). Zur pathologischen anatomie des Nervensystems beim herpes zoster. *Zentralbl. Gesamte Neurol. Psych.*, **89**, 171–212.

Wolf, S. M. (1974). Decreased cerebrospinal fluid glucose level in herpes zoster meningitis. *Arch. Neurol.*, **30**, 109.

11

Neurological aspects of human African trypanosomiasis

Jorge L. M. de Atouguia and Peter G. E. Kennedy

Introduction

Human African trypanosomiasis, also known as sleeping sickness, is caused by protozoan parasites of the *Trypanosoma* species and occurs in 36 African countries, between latitudes 14° North and 29° South. In general, the localization is determined by the distribution of the tsetse fly vectors. However, sleeping sickness is a focal disease, and there are areas where the vectors are present but there is no transmission (Cruz Ferreira, 1973). It is estimated that 50 million people are at risk of contracting the disease (World Health Organization, 1986). The reported annual incidence of human cases has increased year after year (from between 6000 to 10 000 in 1984 (Spencer, 1984) to 20 000 in 1986 (World Health Organization, 1986) and 25 000 in 1993 (Kuzoe, 1993)), although the presumed incidence is between 200 000 and 300 000 new human cases each year (Kuzoe, 1993). Sleeping sickness is considered to be a major health problem in many African countries. Epidemics are not uncommon, usually resulting from an increase in man–fly contact from population movements, changes in vegetation or climate, interruption of systematic medical surveillance, introduction of new virulent strains of the parasite, or, in some instances, a natural periodicity, perhaps related to the susceptibility of humans. The most recent outbreaks occurred in Kenya and Uganda during 1980, but the actual situation in West Africa, namely in Angola and in the Democratic Republic of Congo, is explosive (Cattand, 1994). Animal trypanosomiasis is also an important economic and social problem: due to the disease, vast areas of Africa cannot be used to breed domestic animals, namely cattle, goats, camels and horses (Figure 11.1).

Transmission and life cycle

The vector is the genus *Glossina* which contains more than 20 species of tsetse fly, all restricted to Africa. Only a few, however, are of importance in the

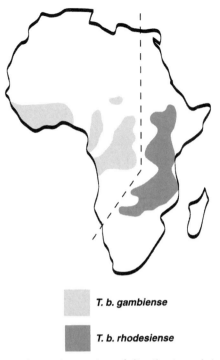

T. b. gambiense

T. b. rhodesiense

Figure 11.1   Diagrammatic representation of distribution of the two types of human African trypanosomiasis in Africa (modified, with permission, from WHO).

transmission of sleeping sickness. Both sexes feed on mammalian blood (Cruz Ferreira, 1973) and inflict painful bites (Manson-Bahr and Apted, 1982). Tsetse flies are viviparous and produce mature larvae that pupate after burrowing into sandy soil (Glasgow, 1970). They live in hot, dark, moist places in proximity of blood meals. The flies that transmit Gambian (West African) and Rhodesian (East African) disease have different ecological requirements that relate to the epidemiological differences between the two types (Manson-Bahr and Apted, 1982). In natural conditions, between 2 and 10% of the flies are infected in an endemic area. A fly remains infective for life (Cruz Ferreira, 1973).

The trypanosomes are transmitted cyclically by blood-sucking flies of the genus *Glossina* (Figure 11.2). Trypomastigotes are ingested during the blood meal. Only short stumpy trypanosomes and those with intermediate morphology are infective to the fly (Vickerman and Tetley, 1978). Morphological changes in the trypanosomes in the anterior midgut of the tsetse fly include elongation of the post-kinetoplast portion of the body as the simple mitochondrion enlarges and becomes branched. At the same time, glycosomes change from spherical to elongated structures (Vickerman, 1985). As the trypanosomes change, there is a switch of energy source: glucose to proline, the source of energy to the tsetse fly (Hatson, 1975) and a change from aerobic to anaerobic respiration (Bowman and Flynn, 1976). In the midgut of the fly, the

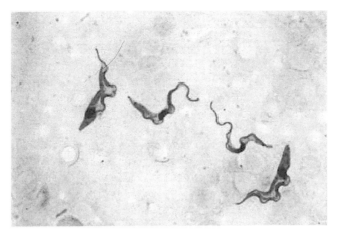

Figure 11.2 Blood slide which has been stained with Giemsa's staining showing trypanosomes in the blood.

ingested blood forms lose their variant surface antigenic coat and begin to multiply (Steiger, 1973). Long, slender forms are produced which then move to the salivary glands and form epimastigotes. In turn, these epimastigotes change into short, stumpy, infective metacyclic trypanosomes (Vickerman, 1985), which enter the bite wound through the hypopharynx. Flies become infective 18–35 days (usually approximately 21 days) after feeding on an infected host, depending on the temperature and the humidity. The intratsetse cycle is complex and is probably only completed in less than one in 10 tsetse flies.

Mechanical transmission can theoretically occur when any biting fly, including the tsetse fly, probes an infected host, is disturbed while feeding and, before the blood on the mouth parts has dried, bites again, inoculating trypanosomes in the second host (Cruz Ferreira, 1973). The epidemiological significance of this mode of transmission is unknown (Gouteux et al., 1988). Congenital transmission has been reported but is rare (Rosário Pinto, 1960; Buyst, 1973; Triolo, 1990). Transmission by blood transfusion is also possible but unusual (Spencer, 1984).

The two types of human African trypanosomiasis

West African (Gambian) trypanosomiasis and East African (Rhodesian) trypanosomiasis are epidemiologically and clinically distinct (Cruz Ferreira, 1973). Overlap of distribution occurs in several areas.

West African (Gambian) trypanosomiasis

Gambian trypanosomiasis is caused by *Trypanosoma (Trypanozoon) brucei gambiense*. The disease is a rural one because of the characteristics of the vector and reservoir. The vectors are the 'riverine' tsetse flies *Glossina palpalis*,

G. tachinoides and *G. fuscipes* (Manson-Bahr and Apted, 1982). The principal habitat of these tsetse flies is dense vegetation along rivers and forests, where proper conditions of temperature, moisture, and light are combined with the availability of blood meals (Glasgow, 1970). The distribution is focal (Morris, 1962; Cruz Ferreira, 1973), and these flies readily adapt to whatever source of food is available. Humans are the preferred host and are frequently bitten at water sites, particularly during the dry season, when only holes of water are left, thereby concentrating man–fly contact (Willett, 1963). Humans and peridomestic animals, namely pigs (Gouteux and Malonga, 1985), dogs and goats, are the most important reservoirs (Kageruka, 1989; Noireau *et al.*, 1989). The incidence of the disease is not determined by sex, age, or race characteristics, but only by the risk of exposure (Cruz Ferreira, 1973). The long incubation period and chronicity of the disease reflect the high degree of adaptation of the parasite to humans as a host and are important in transmission. Many infected individuals are almost symptom-free. These human asymptomatic carriers can infect flies, in spite of very low parasitae-mias, and may play a role in the spread of the disease (Cruz Ferreira, 1973; Ricosse *et al.*, 1973).

East African (Rhodesian) trypanosomiasis

East African sleeping sickness is caused by *Trypanosoma (Trypanozoon) brucei rhodesiense* and is transmitted by *G. morsitans, G. pallidipes* and *G. swynnertoni* (Manson-Bahr and Apted, 1982), tsetse flies which are widely distributed through the woodland and thickets of East African lakes and savannah (Glasgow, 1970). These tsetse flies are less flexible in their choice of blood meals than the *G. palpalis* group (Ashcroft, 1959). The disease is a zoonosis, and the most important reservoirs are antelope, particularly bushbuck (*Tragelaphus scriptus*) and hartebeest (*Alcephalus* sp.). Cattle are the domestic reservoirs (Onyango *et al.*, 1966). Many other animals can become infected but are not effective as reservoirs because either parasitaemia is transient or the animal quickly succumbs to the disease (Ashcroft, 1959).

The dependence of the *G. morsitans* group of tsetse flies on the game means that they are generally confined to country regions away from human habitation. Thus, Rhodesian sleeping sickness is an occupational hazard, relatively frequent in fishermen, hunters and game wardens (Cruz Ferreira, 1973; Mbulamberi, 1989a). Humans become infected by travelling into fly-infested country or when vegetation and humidity favour the establishment of man–fly contact close to homesteads (Mbulamberi, 1989a). Sporadic cases are often seen, and the disease is a special threat to visitors to the game reserves of East Africa. Age, sex, and race have no influence on the risk of infection except as they relate to exposure (Willett, 1963). The acute nature of the disease and the risk of spread from an enzoonotic focus imply that epidemics are always possible (World Health Organization, 1986).

The use of land, the presence of game or cattle, and glossina are not compatible, and vast areas of Africa are unused because of the presence of tsetse flies (Travassos Santos Dias, 1988).

Current status of human trypanosomiasis in Africa

The history of sleeping sickness has been characterized by waves of epidemics, resurgences, and outbreaks. Nevertheless, sleeping sickness was brought practically under control in the early 1950s, in West and Central Africa, through systematic surveillance of the population at risk and in East Africa, mainly by vector control. Social and political changes, failure of national health authorities to give due attention to sleeping sickness control, civil and political unrest, lack of adequate resources, and competing national health priorities, have resulted in epidemics and resurgence of many old foci of disease, and the appearance of new ones (Kuzoe, 1993). Reports from endemic areas show explosive situations in several African countries: in the Democratic Republic of Congo, prevalences have reached 70% in a large region east of Kinshasa, with a global prevalence of 3–5% (i.e. 200 000 infected persons) (Cattand, 1994); in Angola, the global prevalence is now 4–6%. In some villages, half the population is infected, and some previously extinct foci, such as the Quiçama foci, south of Luanda, have reappeared, and are very active (Josinande Théophile, personal communication); in Uganda and Tanzania, the prevalence of the disease in some regions is around 5%; in Congo and in Burkina Faso hundreds of new cases have been diagnosed (Cattand, 1994). The list of active foci is long. Unfortunately, for political, social and economical reasons, most of these foci are not getting adequate attention, and the current situation of human African trypanosomiasis is deteriorating very quickly.

Clinical manifestations of human African trypanosomiasis

(Table 11.1)

Sleeping sickness is characterized clinically by the development of a lesion at the site of the infected tsetse bite, followed by parasitaemia, fever, and haemolymphatic involvement and then by CNS invasion, with meningoencephalitis and death. Clinical manifestations may vary greatly and are not pathognomonic (Dutertre, 1968; Foulkes, 1981; Mbulamberi, 1989b; Jannin et al., 1993). Rhodesiense disease is usually an acute disease with chancre, fever, early CNS involvement (within 3–4 weeks), no clear distinction between early and late stages, often prominent cardiac involvement, and death within weeks to months (Dutertre, 1968; Apted, 1970a). In contrast, Gambian sleeping sickness is characterized by prominent involvement of lymph glands, late CNS symptoms and signs, and a chronic progressive course that may last months to years before death ensues (Dutertre, 1968; Apted, 1970a).

Non-neurological features

Chancre

A primary lesion (the trypanosomal chancre) may develop within 5–15 days at the site of the tsetse fly bite. Shorter and longer incubation periods have been

Table 11.1 Clinical features of African trypanosomiasis (both stages) in European patients (based on Duggan and Hutchington, 1966).

	Percentage
Constitutional signs and symptoms	
fever	74.3
debility	38.5
headache	24.5
oedema	24.5
anaemia	19.6
Cutaneous signs	
rash	50
chancre	22.6–45.8
pruritus	?
Cardiovascular signs	
tachycardia	36.6
Gastrointestinal signs	
hepatomegaly	23.8
splenonegaly	23.8
Central nervous system symptoms and signs	
somnolence	37.8
hyperaesthesia	26.6
tremor, abnormal movements	25.7
psychiatric symptoms	20.1
ataxia	16.6
slurred speech	10.6
Other symptoms or signs	
lymphadenopathy	50

described (Apted, 1970a; Foulkes, 1981). The chancre starts as a small subcutaneous nodule, and develops into a painful, circumscribed, rubbery, indurated, dusky-red papule, usually 2–5 cm in diameter but, in some cases, reaching 10 cm or more (Willett, 1966). The lesion can be described as a 'furuncle without head' (Blin and Kernéis, 1916; Vernier, 1953; Reynaud *et al.*, 1963) and resembles, on palpation, an early subcutaneous cellulitis without its tenderness, never developing a fluctuant centre (Willett, 1966). It can be found in the trunk, arms but mainly in the legs (Robertson and Baker, 1958; Duggan and Hutchington, 1966; Mbulamberi, 1989b) and subsides spontaneously after 2–3 weeks. After the disappearance of the reaction, the skin at the site of inoculation remains discoloured, the colour varying from pink to dusky-red, and fine superficial desquamation occurs (Fairbairn, 1956; Willett, 1966). The frequency of the primary lesion is variable (Bertrand *et al.*, 1973a), but it occurs more often in non-immune individuals (Gelfand, 1966; Foulkes, 1981) and may be more common in *Trypanosoma b. rhodesiense* infection (Duggan and Hutchington, 1966). The lesions may be associated with local lymph gland enlargement (Reynaud *et al.*, 1963). Prominent cellulitis may occur and mask the chancre.

Early stage (haemolymphatic involvement)

Within a few hours to days after the appearance of the chancre or, if there is no chancre, within 1–3 weeks after the infection bite has occurred, trypanosomes invade the blood stream, the lymph nodes and the tissues. Non-immune cases tend to have an acute onset. In West Africa the onset may be more gradual, and several years may pass before the evidence of clinical symptoms. Symptoms and signs are non-specific, irregular, and inconsistent. All the usual features of ill-health, namely malaise, persistent headache, fatigue, dizziness, joint pains, weight loss and weakness, may be present. The main symptoms and signs during this stage are as follows:

Fever. The first symptom is usually an attack of high fever, accompanied by a frontal or temporal headache, and sometimes rigors and/or vomiting (Apted, 1970a). The fever is remittent, sometimes high, other times low, without a clear pattern (Graf, 1929). Each attack may last from one day to a week (Apted, 1970a; Weinberg *et al.*, 1989), and attacks may be separated by intervals of a few days to a month or more throughout the infection (Duggan and Hutchington, 1966). The patient usually does not seek medical help at this time.

Following the initial febrile episode, the early stage of the disease is characterized by intermittent bouts of fever separated by remissions during which the patient feels well. It is quite common for these clinical manifestations to be interpreted as a malaria episode, and the patient treated with antimalarial drugs (Reynaud *et al.*, 1963; Dutertre, 1968; Boa *et al.*, 1988; Mbulamberi, 1989b) or as a bacterial infection, and treated with antibiotics (Weinberg *et al.*, 1989).

Lymph gland involvement. Generalized lymph node enlargement occurs as the disease progresses. In Gambian disease, the supraclavicular and posterior cervical lymph nodes are often enlarged (Kellersberger, 1933; Duggan and Hutchington, 1966). Very characteristic of Gambian disease is visible enlargement of the glands of the posterior cervical triangle (Winterbottom's sign). Classically, the lymph nodes are discrete, freely movable, non-tender, rubbery, without periadenitis and painless (Duggan and Hutchington, 1966; Apted, 1970a). Suppuration does not occur (Dutertre, 1968). Progression of the disease leads to fibrosis (Cruz Ferreira and Lehmann de Almeida, 1950; Bertrand *et al.*, 1973a).

Spleen and liver involvement. The spleen may be mildly enlarged and soft, but this is so common in other tropical diseases, especially malaria, that it is not of great help in the diagnosis (Dutertre, 1968; Apted, 1970a). There is a discrete liver involvement in sleeping sickness, sometimes clinically apparent, but in most cases the liver changes are functional rather than morphological (Duggan, 1959). The development of jaundice (Le Bras *et al.*, 1973; Foulkes, 1981) is unusual and must be distinguished from jaundice occurring as a result of haemolysis (Duggan and Hutchington, 1966).

Skin involvement. An irregular, evanescent annular rash may appear (Dutertre, 1968, Apted, 1970a, Cook, 1991). A large proportion of the macules develop a central area of normal-coloured skin, giving the rash a circinate or serpiginous outline (Cooke *et al.*, 1937; Duggan and Hutchington, 1966, Cook, 1991). This rash is most commonly observed in the trunk, shoulders, and thighs as scattered, oval, pinkish, erythematous areas often 8–12 cm in diameter with clear centres (Apted, 1970a). Cold, heat or sweating may accentuate it. There is no itching, but a sensation of formication may be described (Apted, 1970a). The rash, which is not correlated with the fever episodes, often fades and reappears several times over a period of weeks, (Grau Junyent *et al.*, 1988) a feature which may account for its being noted in only a proportion of cases (Dutertre, 1968). Duggan and Hutchington (1966) considered the trypanosomal rash, in its typical form, as the most specific of all the clinical signs of early sleeping sickness in the European.

Pruritus is observed in 40% (Cruz Ferreira and Lehmann de Almeida, 1950), and almost 50% of the cases (Boa *et al.*, 1988). It is, however, difficult to attribute this sign to the sleeping sickness itself, as there are multiple infections that may be responsible for it, including filarial infections (Dutertre, 1968). However, Cruz Ferreira and Lehmann de Almeida (1950) suggest that pruritus in a patient without scabies is strongly suggestive of trypanosomiasis. Painful local oedema of the face, more evident in the eyelids and periorbital areas, hands, feet, and joint regions, are frequent and transient, in the early stage, occurring in 15% of patients (Cruz Ferreira and Lehmann de Almeida, 1950). The peripheral oedema of the later stages, seen especially in the legs, is associated with wasting, avitaminosis, cardiac insufficiency (Cruz Ferreira and Lehmann de Almeida, 1950) and anaemia (Apted, 1970a).

Cardiovascular system. Tachycardia in the absence of fever may be a very early sign of cardiac involvement (Buchanan, 1929; Cruz Ferreira and Lehmann de Almeida, 1950; Duggan and Hutchington, 1966). Heart damage, in a proportion of patients, is evident almost from the onset of the disease (Apted, 1970a). Other clinical manifestations of cardiovascular system involvement include lower intensity of heart sounds as well as cardiac murmurs (Buchanan, 1929; Bertrand *et al.*, 1973b), myocarditis with congestive heart failure (Manson-Bahr and Charters, 1963; Duggan and Hutchington, 1966; Collomb and Bartoli, 1967; De Raadt and Kotten, 1968), pericarditis (Bertrand *et al.*, 1973b), pericardial effusions (Hawking and Greenfield, 1941; Manson-Bahr and Charters, 1963; Kotten and De Raadt, 1969) and pancarditis (Collomb and Bartoli, 1967). Electrocardiographic studies have revealed not only lengthening of the P-Q segment (Collomb and Bartoli, 1967), and flattening or inversion of the T wave (Collomb and Bartoli, 1967; Bertrand *et al.*, 1967), but also, in a few patients, a conduction defect (Bertrand *et al.*, 1967, 1968) and cardiac ischaemia. Radiologically, the heart frequently appears enlarged, sometimes grossly (Manson-Bahr and Charters, 1963; Bertrand *et al.*, 1967). Cardiovascular abnormalities usually disappear after successful treatment.

Endocrine dysfunction. In women, sterility, menstrual disorders and high abortion rates are the main manifestations of endocrine dysfunction (Cruz Ferreira and Lehmann de Almeida, 1950). Menstruation arrest is more common in the advanced stages, but may appear at the onset of the disease. After treatment, menstrual function often returns to normal. Abortion has been shown to be associated with uterine hypoplasia secondary to defective hormonal secretions (Ridet, 1953). In addition, premature births, stillbirths and perinatal deaths frequently occur in infected women (Apted, 1970a). Also recorded is the loss of skin hair and atrophy of the sexual organs (Cruz Ferreira and Lehmann de Almeida, 1950; Noireau *et al.*, 1988).

In men, loss of libido and impotence are the most common clinical symptoms (Cruz Ferreira and Lehmann de Almeida, 1950). Also described, in the later stages of the disease, are gynaecomastia, feminine distribution of fat and myxoedematous infiltration of subcutaneous tissues (Cruz Ferreira and Lehmann de Almeida, 1950), giving the appearance of a very well-nourished person – the 'forme bouffie' described by the French authors (Noireau *et al.*, 1988). Loss of skin hair, reduction of testicular volume (Noireau *et al.*, 1988) and orchitis have also been recorded (Apted, 1970a).

Eye involvement. There have been several reports of eye disease caused by trypanosomiasis. The symptoms and signs include iritis (Nattan-Larrier and Monthus, 1908), cyclitis (Morax and Kérandel, 1908), iridocyclitis, keratitis, conjunctivitis (Hissette, 1932), circumcorneal injection and photophobia (Apted, 1970a). Duggan and Hutchington, (1966) in their study regarding 109 Europeans, described eye changes in 11, namely keratitis, papilloedema, optic neuritis and choroidal atrophy, with one case progressing to complete blindness. The progressive visual deficit leading to blindness in one case has also been described by Cruz Ferreira and Lehmann de Almeida (1950) in their study regarding 500 *T. b. gambiense* patients in Portuguese Guinea.

Eye lesions are very rare and, when they are detected, it has not been proven that trypanosomiasis actually plays a part in their causation (Apted, 1970a). Also reported in trypanosomiasis patients, but not directly caused by trypanosomes, are choroiditis, choroidoretinitis (Hissette, 1932), papilloedema secondary to the meningeal reaction, optic atrophy secondary to Atoxyl or tryparsamide treatment (Van den Branden and Appelmans, 1934; Cruz Ferreira and Lehmann de Almeida, 1950), diplopia, and paralytic strabismus due to nervous system involvement (Apted, 1970a).

Neurological features (Table 11.2)

Early mental and neurological symptoms and signs

Irritability, insomnia, loss of ability to concentrate, personality change, and even somnolence are characteristic early features (Giordano, 1973), especially in non-Africans (Duggan and Hutchington, 1966). These symptoms may be present long before there are detectable changes in the cerebrospinal fluid and are not diagnostic of CNS involvement. Deep hyperaesthesia – Kérandel's sign

Table 11.2   Central nervous system involvement in late-stage human trypanosomiasis.

Mental disturbances	Motor system disturbances	Sensory system involvement	Abnormal reflexes
Indifference	Tremors of tongue and fingers	Hyperaesthesia	Pout
Lassitude	Muscular fasciculation	Generalized pruritus	Palmo-mental
Irritability	Choreiform or oscillatory movements	Paraesthesia	Babinski
Anxiety	Increased muscular tonicity Increased muscular rigidity	Anaesthesia	
Agitation/mania episodes	Slurred speech		
Uncontrolled sexual impulses	Cerebellar ataxia		
Violent mood	Paralysis of one or more muscular groups		
Delirium and hallucinations	Neuritis/polyneuritis		
Increased suicidal tendencies			

(Martin and Darré, 1908; Kérandel, 1910) or 'signe de la clé' (key's sign), described by Heckenroth and Ouzilleau in 1907 (Nozais, 1988) – is reported to occur in 23% of Europeans (Duggan and Hutchington, 1966), but is uncommon in Africans (Apted, 1970a), and results in delayed, intense pain when soft tissues are compressed, e.g. by a sharp blow or squeeze (Martin and Darré, 1908; Blin and Kernéis, 1916).

Late stage (central nervous system involvement)

Involvement of the CNS may occur within weeks to a few months during the clinical course in Rhodesian disease, or may not develop until months or, more commonly, years after, in the Gambian disease (Apted, 1970a). Onset of this CNS stage is usually insidious, with a gradual and progressive evolution. Neurological involvement presents with a variety of symptoms and signs, depending on the topographical distribution of the nervous lesions (Cruz Ferreira and Lehmann de Almeida, 1950; Giordano *et al.*, 1977). Headache is a frequent symptom in the late stage of the infection, being characteristically severe and continuous, with episodic aggravation, followed by transitory less severe periods (Cruz Ferreira and Lehmann de Almeida, 1950). Headache may be an isolated symptom (Antoine, 1977).

The most frequent clinical picture includes mental, sleep and motor disturbances, the latter mainly of extrapyramidal type (Antoine, 1977). Also described are a frontal syndrome, neuroendocrine dysfunction, vestibular, cerebellar, pyramidal and meningeal syndromes (Nkanga *et al.*, 1988).

Mental disturbances. The clinical manifestations are not characteristic, and early changes may be subtle, involving alterations in personality and behaviour (Gelfand, 1947; Cruz Ferreira and Lehmann de Almeida, 1950; Nkanga *et al.*, 1988).

The common presenting symptom is gradually increasing indifference and lassitude (Gelfand, 1947; Van Bogaert and Janssen, 1957). Irritability, anxiety, indifference, agitation and manic episodes sometimes with euphoria (Cruz Ferreira and Lehmann de Almeida, 1950; Dutertre, 1968), uncontrolled sexual impulses (Antoine, 1977), violent mood, delirium and hallucinations (Van Bogaert and Janssen, 1957) are common. Suicidal tendencies with successful suicide attempts have also been described (Duggan and Hutchington, 1966).

Some sleeping sickness patients are primarily hospitalized in mental hospitals, on psychiatric grounds (Antoine, 1977). Robertson and Baker (1958) described a case of schizophrenic-like manifestations, and Duggan and Hutchington (1966) reported the development of psychosis in 36% of patients in their study on sleeping sickness in Europeans.

Motor system involvement. Tremors in a distal distribution, mainly of the tongue and fingers, are very common (Cruz Ferreira and Lehmann de Almeida, 1950; Giordano, 1973; Antoine, 1977). Fasciculations of the muscles of the limbs, face, lips, and tongue, choreiform or oscillatory movements of the arms, head, neck, and trunk, and increasing tonicity or muscular rigidity have also been described (Giordano, 1973; Nkanga *et al.*, 1988).

Speech becomes indistinct and difficult to understand (Kellersberger, 1933). There is usually a considerable element of cerebellar ataxia, leading to problems with walking (Cruz Ferreira and Lehmann de Almeida, 1950; Van Bogaert and Janssen, 1957). Focal lesions, or the effects of pressure, may cause paralysis of one or more groups of muscles, occasionally transient but more usually permanent, and various forms of neuritis or polyneuritis may develop (Cruz Ferreira and Lehmann de Almeida, 1950; Apted, 1970a; Antoine, 1977). Paralysis mainly affects the lower limbs, and is related to spinal cord involvement or is the consequence of a polyneuritis (Van Bogaert and Janssen, 1957). There are reports of paralysis of other muscle groups (Martin and Darré, 1908; Kellersberger, 1933; Gelfand, 1947). Hemiplegic forms of sleeping sickness have been described (Cruz Ferreira and Lehmann de Almeida, 1950; Antoine, 1977; Nkanga *et al.*, 1988). From 1963 to 1987, 14 cases of this have been reported in the literature to date (Sonan *et al.*, 1988).

Sleep disturbances. These include loss of attention, distractibility and narcoleptic crises (Giordano, 1973). These narcoleptic crises, defined as an uncontrollable urge to sleep, may overtake the patient anywhere and any time. Daytime somnolence is prominent, often alternating with the insomnia at night (Cruz Ferreira and Lehmann de Almeida, 1950; Antoine, 1977; Nkanga *et al.*, 1988). This uncontrollable urge to sleep in the final stage is almost continuous, the patient drifting into sleep while talking or in the middle of an action or movement (Kellersberger, 1933; Cruz Ferreira and Lehmann de Almeida, 1950; Duggan and Hutchington, 1966).

Sensory system involvement. The most frequent manifestation is unpleasant or painful hyperaesthesia (Giordano *et al.*, 1977). Paraesthesia and anaesthesia are uncommon (Cruz Ferreira and Lehmann de Almeida, 1950; Bertrand *et al.*, 1973b), but there are cases where they are the first symptoms of the disease (Martin and Darré, 1908).

Intense, generalized, pruritus has been considered as an important sensory system symptom (Bertrand *et al.*, 1973b; Giordano, 1973; Giordano *et al.*, 1977; Boa *et al.*, 1988). However, other aetiologies may also be responsible for pruritus, namely parasitic infections, mainly of filarial origin, and psychiatric disturbances.

Abnormal reflexes. Positive pout and palmo-mental reflexes are the most frequent abnormal findings (Giordano, 1973; Giordano *et al.*, 1977; Boa *et al.*, 1988; Mbulamberi, 1989b). They have different intensities, the pout reflex varying from the weak contraction of the mentum muscles to the elevation of the lower lip after a light percussion of the upper peribuccal area, and the palmo-mental reflex varying from a weak but repetitive contraction of the same chin area to an intense contraction of the mentum muscles after the stimulation of the thumb palmar region or thenar eminence (Boa *et al.*, 1988). These reflexes are not pathognomonic of sleeping sickness (Antoine, 1977), and can be elicited in 30% of normal people (Giordano *et al.*, 1977), but may be considered as the first neurological signs to be found in a late stage sleeping sickness patient (Boa *et al.*, 1988; Nkanga *et al.*, 1988). The Babinski reflex is described, but in most series is less frequent than the pout and palmo-mental positive reflexes (Nkanga *et al.*, 1988; Mbulamberi, 1989b).

Final stage

Further neurological abnormalities appearing in the final stage of the disease include epileptiform seizures, sometimes followed by local paralysis (Giordano, 1973; Antoine, 1977), urinary and faecal incontinence, euphoria, mania and somnolence. The patient becomes indifferent to his environment. Backache, neck stiffness, and papilloedema, reflecting cerebral oedema (Zola *et al.*, 1994) may also be present.

The final stage is one of progressive mental deterioration and classic sleeping sickness. There is intolerable pruritus, generalized wasting, and dribbling of saliva. The patient is difficult to arouse and lies immobile in the hut or hospital bed. Initially, the patient can be aroused to take food and water, but he never speaks or takes food spontaneously. Later, coma ensues. Death results from the sleeping sickness itself, intercurrent infection, or malnutrition (Kellersberger, 1933). In acute Rhodesian disease, death often occurs before CNS symptoms and signs develop, perhaps as the result of cardiac arrhythmia or cardiac failure from pancarditis (Apted, 1970a).

Presentation in paediatric age group

Children are not usually infected under normal circumstances, mainly because of their decreased risk of exposure. The infection is reported less in age groups below 5 years (Rey *et al.*, 1964). However, African trypanosomiasis in children is often fulminant, with early CNS involvement (Ngandu-Kabeya, 1976; Triolo *et al.*, 1985).

The most frequent symptoms and signs show regional variations, and include fever, lymphadenopathy (relatively uncommon in younger children), anaemia, hepatomegaly, splenomegaly, meningeal signs, dullness, lethargy, and behavioural changes (Ngandu-Kabeya, 1976; Triolo *et al.*, 1985; Kazumba *et al.*, 1993). The diagnosis is often delayed, and the child presents with psychomotor retardation, seizures and/or coma. In non-endemic areas, diagnosis is often accidental, trypanosomes being found in the blood, CSF or lymph node aspirate or tissue collected for other clinical studies (Satge *et al.*, 1964; Borges *et al.*, 1992). There is a high risk of neurological sequelae involving not only the sensory and motor systems, but also mental and intellectual involvement (Triolo *et al.*, 1985; Medina *et al.*, 1986; Kazumba *et al.*, 1993).

Congenital trypanosomiasis

This is an uncommon situation, and has been reported mainly from *Trypanosoma b. gambiense* areas (Burke *et al.*, 1973). Its higher occurrence in these areas is related to the long infection period, the frequency of pregnancy and the trypanosomes' ability to cross the placental barrier (Pepin *et al.*, 1989a). Reports of congenital trypanosomiasis caused by *Trypanosoma b. rhodesiense* are mainly from Zambia (Buyst, 1973; Buyst, 1976). Most of the cases are clinically silent. When they exist, the most common clinical manifestations of congenital trypanosome infection include decrease in body weight (Darré *et al.*, 1937; Rosário Pinto, 1960; Triolo, 1990), cessation of breast feeding (Davelloose, 1971), hepatosplenomegaly (Triolo *et al.*, 1985) or splenomegaly alone (Triolo *et al.*, 1985; Triolo, 1990). Hydrocephalus has also been described (Darré *et al.*, 1937). In more severe cases death occurs just after birth. Undiagnosed infections which develop without treatment may present with fever, convulsions (Triolo *et al.*, 1985) and raised intracranial pressure (Davelloose, 1971).

Concurrent diseases

Malaria (Cruz Ferreira and Lehmann de Almeida, 1950), filariasis caused by *Dipetalonema perstans* (Blair, 1939) and *Wuchereria bancrofti* (Cruz Ferreira and Lehmann de Almeida, 1950), as well as onchocercosis, and intestinal helminthic infections (Buchanan, 1929; Cruz Ferreira and Lehmann de Almeida, 1950) are the most common infections associated with human African trypanosomiasis. The frequency of these diseases is related to their prevalence in the particular geographical area, and are not the consequence of a special susceptibility to these conditions provoked by the trypanosome infection *per se*.

An association of human immunodeficiency virus (HIV) infection and human African trypanosomiasis has been suggested, and is a cause for concern (Estambale and Knight, 1992). Studies of both *Trypanosoma b. gambiense* (Noireau *et al.*, 1987; Louis *et al.*, 1991; Pépin *et al.*, 1992a) and *Trypanosoma b. rhodesiense* (Mbulamberi, 1989b; Okia *et al.*, 1994) infection did not show any change in the epidemiology of human African trypanoso-miasis in relation to HIV infection in the region, although further detailed studies are needed to determine whether HIV infection itself influences the clinical course of human African trypanosomiasis (Meda *et al.*, 1995). Exacerbation of trypanosome infection and the development of encephalo-pathy after melarsoprol treatment with concurrent coxsackie B virus infection (Janssens *et al.*, 1960), tropical pyomyositis associated with *Trypanosoma b. rhodesiense* infection (Weinberg *et al.*, 1989), associated bacterial meningitis (Haller *et al.*, 1986), tuberculosis and lepra (Cruz Ferreira and Lehmann de Almeida, 1950), and other bacterial and viral infections (Triolo *et al.*, 1985) have all been reported, but are isolated cases. There is no evidence of a particular disease associated with human African trypanosomiasis. Children with human African trypanosomiasis are more susceptible to malaria, mainly the first episode, which is usually fatal, as well as chickenpox, German measles, and whooping cough (Triolo *et al.*, 1985).

Diagnosis and differential diagnosis of human African trypanosomiasis

Being clinically very difficult, the diagnosis depends on the geographical pattern of disease, and on the demonstration of the trypanosomes from the chancre, in the blood, in aspirate from enlarged lymph nodes, or in the CSF. Serological tests are helpful in epidemiological surveys but are not diagnostic. Lumbar puncture should be performed in all patients, both those with suspected and those with proven haemolymphatic disease (see later). The specific laboratory diagnosis of Human African Trypanosomiasis is made with the aid of a variety of specific diagnostic tests, e.g. actual demonstration of the parasite, antigen detection, antibody detection and DNA detection. These will be discussed later.

Clinical diagnosis

The clinical manifestations are non-specific and the chronic evolution of the Gambian disease, with periodic outbreaks of fever resembling malaria and usually treated with antimalarial drugs, can make the clinical diagnosis very difficult. The effects of the treatment for malaria usually reduce the fever and the patient may return to normal activity until development of the next fever which will be treated in the same way. This situation is likely to be repeated several times until neurological/psychological symptoms appear. Only then is the diagnosis of sleeping sickness likely to be suspected clinically. Rhodesian disease, usually without CNS signs and symptoms, is even more difficult to diagnose clinically, which is usually only possible with the onset of the cardiac manifestations in the terminal phase of the disease. Therefore, a high index of suspicion is necessary, particularly in patients presenting in non-endemic areas.

Differential diagnosis

In sleeping sickness endemic areas the differential diagnosis is not a great problem, since the constant suspicion that almost any condition may be due to or related to a trypanosome infection leads experienced clinicians almost automatically to carry out additional tests to confirm the diagnosis. In non-endemic areas, however, diagnosis is often delayed, for it is natural to consider first more familiar conditions such as malaria, tuberculosis, typhoid fever, lymphomas, infectious mononucleosis, brucellosis and HIV infection. The following specific features can now be considered.

Chancre

The typical trypanosomal chancre is unique, but there may be a diagnostic problem if it is fading or if a less typical lesion is present; furuncles and insect bites from insects other than tsetse flies may also cause diagnostic confusion.

Fever

In most of the patients the first provisional diagnosis is malaria, which is consistent with the intermittent character of the febrile episodes of sleeping sickness patients. It has been suggested that tropical febrile episodes which do not respond to antimalarials should be investigated for alternative causes of fever (Duggan and Hutchington, 1966), but the occurrence of drug-resistant malaria is now very common increasing the likelihood of overlooking a trypanosomal fever. Other causes of fever in patients in or from a sleeping sickness area include typhoid and paratyphoid fever, relapsing fever, visceral leishmaniasis, infectious mononucleosis, tick typhus, and brucellosis. Hodgkin's disease, with associated lymphadenopathy and Pel-Ebstein fever also enters the differential diagnosis, as well as other non-Hodgkin's lymphomas. Febrile and adenopathic manifestations during HIV infection or associated diseases is an increasingly frequent differential diagnosis. The possibility of a dual infection, such as malaria and trypanosomiasis, or HIV and trypanosome infection, also has to be borne in mind.

Trypanosomal rash

Although some authors consider this skin lesion as a pathognomonic lesion of human African trypanosomiasis (Apted, 1970a), urticarial and drug rashes, and even some leprosy skin lesions, may cause some diagnostic doubts. The occurrence of a streptococcal skin infection, in the form of an erysipelas, is not uncommon, and must be distinguished from the trypanosomal rash (Duggan and Hutchington, 1966).

Lymph node enlargement

The enlarged glands may be thought to be due to glandular tuberculosis, lymphomas, infectious mononucleosis, HIV infection, or even fungal infections, such as African histoplasmosis. It must be remembered, however, that in the African patient particularly, the lymph nodes may be chronically enlarged from repeated bacterial or parasitic infections.

Neuropsychiatric manifestations

The misinterpretation of the late signs of nervous system involvement may have far-reaching results. Neurosyphilis (Gallais and Ranque, 1953), tuberculous meningitis, viral encephalitis and other causes of meningoencephalitis with a mononuclear response, cerebral tumour, HIV-associated CNS infection such as cryptococcal meningitis, toxoplasmosis, cerebral lymphoma and progressive multifocal leucoencephalopathy, may all cause difficulties in the differential diagnosis, as well as all possible causes of coma.

Parkinson's disease may be mimicked by a shuffling gait, muscular rigidity, tremors of the tongue and muscles, and slurred speech. Sleeping sickness must also be considered as a possible cause of mental illness, and a large number of patients are hospitalized in a psychiatric ward, with provisional diagnoses such as neuraesthenia, dementia, psychosis, schizophrenia and alcoholism (Duggan and Hutchington, 1966).

Wasting

The wasting is associated with the later stages of the Gambian infection and also sometimes with the early stages of the Rhodesian disease. Tuberculosis, hookworm infection (sometimes coexisting with sleeping sickness) and HIV infection are the most important diseases entering the differential diagnosis.

Investigations

Haematology and biochemistry

The main abnormalities associated with sleeping sickness that are revealed by laboratory tests include anaemia, increased erythrocyte sedimentation rate (Almeida Franco, 1960), rouleau formation of the red blood cells, thrombocytopenia (Trincão and Gouveia, 1951), complement and coagulation disorders. The anaemia is mainly haemolytic, due to erythrophagocytosis by the mononuclear phagocyte system (MPS), but impaired erythropoiesis may also play a role in the aetiology of the anaemia.

Other laboratory abnormalities include abnormal liver function and increased plasma kinins. Laboratory features of disseminated intravascular coagulation (DIC) may be prominent (Cook, 1991). None of these changes, however, is pathognomonic (Cook, 1991). The most characteristic laboratory feature is increased serum and CSF (after CNS invasion) IgM (Clerc et al., 1973). White cells, mainly mononuclear, are also present in the CSF. Morular cells of Mott may be seen. Anaemia, abnormal liver function tests, thrombocytopenia and DIC are more marked in Rhodesian disease than in Gambian disease. Immune complexes, IgM heterophile antibodies and a wide range of other antibodies resulting from autoimmune responses and polyclonal B cell activation may also be present. Endocrine abnormalities include decreased levels of oestradiol in women and testosterone in men, without decrease of pituitary gondatrophins, leading to secondary hypogonadism, decrease in T3 and FT3 (free fraction) (Hublart et al., 1988) as well as combined central and peripheral adrenal insufficiency with suppressed peak cortisol levels (Heppner et al., 1995).

Specific neurological investigations

Neuroradiology

There are few reports of the utility of computerized tomographic (CT) scanning or magnetic resonance imaging (MRI) techniques in the diagnosis and follow up of patients with human African trypanosomiasis. Although at the CNS parasite invasion and development stage radiological abnormalities are very unlikely to be detectable by CT or MRI (Sabbah et al., 1997), pathological aspects may still be observed subsequently with the evolution of the disease. However, because there are no preferential CNS sites for the localization of the trypanosomes, pathognomonic CT or MRI images have not been described. Existing reports refer to asymmetrical heterogeneous hypodensities of the centrum semiovale, cerebral oedema and demyelination (Poisson et al., 1980; Medina et al., 1986) on CT scanning. MRI has revealed lesions of the basal nuclei, brainstem and white matter (Serrano-Gonzalez et al., 1996) sometimes suggesting leucoencephalitis (Spinazzola et al., 1989). MRI can also be important in post-treatment assessment (Figure 11.3), and reported cases of treated human African trypanosomiasis in which the MRI was performed in the follow-up stage showed the disappearance of the lesions (Serrano-Gonzalez et al., 1996; Sabbah et al., 1997).

Electroencephalography

Electroencephalogram (EEG) and polysomnographic techniques have been used by several clinical research groups in patients with sleeping sickness (Buguet et al., 1994). Studies of the sleep–wake patterns in sleeping sickness patients have shown that, although dampened, the waking process remains responsive and slows down only during the late stage of meningoencephalitis (Tapie et al., 1996). However, there are no pathognomonic patterns. Hamon

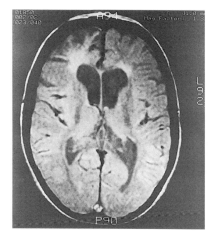

Figure 11.3   MRI scan (proton density) of a 13-year-old patient with CNS trypanosomiasis 3 years after successful completion of multiple treatment regimens for numerous
relapses of the disease. Note the ventricular enlargement (especially of the frontal horns)
as well as diffuse white matter changes which are prominent in the right frontal and
periventricular regions.

and collaborators (1993) identified three unusual EEG patterns. The first type,
apparently indicative of early cerebral impairment, had a sustained low-voltage
background similar to that seen during light sleep. The second type, seen in
cases with acute cerebral involvement but without focal seizures, showed
paroxysmal waves. The third EEG pattern consisted of various types of delta
wave and rapid intermittent high-voltage delta bursts between periods of
lower-voltage delta activity (as often seen in meningoencephalitis). In this
third profile, all types of delta wave were of higher voltage than the spike
and wave complexes (Hamon *et al.*, 1993, 1995). Even when no definite
correlation has been established between the severity of the disease, the results
of clinical tests, and waking EEG patterns, it has been suggested that the three
types of EEG profile may be indicative of the degree of cerebral involvement
(Hamon *et al.*, 1993). If EEG or polysomnographic studies are made during
successful treatment, the recordings gradually return to fast rhythms, and the
tracings return to normal shortly after completion of therapy. However, if there
is an incomplete response to chemotherapy, these techniques are likely to show
a variety of abnormalities compatible with the cerebral disease. This possibility
of indirectly evaluating the results of treatment has led some authors to
recommend monitoring the progress of treated human African trypanosomiasis
patients by EEG or polysomnographic recording in a sleep laboratory (Hamon
and Camara, 1992; Montmayeur *et al.*, 1994).

Lumbar puncture

Once the infection has been detected in the lymph or blood, the CSF has to be
examined for markers characterizing the meningoencephalitic stage of the

disease. This is an important step in the diagnostic procedure having important implications for the choice of chemotherapeutic agents and regimens to be employed. The finding of trypanosomes in the CSF is a strong indication that the CNS has become involved. In a patient in the late stage of the disease the CSF examination shows pleocytosis, with the lymphocyte count between 10 and 1000/µl, and a protein content usually between 40 and 200 mg/100 ml. IgM is very high, and is a good marker of CNS involvement. Morular cells of Mott may be seen in advanced cases. Trypanosomes are not very easy to find, and concentration techniques must be used. A single or double centrifugation of CSF (at 1500G for 10 minutes) with the observation of the deposit may be the best method to observe the trypanosomes.

Specific laboratory diagnostic tests

Direct demonstration of the parasite

The finding of a single trypanosome gives diagnostic certainty but the parasitaemia is often so low that repeated and time consuming examination may be required. Trypanosomes may be found in the chancre before their appearance in the peripheral blood. The chancre is punctured and a drop of the serous exudate is then examined for motile trypanosomes as a wet preparation (Gelfand, 1966). Wet lymph examination is a valuable routine test (Henry *et al.*, 1981; Wéry and Mulumba, 1989) but has important limitations due to the frequent absence of swollen glands in trypanosomiasis patients (Van Meirvenne, 1992). Examination of stained thick and thin peripheral blood films is a sensitive method of detection of *T. b. rhodesiense*. Giemsa is the most appropriate stain, but Wright's and Leishman's stains may also be used. Microscopic examination of blood is less useful in identifying *T. b. gambiense* because these parasites are very scarce in the peripheral circulation (Stanghellini and Roux, 1984). The blood is more often positive in the early stages of the infection. It is advisable to examine consecutive daily specimens, each day over a 12-day period, because parasitaemia occurs in waves and may be below detectable levels at any particular time (World Health Organization, 1986). The possibility of platelet abnormalities resulting in false-positive trypanosome identification, although very rare, should be borne in mind when examining thin peripheral blood films (Frean and Bush, 1993).

Several methods using concentration techniques can increase the accuracy of blood examination, but all of these methods differ in sensitivity, the time needed for reading the result, cost price and centrifugation requirements (Lumsden *et al.*, 1981). The selective haemolytic action of some agents such as SDS can also be exploited to facilitate blood examination (Van Meirvenne, 1992).

Bone marrow examination for haematological studies (Trincão and Gouveia, 1951; Trincão and Parreira, 1957) or for detecting trypanosomes (Cruz Ferreira and Lehmann de Almeida, 1950; Pinto *et al.*, 1952) is a very sensitive technique (Shi-hua, 1985; Wéry and Mulumba, 1989) but should be reserved for exceptional circumstances.

To detect trypanosomes in the cerebrospinal fluid a double step centrifugation starting in a tube and ending in a capillary (Doucet, 1973; Stanghellini and Roux, 1984) is the most sensitive technique (Cattand *et al.*, 1988).

Regarding *in vitro* culture, quite promising results have recently been obtained with a kit for *in vitro* isolation of trypanosomes (KIVI), which allows direct introduction of patients' blood into culture medium, with the subsequent transformation to, and multiplication of, procyclic trypanosomes (Aerts *et al.*, 1992). More than just a clinical diagnostic tool, the KIVI takes 2–4 weeks to show a positive result, and it is an important epidemiological method for characterization of trypanosome populations in different areas (McNamara *et al.*, 1995).

Antibody detection

Tests for detection of trypanosome antibodies include direct agglutination (Gray, 1967), complement-fixation (Schoenaers *et al.*, 1953), passive haemagglutination (PA or IHA) (Woo and Soltys, 1972), capillary agglutination (CA) (Ross, 1971), gel diffusion (Mattern *et al.*, 1967), capillary haemagglutination (Boné and Charlier, 1975), enzyme-linked immunosorbent assay (ELISA) (Voller *et al.*, 1975) and the procyclic agglutination trypanosome test (PATT) (Pearson *et al.*, 1986; Liu *et al.*, 1989). In a comparative trial of serological tests, organized by WHO, which included ELISA, capillary haemagglutination, and gel diffusion, ELISA had the higher rate of detection of positive samples (World Health Organization, 1976).

Immunofluorescence (IFA) (Lucasse, 1964; Courtois and Bideau, 1966) with its adaptation to field studies (Wéry *et al.*, 1970; Duvallet and Saliou, 1978; Duvallet *et al.*, 1978) and, more recently, the card agglutination trypanosomiasis test (CATT) (Magnus *et al.*, 1978) are the most employed tests for the detection of trypanosome antibodies.

A breakthrough is to be expected from the introduction of perfectly defined recombinant or synthetic antigens. Recently an innovative assay detecting antibodies to parasite enzymes has been introduced (Van Meirvenne, 1992).

Reliable laboratory and field tests, including several systems using defined variable antigens, already exist for *T. b. gambiense* and have been proven to be indispensable tools for mass surveys. Similar tests allowing even earlier detection of *T. b. rhodesiense* infections remain to be developed.

Most antibody tests can be applied to serum, plasma, wet or dry blood and CSF. If needed, the sensitivity and specificity of the assay can be adjusted to some extent by varying dilutions, conjugates and cut-off values. False negative results are to be expected at a very early stage of the infection. False or unexplainable positives may be due to various cross-reactions, malaria may be a complicating factor, as well as leishmaniosis, toxoplasmosis (Seah and Gabrielan, 1972; Poupin *et al.*, 1983), and Chagas disease (Voller, 1977). An unknown history of treated trypanosomiasis or abortive infections with other trypanosome species may also lead to misleading results.

Antigen detection

Serodiagnostic techniques detecting circulating antibodies may indicate past as well as active infections, while antigen detection methods should theoretically indicate current infections. A first generation of antigen detection tests already exists. These are mainly enzyme-linked immunosorbent assay (ELISA) systems using polyclonal or monoclonal antibodies to whole lysates of procyclic trypanosomes (Liu and Pearson, 1987) or one or more invariable intracellular or surface antigens (Nantulya *et al.*, 1989). These sandwich antibody antigen capture ELISA for the detection of Trypanosoma infections have been described and used in animal (Liu *et al.*, 1988; Nantulya *et al.*, 1992a) and human studies (Liu *et al.*, 1989; Nantulya *et al.*, 1992b). A multiple antigen detection dipstick colloidal dye immunoassay (DIA), which is easier to use, has been tested in cattle with promising results (Kashiwazaki *et al.*, 1994). Simple latex agglutination tests are also being developed and there is hope that highly effective field assays will become available to complement parasite and antibody detection tests (Van Meirvenne, 1992).

DNA detection

The idea of developing a sensitive test for detection of specific trypanosomal DNA has proven to be realistic. Polymerase chain reaction (PCR) represents a powerful new technology with a variety of field applications. The first PCR test to be developed identifies a 177 base pair (bp) trypanosome repetitive DNA element from *T. brucei brucei* infected animals (Moser *et al.*, 1989). This test may have limitations, revealing PCR DNA positivity in blood and brains of cured *T. brucei*-infected mice and blood and CSF of early-stage *T. gambiense*-infected cured humans (J. Burke, personal communication). More recently, a new PCR test to detect the expression of a trypanosome phosphoglycerate (PGK) housekeeping gene has been developed. This PGK cDNA amplification test has been tested in an animal model system and also in humans with promising results (J. Burke, personal communication). Amplification methods using minicircle kDNA probes by conventional PCR (Mathieu-Daudé *et al.*, 1994) or nested PCR (Schares and Mehlitz, 1996) are currently under evaluation. The decision to utilize PCR diagnostic assays in parasitological studies depends upon addressing several issues, including cost, technical capabilities, and clinical and epidemiological utility (Barker, 1994).

Pathogenesis of human African trypanosomiasis

General pathogenesis

The pathogenesis of human African trypanosomiasis is still incompletely understood. Available information is mainly from animal trypanosomiasis or studies in experimental animals (Poltera, 1980). Most theories implicate immunopathological processes (Seed *et al.*, 1983). The African trypanosome survives in the mammalian host by periodically altering its surface antigenic coat, thereby aborting the developing of a complete immune response of the host (Cook, 1991). These variant antigenic types mark the identity of different subpopulations of trypanosomes; acquired immunity is thus type-specific only. Therefore, sleeping sickness is characterized by recurring parasitaemia, with each new wave of parasites representing the development of an immunologically distinct antigenic variant and a corresponding antibody response (World Health Organization, 1986). Pronounced immunological changes occur during the course of the disease. In the acute phase, there is marked reactivity of the lymphoid tissue with predominant plasma cells. A classic immunological feature of human African trypanosomiasis at this stage is the production of large amounts of immunoglobulins, reflecting a non-specific polyclonal B lymphocyte activation (Kazyumba et al., 1986).

Immune complexes formed between variant antigens and antibodies, frequently associated with complement, have been demonstrated in the circulation (Fruit et al., 1977; Greenwood and Whittle, 1980), but there is no evidence of deposits in target organs (Whittle et al., 1980). Hypocomplementaemia, high levels of cryoglobulins containing IgM and C3 (Greenwood and Whittle, 1976), and increased immunoconglutinin levels (Pautrizel et al., 1962) are common features and both the complement pathway and the kinin system are activated (Boreham, 1970). Later, the immune system becomes depleted of lymphocytes and plasma cells, which are replaced by macrophages. Serum levels of immunoglobulin M (IgM), although highest in the early stage of the infection, are still elevated in most patients with advanced disease (Whittle et al., 1977), but little of the IgM produced is specific antitrypanosome antibody (Greenwood and Whittle, 1980). The production of autoantibodies has been reported, and is related not only to the polyclonal B cell activation but also to specific stimulation by autoantigens or by cross-reacting antigens (Hunter and Kennedy, 1992). These autoantibodies, directed against antigenic components of red cells, brain, and heart, can cause damage in those organs (Greenwood and Whittle, 1980, Cook, 1991). Heterophile antibody, rheumatoid-factor-like substance, anti-DNA, anti-galactocerebroside (Amevigbe et al., 1992), and anti-tryptophan-like epitopes antibodies (Okomo-Assoumou et al., 1995) are also produced. A stage of relative immunosuppression develops. Impairment of both cellular and humoral immunity occurs (Cook, 1991) as evidenced by a reduced reaction to a variety of skin test antigens and diminished response to bacterial and viral vaccines (Greenwood et al., 1973).

Anaemia can be severe, and the resulting anoxia could contribute to tissue destruction. The urticaria and pruritus that are sometimes present could be caused by a type I immediate hypersensitivity reaction directed toward the trypanosomes (Greenwood and Whittle, 1980). However, the classic clinical and pathological features of this disease cannot be readily explained by any of the four types of immunological reactions. A direct role for a toxin produced by the organism (Seed, 1969) or an antigenic substance released after its destruction by the immune system has not been proved (Greenwood and Whittle, 1980). The pathological importance of metabolic changes induced by the pharmacologically active substances such as kinins that are known to be increased in the disease is also unclear (Boreham, 1968, 1970; Boreham and Goodwin, 1970).

CNS pathogenesis and pathology

CNS involvement occurs by early trypanosome invasion of areas lacking the blood–brain barrier or blood–nerve barrier (Schultzberg et al., 1988), and results in meningoencephalitis or meningomyelitis. Perivascular infiltration of mononuclear cells and occasional morular cells (Poltera, 1980) together with marked cell proliferation is present and is prominent in the pia and arachnoid of the brain and spinal cord (Van Bogaert and Janssen, 1957; Brown and Voge, 1982; Cook, 1991). There is also involvement of the choroid plexus (Calwell, 1937; Poltera, 1980), and oedema, haemorrhages, and granulomatous lesions are present within the brain (Cook, 1991). Thrombosis as a result of endarteritis is a major cause of cerebral degeneration (Cook, 1991). Two cellular abnormalities suggestive of sleeping sickness which may be found are lymphophagocytosis and the so-called morular or Mott cells. The latter are modified plasma cells (up to $20\,\mu m$ in diameter) with large eosinophilic inclusions that have been shown to consist of immunoglobulins (Mattern, 1962, Cook, 1991). Mott cells may be responsible for the local production of IgM in the cerebrospinal fluid. These cells have also been found in other organs, but are not pathognomonic of human African trypanosomiasis. Demyelination may also play a role (Dutertre, 1968), but appears to be only minimal (Cook, 1991). During the course of the disease, the meninges become progressively infiltrated with lymphocytes (especially B cells), plasma cells and morular cells. The same infiltration occurs around the blood vessels, forming perivascular cuffing (Adams et al., 1986). Both the cuffs and the surrounding brain parenchyma contain activated microglial cells and astrocytes (Pentreath, 1989). A diffuse white-matter degeneration has been described, but there are no structural nerve-cell alterations (Bentivoglio et al., 1994)

Trypanosomes release a molecule which triggers the CD8+ T cell to produce IFN-gamma, which has been reported to have a growth-enhancing effect on the trypanosomes. This molecule has been termed as trypanosome-derived lymphocyte triggering factor (TLTF) (Bentivoglio et al., 1994). The observed polyclonal proliferation of B lymphocytes in lymph nodes, brain, and heart could lead to tissue damage (Greenwood and Whittle, 1980). Prostaglandin D_2 (PGD_2) levels have been found to be markedly elevated in the CSF of late-stage patients, which may in part account for the increased somnolence and the immunosuppression within the CNS (Greenwood, 1974; Pentreath et al., 1990). Raised endotoxin levels may also contribute to the pathology in sleeping sickness (Greenwood, 1974; Pentreath et al., 1996., 1997).

Post-treatment reactive encephalopathy

Treatment of human African trypanosomiasis may precipitate different neurological complications. The post-treatment reactive encephalopathy (PTRE), also called reactive arsenical encephalopathy (RAE), and usually associated with the use of the arsenical drug melarsoprol (Robertson, 1963), is the most severe neurological complication, being fatal in up to 10% of all cases of late-stage disease (Haller et al., 1986). Clinically, the initial symptoms of reactive encephalopathy may be sudden, or the condition may develop slowly, with fever, headache and dizziness, tremor, slurred speech, followed by mental dullness and confusion, staggering gait or restlessness. Incontinence, convulsions or loss of consciousness are common in more severe cases, and precede the coma. The PTRE is not exclusively associated with melarsoprol treatment, and can occur with other drugs, including diminazene aceturate (De Raadt, 1966) or Mel W (Collomb et al., 1964). Less severe neurological complications such as convulsions and paresis have been observed with eflornithine (J. Atouguia, personal observation).

Pathologically, the CNS lesions found during the PTRE represent an exacerbation of the brain lesions of late-stage trypanosomiasis, namely the cellular infiltrates, perivascular cuffs consisting mainly of macrophages and lymphocytes, and the astrocyte activation in the white matter (Adams et al., 1986) which can progress to an acute haemorrhagic leucoencephalopathy (Adams et al., 1986; Haller et al., 1986).

The pathophysiological mechanisms possibly involved in CNS trypanosomiasis, and in the PTRE, include the existence of parasite antigens within the CNS and their attachment to glial cells which then become targets for destruction by the immune system (Pépin and Milord, 1991), autoimmunity (Poltera, 1980), immune complex deposition (Lambert et al., 1981) arsenical toxicity (Hurst, 1959) and subcurative treatment (Hunter et al., 1992). These various mechanisms are not necessarily mutually exclusive.

The use of more sophisticated diagnostic techniques, which unfortunately exist only in well-equipped medical centres outside Africa, may contribute to the detailed elucidation of the PTRE. Thus, Sabbah and colleagues (1997) have described the use of MRI in a patient who developed a clinically typical PTRE after a second series of melarsoprol injections. T2-weighted MRI showed no oedema, but focal bilateral high signal areas in the white matter. Thus, a PTRE was thought to be excluded and a third course of treatment was undertaken. The lesions progressively disappeared and the patient recovered (Sabbah et al., 1997).

The use of corticosteroids before and during treatment for the prevention of treatment-induced encephalopathy is still controversial. Although some authors have shown that their use does not increase the risk of treatment failure (Pépin et al., 1994) and reported good results with a dose of 1 mg/kg/day (40 mg maximum) of prednisolone (Pepin et al., 1985, 1989b, 1995), others are more sceptical about the corticosteroids' efficacy as a preventive drug either in Trypanosoma gambiense (Whittle and Pope, 1972; Bertrand et al., 1974) or in Trypanosoma rhodesiense infections (Foulkes, 1975; Arroz, 1987). Because of these different results, there are still no definitive guidelines for the use of corticosteroids before and during the trypanosomiasis treatment, but their use is strongly recommended in the management of the encephalopathy (World Health Organization, 1986).

Drug treatment and follow up

Current therapy of human African trypanosomiasis is based on the availability of five drugs. In fact, most of the drugs still in use were developed in the first half of the century (e.g. suramin, pentamidine, nitrofurans and arsenicals) (Van Nieuwenhove, 1992) and some of them would not pass current standards for drug safety (Fairlamb, 1990). Diminazene aceturate (Berenil), developed in the mid-1950s as a cattle trypanocide, has been successfully used in the treatment of human trypanosomiasis in several countries, but has never been registered for human treatment (Van Nieuwenhove, 1992). Drug development in recent times has been slow and insufficient. The introduction of a-difluoromethylornithine (DFMO or eflornithine) for the treatment of late-stage Gambian sleeping sickness (Van Nieuwenhove *et al.*, 1985) was not the result of specific trypanosomiasis drug research. Eflornithine was primarily developed as an anti-tumour proliferation agent (Sunkara *et al.*, 1987), and to modulate cell differentiation (Heby *et al.*, 1987). Although the clinical trials of DFMO in such diseases were very disappointing (Schechter *et al.*, 1987), good results were obtained in the treatment of experimental trypanosome infections, and DFMO was approved for human African trypanosomiasis. More recently, nifurtimox, largely employed in the treatment of *Trypanosoma cruzi* infections, has been tried in human African trypanosomiasis with some success (Janssens and De Muynck, 1977; Moens *et al.*, 1984; Van Nieuwenhove, 1992).

Current choices for the therapy of human African trypanosomiasis, in the early stage, are pentamidine, exclusively for *Trypanosoma gambiense* infections, and suramin or diminazene aceturate for early stage *Trypanosoma rhodesiense*. In the late stage, melarsoprol (which crosses the blood–brain barrier) or eflornithine are used and, as second choice drugs, usually for melarsoprol relapses (arsenic-resistant trypanosomes) the nitrofurans, nitrofurazone and nifurtimox. It should be emphasized that melarsoprol is *only* used in the late stage when the CNS has become involved (Cook, 1991).

Suramin

Suramin must be administered parenterally. Following its intravenous administration, a high concentration is achieved in the plasma. This falls fairly rapidly for a few hours, then more slowly for a few days, after which a low concentration is maintained for as long as 3 months. The common dosage is 20 mg/kg of body weight/injection (World Health Organization, 1986), up to a maximum of 1000 mg/injection. It is advisable to employ a small dose of 4 mg/kg initially to test for sensitivity, after which the normal dose is given on days 1, 3, 7, 14, and 21 (Apted, 1970b), or every 5–7 days (World Health Organization, 1986). The course usually comprises five injections and should not exceed seven (World Health Organization, 1986) or when the total dose has reached 5 g (Apted, 1970b). Local circumstances will often dictate the choice of a particular schedule: weekly doses may be given for an additional 5 weeks. The most important secondary effect of suramin in kidney damage, which is usually mild (Apted, 1970b). Its mode of action is not completely understood. Two mechanisms may be involved: suramin blocks the binding of various growth factors to their corresponding cell-surface receptors; and suramin is taken up by cells, where it inhibits protein kinase C, nucleic acid polymerases, and nuclear DNA topoisomerase II (reviewed by Baumann and Strassmann, 1993). The last mechanism may be involved in the trypanocidal action of suramin.

Pentamidine

One of the main advantages of pentamidine over suramin is the shortness of the course, a mere 7–10 days instead of 3–4 weeks. The dose, for each injection, is 3–4 mg/kg of body weight. The drug is given intramuscularly, one injection every day for 7–10 days, preferably for 10 days, unless local experience dictates otherwise (Apted, 1970b). Care must be taken with the calculation of the appropriate dose of pentamidine, depending on whether the salt or the base is used to determine dosage (Arnott et al., 1992).

The postulated mechanisms of action of pentamidine include its possible interference with the action and synthesis of polyamines, inhibiting S-adeno-sylmethionine decarboxylase (AdoMetDC) (Bitonti et al., 1986a), the promotion of a marked increase of the amino acid lysine (Berger et al., 1993) and its inhibition of plasma-membrane Ca^{2+}-ATPase of the parasites (Benaim et al., 1993). Pentamidine may be less effective in T. rhodesiense infections than in those caused by T. gambiense despite some reports of therapeutic success of pentamidine in early-stage cases of rhodesiense trypanosomiasis (Andrade Silva, 1957; Apted, 1980). This lack of sensitivity of T. rhodesiense to pentamidine may be related to lower rates of pentamidine transport and uptake (Damper and Patton, 1976). Suramin should be used in these infections, with pentamidine as a valuable second drug for the treatment of patients in whom suramin is not appropriate, such as those with kidney damage or those who develop a severe albuminuria during the course of treatment with suramin.

The intravenous injection of pentamidine is often followed quickly by alarming side-effects which include breathlessness, tachycardia, dizziness or fainting, headache, and vomiting. These reactions are probably related to the sharp fall in blood pressure that follows too rapid intravenous administration of the drug (Saunders et al., 1944; Harding, 1945), and they may be due in part to the release of histamine (Apted, 1970b; Rollo, 1975). Because pentamidine is better tolerated by intramuscular injection this route is to be preferred (Pille, 1953). Pain and inflammatory reaction of the skin at the site of injection are frequent (Walzer et al., 1974). Necrosis is rare, but can lead to septic reactions that are usually fatal (Jonchère, 1951). Hypoglycaemia occurs in 5–40% of the patients (Goa and Campoli-Richards, 1987). Paradoxically, hyperglycaemia has been reported following administration of pentamidine (Collomb et al., 1956; Sands et al., 1985). Hypo- and hyperglycaemia may be produced by direct toxicity of pentamidine on the β-cell of the pancreas (Boillot et al., 1985).

Renal dysfunction, usually reversible, has been associated with the use of the drug (Payet and Sankale, 1960; DeVita et al., 1969). Severe renal insufficiency, although rare, has also been reported (Coulaud *et al.*, 1975; Limbos *et al.*, 1977). It has been suggested that renal and pancreatic toxicity, which often occur together (Collomb *et al.*, 1956), may be dose related, occurring in patients with higher pentamidine serum levels (Comtois *et al.*, 1992).

Berenil

Berenil is given as three deep i.m. injections using a 2% solution in sterile 5% glucose, at a dose of 5 mg/kg given at 1- or 2-day intervals (Abaru *et al.*, 1984). This drug (and pentamidine) has been found to be a potent competitive inhibitor of human spermidine/spermine acetyltransferase, an enzyme of polyamine back-conversion (Libby and Porter, 1992). Berenil has not been fully evaluated for its toxicity in humans. There are reports of transient albuminuria but no other local or systemic toxicity in *Trypanosoma brucei gambiense* treated patients (Hutchinson and Watson, 1962) as well as reports on complete cures with no toxicity in *Trypanosoma brucei rhodesiense* patients (Onyango *et al.*, 1970a). Abaru and collaborators (1984), in their retrospective study of 99 cases of *Trypanosoma brucei rhodesiense* infection treated with berenil, concluded that the various transient side-effects observed were no more serious than those produced by suramin. These side-effects included fever accompanied by sweating, nausea and vomiting, increased intensity of headache and backache, malaise, pruritus, and mental disorientation, all occurring after the first injection (Abaru, 1978). Numbness of the legs, pain in the soles of the feet, paralysis and coma (Abaru and Matovu, 1981) were also reported. Recovery from these side-effects, which are not usually permanent, can be very slow; one paralysed patient only recovered completely 90 days after berenil treatment (Abaru *et al.*, 1984). When berenil was used before melarsoprol in the treatment of late-stage human trypanosomiasis the occurrence of encephalopathy was very high (32% for oral berenil and 38% for i.m. berenil) (Onyango *et al.*, 1970b). This correlates with the findings in a mouse model of the PTRE, in which an encephalopathy and paralysis can be provoked by the administration of berenil to mice in the late stage of the disease (Jennings *et al.*, 1989; Hunter *et al.*, 1992; Atouguia *et al.*, 1995). Toxic reactions have been observed in animals treated with berenil, the most important being brain damage reported in dogs (Losos and Crockett, 1969; Ogada, 1970; World Health Organization, 1986), camels (Homeida *et al.*, 1981) and asses (reviewed by Abaru *et al.*, 1984).

Melarsoprol

Melarsoprol is used in late-stage infections. The injection must be given very slowly and *strictly* intravenously, since all product contacting the surrounding tissues leads to severe pain and necrosis (Richet *et al.*, 1959; Rive *et al.*, 1973).

The classical treatment protocol for late-stage trypanosomiasis uses intravenous injections of 3.6 mg/kg melarsoprol (5.5 ml/injection maximum) and the number of courses is based on the number of cells in the CSF as follows: less than 20 cells: one course of three injections (one each day); more than 20 and less than 100 cells: two courses of three injections with 1-week interval; more than 100 cells: three courses of three injections with 1-week interval between each course; repeated treatments: four courses of three injections with 1-week interval between each course. Different treatment regimens have been proposed and are in use in Africa. The dosage and duration of therapy differ considerably between centres; some use maximum daily doses while others prefer progressively increasing doses (Bertrand *et al.*, 1974), or even an individually calculated dose depending on the patient's cardiac risk (Dumas *et al.*, 1976). Most of the treatment protocols include a preliminary treatment with suramin (two (5, 10 mg/kg) or three doses (5, 10 and 20 mg/kg) on alternate days) in *Trypanosoma brucei rhodesiense* infections, and pentamidine (4 mg/kg, 2 days) in *Trypanosoma brucei gambiense* infections (World Health Organization, 1986). Suramin is also used in the Gambian form in some centres, and berenil has also been used as a preliminary treatment, before melarsoprol (Van Nieuwenhove, 1992). Unfortunately, there are no established rules for the treatment of human African trypanosomiasis with melarsoprol, in terms of its dose, its duration, the preliminary treatment with early stage drugs (World Health Organization, 1986), and the use of corticosteroids during melarsoprol treatment (Arroz, 1987; Pepin *et al.*, 1985, 1989b). Following the existing regimens, about 80–90% of patients are cured, but a proportion of those relapsing will be refractory to further treatment with melarsoprol (Rollo, 1975).

The more physiologically important interaction of melarsoprol is with the spermidine-glutathione peptide trypanothione [N^1, N^8-bis(glutathionyl)spermidine], a molecule unique to trypanosomes that substitutes for glutathione in reducing reactive oxygen species from the cell and is essential in maintaining an intracellular reducing environment (Fairlamb and Cerami, 1992; Cunningham *et al.*, 1994). The melarsoprol-trypanothione adduct (Mel T) (Fairlamb *et al.*, 1989) formed in the cytosol of trypanosomes exposed to physiological doses of melarsoprol is unable to perform the essential role of trypanothione (Fairlamb *et al.*, 1992). Mel T is also an active competitive inhibitor of trypanothione reductase which serves to re-oxidize trypanothione thus maintaining the proper cytosolic reducing environment (Fairlamb *et al.*, 1989).

Side-effects are common during treatment with melarsoprol (Robertson, 1963). Just after the first injection malaise, nausea and vomiting, diarrhoea and, almost constantly, fever (Whittle and Pope, 1972) are described in the Rhodesian (Andrade e Silva *et al.*, 1954) and in the Gambian (Rive *et al.*, 1973) forms of the disease. Other more serious immediate reactions include rash, subconjunctival haemorrhages, swelling of the lips and tongue, tachycardia, retrosternal pain and headache (Triolo *et al.*, 1990). These side-effects are usually short, and do not appear following subsequent injections. Some symptoms, however, may appear after the third or fourth injection, and include fever and chills, malaise, headache, nausea and vomiting, albuminuria or oliguria, hiccup, rash, and haemorrhagic signs (Rive *et al.*, 1973).

Reactive encephalopathy (PTRE) is the most severe reaction to melarsoprol therapy, and occurs in 1% (Robertson, 1963) to 11.4% (Pepin *et al.*, 1989) of patients treated with melarsoprol (reviewed by Sina *et al.*, 1977). Its clinical features usually appear between the first and the second course of treatment (Haller *et al.*, 1986), and may be characterized by three different syndromes: fulminant convulsive status, sometimes preceded by minor prodromes such as dizziness or nausea, associated with acute cerebral oedema as shown by papilloedema; rapidly progressive coma, developing within hours, without convulsions or signs of cerebral oedema; and acute mental disturbances, such as aggression, restlessness, confusion, and emotional disorders, lasting for a few days, without neurological signs (Haller *et al.*, 1986). The final clinical feature is a deep comatose state, with sporadic epileptiform convulsions (Sina *et al.*, 1977). Some authors view the clinical picture of the encephalopathy as a non-characteristic coma with isolated signs of arsenical intoxication, the complete picture resembling an acceleration of the terminal stage of human African trypanosomiasis (Marneffe, 1955).

Treatment and care of patients developing encephalopathy include general measures for management of comatose patients, intravenous drip with 5% isotonic glucose, control of body temperature with antipyretics and cold sponging, antiepileptic drugs for convulsions, and treatment of cerebral oedema with mannitol or ACTH, diuretics, adrenaline and corticosteroids (World Health Organization, 1986). The administration of dimercaprol produces little or no benefit (Collomb *et al.*, 1973), and is no longer indicated (World Health Organization, 1986). After recovery from the PTRE treatment may be restarted with a small dose of melarsoprol and increasing this slightly, never giving the complete dose (Collomb *et al.*, 1973), or, alternatively, until it is possible to give a course in full dosage (Robertson, 1963). Even with prompt treatment, this reaction is fatal in more than 50% of the cases (Pépin *et al.*, 1989). Deaths due to this condition, however, have become less frequent with increasing experience in the use of melarsoprol. The reactive encephalopathy occurs more frequently and is more severe in patients with malnutrition, intercurrent infections, fever, and at the extremes of age. It has been suggested that factors such as a fourth series of melarsoprol injections, the number of white cells exceeding 100 in the CSF, and failure to use prednisolone during treatment all predispose to a higher incidence of the PTRE (Pépin *et al.*, 1995).

Other side-effects of melarsoprol treatment include lower limb motor neuropathy, gait disturbances, paralysis and sensory disturbances (Schneider, 1963). A case of tetraparesis (Grau Junyent *et al.*, 1988) and heart abnormalities consisting of cardiac arrhythmia, heart block and cardiac arrest (Apted, 1957) has also been described. Exfoliative dermatitis (Cruz Ferreira and Coutinho da Costa, 1963; Buyst, 1975) also known as arsenical dermatitis, since there are reports of the same condition with other arsenicals, namely melarsen (Butler *et al.*, 1957), agranulocytosis (Ogada and Okach, 1970), and diarrhoea (Sina *et al.*, 1982) have also been reported (Schneider, 1963).

Eflornithine

During the early period of its use, a complete course of eflornithine treatment included intravenous followed by oral administration of the drug. The recommended dose and schedule was 100 mg/kg 6-hourly i.v. for 15 days, followed by 75 mg/kg 6-hourly *per os*, for 21 days. Although some authors suggested that the oral formulation provided as good results as those obtained with the oral/i.v. therapy (De Groof *et al.*, 1992), until the end of the production of the oral compound, different doses and schedules had been used, some using only the oral DFMO, 100 mg/kg 6-hourly for 21 to 45 days, others using exclusively the i.v. formulation, 100 mg/kg 6-hourly for 14 days or 200 mg/kg 12-hourly for 14 days. The actual recommended dose and period of treatment is based on the i.v. formulation, 400 mg/kg/day, preferably divided into four 4 doses, or running continuously for 24 hours, for 14 days. A field trial based on the same dose but with only 7 days of treatment is still under evaluation (World Health Organization, 1995). When used in patients who have relapsed from a first treatment the results were very encouraging, with a failure rate of only 6.5% in 47 patients (Khonde *et al.*, 1997). Studies on the pharmacokinetics of eflornithine suggest the use of a higher dose, based on body surface area rather than on weight, for treating *T. gambiense* late-stage infection in children (Milord *et al.*, 1993).

Eflornithine is a catalytic enzyme-activated irreversible inhibitor of ornithine decarboxylase (ODC), the lead enzyme in the synthesis of the polyamines putrescine, spermidine and, in mammals, spermine, (Bey *et al.*, 1987) which are essential for cell division and differentiation. Studies in animal models using DFMO treatment have shown a significant depletion of whole brain putrescine and spermidine levels, whereas spermine levels remained unchanged (Gerrish *et al.*, 1993). Eflornithine also inhibits trypanosome DNA and protein synthesis (Bacchi *et al.*, 1983; Bitonti *et al.*, 1988). The physiological consequence of these actions for the trypanosomes is the transformation of the long-slender forms into the non-dividing, short-stumpy forms (Feagin *et al.*, 1986; Giffin *et al.*, 1986). This non-dividing form is incapable of changing its variant surface glycoprotein coat and can eventually be eliminated by the host immune response. Thus, a competent host immune response is required for elimination of the parasites after DFMO treatment (deGee *et al.*, 1983; Bitonti *et al.*, 1986b).

The most important side-effects are anaemia, leucopenia and thrombocytopenia (Pepin *et al.*, 1987; Eozenou *et al.*, 1989; Milord *et al.*, 1992), and some patients may therefore require blood transfusions (an often difficult procedure in rural hospitals in Africa). Other adverse effects include diarrhoea, nausea, vomiting, abdominal pain and anorexia, which appear to be related to the oral administration of the drug (Kazyumba *et al.*, 1988). Bilateral high-frequency hearing loss is common during treatment. Alopecia may start near the end of DFMO therapy, and may persist for months (J. Atouguia, personal observations). An increase in the number of infections, particularly abscesses, has been reported (Kazyumba *et al.*, 1988). In some late-stage HAT patients convulsions (Pepin *et al.*, 1987; Milord *et al.*, 1992) and hemiparesis (J. Atouguia, personal observations) may occur. The association of convulsions and anaemia with higher drug levels and previous melarsoprol therapy has also been reported (Milord *et al.*, 1993). All adverse effects associated with eflornithine treatment are generally reversible after decreasing the dose or stopping treatment. Eflornithine is not currently available because of production problems.

Nifurtimox

This drug is given orally. It is mainly used in Chagas' disease, and there is no standard dose and treatment period for sleeping sickness. Depending on the clinical trial, different doses and schedules have been adopted: 6 mg/kg/day during 40–120 days (Janssens and De Muynck, 1977), 4–5 mg/kg three times a day during 60 days (Moens *et al.*, 1984), 5 mg/kg three times a day during 60 days (Pepin *et al.*, 1989c), 5 mg/kg three times a day for 15–45 days (Van Niewenhove and Declercq, 1981; Van Niewenhove, 1988, 1992), 5 mg/kg three times a day for 14–21 days (Van Niewenhove, 1992) and 10 mg/kg three times a day for 30 days (Pepin *et al.*, 1992b). When children had to be treated, they received a higher dose, 20 mg/kg/day divided in three doses, for the same duration as the adults.

Little is known of nifurtimox's mode of action in the *T. brucei* group. It has been suggested that the drug blocks the removal of peroxides which occur during the transformation of the dithiol form into the disulfide form of trypanothione (Fairlamb, 1990).

Nifurtimox is not well tolerated. In humans, the incidence of undesirable side effects has been high and from 40 to 70% of patients have been affected. Children appear to tolerate the drug better than adults. Gastrointestinal discomfort, nausea, vomiting and epigastric pain are frequent, and these side-effects are responsible for refusal and cessation of treatment. Some CNS complications may be severe, and include vertigo, convulsions, status epilepticus, psychotic reactions and cerebellar syndrome. Other side-effects include peripheral polyneuropathy, anorexia and weight loss, and skin rashes. Nifurtimox may also exacerbate existing symptoms. Acute haemolytic anaemia can occur in G-6-PD-deficient individuals. The frequency and severity of the complications tend to increase with the dose and duration of treatment, but they are generally rapidly reversible after stopping the drug (Van Niewenhove, 1992). Gastric upset resulting from drug administration may be alleviated by simultaneous administration of aluminium hydroxide preparations. Phenobarbital provides symptomatic control of the drug's effects on the CNS (Rollo, 1975). Due to the gastrointestinal discomfort some patients avoid swallowing the tablets so rigorous supervision of drug intake is essential in nifurtimox treatment.

New therapeutic approaches

These include: *the development of new drugs*, such as the nitroimidazole megazole, a new compound with trypanocidal action under active investigation (Enanga *et al.*, 1997); *the development of new regimens*, using new melarsoprol (Burri *et al.*, 1995) and eflornithine (World Health Organization 1995; Khonde *et al.*, 1997) therapeutic regimens; *the development of drug combinations*, e.g. metronidazole with suramin (Arroz and Djedje 1988; Foulkes 1996), eflornithine with suramin (Taelman *et al.*, 1996), and eflornithine combined with melarsoprol (Simarro and Asumu 1996); and *the development of new formulations* based on experimental work in a mouse model which has showed promising results with the topical melarsoprol gel therapy (Atouguia *et al.*, 1995), alone or in combination with the nitrofuranes and the nitroimidazoles (Jennings *et al.*, 1996).

Follow up

Follow up of a treated patient is mandatory to prevent relapses, and must be continued for at least 2 years after the end of treatment (World Health Organization, 1986). There are no definitive criteria to establish that a patient is completely cured. Immediately following treatment, and after documenting an improvement of the clinical features, the most important criterion is the disappearance of parasites from the blood and, in late stage patients, from the CSF (Apted, 1970b). This evaluation must be done by a direct method, preferably m-AECT for the blood examination, and double centrifugation for CSF.

Immediately after treatment antibody levels are still high, but should still be measured for future reference. It has been reported that CSF cell counts and protein levels at this stage may show higher values than before when on arsenical treatment (Janssens, 1977) – the French speaking authors called it 'orage liquidien', or 'CSF storm' – and should not be considered as markers of unsuccessful treatment or relapse. These abnormal CSF cells and proteins values can be observed until 9 months after the arsenical treatment (Ginoux *et al.*, 1984), and have not been reported with other drugs or with Rhodesiense infections.

Studies using antigen detection for the follow up of treated patients have shown inconsistent results (Olaho-Mukani *et al.*, 1994). The PCR technique, which looks promising in experimental studies (J. Burke, personal communication) and in the diagnosis of animal trypanosomiasis (Desquesnes, 1997), should in principle prove very useful after the treatment: a treated patient with a negative PCR would indicate successful chemotherapy, and obviate the need for a 2-year follow up. However, existing trypanosome-PCR techniques are still under evaluation, and there are no reports of its use in the follow up of human trypanosomiasis.

Six-monthly clinical and laboratory evaluations for a period of 2 years are proposed for effective follow up. On these occasions a clinical examination is performed, blood is collected and analysed for the presence of trypanosomes, and the levels of IgM and trypanosome antibodies measured. In late-stage treated patients the CSF is also collected and examined, and screened for parasites, increased number of cells, higher values of protein levels, and also levels of IgM and trypanosome antibodies. Direct blood and CSF examination for parasites should be negative, and IgM and trypanosome antibody titres should have returned to normal values between 6 and 12 months following successful treatment. If, 2 years after the end of the treatment, parasitological, serological and biochemical parameters are normal, the patient is considered to be cured. At present, there is no method which can distinguish between a relapse and a reinfection (Van Meirvenne, 1992).

Prognosis and neurological sequelae

An infected person will always develop the disease. In the Gambiense form of the disease several years may pass between the infection and the first clinical manifestations. The Rhodesiense form of the disease has a more acute clinical picture (Wéry, 1991). It is assumed that every untreated patient will develop early-stage infection followed by the invasion of the CNS by the trypanosomes and the consequent neurological infection. Death invariably occurs in untreated cases (Cegielsky and Dusack, 1991).

The prognosis of human African trypanosomiasis is good when the patient is correctly treated with pentamidine or suramin in the early stage of the disease. Patients in the late stage of the disease with severe CNS involvement are difficult to treat, and may be left with neurological sequelae, which usually include the persistence of the neurological abnormalities found prior to treatment (Kazumba *et al.*, 1993), or the exacerbation or appearance of new symptoms or signs during or after the treatment (Collomb and Miletto, 1957). The most common psychiatric sequelae include intellectual problems (fatiguability and lack of concentration), sexual (increase or decrease of the libido) and personality changes, and also depressive and psychotic clinical features (Collomb and Miletto, 1957). The most frequent neurological sequelae include hemiplegia, ataxic gait, involuntary movements, and convulsions (Kazumba *et al.*, 1993; J. Atouguia, personal observations). Most of these neurological sequelae have been reported in children (Triolo *et al.*, 1985) and in Europeans (Collomb and Miletto, 1957). They are usually transient, and the patient, with appropriate treatment, will usually recover within 6 months to 1 year. Patients who have undergone several late-stage treatment regimens due to relapses, with the disease showing a progressive and chronic pattern, have more frequent and permanent sequelae (J. Atouguia, personal observation).

References

Abaru, D. E. (1978). Reactions seen in human trypanosomiasis patients treated with berenil. *ICOPA V*, Warsaw, 1978, Section D, p. 86.

Abaru, D. E. and Mantovu, F. S. (1981). Berenil in the treatment of early stage human trypanosomiasis cases. In: *Proceedings, 17th meeting, International Scientific Council for Trypanosomiasis Research and Control, Arusha, Tanzania*, OAU/STRC Publication 112, pp. 194–198.

Abaru, D. E., Liwo, D. A., Isakina, D. and Okori, E. E. (1984). Retrospective long-term study of effects of Berenil by follow-up of patients treated since 1965. *Tropenmed. Parasitol.*, 35, 148–150.

Adams, J. H., Haller, L., Boa, F. Y. *et al.* (1986). Human African trypanosomiasis (*T. b. gambiense*): a study of 16 fatal cases of sleeping sickness with some observations on acute reactive arsenical encephalopathy. *Neuropathol. Appl. Neurobiol.*, **12**, 81–94.

Aerts, D., Truc, P., Penchenier, L. *et al.* (1992). A kit for in vitro isolation of trypanosomes in the field: first trial with sleeping sickness patients in the Congo Republic. *Trans. Roy. Soc. Trop. Med. Hyg.*, **86**, 394–395.

Almeida Franco, L. T. (1960). A velocidade de sedimentação dos eritrócitos na tripanossomíase humana (*T. gambiense*). *An. Inst. Med. Trop.*, **17**, 967–1008.

Amevigbe, M. D. D., Jauberteau-Marchan, M. O., Bouteille, B. *et al.* (1992). Human African trypanosomiasis: presence of antibodies to galactocerebrosides. *Am. J. Trop. Med. Hyg.*, **47**, 652–662.

Andrade e Silva, M. A. (1957). The value of drugs commonly used in the treatment of *T. rhodesiense* sleeping sickness. *An. Inst. Med. Trop.*, **14**, 159–177.

Andrade e Silva, M. A., Caseiro, A., Carmo, R. P. and Basto, A. X. (1954). Arsobal in the treatment of Rhodesian sleeping sickness. *An. Inst. Med. Trop.*, **11**, 261–285.

Antoine, Ph. (1977). Étude neurologique et psychologique de malades trypanosomés et leur evolution. *Ann. Soc. Belge Méd. Trop.*, **57**, 227–247.

Apted, F. I. C. (1957). Four years' experience of melarsen oxide/bal in the treatment of late-stage Rhodesian sleeping sickness. *Trans. Roy. Soc. Trop. Med. Hyg.*, **51**, 75–86.

Apted, F. I. C. (1970a). Clinical manifestations and diagnosis of sleeping sickness. In: *The African Trypanosomiases*, (H. W. Mulligan, ed.). London: George Allen & Unwin. pp. 661–683.

Apted, F. I. C. (1970b) Treatment of human trypanosomiasis. In: *The African Trypanosomiases*, (H. W. Mulligan, ed.). London: George Allen & Unwin. pp. 684–710.

Apted, F. I. C. (1980) Present status of chemotherapy and chemoprophylaxis of human trypanosomiasis in the eastern hemisphere. *Pharmacol. Ther.*, **11**, 391–413.

Arnott, M. A., Cairns, D. and Hay, J. (1992). Pentamidine in blood. *Trans. Roy. Soc. Trop. Med. Hyg.*, **86**, 460.

Arroz, J. O. L. (1987). Melarsoprol and reactive encephalopathy in *Trypanosoma brucei rhodesiense*. *Trans. Roy. Soc. Trop. Med. Hyg.*, **81**, 192.

Arroz, J. and Djedje, M. (1988). Suramin and metronidazole in the treatment of *Trypanosoma brucei rhodesiense*. *Trans. Roy. Soc. Trop. Med. Hyg.*, **82**, 421.

Ashcroft, M. T. (1959). A critical review of the epidemiology of human trypanosomiasis in Africa. *Trop. Dis. Bull.*, **56**, 1073–1093.

Atouguia, J. M., Jennings, F. W. and Murray, M. (1995). Successful treatment of experimental murine *Trypanosoma brucei* infection with topical melarsoprol gel. *Trans. Roy. Soc. Trop. Med. Hyg.*, **89**, 531–533.

Bacchi, C. J., Garofalo, J., Mockenhaupt, D. *et al.* (1983). *In vitro* effects of alpha-DL-difluoromethylornithine on the metabolism and morphology of *Trypanosoma brucei brucei*. *Mol. Biochem. Parasitol.*, **7**, 209–225.

Barker, R. H. JR (1994). Use of PCR in the field. *Parasitol. Today*, **10**, 117–119.

Baumann, H. and Strassmann, G. (1993). Suramin inhibits the stimulation of acute phase plasma protein genes by IL-6-type cytokines in rat hepatoma cells. *J. Immunol.*, **151**, 1456–1462.

Benaim, G., Lopez-Estrano, C., Docampo, R. and Moreno, S. N. J. (1993). A calmodulin-stimulated Ca^{2+} pump in plasma-membrane vesicles from *Trypanosoma brucei*; selective inhibition by pentamidine. *Biochem. J.*, **296**, 759–763.

Bentivoglio, M., Grassi-Zucconi, G., Olsson, T. and Kristensson, K. (1994). *Trypanosoma brucei* and the nervous system. *Trends Neurosci.*, **17**, 325–329.

Berger, B. J., Carter, N. S. and Fairlamb, A. H. (1993). Characterisation of pentamidine-resistant *Trypanosoma brucei brucei*. *Mol. Biochem. Parasitol.*, **69**, 289–298.

Bertrand, Ed., Baudin, L., Vacher, P. *et al.* (1967). L'atteinte du coeur dans 100 cas de tripanosomiase africaine à *Trypanosoma gambiense*. *Bull. Soc. Pathol. Exot.*, **60**, 360–369.

Bertrand, Ed., Sentilhes, L., Baudin, L. *et al.* (1968). Troubles de conduction cardiaque dans la trypanosomiase humaine africaine à *Trypanosoma gambiense*. *Bull. Soc. Pathol. Exot.*, **61**, 613–617.

Bertrand, Ed., Serie, F., Kone, I. *et al.* (1973a). Symptomatologie générale de la trypanosomiase humaine africaine au moment du dépistage. *Méd. Afrique Noire*, **20**, 303–314.

Bertrand, Ed., Serie, F., Rive, J. *et al.* (1973b). La symptomatologie cardio-vasculaire dans la trypanosomiase humaine africaine à *Trypanosoma gambiense* (à propos de 187 malades). *Mèd. Afrique Noire*, **20**, 327–339.

Bertrand, Ed., Serie, F., Rive, J. *et al.* (1974). Les traitements d'attaque de la trypanosomiase humaine Africaine: problèmes et suggestions. *Méd. Trop.*, **34**, 445–494.

Bey, P., Danzin, C. and Jung, M. (1987). Inhibition of basic amino acid decarboxylases involved in polyamine biosynthesis. In: *Inhibition of Polyamine Metabolism: Biological Significance and Basis for New Therapies*, (P. P. McCann and A. Sjoerdsma, eds). Orlando: Academic Press. pp. 1–31.

Bitonti, A. J., Dumont, J. A. and McCann, P. P. (1986a). Characterization of *Trypanosoma brucei brucei* S-adenosylmethionine decarboxylase and its inhibition by Berenil, pentamidine and methylglyoxal bis(guanylhydrazone). *Biochem. J.*, **237**, 685–689.

Bitonti, A. J., McCann, P. P. and Sjoerdsma, A. (1986b). Necessity of antibody response in the treatment of African trypanosomiasis with alpha-difluoromethylornithine. *Biochem. Pharmacol.*, **35**, 331–334.

Bitonti, A. J., Cross-Doersen, D. E. and McCann, P. P. (1988). Effect of alpha-difluoromethylornithine on protein synthesis and synthesis of the variant-specific glycoprotein (VSG) in *Trypanosoma brucei brucei*. *Biochem. J.*, **250**, 295–298.

Blair, D. M. (1939). Human trypanosomiasis in Southern Rhodesia 1911–1938. *Trans. Roy. Soc. Trop. Med. Hyg.*, **32**, 729–742.

Blin, G. and Kernéis, J. (1916). Note concernant le premier cas de maladie du sommeil constaté chez un Européen en Guinée Française. *Bull. Soc. Pathol. Exot.*, **9**, 231–234.

Boa, Y. F., Traore, M. A., Doua, F. *et al.* (1988). Les différents tableaux cliniques actuels de la trypanosomiase humaine Africaine a *T. b. gambiense*. Analyse de 300 dossiers du foyer de Daloa, Côte-D'Ivoire. *Bull. Soc. Pathol. Exot.*, **81**, 427–444.

Boillot, D., Veld, P., Sai, P. *et al.* (1985). Functional and morphological modifications induced in rat islets by pentamidine and other diamidines in vitro. *Diabetologia*, **28**, 359–364.

Boné, G. J. and Charlier, J. (1975). L'hémaglutination indirecte en cappillaire. Une méthode de diagnostic de la trypanosomiase applicable sur le terrain. *Ann. Soc. Belge Méd. Trop.*, **55**, 559–569.

Boreham, P. F. L (1968). Immune reactions and kinnin formation in chronic trypanosomiasis. *Br. J. Pharmacol. Ther.*, **32**, 493–504.

Boreham, P. F. L (1970). Kinnin release and immune reaction in human trypanosomiasis caused by *Trypanosoma rhodesiense*. *Trans. Roy. Soc. Trop. Med. Hyg.*, **64**, 394–400.

Boreham, P. F. L and Goodwin, L. G. (1970). The release of kinnin as a result of antigen antibody reactions in trypanosomiasis. *Pharmacol. Res. Commun.*, **1**, 144–145.

Borges, F., Romão, T., Atouguia, J. and Champalimaud, J. L. (1992). Tripanossomose africana: um caso clínico. 1ᵃˢ Jornadas de Doenças Infecciosas e de Medicina Tropical, Instituto de Higiene e Medicina Tropical, Lisboa, 1992.

Bowman, I. B. R. and Flynn, I. W. (1976). Oxidative metabolism of trypanosomes. In: *Biology of Kinetoplastida*, (W. H. R. Lumsden and D. A. Evans, eds). Vol. I. London: Academic Press. pp. 435–476.

Brown, W. J. and Voge, M. (1982). *Neuropathology of Parasitic Infections*. Oxford: Oxford University Press, p. 240.

Buchanan, J. C. R. (1929). Some clinical aspects of trypanosomiasis rhodesiensis. *Trans. Roy. Soc. Trop. Med. Hyg.*, **23**, 81–88.

Buguet, A., Bert, J., Tapie, P. *et al.* (1994). Distribution du sommeil et de la veille dans la trypanosomose humaine africaine. *Bull. Soc. Pathol. Exot.*, **87**, 362–367.

Burke, J. A. M. E., Bengosi, K. and Diantete, N. L. (1973). Un cas de trypanosomiase africaine (*T. gambiense*) congénitale. *Ann. Soc. Belge Méd. Trop.*, **54**, 1–5.

Burri, C., Blum, J. and Brun, R. (1995). Alternative application of melarsoprol for treatment of *T. b. gambiense* sleeping sickness. *Ann. Soc. Belge Méd. Trop.*, **75**, 65–71.

Butler, G. C., Duggan, A. J. and Hutchinson, M. P. (1957). Melarsen in the treatment of *Trypanosoma gambiense* infection in man. *Trans. Roy. Soc. Trop. Med. Hyg.*, **51**, 69–74.

Buyst, H. (1973). Pregnancy complications in Rhodesian sleeping sickness. *East African Med. J.*, **50**, 19–21.

Buyst, H. (1975). The treatment of *T. rhodesiense* sleeping sickness with special reference to its physio-pathological and epidemiological basis. *Ann. Soc. Belge Méd. Trop.*, **55**, 95–104.

Buyst, H. (1976). The treatment of congenital trypanosomiasis. *Trans. Roy. Soc. Trop. Med. Hyg.*, **70**, 163–164.

Calwell, H. G. (1937). The pathology of the brain in Rhodesian trypanosomiasis. *Trans. Roy. Soc. Trop. Med. Hyg.*, **30**, 611–624.

Cattand, P. (1994). Trypanosomiase humaine africaine. Situation épidémiologique actuelle, une recrudescence alarmante de la maladie. *Bull. Soc. Path. Ex.*, **87**, 307–310

Cattand, P., Miézan, B. P. and De Raadt, P. (1988). Human African trypanosomiasis: use of double centrifugation of cerebrospinal fluid to detect trypanosomes. *Bull. World Hlth Org.*, **66**, 83–86.

Cegielsky, J. P. and Dusack, D. T. (1991). Protozoal infections of the central nervous system. In: *Infections of the Central Nervous System*. (W. M. Scheld, R. J. Whitley and D. T. Dusack, eds). New York: Raven Press. pp. 767–800.

Clerc, M., Rive, J., Le Bras, M. *et al.* (1973). Rapport sur l interêt des immunoglobulines pour le diagnostic de la trypanosomiase. *Méd. Afrique Noire*, **20**, 357–376.

Collomb, H., Miletto, G. and Levron, M. (1956). Troubles de la glycorégulation et diamidines. (À propos de trois observations de diabète après traitement par la Lomidine). *Méd. Trop.*, **16**, 786.

Collomb, H. and Miletto, G. (1957). Les séquelles de la trypanosomiase humaine africaine. *Bull. Soc. Path. Exot.*, **50**, 573–585.

Collomb, H., Ayats, H. and Martino, P. (1964). Les causes de décès das la Trypanosomiase humaine africaine. *Bull. Soc. Méd. Afrique Noire Langue Fran.*, **9**, 54–59.

Collomb, H. and Bartoli, D. (1967). Le coeur dans la trypanosomiase humaine africaine à *Trypanosoma gambiense*. *Bull. Soc. Pathol. Exot.*, **60**, 142–156.

Collomb, H., Dumas, M. and Girard, P-L. (1973). Trypanocides, indications cliniques. *Méd. Afrique Noire*, **20**, 837–844.

Comtois, R., Pouliot, J., Vinet, B. *et al.* (1992). Higher pentamidine levels in AIDS patients with hypoglycemia and azotemia during treatment of *Pneumocystis carinii* pneumonia. *Am. Rev. Resp. Dis.*, **146**, 740–745.

Cook, G. C. (1991). Protozoan and helminthic infections. In: *Infections of the Central Nervous System*, (H. P. Lambert, ed.) Philadelphia: BC Decker Inc. pp. 264–282.

Cooke, W. E., Gregg, A. L. and Manson-Bahr, P. H. (1937). Recent experiences of mild or symptomless infections with *Trypanosoma gambiense* from the Gold Coast and Nigeria. *Trans. Roy. Soc. Trop. Med. Hyg.*, **30**, 461–466.

Coulaud, J., Caquet, R., Froli, G. *et al.* (1975). Atteintes rénale et pancréatique sévères au cours d'un traitement par la pentamidine d'une tripanosomiase africaine. *Ann. Méd. Int. (Paris)*, **126**, 665–669.

Courtois, D. and Bideau, J. (1966) L'immunofluorescence appliquée au diagnostic de la trypanosomiase humaine Africaine. Valeur comparative avec le titrage de l'immunoglobuline IgM. *Bull. Soc. Pathol. Exot.*, **59**, 809–817.

Cruz Ferreira, F. (1973). Tripanossomíase africana. In: *Epidemiologia e profilaxia das doenças infecciosas e parasitárias*. Lisboa: Junta de Investigação do Ultramar. pp. 361–380.

Cruz Ferreira, F. and Lehmann de Almeida, C. (1950). Sobre a sintomatologia clínica da doença do sono. *Gaz. Méd. Port.*, **3**, 769–788.

Cruz Ferreira, F. S. and Coutinho da Costa, F. M. (1963). Resultados do tratamento da tripanosomiase humana Africana com o Arsobal. *Gaz. Méd. Port.*, **16**, 239–246.

Cunningham, M. L., Zvelebil, Marketa J. J. M. and Fairlamb, A. H. (1994). Mechanism of inhibition of trypanothione reductase and glutathione reductase by trivalent organic arsenicals. *Eur. J. Biochem.*, **221**, 285–295.

Damper, D. and Patton, C. L. (1976). Pentamidine transport and sensitivity in *brucei*-group trypanosomes. *J. Protozool.*, **23**, 349–356.

Darré, H., Mollaret, P., Tanguy, Y. and Mercier, P. (1937). Hydrocéphalie congénitale par trypanosomiase hereditaire. Démonstration de la possibilité du passage transplacentaire dans l'espèce humaine. *Bull. Soc. Pathol. Exot.*, **30**, 159–176.

Davelloose, P. (1971). Un cas de trypanosomiase africaine congénitale. *Ann. Soc. Belge Méd. Trop.*, **52**, 63.

De Gee, A. L., McCann, P. P. and Mansfield, J. M. (1983). Role of antibody in the elimination of trypanosomes after DL-alpha-difluoromethylornithine chemotherapy. *J. Parasitol.*, **69**, 818–822.

De Groof, D., Bruneel, H., Musumari, T. S. and Ruppol, J. F. (1992). Treatment of sleeping disease caused by *Trypanosoma brucei gambiense* with α-difluoro-methylornithine (DFMO) in a rural hospital in Zaire. *Méd. Trop.*, **52**, 369–375.

De Raadt, P. (1966). Reactive encephalopathy occurring as a complication during treatment of *Trypanosoma rhodesiense* infections with non-arsenical drugs. *East African Trypanosome Research Organisation Report*, 1966, pp. 85–86.

De Raadt, P. and Kotten, J. W. (1968). Myocarditis in *T. rhodesiense* infections. *Trans. Roy. Soc. Trop. Med. Hyg.*, **62**, 121.

Desquesnes, M. (1997). Evaluation of a simple PCR technique for the diagnosis of *Trypanosoma vivax* infection in the serum of cattle incomparison to para-sitological techniques and antigen-enzyme-linked immuno sorbent assay. *Acta Trop.*, **65**, 139–148.

DeVita, V. T., Emmer, M., Levine, A. *et al.* (1969). *Pneumocystis carinii* pneumonia. *N. Engl. J. Med.*, **280**, 287–291.

Doucet, J. (1973). La trypanosomiase: diagnostic parasitologique. *Méd. Afrique Noire*, **20**, 283–288.

Duggan, A. J. (1959). An approach to clinical problems of Gambian sleeping sickness. *J. Trop. Med. Hyg.*, **62**, 268–274.

Duggan, A. J. and Hutchington, M. P. (1966). Sleeping sickness in Europeans: a review of 109 cases. *J. Trop. Med. Hyg.*, **69**, 124–131.

Dumas, M., Girard, P-L. and N'diaye, I. P. (1976). Traitement de la trypanosomiase humaine africaine en milieu hospitalier. *Méd. Afrique Noire*, **23**, 39–41.

Dutertre, J. (1968). La trypanosomiase humaine africaine. I. Generalités historique. *Méd. Afrique Noire*, **4**, 147–157.

Duvallet, G. and Saliou, P. (1978). Organization du despistage de la trypanosomiase humaine en Afrique de l'ouest. *Med. Trop.*, **38**, 533–536.

Duvallet, G., Saliou, P. and Rey, J-L. (1978). Fiabilité de la reaction d'immunofluorescence indirecte pour le diagnostic de la trypanosomiase humaine africaine. *Med. Trop.*, **38**, 513–518.

Enanga, B., Labat, C., Boudra, H. *et al.* (1997). Simple high-performance liquid chromatographic method to analyse megazol in human and rat plasma. *J. Chromatogr. B: Biomed. Appl.*, **696**, 261–266.

Eozenou, P., Jannin, J., Ngampo, S. *et al.* (1989). Essai de traitement de la trypanosomiase a *Trypanosoma brucei-gambiense* par l'eflornithine en République Populaire du Congo. *Méd. Trop.*, **49**, 149–154.

Estambale, B. B. A. and Knight, R. (1992). Protozoan and HIV-1 infection: a review. *East Afr. Med. J.*, **69**, 373–377.

Fairbairn, H. (1956). The infectivity to man of syringe-passaged strains of *Trypanosoma rhodesiense* and *T. gambiense*. *Ann. Trop. Med. Parasitol.*, **50**, 167–171.

Fairlamb, A. H. (1990). Future prospects for the chemotherapy of human trypanosomiasis. 1. Novel approaches to the chemotherapy of trypanosomiasis. *Trans. Roy. Soc. Trop. Med. Hyg.*, **84**, 613–617.

Fairlamb, A. H., Henderson, G. B. and Cerami, A. (1989). Trypanothione is the primary target for arsenical drugs against African trypanosomes. *Proc. Nat. Acad. Sci. USA*, **86**, 2607–2611.

Fairlamb, A. H. and Cerami, A. (1992). Metabolism and functions of trypanothione in kinetoplastida. *Ann. Rev. Microbiol.*, **46**, 695–729.

Fairlamb, A. H., Carter, N. S., Cunningham, M. and Smith, K. (1992). Characterisation of melarsen-resistant *Trypanosoma brucei brucei* with respect to cross-resistance to other drugs and trypanothione metabolism. *Mol. Biochem. Parasitol.*, **53**, 213–222.

Feagin, J. E., Jasmer, D. P. and Stuart, K. (1986). Differential mitochondrial gene expression between slender and stumpy bloodforms of *Trypanosoma brucei*. *Mol. Biochem. Parasitol.*, **20**, 207–214.

Foulkes, J. R. (1975). An evaluation of prednisolone as a routine adjunct to the treatment of *Trypanosoma rhodesiense*. *J. Trop. Med. Hyg.*, **78**, 72–74.

Foulkes, J. R. (1981). Human trypanosomiasis in Africa. *Br. Med. J.*, **283**, 1172–1174.

Foulkes, J. R. (1996). Metronidazole and suramin combination in the treatment of arsenical refractory rhodesian sleeping sickness – a case study. *Trans. Roy. Soc. Trop. Med. Hyg.*, **90**, 422.

Frean, J. A. and Bush, J. B. (1993). False-positive trypanosome identification. *Sth Afr. Med. J.*, **83**, 222–223.

Fruit, J., Santoro, D., Afchain, G. *et al.* (1977). Les immunocomplexes circulants dans la trypanosomiase africaine humaine et experimentale. *Ann. Soc. Belge Méd. Trop.*, **57**, 257–266.

Gallais, P. and Ranque, J. (1953). Trypanosomiase et syphillis. Interet du test de Nelson dans la trypanosomiase. *Méd. Trop.*, **13**, 857–858.

Gelfand, M. (1947). Transitory neurological signs in sleeping sickness. *Trans. Roy. Soc. Trop. Med. Hyg.*, **41**, 255–258.

Gelfand, M. (1966). The early clinical features of rhodesian trypanosomiasis with special reference to the 'chancre' (local reaction). *Trans. Roy. Soc. Trop. Med. Hyg.*, **60**, 376–379.

Gerrish, K. E., Fuller, D. J. M., Gerner, E. W. and Gensler, H. L. (1993). Inhibition of DFMO-induced audiogenic seizures by chlordiazepoxide. *Life Sci.*, **52**, 1101–1108.

Giffin, B. F., McCann, P. P., Bitonti, A. J. and Bacchi, C. J. (1986). Polyamine depletion following exposure to DL-alpha-difluoromethylornithine both *in vivo* and *in vitro* initiates morphological alterations and mitochondrial activation in a monomorphic strain of *Trypanosoma brucei brucei*. *J. Protozool.*, **33**, 238–243.

Ginoux, P. Y., Lancien, J., Frezil, J. L. and Bissadidi, N., (1984). Les échecs du traitement de la trypanosomiase a *T. gambiense* au Congo. *Med. Trop.*, **44**, 149–154.

Giordano, C. (1973). Les signes neurologiques et électro-encephalographiques de la trypanosomiase humaine africaine. *Méd. Afrique Noire*, **20**, 317–324.

Giordano, C., Clerc, M., Doutriaux, C. *et al.* (1977). Le diagnostique neurologique au cours des différentes phases de la trypanosomiase humaine Africaine. *Ann. Soc. Belge Méd. Trop.*, **57**, 213–225.

Glasgow, J. P. (1970). The genus *Glossina*. Introduction. In: *The African Trypanosomiases*, (H.W. Mulligan, ed.). London: George Allen & Unwin. pp. 225–242.

Goa, K. L. and Campoli-Richards, D. M. (1987). Pentamidine isethionate. A review of its antiprotozoal activity, pharmacokinetic properties and therapeutic use in *Pneumocystis carinii* pneumonia. *Drugs*, **33**, 242–258.

Gouteux, J. P. and Malonga, J. R. (1985). Enquête socio-entomologique dans le foyer de trypanosomiase humaine de Yamba. *Méd. Trop.*, **45**, 259–263.

Gouteux, J. P., Noireau, F., Malonga, J. R. and Frézil, J. L. (1988). 'Effect de case' et 'contamination familiale' dans la maladie du sommeil: essay d'interpretation du phénoméne. *Ann. Parasitol. Hum. Comp.*, **68**, 315–333.

Graf, H. (1929). Report on four cases of trypanosomiasis occurring in Europeans of the British Cameroons. *Trans. Roy. Soc. Trop. Med. Hyg.*, **23**, 95–100.

Grau Junyent, J. M., Rozman, M., Corachán, M. *et al.* (1988). An unusual course of West African trypanosomiasis in a Caucasian man. *Trans. Roy. Soc. Trop. Med. Hyg.*, **81**, 931–932.

Gray, A. R. (1967). Some principles of the immunology of trypanosomiasis. *Bull. World Hlth Org.*, **37**, 177–193.

Greenwood, B. M. (1974). Possible role of a B-cell mitogen in hypergammaglobulinaemia in malaria and trypanosomiasis. *Lancet*, **1**, 435–436.

Greenwood, B. M., Whittle, H. C. and Molyneux, D. H. (1973). Immunosupression in Gambian trypanosomiasis. *Trans. Roy. Soc. Trop. Med. Hyg.*, **67**, 846–850.

Greenwood, B. M. and Whittle, H. C. (1976). Complement activation in patients with Gambian sleeping sickness. *Clin. Exp. Immunol.*, **24**, 133–138.

Greenwood, B. M. and Whittle, H. C. (1980). The pathogenesis of sleeping sickness. *Trans. Roy. Soc. Trop. Med. Hyg.*, **74**, 716–725.

Haller, L., Adams, H., Merouze, F. and Dago, A. (1986). Clinical and pathological aspects of human African trypanosomiasis (*T. b. gambiense*) with particular reference to reactive arsenical encephalopathy. *Am. J. Trop. Med. Hyg.*, **35**, 94–99.

Hamon, J. F. and Camara, P. (1992). Étude electroencephalographique chez des trypanosomes en phase meningoencephalitique de la trypanosomiase humaine africaine à *Trypanosoma brucei gambiense* avant et après un traitement a la DL-alphadifluoromethylornithine hydrochloride monohydratee (DFMO). *Bull. Soc. Pathol. Exot.*, **85**, 378–384.

Hamon, J. F., Camara, P., Gauthier, P. *et al.* (1993). Waking electroencephalograms in the blood-lymph and encephalitic stages of gambian trypanosomiasis. *Ann. Trop. Med. Parasitol.*, **87**, 149–155.

Hamon, J. F., Juan de Mendoza, J. L. and Camara, P. A. (1995). Trypanosomiase: determination de groupes de patients a partir de donnees cliniques et electro-encephalographiques. *Neurophysiol. Clin.*, **25**, 196–202.

Harding, R.D. (1945). Late results of treatment of sleeping sickness in Sierra Leone by antrypol, tryparsamide, pentamidine and propamidine singly and in various combinations. *Trans. Roy. Soc. Trop. Med. Hyg.*, **39**, 99–124.

Hatson, H. S. (1975). Studies on the early development of *Trypanosoma brucei* in the vector *Glossina morsitans*. *PhD Thesis*. University of Glasgow.

Hawking, F. and Greenfield, J. G. (1941). Two autopsies on Rhodesiense sleeping sickness: visceral lesions and significance of changes in cerebrospinal fluid. *Trans. Roy. Soc. Trop. Med. Hyg.*, **35**, 155–164.

Heby, O., Luk, G. D. and Schindler, J. (1987). Polyamine synthesis inhibitors act as both inducers and suppressors of cell differentiation. In: *Inhibition of Polyamine Metabolism*, (P. P. McCann, A. E. Pegg and A. Sjoerdsma, eds). Orlando: Academic Press. pp. 165–186.

Henry, M. C., Kageruka, P., Ruppol, J. F. *et al.* (1981). Evaluation du diagnostic sur le terrain de la trypanosomiase a *Trypanosoma brucei gambiense*. *Ann. Soc. Belge Med. Trop.*, **61**, 79–92.

Heppner, C., Petzke, F., Arlt, W. *et al.* (1995). Adrenocortical insufficiency in Rhodesian sleeping sickness is not attributable to suramin. *Trans. Roy. Soc. Trop. Med. Hyg.*, **89**, 65–68.

Hissette, J. (1932). Considerations pratiques sur des accidents oculaires de la trypano-somiase ou de son traitement. *Ann. Soc. Belge Méd. Trop.*, **12**, 531–538.

Homeida, A. M., El Amin, E. A., Adam, S. E. I. and Mahmoud, M. M. (1981). Toxicity of diminazene aceturate (Berenil) to camels. *J. Comp. Pathol.*, **91**, 355–360.

Hublart, M., Lagouche, L., Racadot, A. *et al.* (1988). Fonction endocrine et trypano-somiase Africaine. *Bull. Soc. Pathol. Exot.*, **81**, 468–476.

Hunter, C. A. and Kennedy, P. G. E. (1992). Immunopathology in central nervous system human African trypanosomiasis. *J. Neuroimmunol.*, **36**, 56–61.

Hunter, C. A., Jennings, F. W., Adams, J. H. *et al.* (1992). Subcurative chemotherapy and fatal post-treatment reactive encephalopathies in African trypanosomiasis. *Lancet*, **339**, 956–958.

Hurst, E. W. (1959). The lesions produced in the central nervous system by certain organic arsenical compounds. *J. Pathol. Bacteriol.*, **77**, 523–533.

Hutchinson, M. P. and Watson, H. J. C. (1962). Berenil in the treatment of Trypanosoma gambiense infection in man. *Trans. Roy. Soc. Trop. Med. Hyg.*, **56**, 227.

Jannin, J., Mouliat-Pelat, J. P., Chanfreau, B. *et al.* (1993). Trypanosomiase humaine africaine: étude d'un score de présomption de diagnostic au Congo. *Bull. Org. Mond. Santé*, **71**, 215–222.

Janssens, P. G. (1977). Quatre décennies de la maladie du sommeil. *Ann. Soc. Belge Med. Trop.*, **57**, 191–200.

Janssens, P. G., Van Bogaert, L., Michiels, A. and Van de Steen, R. (1960). Trypanosomiase africaine, affection virale, mel B et encéphalite. *Ann. Soc. Belge Med. Trop.*, **40**, 759–769.

Janssens, P. G. and De Muynck, A. (1977). Clinical trials with 'Nifurtimox' in african trypanosomiasis. *Ann. Soc. Belge Med. Trop.*, **57**, 475–479.

Jennings, F. W., McNeil, P. E., Ndung'u, J. M. and Murray, M. (1989). Trypanoso-miasis and encephalitis: possible aetiology and treatment. *Trans. Roy. Soc. Trop. Med. Hyg.*, **83**, 518–519.

Jennings, F. W., Atouguia, J. M. and Murray, M. (1996). Topical chemotherapy for experimental murine African CNS-trypanosomiasis: the successful use of the arsenical, melarsoprol, combined with the 5-nitroimidazoles, fexinidazole or MK-436. *Trop. Med. Int. Hlth*, **5**, 590–598.

Jonchère, H. (1951). Traitement par les diamidines de la phase lymphatico-sanguine de la trypanosomiase humaine en A. O. F. *Bull. Soc. Pathol. Exot.*, **44**, 603–625.

Kageruka, P. (1989). Reservoir animal de *Trypanosoma* (*Trypanozoon*) *brucei gam-biense* in Afrique Centrale. *Ann. Soc. Belge Méd. Trop.*, **69**, 155–163.

Kashiwazaki, Y., Snowden, K., Smith, D. H. and Hommel, M. (1994). A multiple antigen detection dipstick colloidal dye immunoassay for the field diagnosis of trypanosome infections in cattle *Vet. Parasitol.*, **55**, 57–69

Kazumba, M., Kazadi, K. and Mulumba, M. P. (1993). Caracteristiques de la trypanosomiase de l'enfant. A propos de 19 observations effectuées au CNPP, Cliniques Universitaires de Kinshasa, Zaire. *Ann. Soc. Belge Méd. Trop.*, **73**, 253–259.

Kazyumba, G., Berney, M., Brighouse, G. *et al.* (1986). Expression of the cell repertoire and autoantibodies in human African trypanosomiasis. *Clin. Exp. Immunol.*, **65**, 10–18.

Kazyumba, G. I., Ruppol, J. F., Tshefu, A. K. and Nkanga, N. (1988). Arsénorésistance et difluorométhylornithine dans le traitement de la trypanosomiase humaine Africaine. *Bull. Soc. Pathol. Exot.*, **81**, 591–594.

Kellersberger, E. R. (1933). African sleeping sickness. A review of 9000 cases from a Central African clinic. *Am. J. Trop. Med.*, **13**, 211–236.

Kérandel, P. (1910). Un cas de trypanosomiase chez un médecin. *Bull. Soc. Pathol. Exot.*, **3**, 642–662.

Khonde, N., Pépin, J. and Mpia, B. (1997). A seven days course of eflornithine for relapsing *Trypanosoma brucei gambiense* sleeping sickness. *Trans. Roy. Soc. Trop. Med. Hyg.*, **91**, 212–213.

Kotten, J. W. and De Raadt, P. (1969). Myocarditis in *Trypanosoma rhodesiense* infections. *Trans. Roy. Soc. Trop. Med. Hyg.*, **63**, 485–489.

Kuzoe, F. A. (1993). Current situation of African trypanosomiasis. *Acta Trop.*, **54**, 153–162.

Lambert, P. H., Berney, M. and Kazyumba, G. L. (1981). Immune complexes in serum and cerebrospinal fluid in sleeping sickness. Correlation with polyclonal B-cell activation and with intracerebral immunoglobulin synthesis. *J. Clin. Invest.*, **67**, 77–85.

Le Bras, M., Clerc, M., Loubiere, R. *et al.* (1973). Aspects de la symptomatologie hépatique au cours de la trypanosomiase humaine africaine. *Méd. Áfrique Noire*, **20**, 343–353.

Libby, P. R. and Porter, C. W. (1992). Inhibition of enzymes of polyamine back-conversion by pentamidine and berenil. *Biochem. Pharmacol.*, **4**, 830–832.

Limbos, P., Thomas, H., Beelaerts, W. and Van Caesbroeck, D. (1977). Insuffisance renale au cours du traitement de la trypanosomiase a *T. rhodesiense* par la Pentamidine. *Ann. Soc. Belge Med. Trop.*, **57**, 495–500.

Liu, M. K. and Pearson, T. W. (1987). Detection of circulating trypanosomal antigens by double antibody ELISA using antibodies to procyclic trypanosomes. *Parasitology*, **95**, 277–290.

Liu, M. K., Pearson, T. W., Sayer, P. D. *et al.* (1988). Serodiagnosis of African sleeping sickness in vervet monkeys by detection of parasite antigens. *Acta Trop.*, **45**, 321–330.

Liu, M. K., Cattand, P., Gardiner, I. C. and Pearson, T. W. (1989). Immunodiagnosis of sleeping sickness due to *Trypanosoma brucei gambiense* by detection of anti-procyclic antibodies and trypanosome antigens in patient's sera. *Acta Trop.*, **46**, 257–266.

Losos, G. J., and Crockett, E. (1969). Toxicity of Berenil in dogs. *Vet. Rec.*, **8**, 196.

Louis, J. P., Mouliat-Pelat, J. P., Jannin, J. *et al.* (1991). Absence of epidemiological inter-relations between HIV infection and African human trypanosomiasis in Central Africa. *Trop. Med. Parasitol.*, **42**, 155.

Lucasse, Chr. (1964). Fluorescent antibody test as applied to cerebrospinal fluid in human sleeping sickness. *Bull. Soc. Pathol. Exot.*, **57**, 283–292.

Lumsden, W. H. R., Kimber, C. D., Dukes, P. *et al.* (1981). Field diagnosis of sleeping sickness in the Ivory Coast. I. Comparison of the miniature anion-exchange/

centrifugation technique with other protozoological methods. *Trans. Roy. Soc. Trop. Med. Hyg.*, 75, 242–250.

Magnus, E., Vervoort, T. and Van Meirvenne, N. (1978). A card-agglutination test with stained trypanosomes (C.A.T.T.) for the serological diagnosis of *T. b. gambiense* trypanosomiasis. *Ann. Soc. Belge Med. Trop.*, 58, 169–176.

Manson-Bahr, P. E. C. and Charters, A. D. (1963). Myocarditis in African trypanosomiasis. *Trans. Roy. Soc. Trop. Med. Hyg.*, 57, 119–121.

Manson-Bahr, P. E. C. and Apted, F. I. C. (1982). African trypanosomiasis. In: *Manson's Tropical Diseases*, 18th edn, (P. E. C. Manson-Bahr and F. I. C. Apted, eds). London: Baillière-Tindall.

Marneffe, J. (1955). Observation d'un foyer de trypanosomiase rhodesiense en Urundi. Historique et aspect géographique. Clinique – traitement – prophylaxie – 1954–1955. *Ann. Soc. Belge Med. Trop.*, 35, 357–388.

Martin, L. and Darré (1908). Sur les symptômes nerveux du début de la maladie du sommeil. *Bull. Soc. Pathol. Exot.*, 1, 15–18.

Mathieu-Daudé, F., Bicart-See, A., Bosseno, M-F. *et al.* (1994). Identification of *Trypanosoma brucei gambiense* group I by a specific kinetoplast DNA probe. *Am. J. Trop. Med. Hyg.*, 50, 13–19.

Mattern, P. (1962). Beta-2-macroglobulinorachie importante chez les malades atteints de trypanosomiase Africaine. *Ann. Inst. Pasteur*, 102, 64–72.

Mattern, P., Benz, M. and McGregor, I. A. (1967). Les anticorps précipitants présents dans le sang et dans le liquide céphaloraquidien de malades atteints de trypanosomiase humaine africaine a *T. gambiense. Ann. Inst. Pasteur*, 112, 105.

Mbulamberi, D. B. (1989a). Possible causes leading to an epidemic outbreak of sleeping sickness: facts and hypothesis. *Ann. Soc. Belge Med. Trop.*, 69 (suppl 1), 173–179.

Mbulamberi, D. B. (1989b). Clinical and laboratorial features of late stage rhodesian sleeping sickness in South Eastern Uganda. *International Scientific Council for Trypanosomiasis Research and Control. 20th Meeting. Mombasa, Kenya*, (OAU/STRC, 1989, no 115). pp. 234–244.

McNamara, J. J., Bailey, J. W., Smith, D. H. *et al.* (1995). Isolation of *Trypanosoma brucei gambiense* from northern Uganda: evaluation of the kit for in vitro isolation (KIVI) in an epidemic focus. *Trans. Roy. Soc. Trop. Med. Hyg.*, 89, 388–389.

Meda, H. A., Doua, F., Laveissière, C. *et al.* (1995). Human immunodeficiency virus infection and human African trypanosomiasis: a case-control study in Côte d'Ivoire. *Trans. Roy. Soc. Trop. Med. Hyg.*, 89, 639–643.

Medina, E. A., Ventura F. A. and Champalimaud, J. L. (1986). Computer assisted tomographic findings in a patient with African trypanosomiasis. *J. Trop. Med. Hyg.*, 89, 75–77.

Milord, F., Pepin, J., Loko, L. *et al.* (1992). Efficacy and toxicity of eflornithine for the treatment of *Trypanosoma brucei gambiense* sleeping sickness. *Lancet*, 340, 652–655.

Milord, F., Loko, L., Ethier, L. *et al.* (1993). Eflornithine concentrations in serum and cerebrospinal fluid of 63 patients treated for *Trypanosoma brucei gambiense* sleeping sickness. *Trans. Roy. Soc. Trop. Med. Hyg.*, **87**, 473–477.

Moens, F., De Wilde, M. and Ngato, K. (1984). Essai de traitment au nifurtimox de la trypanosomiase humaine africaine. *Ann. Soc. Belge Med. Trop.*, **64**, 37–43.

Montmayeur, A., Brosset, C., Imbert, P. and Buguet, A. (1994). Cycle veille-sommeil au decours d'une trypanosomose humaine africaine à *Trypanosoma brucei rhodesiense* chez deux parachutistes francais. *Bull. Soc. Pathol. Exot.*, **87**, 368–371.

Morax, V. and Kérandel, P. (1908) Un cas de cyclite dans la trypanosomiase humaine. *Bull. Soc. Pathol. Exot.*, **1**, 398-401.

Morris, K. R. S. (1962). The epidemiology of sleeping sickness in East Africa. *Trans. Roy. Soc. Trop. Med. Hyg.*, **56**, 316–338.

Moser, D. R., Cook, G. A., Ochs, D. E. *et al.* (1989). Detection of *Trypanosoma congolense* and *Trypanosoma brucei* subspecies by DNA amplification using the polymerase chain reaction. *Parasitology*, **99**, 57–66.

Nantulya, V. M., Lyndqvist, K. J., Diall, O. and Olaho-Mukani (1989). Two simple antigen-detection enzyme immunoassays for the diagnosis of *Trypanosoma evansi* infection in the dromedary camel (*Camelus dromedarius*). *Trop. Med. Parasitol.*, **40**, 415–418.

Nantulya, V. M., Lyndqvist, K. J., Stevenson, P. and Mwangi, E. K. (1992a). Application of a monoclonal antibody-based antigen detection enzyme-linked immunosorbent assay (antigen ELISA) for field diagnosis of bovine trypanosomiasis at Nguruman, Kenya. *Ann. Trop. Med. Parasitol.*, **86**, 225–230.

Nantulya, V. M., Doua, F. and Molisho, S. (1992b). Diagnosis of *Trypanosoma brucei gambiense* sleeping sickness using an antigen detection enzyme-linked immunosorbent assay. *Trans. Roy. Soc. Trop. Med. Hyg.*, **86**, 42–45.

Nattan-Larrier, L. and Monthus, A. (1908). Iritis et trypanosomiase chez l'homme. *Bull. Soc. Pathol. Exot.*, **1**, 277–280.

Ngandu-Kabeya, G. (1976). Étude de la symptomatologie de la trypanosomiase africaine chez l enfant (a propos de 24 observations). *Ann. Soc. Belge Méd. Trop.*, **56**, 85–93.

Nkanga, N. G., Kazadi, K., Kazyumba G. L. and Dechef, G. (1988). Signes cliniques neurologiques de la trypanosomiase humaine Africaine au stade méningo encéphalitique (a propos de 23 cas). *Bull. Soc. Pathol. Exot.*, **81**, 449–458.

Noireau, F., Brun-Verzinet, F., Larouze, B. *et al.* (1987). Absence of relationship between human deficiency virus 1 and sleeping sickness. *Trans. Roy. Soc. Trop. Med. Hyg.*, **81**, 1000.

Noireau, F., Apembet, J. D. and Frézil, J. L. (1988). Revue clinique des troubles endocriniens observés chez l'adulte trypanosome. *Bull. Soc. Pathol. Exot.*, **81**, 464–467.

Noireau, F., Paindavoine, P., Lemesre, J. L. *et al.* (1989). The epidemiological importance of the animal reservoir of *Trypanosoma gambiense* in the Congo. 2. Characterization of the *Trypanosoma brucei* complex. *Tropenmed. Parasitol.*, **40**, 9–11.

Nozais, J. P. (1988). Mais où est donc passée la ≪clé≫ de Kérandel? *Bull. Soc. Pathol. Exot.*, **81**, 477–479.

Ogada, T. (1970). Toxicity of intramuscular berenil in dogs. In: *EATRO Annual Report for 1969*, pp. 121–123.

Ogada, T. and Okach, R. W. (1970). Mel B induced agranulocytosis. In: *EATRO Annual Report for 1969*, pp. 135–136.

Okia, M., Mbulamberi, D. B. and De Muynck, A. (1994). Risk factors assessment for *T. b. rhodesiense* sleeping sickness acquisition in S. E. Uganda. A case control study. *Ann. Soc. Belge Méd. Trop.*, **74**, 105–112.

Okomo-Assoumou, M.C., Geffard, M., Daulouede, S. *et al.* (1995). Circulating antibodies directed against tryptophan-like epitopes in sera of patients with human African trypanosomiasis. *Am. J. Trop. Med. Hyg.*, **52**, 461–467.

Olaho-Mukani, W., Nyang'ao, J. M., Ngaira, J. M. *et al.* (1994). Immunoassay of circulating trypanosomal antigens in sleeping sickness patients undergoing treatment. *J. Immunoassay*, **15**, 69–77.

Onyango, R. J., Van Hoeve, K. and De Raadt, P. (1966). The epidemiology of *Trypanosoma rhodesiense* sleeping sickness in Alego location, Central Nyanza, Kenya – Evidence that cattle may act as reservoir hosts of the trypanosome infective to man. *Trans. Roy. Soc. Trop. Med. Hyg.*, **60**, 175–182.

Onyango, R. J., Bailey, N. M., Okach, R. W. *et al.* (1970a). The use of Berenil for the treatment of early cases of human trypanosomiasis. In: *EATRO Annual Report for 1969*, pp. 120–121.

Onyango, R. J., Bailey, N. M., Okach, R. W. *et al.* (1970b). Encephalopathy during treatment of human trypanosomiasis. In: *EATRO Annual Report for 1969*, pp. 136–139.

Pautrizel, R., Durret, J., Tribouley, J. and Ripert, C. (1962). Application de la réaction de conglutination au diagnostic sérologique des trypanosomes. *Bull. Soc. Pathol. Exot.*, **55**, 391–397.

Payet, M. and Sankale, M. (1960). Hyperazotémies transitoires consécutives au traitement de la trypanosomiase humaine africaine par les diamidines. *Bull. Soc. Pathol. Exot.*, **53**, 690–696.

Pearson, T. W., Liu, M., Gardiner, I. C. *et al.* (1986). Use of procyclic trypanosomes for detection of antibodies in sera from vervet monkeys infected with *Trypanosoma rhodesiense*: an immunodiagnostic test for African sleeping sickness. *Acta Trop.*, **43**, 391–399.

Pentreath, V. W. (1989). Neurobiology of sleeping sickness. *Parasitol. Today*, **5**, 215–218.

Pentreath, V. W., Rees, K., Owolabi, O. A. *et al.* (1990). The somnogenic T lymphocyte suppressor prostaglandin D_2 is selectively elevated in cerebrospinal fluid of advanced sleeping sickness patients. *Trans. Roy. Soc. Trop. Med. Hyg.*, **84**, 795–799.

Pentreath, V. W., Alafiatayo, R. A., Crawley, B. *et al.* (1996). Endotoxins in the blood and cerebrospinal fluid of patients with African sleeping sickness. *Parasitology*, **112**, 67–73.

Pentreath, V. W., Alafiatayo, R. A., Barclay, G. R. *et al.* (1997). Endotoxin antibodies in African sleeping sickness. *Parasitology*, **114**, 361–365.

Pepin, J., Tetreault, L. and Gervais, C. (1985). Utilisation des corticosteroides oraux dans le traitement de la trypanosomiase humaine africaine: une enquete retrospective a Nioki, Zaire. *Ann. Soc. Belge Méd. Trop.*, **65**, 17–29.

Pepin, J. Milord, F. Guern, C. and Schechter, P. J. (1987). Difluoromethylornithine for arseno-resistant *Trypanosoma brucei gambiense* sleeping sickness. *Lancet*, **iii**, 1431–1433.

Pepin, J., Guérin, C., Milord, F. *et al.* (1989a). Utilization de la difluoromethylornithine dans la trypanosomiase congénitale à *Trypanosoma brucei gambiense*. *Méd. Trop.*, **49**, 83–85.

Pepin, J., Milord, F., Guern, C. *et al.* (1989b). Trial of prednisolone for prevention of melarsoprol-induced encephalopathy in gambiense sleeping sickness. *Lancet*, **i**, 1246–1250.

Pepin, J., Milord, F., Mpia, B. *et al.* (1989c). An open clinical trial of nifurtimox for arseno-resistant *Trypanosoma brucei gambiense* sleeping sickness in central Zaïre. *Trans. Roy. Soc. Trop. Med. Hyg.*, **83**, 514–517.

Pépin, J. and Milord, F. (1991). African trypanosomiasis and drug induced encephalopathy: risk factors and pathogenesis. *Trans. Roy. Soc. Trop. Med. Hyg.*, **85**, 222–224.

Pépin, J., Ethier, L., Kazadi, C. *et al.* (1992a). The impact of human immunodeficiency virus infection on the epidemiology and treatment of *Trypanosoma brucei gambiense* sleeping sickness in Nioki, Zaire. *Am. J. Trop. Med. Hyg.*, **47**, 133–140.

Pépin, J., Milord, F., Meurice, F. *et al.* (1992b). High-dose nifurtimox for arseno-resistant *Trypanosoma brucei gambiense* sleeping sickness: an open trial in central Zaire. *Trans. Roy. Soc. Trop. Med. Hyg.*, **86**, 254–256.

Pépin, J., Milord, F., Khonde, A. N. *et al.* (1994). Gambiense trypanosomiasis: frequency of, and risk factors for, failure of melarsoprol therapy. *Trans. Roy. Soc. Trop. Med. Hyg.*, **88**, 447–452.

Pépin, J., Milord, F., Khonde, A. N. *et al.* (1995). Risk factors for encephalopathy and mortality during melarsoprol treatment of *Trypanosoma brucei gambiense* sleeping sickness. *Trans. Roy. Soc. Trop. Med. Hyg.*, **89**, 92–97.

Pille, G. (1953). Considérations pharmacologiques sur les diamidines et leur utilisation dans la trypanosomiase. *Méd. Trop.*, **13**, 859–869.

Pinto, A.R., Parreira, F. and Almeida Franco (1952). A mielocultura na doença do sono. *Bol. Cult. Guiné Port.*, **26**, 245–247.

Poisson, M., Bleibel, J. M., Regnier, A. *et al.* (1980). Formes pseudo-tumorales de la trypanosomiase africaine à *Trypanosoma gambiense*. Étude clinique et tomo-densitometrique. *Sem. Hop.*, **56**, 1979–1982.

Poltera, A. A. (1980). Immunopathological and chemotherapeutic studies in experimental trypanosomiasis with special reference to the heart and brain. *Trans. Roy. Soc. Trop. Med. Hyg.*, **74**, 706–715.

Poupin, F., Cailliez, M., Petithory, J. C. and Savel, J. (1983). Le diagnostic sero-immunologique de la trypanosomose africaine humaine: reactions croisees au cours de diverses parasitoses et hyperglobulinemies. *Bull. Soc. Pathol. Exot.*, **76**, 393–405.

Rey, M., Diop Mar, I., Hocquet, P. *et al.* (1964). Trypanosomiase nerveuse chez deux enfants de 3 ans. *Bull. Soc. Méd. Afrique Noire Langue Franç.*, **9**, 271–277.

Reynaud, R., Revil, H. and Mattern, P. (1963). Deux cas européens de trypanosomiase contractée aux environs de Dakar. *Bull. Soc. Méd. Afrique Noire Langue Franç.*, **8**, 426–432.

Ricosse, J. H., Challier, A., Le Mao, G. *et al.* (1973). L'épidémiologie actuelle de la trypanosomiase humaine africaine et les problémes qu'elle pose. *Méd. Afrique Noire*, **20**, 291–300.

Richet, P., Lotte, M. and Foucher, G. (1959). Resultats des traitements de la trypanosomiase humaine a 'T. gambiense' par le mel B ou l'arsobal. *Méd. Trop.*, **19**, 250–265.

Ridet, J. (1953). Étude des troubles du cycle menstruel chez la femme trypanosomée a l'aide de frottis vaginaux (étude preliminaire). *Méd. Trop.*, **13**, 514–519.

Rive, J., Serie, F., Kone, I. and Bertrand, Ed. (1973). Considérations sur le traitement de la trypanosomiase humaine africaine à *Trypanosoma gambiense. Méd. Afrique Noire*, **20**, 379–387.

Robertson, D. H. H. (1963). The treatment of sleeping sickness (mainly due to *Trypanosoma rhodesiense*) with melarsoprol. I. Reactions observed during treatment. *Trans. Roy. Soc. Trop. Med. Hyg.*, **57**, 122–133.

Robertson, D. H. H. and Baker, J. R. (1958). Human trypanosomiasis in south-east Uganda. I. A study of the epidemiology and present virulence of the disease. *Trans. Roy. Soc. Trop. Med. Hyg.*, **52**, 337.

Rollo, I. M. (1975). Miscellaneous drugs used in the treatment of protozoal infections. In: *The Pharmacological Basis of Therapeutics*, (L. S. Goodman and A. Gilman, eds). New York: MacMillan Publishing Co. Inc. pp. 1081–1089.

Rosário Pinto, A. C. (1960). Um caso de doença do sono congénita. *An. Inst. Med. Trop.*, **17**, 1195–1200.

Ross, J. P. J. (1971). The deduction of circulating trypanosomal antibodies by capillary tube agglutination test. *Ann. Trop. Med. Parasitol.*, **65**, 327–333.

Sabbah, P., Brosset, C., Imbert, P. *et al.* (1997). Human African trypanosomiasis: MRI. *Neuroradiology*, **39**, 708–710.

Sands, M., Kron, M. A. and Brown, R. B. (1985). Pentamidine: a review. *Rev. Infect. Dis.*, **7**, 625–634.

Satge, P., Lariviere, M., Mattern, P. *et al.* (1964). A propos d'un cas de trypanosomiase africaine chez un nourrisson. *Bull. Soc. Méd. Afrique Noire Langue Franç.*, **9**, 278–284.

Saunders, G. F. T., Holden, J. R. and Hughes, M. H. (1944). Second report on the treatment of trypanosomiasis by pentamidine. *Ann. Trop. Med. Parasitol.*, **38**, 159–168.

Schares, G. and Mehlitz, D. (1996). Sleeping sickness in Zaire: a nested polymerase chain reaction improves the identification of *Trypanosoma (Trypanozoon) brucei gambiense* by specific kinetoplast DNA probes. *Trop. Med. Int. Hlth*, 1, 59–70.

Schechter, P. J., Barlow, J. L. R. and Sjoerdsma, A. (1987). Clinical aspects of inhibition of ornithine decarboxylase with emphasis on therapeutic trials of eflornithine (DFMO) in cancer and protozoan diseases. In: *Inhibition of Polyamine Metabolism*, (P. P. McCann, A. E. Pegg and A. Sjoerdsma, eds). Orlando: Academic Press. pp. 345–364.

Schneider, J. (1963). Traitement de la trypanosomiase africaine humaine. *Bull. World Hlth Org.*, 28, 763–786.

Schoenaers, F., Neujean, G. and Evens, F. (1953). Valeur pratique de la réaction de fixation du complément dans la maladie du sommeil. *Ann. Soc. Belge Méd. Trop.*, 33, 141–148.

Schultzberg, M., Ambatsis, M., Samuelsson, E.-B. *et al.* (1988). Spread of *Trypanosoma brucei* to the nervous system: early attack on circumventricular organs and sensory ganglia. *J. Neurosci. Res.*, 21, 56–61.

Seah, S. K. and Gabrielan, S. (1972). Toxoplasmosis and African trypanosomiasis. *Trans. Roy. Soc. Trop. Med. Hyg.*, 66, 807–808.

Seed, J. R. (1969). *Trypanosoma gambiense* and *T. lewisi*: increased vascular permeability and skin lesions in rabbits. *Exp. Parasitol.*, 26, 214–223.

Seed, J. R., Hall, J. E. and Price, C. C. (1983). A physiological mechanism to explain pathogenesis in African trypanosomiasis. *Contr. Microbiol. Immunol.*, 7, 83–94.

Serrano-Gonzalez, C., Velilla, I., Fortuno, B. *et al.* (1996). Neuroimagen y eficacia del tratamiento en la tripanosomiasis africana avanzada. *Rev. Neurol.*, 24, 1554–1557.

Shi-hua, W. (1985). African trypanosomiasis in southern Sudan. Report of 77 cases. *Chinese Med. J.*, 98, 37–41.

Simarro, P. P. and Asumu, P. N. (1996). Gambian trypanosomiasis and synergism between melarsoprol and eflornithine: first case report. *Trans. Roy. Soc. Trop. Med. Hyg.*, 90, 315.

Sina, G., Triolo, N., Trova, P. and Clabaut, J. M. (1977). L'encephalopathie arsenicale lors du traitement de la trypanosomiase humaine africaine a *T. gambiense* (à propos de 16 cas). *Ann. Soc. Belge Méd. Trop.*, 57, 57–74.

Sina, G. C., Triolo, N., Cramet, B. and Suh Bandu, M. (1982). L'adrenaline dans la prevention et le traitement des accidents de l'arsobaltherapie. A propos de 776 cas de trypanosomiase humaine africaine a *T. gambiense* traités dans les formations sanitaires de Fontem (R. U. du Cameroun). *Méd. Trop.*, 42, 531–536.

Sonan, T., Giordano, C., Boa, F. and Dumas, M. (1988). Formes hémiplégiques de la trypanosomiase humaine Africaine. *Bull. Soc. Pathol. Exot.*, 81, 459–463.

Spencer, H. C. (1984). African trypanosomiasis. In: *Hunter's Tropical Medicine*, 6th edn, (G. T. Strickland, ed.). Philadelphia: W. B. Saunders Company, pp. 553–565.

Spinazzola, F., D'Amato, C., De Felici, A. *et al.* (1989). Plasmapheresis for late-stage trypanosomiasis. *Lancet*, **1**, 1200.

Stanghellini, A. and Roux, J. F. (1984). Techniques de despistage et de diagnostic de la trypanosomose humaine africaine. *Med. Trop.*, **44**, 361–367.

Steiger, R. F. (1973). On the ultrastructure of *Trypanosoma (Trypanzoon) brucei* on the course of its life cycles and some related aspects. *Acta Trop.*, **30**, 64–68.

Sunkara, P. S., Baylin, S. B. and Luk, G. D. (1987). Inhibition of polyamine biosynthesis: cellular and *in vivo* effects on tumor proliferation. In: *Inhibition of Polyamine Metabolism*, (P. P. McCann, A. E. Pegg and A. Sjoerdsma, eds). Orlando: Academic Press, pp. 121–140.

Taelman, H., Clerinx, J., Bogaerts, J. and Vervoort, T. (1996). Combination treatment with suramin and eflornithine in late stage rhodesian trypanosomiasis: case report. *Trans. Roy. Soc. Trop. Med. Hyg.*, **90**, 572–573.

Tapie, P., Buguet, A., Tabaraud, F. *et al.* (1996). Electroencephalographic and polygraphic features of 24-hour recordings in sleeping sickness and healthy African subjects. *J. Clin. Neurophysiol.*, **13**, 339–344.

Travassos Santos Dias, J. A. T. (1988). Os aldeamentos rurais como sistema a preconizar nas áreas endémicas de doença-do-sono. *Garcia da Horta, Série Zool.*, **15**, 138–144.

Trincão, C. and Gouveia, E., (1951). The blood and bone marrow pattern in sleeping sickness in Portuguese Guinea. *Am. J. Trop. Med.*, **31**, 335–340.

Trincão, C. and Parreira, F. (1957). A cultura *in vitro* dos megacariocitos na doença do sono. *Ana. Inst. Med. Trop.*, **14**, 105–109.

Triolo, N. (1990). A case of coma due to Arsobal in a newborn affected with congenital trypanosomiasis gambiense. *Ther. Infect. Dis.*, **5**, 165–166.

Triolo, N., Trova, P., Fusco, C. and Le Bras, J. (1985). Bilan de 17 années d'étude de la trypanosomiase humaine africaine a *T. gambiense* chez les enfants de 0 a 6 ans. A propos de 227 cas. *Méd. Trop.*, **45**, 251–257.

Triolo, N., Parody, A., Fiorucci, G. and Bazzoli, A. (1990). Side-effects caused by arsobal therapy in 2,052 patients treated in Fontem Hospital (Cameroun) from 1970 to 1989. *Ther. Infect. Dis.*, **5**, 113–128.

Van Bogaert, L. and Janssen, P. (1957). Contribuition à l'étude de la neurologie et neuropathologie de la trypanosomiase humaine. *Ann. Soc. Belge Méd. Trop.*, **37**, 379–412.

Van den Branden, F. and Appelmans, M. (1934). Les troubles visuels dans la trypanosomiase humaine. *Ann. Soc. Belge Méd. Trop.*, **14**, 91–107.

Van Meirvenne, N. (1992). Diagnosis of human African trypanosomiasis. *Ann. Soc. Belge Mèd. Trop.*, **72** (suppl. 1), 53–56.

Van Niewenhove, S. and Declercq, J. (1981). Nifurtimox (Lampit) treatment in late stage of gambiense sleeping sickness. In: *Proceedings, 17th meeting, Inter-*

national Scientific Council for Trypanosomiasis Research and Control, Arusha, Tanzania, OAU/STRC Publication 112, pp. 206–208.

Van Nieuwenhove, S. (1988). Nifurtimox au stade tardif de la maladie du sommeil à *T. gambiense* réfractaire aux arsénicaux. *Bull. Soc. Pathol. Exot. Fil.*, **81**, 650.

Van Nieuwenhove, S. (1992). Advances in sleeping sickness therapy. *Ann. Soc. Belge Méd. Trop.*, **72** (suppl. 1), 39–51.

Van Nieuwenhove, S., Schechter, P. J., Declercq, J. *et al.* (1985). Treatment of Gambiense sleeping sickness in the Sudan with oral DFMO (DL-α-difluoromethylornithine), an inhibitor of ornithine decarboxylase; first field trial. *Trans. Roy. Soc. Trop. Med. Hyg.*, **79**, 692–698.

Vernier, J. (1953). La Tsé-Tsé et moi. *Méd Trop.*, **13**, 210–212.

Vickerman, K. (1985). Developmental cycles and biology of pathogenic trypanosomes. *Br. Med. Bull.*, **41**, 105–114.

Vickerman, K. and Tetley, L. (1978). Biology and ultrastructure of trypanosomes in relation to pathogenesis. In: *Pathogenicity of Trypanosomes. Proceedings of a workshop held at Nairobi, Kenya, 20–23 November 1978*, (G. Losos and A. Chouinard, eds). Ottawa, Ont: IDRC, pp. 23–31.

Voller, A. (1977). Serology of African trypanosomiasis. *Ann. Soc. Belge Méd. Trop.*, **57**, 273–280.

Voller, A., Bidwell, D. E. and Bartlett, A. (1975). A serological study on human *T. rhodesiense* infection using a microsale ELISA. *Tropenmed. Parasitol.*, **26**, 247–251.

Walzer, P. D., Perl, D.P., Krogstad, D. J. *et al.* (1974). *Pneumocystis carinii* pneumonia in the United States. Epidemiologic, diagnostic and clinical features. *Ann. Int. Med.*, **80**, 83–93.

Weinberg, J. R., Wright, P. A. and Cook, G. C. (1989). Tropical pyomyositis associated with *Trypanosoma brucei rhodesiense* infection in a Europid. *Trans. Roy. Soc. Trop. Med. Hyg.*, **83**, 77–79.

Wéry, M. (1991). Therapy for African trypanosomiasis. *Curr. Op. Infect. Dis.*, **4**, 838–843.

Wéry, M., Wéry-Paskoff, S. and Van Wettere, P. (1970). The diagnosis of human African trypanosomiasis (*T. gambiense*) by the use of fluorescent antibody test. 1. Standardization of an easy technique to be used in mass surveys. *Ann. Soc. Belge Méd. Trop.*, **50**, 613–634.

Wéry, M. and Mulumba, M. P. (1989). Detection of *Trypanosoma brucei gambiense* in the host and alternative sleeping sickness diagnostic approaches. *Ann. Soc. Belge Méd. Trop.*, **69**, 181–187.

Whittle, H. C. and Pope, H. M. (1972). The febrile response to treatment in Gambian sleeping sickness. *Ann. Trop. Med. Parasitol.*, **66**, 7–14.

Whittle, H., Greenwood, B. M., Bidwell, D. E. *et al.* (1977). IgM and antibody measurement in the diagnosis and management of Gambian trypanosomiasis. *Am. J. Trop. Med. Hyg.*, **26**, 1129–1134.

Whittle, H., Greenwood, B. M. and Mohammed, I. (1980). Immune complexes in Gambian sleeping sickness. *Trans. Roy. Soc. Trop. Med. Hyg.*, **74**, 833–834.

Willett, K. C. (1963). Some principles of the epidemiology of human trypanosomiasis in Africa. *Bull. World Hlth Org.*, **28**, 645–652.

Willett, K. C. (1966). The 'trypanosome chancre' in Rhodesian sleeping sickness. *Trans. Roy. Soc. Trop. Med. Hyg.*, **60**, 689–690.

Woo, P. T. K. and Soltys, M. A. (1972). Indirect hemagglutination and charcoal agglutination tests in the diagnosis of African sleeping sickness. *Zeits. Tropenmed. Parasitol.*, **23**, 166–172.

World Health Organization (1976). Parallel evaluation of serological tests applied to African trypanosomiasis. *Bull. World Hlth Org.*, **54**, 141–147.

World Health Organization (1986). Epidemiology and control of African trypanosomiasis. *Report of a WHO Expert Committee, Technical Report Series*, **739**, 1–125

World Health Organization (1995). Tropical Diseases Research. Progress 1975–94, Highlights 1993–1994. *Twelfth Programme Report of the UNDP/World Bank/ WHO Special Programme for Research and Training in Tropical Diseases (TDR)*. Geneva: World Health Organization.

Zola, J. M., Wassoumbou-Loubienga, S., Goma, G. C. and Mouanga-Yidika, G. (1994). Meningo-encephalite aigué a *Trypanosoma brucei gambiense* revelée par un oedeme papillaire. *Bull. Soc. Pathol. Exot.*, **87**, 312–314.

12
Neurosyphilis
Christina M. Marra

Introduction

Most of what we know about neurosyphilis is based on the work of H. Houston Merritt and other syphilologists that was conducted in the first half of this century. This chapter reviews early studies on neurosyphilis and uses them to frame a current discussion of pathogenesis, diagnosis and treatment of this disorder. These topics are particularly timely because neurosyphilis is most common in persons infected with the human immunodeficiency virus type-1 (HIV) and HIV impacts the clinical course and treatment response of syphilis and neurosyphilis.

Clinical manifestations and pathology of neurosyphilis

Neurosyphilis has been traditionally categorized into discrete syndromes, each occurring at a typical time after primary infection. These include asymptomatic neurosyphilis, meningitis, meningovasculitis, general paresis and tabes dorsalis. A brief clinical summary of each syndrome is shown in Table 12.1. An appreciation of the common underlying pathology for all these syndromes is a useful aid in understanding their clinical and laboratory presentations.

Treponema pallidum invades the central nervous system CNS early in the course of infection and elicits meningeal inflammation (Ravant, 1903; Wile and Stokes, 1914; Fildes *et al.*, 1918; Moore, 1922; Mills, 1927; Lukehart *et al.*, 1988; Rolf *et al.*, 1997). Most patients are able to clear the organism from the CNS, but it persists in about 30% of individuals and neurological complications may develop weeks to decades later (Ravant, 1903). Chronic meningeal inflammation is a feature of all forms of neurosyphilis and is the underlying pathological change that provides a unifying classification scheme as shown in Table 12.2. Clinically, meningitis is most prominent in the forms of neuro-syphilis that occur early after primary infection, while parenchymal manifestations are more commonly seen late after primary infection. In some instances the meningeal component is evident only at necropsy. However, an individual patient may manifest both meningeal and parenchymal features.

Table 12.1 Clinical classification of neurosyphilis.

Asymptomatic

These patients have CSF abnormalities due to CNS invasion by *T. pallidum*, but remain clinically well. This syndrome may occur at any time after infection, but is most common in the first few years of infection. Patients with asymptomatic neurosyphilis are at risk for development of symptomatic neurosyphilis and should be treated with penicillin regimens recommended for neurosyphilis to prevent this progression.

Meningeal

These patients have clinical evidence of meningitis with headache, stiff neck, nausea and vomiting. Cranial nerves may be involved and hydrocephalus may develop. This syndrome is most common within the first year of infection. Therapy results in clinical improvement.

Meningovascular

These patients present with a stroke most commonly in the distribution of the middle cerebral artery. Other vascular distributions, including the spinal cord, may be involved. Symptoms of meningitis may also be present. Peak incidence is 7 years after primary infection. Therapy usually results in clinical improvement, although residual deficits are common.

General paresis

Early in their course, these patients display forgetfulness and personality changes. Over time they may develop psychiatric symptoms. All eventually progress to frank dementia, often with pupillary abnormalities, hypotonia and intention tremor. Onset is usually 10–20 years after primary infection with a range of 2 to 30+ years. Treatment may halt progression of the disease but does not usually result in clinical improvement.

Tabes dorsalis

These patients present with sensory loss, ataxia, lancinating pains and bowel and bladder dysfunction. This syndrome has the longest latent period between primary infection and onset of symptoms with an average of 20 years and a range of 3 to 50 years. Treatment may halt progression of the disease but does not usually result in clinical improvement.

Table 12.2 Pathological classification scheme for neurosyphilis and per cent of patients with syphilis in the pre-antibiotic era that developed each form of neurosyphilis.

Meningeal
Asymptomatic (25–30%)
Symptomatic
  Meningitis (0.5%)
  Cranial neuritis (0.2%)
  Polyradiculitis (rare)
  Gumma (rare)
  Hypertrophic meningitis (rare)
  Meningomyelitis (1%)
  Meningovasculitis (3%)

Meningeal and parenchymal
Meningoencephalitis (general paresis) (5%)
Tabes dorsalis (9%)
Gumma (rare)

Meningeal neurosyphilis

Asymptomatic neurosyphilis

Asymptomatic neurosyphilis refers to the situation where the CSF is abnormal because of CNS *T. pallidum* infection but there are no clinical signs or symptoms. CSF abnormalities can be seen at any time after acquisition of *T. pallidum*, but probably peak during the second year after infection (Fordyce and Rosen, 1921; Moore, 1922). With time, the proportion of patients with CSF abnormalities or asymptomatic neurosyphilis declines relative to the total number of patients with neurosyphilis because previously asymptomatic patients become symptomatic or because of spontaneous sterilization of the CSF, or both (O'Leary *et al.*, 1937). For example, Merritt and coworkers observed asymptomatic neurosyphilis in only 9.5% of 2263 patients examined in the neurosyphilis outpatient department of the Boston City Hospital, consistent with the fact that 90% of patients were seen more than 5 years after primary infection (Merritt *et al.*, 1946).

The frequency of specific CSF abnormalities reported in asymptomatic neurosyphilis varies with the duration of syphilis infection. Moore (1922) reported that 87% of his patients with asymptomatic neurosyphilis who had been infected for less than 1 year had >5 CSF white blood cells (WBC)/µl and only 48% had reactive CSF Wassermann tests; the Wassermann test is the predecessor of today's Venereal Disease Research Laboratory (VDRL) test. In contrast, Merritt *et al.* (1946) found that only 40% of their patients with asymptomatic neurosyphilis had >5 CSF WBC/µl but 84% had reactive CSF Wassermann reactions. These results demonstrate that CSF pleocytosis is more common in early asymptomatic neurosyphilis and that reactivity of CSF non-treponemal serological tests occurs later.

Pathology of asymptomatic neurosyphilis

Pathological data in asymptomatic neurosyphilis are limited because patients rarely die with this form of disease. The changes described are similar to, but perhaps less extensive than, those seen in symptomatic neurosyphilis and are mostly limited to the meninges with infiltration of lymphocytes and plasma cells. There may be concomitant involvement of nerve roots, blood vessels or parenchyma. Ependymitis may also be seen.

Symptomatic neurosyphilis

Symptoms associated with meningeal syphilis include headache, confusion, nausea and vomiting, and stiff neck. In addition, cranial nerves, or rarely, spinal roots, may be affected as manifested by cranial neuropathy or poly-radiculopathy. Meningitis may cause arteritis of small, medium or large blood vessels, producing ischaemia or infarction of brain or spinal cord, or meningitis may obstruct the CSF pathways and produce hydrocephalus. Focal meningeal inflammation may lead to the formation of hypertrophic meningitis or gummata that exert pressure on adjacent structures. Seizures may occur as a result of cortical irritation by meningitis, stroke or gumma.

Meningitis affecting the brain

Merritt and Moore reported the largest series of cases of symptomatic or acute meningitis in 1935. All 80 patients had historical or clinical evidence of syphilis and clinical evidence of meningitis. All but one patient had CSF pleocytosis; this patient had a reactive CSF Wassermann test. The authors stated that syphilitic meningitis was rare, and in a subsequent publication Merritt (1940) estimated that it occurred in less than 0.5% of individuals with syphilis. As in previous reports (Wile and Stokes, 1914; Moore, 1922, 1929), Merritt and Moore found that symptomatic meningitis was more commonly seen in patients who had been inadequately or incompletely treated for early syphilis. Merritt and Moore (1935) subdivided their cases into three groups: syphilitic hydrocephalus, meningitis of the vertex and basilar meningitis. Patients in all three groups had meningeal signs, nausea, and vomiting. Additionally, syphilitic hydrocephalus included papilloedema; meningitis of the vertex included convulsions, focal findings or confusion; and basilar meningitis included cranial nerve abnormalities. These groups were not mutually exclusive.

Overall, two-thirds of cases occurred within a year of primary infection (range 2 months to 26 years), and in 7.5% the rash of secondary syphilis was still present. The blood Wassermann test was positive in only 64% of cases. The mean CSF WBC was 434/μl; CSF protein was greater than 45 mg/dl in 88% with a mean of 110 mg/dl; CSF glucose content was less than 50 mg/dl in 55% with a mean of 49 mg/dl; and the CSF Wassermann test was reactive in 91% at initial or follow-up examination. The low prevalence of reactive serum Wassermann tests in this series is surprising but is most likely explained by previous treatment in many patients.

Table 12.3 outlines the prevalence of cranial nerve involvement in patients with acute syphilitic meningitis compiled by Merritt and coworkers (Merritt and Moore, 1935; Merritt et al., 1946) from their experience and from the literature. Involvement of the facial and auditory nerves was most common, followed by involvement of the optic nerve with decreased visual acuity presumably due to optic neuritis. Although the authors did not specifically address other ocular abnormalities seen with syphilitic meningitis, their data suggest that these may have been present. They state that 'choked discs', or papilloedema, was seen in 59% of cases, yet in some instances the CSF pressure was normal. Optic perineuritis may be seen in the setting of syphilitic meningitis (Rush and Ryan, 1981; Toshniwal, 1987). Both optic neuritis and optic perineuritis are characterized by an elevated disc and normal CSF pressure. Unlike the case in optic neuritis, visual acuity is preserved in optic perineuritis, probably because inflammation is localized to the optic nerve sheath and spares the nerve itself. Chorioretinitis, retinal vasculitis and neuroretinitis can also accompany syphilitic meningitis (Folk et al., 1983; Mendelsohn and Jampol, 1984; Arruga et al., 1985; Halperin et al., 1989).

Table 12.3   Cranial nerve involvement in acute syphilitic meningitis.

	Cranial nerve	Per cent involved
I	Olfactory	1.5
II	Optic	27
III	Oculomotor	24
IV	Trochlear	2.6
V	Trigeminal	12
VI	Abducens	22
VII	Facial	41
VIII	Auditory	42
IX, X	Glossopharyngeal, vagus	6.0
XI	Spinal accesory	0.5
XII	Hypoglossal	3.6

Adapted from Merritt et al. (1946).

Uveitis may be seen alone or with meningitis, and subclinical involvement of the anterior chamber of the eye may occur in as many as one-half of patients with secondary syphilis (Zwink and Dunlop, 1976). Moore published the largest series of patients with syphilitic uveitis in 1931 (Moore and Gieske, 1931). He showed that, like syphilitic meningitis, uveitis occurred more commonly in patients inadequately treated for early syphilis and uveitis was more often associated with meningitis in that circumstance.

Some authors have suggested that patients in Merritt and coworkers' series of syphilitic meningitis may have been misdiagnosed, and that those with negative CSF serology probably represent cases of viral meningitis with an incidentally reactive blood serology (Simon, 1985). Certainly, viral meningitis was not recognized by the authors in their differential diagnosis. This diagnostic uncertainty plagues the interpretation of most literature on neuro-syphilis and is difficult to resolve. Nonetheless, it seems likely that most cases were correctly diagnosed; the high prevalence of CSF Wassermann reactivity and of cranial nerve abnormalities would be unusual in viral meningitis. More problematic are reports of isolated cranial nerve abnormalities attributed to CNS infection by *T. pallidum* in the absence of CSF abnormalities (Wile and Stokes, 1914; Moore, 1929). Merritt found these reports to be unconvincing, and it seems likely that many such cranial nerve palsies, especially those involving cranial nerves III and VI, were secondary to other causes such as diabetes or hypertension. However, optic neuritis, eighth nerve deafness and even some cases of Menière's disease can be due to infection with *T. pallidum* localized to the optic nerve or the temporal bone without evidence of CSF involvement (Lorentzen, 1967; Becker, 1979; McNulty and Fassett, 1981; Hughes and Rutherford, 1986; Smith and Canalis, 1989; Pulec, 1997). In many cases response to high-dose penicillin supports a treponemal aetiology.

Meningitis affecting the spinal cord

Syphilitic meningitis may uncommonly affect the spinal cord, presenting as meningomyelitis or hyperplastic pachymeningitis, although these entities are rarely seen without evidence of involvement of other regions of the nervous system. Adams and Merritt (1944) described 15 cases of meningomyelitis and one case of hyperplastic meningitis among 2231 syphilis cases seen at Boston City Hospital. Symptoms and signs in these patients included back pain, sensory loss, incontinence, leg weakness, and muscle atrophy. In this small series, the CSF findings were similar to those described in meningitis involving the brain. Occasional cases of syphilitic meningomyelitis (Fisher and Poser, 1977; Agdal *et al.*, 1980; Silber, 1989; Strom and Schneck, 1991; Berger, 1992; Gentile *et al.*, 1998) and polyradiculopathy without other evidence of spinal cord involvement are reported in modern times (Lanska *et al.*, 1988; Byrne *et al.*, 1991; Stepper *et al.*, 1998).

Pathology of meningeal neurosyphilis

The pathological changes seen in syphilitic meningitis are perivascular infiltration of meninges with lymphocytes, plasma cells, and occasional neutrophils. This inflammatory reaction may also affect the ependyma. With time, the inflammatory reaction may lead to fibrosis. Inflammation of vessel walls may cause arteritis and vascular occlusion. A combination of inflammation, fibrosis and vascular occlusion is responsible for the cranial neuropathies and radiculopathies seen in syphilitic meningitis.

Gumma

Rarely, localized syphilitic meningitis can produce a circumscribed mass of granulation tissue termed a gumma (Adams and Merritt, 1944; Merritt *et al.*, 1946; Standaert *et al.*, 1991; Case records of the Massachusetts General Hospital, 1991; Berger *et al.*, 1992; Roeske and Kennedy, 1996; Suarez *et al.*, 1996). These commonly arise from the pia mater, and may invade the substance of the brain and spinal cord; parenchymal gummata may rarely be found without concomitant pial involvement. Merritt and coworkers reported CSF findings in four cases of CNS gumma; three had CSF pleocytosis and all had a reactive CSF Wassermann test (Adams and Merritt, 1944; Merritt *et al.*, 1944). Reactive CSF serological tests need not be present however, and cases of biopsy-proven cerebral gummata with negative CSF-VDRL have been reported (Kaplan *et al.*, 1981; Fleet *et al.*, 1986). Despite the fact these lesions may resolve with steroid therapy (Fleet *et al.*, 1986; Case records of the Massachusetts General Hospital, 1991), patients should also be treated with penicillin regimens recommended for neurosyphilis (Berger *et al.*, 1992; Roeske and Kennedy, 1996; Suarez *et al.*, 1996).

Meningovasculitis of the brain

Meningitis may lead to arteritis affecting any intracranial vessel, with thrombosis, ischaemia and infarction. The largest series of patients with meningovascular syphilis was reported by Merritt *et al.* (1946) and was selected from a possible 250 cases. After excluding atherosclerotic cerebrovascular disease, cerebral embolism, other forms of neurosyphilis and other non-syphilitic neurological diseases, 42 cases were available for analysis, representing 3% of all cases of syphilis. Most patients were 30–50 years old, although cases were also identified in children with congenital syphilis. The tendency to describe meningovascular syphilis in younger individuals may be partially explained by exclusion of patients with hypertension and atherosclerotic cerebrovascular disease that occur in an older age group, but is also due to the relatively early occurrence of this complication following primary infection. Merritt and coworkers described development of meningovascular syphilis within months to years after infection, with an average of seven years (Merritt, 1940; Merritt *et al.*, 1946).

In the series reported by Merritt and coworkers (1946), many patients with meningovascular syphilis experienced prodromal symptoms, such as headache, dizziness, and personality changes for days or weeks before the onset of ischaemia or stroke. These symptoms were probably due to concomitant meningitis. Onset of vascular symptoms was abrupt in three-quarters of patients, and hemiplegia or hemiparesis was the most common focal finding, followed by aphasia. These clinical manifestations reflect the fact that the middle cerebral artery and its branches were more frequently affected than any other intracranial vessel.

The blood Wassermann test was reactive in 95% of cases. The CSF WBC count was >10/µl in 63% and the CSF Wassermann was reactive in 81%, however, the selection criteria excluded cases with both negative blood and CSF serologies.

A number of authors prior to Merritt described 'vascular' syphilis occurring in patients with normal spinal fluid (Fordyce and Rosen, 1921; Solomon and Klauder, 1921; Mills, 1927). In an early publication, Merritt himself stated that late vascular lesions could be seen with normal CSF (Merritt, 1940). However, in the 1946 monograph, Merritt and coworkers stated that the aetiology of stroke with a negative CSF serology was likely non-syphilitic. Given that the underlying process in meningovascular syphilis is vasculitis, completely normal CSF would be quite unlikely. The one possible exception to this statement is the case of isolated Nissl-Alzheimer arteritis, which is not characterized by perivascular lymphocytic infiltration (Merritt *et al.*, 1946) (see below). This entity rarely exists alone, but could be responsible for small vessel occlusion in the setting of non-inflammatory CSF.

Angiographic findings in meningovascular syphilis include segmental arterial narrowing, focal narrowing and dilatation ('beading'), and occlusion. These findings may resemble spasm associated with subarachnoid hemorrhage or may mimic other infectious or non-infectious vasculidities (Holmes *et al.*, 1984; Landi *et al.*, 1990). Although atherosclerotic cerebrovascular disease may coexist with syphilitic vasculitis, atherosclerotic cerebrovascular disease tends to involve the common carotid bifurcation and intracavernous internal carotid artery, while syphilitic vasculitis more commonly affects the supraclinoid segment of the internal carotid artery (Vatz *et al.*, 1974). Brain computed tomographic and magnetic resonance imaging show multiple areas of infarction, consistent with diffuse intracranial vasculitis (Gabay *et al.*, 1983; Holland *et al.*, 1986; Brightbill *et al.*, 1995).

Meningovascular syphilis of the spinal cord

Meningovascular syphilis involving the spinal cord is rare. Adams and Merritt (1944) described 16 cases of spinal vascular syphilis seen among 2231 syphilis patients. This form of meningovascular syphilis results from thrombosis of spinal vessels. It presents as an acute transverse myelitis characterized by sudden onset of paralysis and anaesthesia of trunk and legs, usually with a thoracic sensory level as well as loss of sphincter control. CSF findings are identical to those described in meningovascular syphilis affecting the brain. Such cases continue to be reported (Harrigan *et al.*, 1984; Lowenstein *et al.*, 1987; Silber, 1989; Terry *et al.*, 1989; Berger, 1992).

Pathology of meningovascular syphilis

The pathological changes seen in meningovascular syphilis include meningeal inflammation, as previously described, as well as more prominent vascular changes. Heubner arteritis affects large or medium sized arteries and is characterized by infiltration of the adventitia by lymphocytes and plasma cells; these cells may occasionally infiltrate the media and intima, and may occlude the vasa vasorum. Fibroblasts proliferate and thicken the intima. In the late stages there is medial necrosis and replacement by connective tissue. As noted above, Nissl-Alzheimer endarteritis affects small vessels and is characterized by non-inflammatory endothelial and adventitial proliferation that leads to obliteration of the vessel lumen (Merritt *et al.*, 1946).

Parenchymal neurosyphilis

Paresis

Paretic neurosyphilis, also called general paralysis of the insane or dementia paralytica, was estimated by Merritt and coworkers to develop in 5% of cases of syphilis. In their experience it was most commonly seen in individuals 35–50 years of age, and occurred from 5 to 25 years after acquisition of primary infection (Merritt *et al.*, 1946). In a series by Hahn *et al.* (1959), the duration of infection ranged from 2 to more than 30 years, with the majority occurring between 10 and 24 years. Similarly, in a group of untreated patients, duration of infection ranged from 4 to 15 years, with a mean of 10.5 years (Dewhurst, 1969).

The clinical manifestations of paretic neurosyphilis may be subtle in onset and can mimic 'every type of mental disorder' (Merritt *et al.*, 1946). Early in the course of this chronic, progressive, dementing illness, patients display forgetfulness and personality changes. With time, they may develop psychiatric symptoms, such as mania, depression, or psychosis, although the majority simply experience progression of deficits in memory and judgement resulting in frank dementia. In its latest stages, patients become immobile and incontinent; seizures are not uncommon. The most frequent findings on neurological examination of patients with general paresis are pupillary abnormalities, facial and limb hypotonia, intention tremors of the face, tongue and hands, and reflex abnormalities, but early in the course the neurological examination can be normal. Without treatment, death occurs within months to 4 or 5 years, usually secondary to intercurrent infection. If infection is avoided, death most commonly results from uncontrolled seizures or respiratory arrest. The average survival after diagnosis in Merritt and coworkers' experience in the pre-antibiotic era was 2.5 years (Merritt *et al.*, 1946).

Merritt and coworkers found that the CSF was always abnormal in untreated paresis; in 100 cases, mild lymphocytic pleocytosis (10–100 WBC/µl) was seen in 90%, mildly elevated protein (45–100 mg/dl) in 75%, and a strongly positive Wassermann reaction in 100%. Serum serologies were reactive in over 85%. Similarly, in Hahn and coworkers' series (1959) all previously untreated patients had reactive CSF Wassermann tests, and 92% had a reactive serum Wassermann test.

Merritt stated that 'the diagnosis of paretic neurosyphilis is practically never justified in an untreated patient with a consistently negative Wassermann reaction in the cerebrospinal fluid' (Merritt *et al.*, 1946).. Nevertheless, rare cases of pathologically proven meningoencephalitis due to *T. pallidum* in which the CSF non-treponemal serology is non-reactive have been reported (Ch'ien *et al.*, 1970; Burke, 1972).

Pathology of paretic neurosyphilis

The pathological changes in paresis are those of a chronic spirochaetal meningoencephalitis. The brain is atrophic and the meninges are thickened and cloudy. Meningeal and vascular changes are identical to those seen in meningeal neurosyphilis. Additionally, parenchymal involvement with neuronal degeneration and loss, gliosis, and deposition of iron pigment in vessel walls is seen. Spirochaetes can sometimes be identified within grey matter by silver stains (Noguchi and Moore, 1913; Merritt *et al.*, 1946).

Tabes

Tabes dorsalis, also called locomotor ataxia, was the most common form of neurosyphilis described in the pre-antibiotic era, and was evident in 9% of 2231 patients with syphilis seen in the outpatient department of the Boston City Hospital (Merritt *et al.*, 1946). Tabes has the longest latent period between primary infection and onset of symptoms compared to the other manifestations of neurosyphilis, and in Merritt and coworkers' series this ranged from 3 to 47 years, with an average of 21 years (Merritt *et al.*, 1946). The onset of symptoms is typically between the ages of 44 and 60 years, but may occur in adolescence in individuals with congenital syphilis.

The most common symptoms of tabes are lancinating pains, sensory changes, progressive ataxia and bowel and bladder dysfunction. Pupillary abnormalities are the rule, and optic atrophy is common. Lightning or lancinating pains, seen in 75% of 150 cases of tabes collected by Merritt and coworkers (1946), are sudden, brief stabs of pain that may affect the legs, back, arms and face. They may last for minutes to days and occur unpredictably, sometimes separated by long remissions. Some authors have suggested that lancinating pains were not a consequence of syphilis infection, but were due to heavy metal therapy used to treat neurosyphilis in the pre-antibiotic era (Weismann, 1995). Visceral crises occurred in 10–15% of patients with tabes; the most common was the gastric variety, characterized by recurrent attacks of severe epigastric pain, nausea and vomiting. Early sensory changes include paraesthesias or hyperaesthesias in radicular distributions. Later, pain, vibration and tactile sensation become impaired, and reflexes are lost. Sensory ataxia, usually involving the lower more than the upper extremities, was a feature in 42% of Merritt and coworkers' patients (1946). Sensory loss predisposes tabetics to the formation of Charcot joints and trophic ulcers. Bladder dysfunction may occur early with urinary retention and overflow incontinence. A similar process affects the bowel, although faecal incontinence is unusual.

Pupillary abnormalities were described in 94% of the tabes dorsalis cases collected by Merritt and coworkers, and 48% had Argyll Robertson pupils (Merritt et al., 1946). These workers rather strictly defined the Argyll Robertson pupil as a small pupil that does not respond to light but does contract normally to accommodation-convergence, dilates imperfectly to mydriatics, and does not dilate in response to painful stimuli. Thus defined, they believed that Argyll Robertson pupils were specific for neurosyphilis and were most commonly seen in tabetics.

Optic atrophy was seen in 16% of Merritt and coworkers' cases and was also most commonly seen in tabetics (Merritt et al., 1946). Optic atrophy presents with gradual decrease in visual acuity, and examination reveals constriction of the peripheral visual fields, often with central scotomata. Untreated, this disorder progresses to complete blindness over months to years (Hahn, 1957).

The CSF formula in early tabes is similar to that seen in paresis, but with time the meningeal process becomes less active and CSF abnormalities are less evident. Merritt and coworkers examined the CSF of 100 cases of tabes, many of whom had arrested disease. They found that 50% had a normal WBC count ($< 5/\mu l$), 47% had normal protein, and 28% had a negative CSF non-treponemal test. The blood nontreponemal tests were positive in 88%. Overall, two of these 100 cases had normal CSF and non-reactive blood serological tests (Merritt et al., 1946).

Pathology of tabes

In early tabes, the leptomeninges and preganglionic portion of the dorsal roots are infiltrated with lymphocytes and plasma cells. This change is similar to the pathology seen in meningeal neurosyphilis, but is more localized. These inflammatory changes disappear with time and the posterior roots become thin and grey. If optic atrophy is present, similar changes are seen in the optic nerves. The posterior columns of the spinal cord become secondarily atrophic and gliotic, and the overlying arachnoid is slightly opaque and thickened (Merritt *et al.*, 1946). Spirochaetes are rarely demonstrated in dorsal roots or posterior columns. Increased signal in the posterior columns may be seen on T2-weighted magnetic resonance images of the spinal cord (Stepper *et al.*, 1998).

Congenital neurosyphilis

The manifestations and clinical course of congenital neurosyphilis parallel that of acquired disease. CSF abnormalities can be seen in otherwise asymptomatic cases of congenital syphilis (Kingery, 1921), and early and late forms of symptomatic neurosyphilis have similar latent periods. Thus, congenital meningeal neurosyphilis is seen in infancy, and meningovascular disease in the first few years of life. Parenchymal disease usually has its onset around puberty or in early adulthood (Merritt *et al.*, 1946).

Change in spectrum of neurosyphilis in the antibiotic era

Several reports have suggested that the clinical presentation of neurosyphilis differs in the antibiotic era (Kofman, 1956; Joffe *et al.*, 1968; Hooshmand *et al.*, 1972; Heathfield, 1976; Joyce-Clarke and Molteno, 1978). Incomplete forms or 'formes frustes' of neurosyphilis have been described, and are attributed to partial treatment by antibiotics given for unrelated illnesses. Interestingly, Merritt and coworkers described a similar alteration in the natural history of neurosyphilis by intercurrent febrile illnesses (Merritt *et al.*, 1946). The largest series addressing change in clinical findings was reported by Hooshmand and coworkers (1972). They diagnosed neurosyphilis in 241 of 289 (84%) hospitalized patients with reactive serum fluorescent treponemal antibody-absorbed (FTA-ABS) tests. Diagnosis of neurosyphilis was based upon the following criteria: ophthalmologic or neurological findings suggestive of neurosyphilis; or reactive CSF FTA-ABS with >5 CSF WBC/µl and no evidence of bacterial or viral meningitis; or reactive CSF FTA-ABS in patients with progressive neurological symptoms in whom other aetiologies had been excluded and who had either a temporary increase in CSF WBC after treatment with penicillin or significant clinical improvement after treatment with penicillin. Almost half (43%) of these patients were admitted for evaluation of unrelated symptoms, and were incidentally found to have abnormalities on neurological examination that suggested the diagnosis of neurosyphilis. The most common of these were reflex changes, absent ankle jerks, pupillary changes and sensory abnormalities; 24% had adult-onset seizures. Forty-eight per cent of patients in this series had reactive serum non-treponemal serologies, and 57% of 157 patients had reactive CSF-VDRL tests. As in other such reports, the authors concluded 'neurosyphilis, at the present time, presents itself in a most atypical fashion' (Hooshmand *et al.*, 1972). This conclusion seems unjustified for several reasons. Monosymptomatic or 'atypical' cases of neurosyphilis were described in the pre-antibiotic era. The abnormalities most commonly observed by Hooshmand and coworkers and others are non-specific and are seen in many neurological disorders; their coexistence with reactive serum treponemal serologies does not establish causality. Additionally, some studies reporting altered clinical presentations of neurosyphilis have relied on a positive CSF FTA-ABS test to define neurosyphilis. The validity of this approach is unproven (Jaffe *et al.*, 1968; Marra *et al.*, 1995) (see below).

Similarly, a number of authors have argued that late, parenchymal neurosyphilis is less common today than in the pre-antibiotic era, and that meningeal or early neurosyphilis is more common (Hotson, 1981; Burke and Schaberg, 1985). These studies frequently compare a local experience to large series described in the 1940s. Such comparisons are flawed for several reasons: none of the studies are population-based, so reliable denominator data are not available; different laboratory methods and clinical criteria are used for diagnosis; and the studies are not controlled for duration of infection and prior therapy. These drawbacks aside, perhaps the best series to examine this issue is Wolter's comparison of 518 cases of neurosyphilis collected in 1930–1940, and 121 cases of neurosyphilis collected in 1970–1984 from the same neurological clinic of the Academic Hospital of the University of Amsterdam (Wolters, 1987). In this study, the proportion of cases of asymptomatic neurosyphilis diagnosed from 1930 to 1940 (41/577, 7%) was much lower than in 1970–1984 (48/121, 40%). Parenchymal disease occurred in two-thirds of the symptomatic group in 1930–40, but equal proportions of symptomatic meningeal and parenchymal disease were seen in 1970–84. The relative increase in asymptomatic neurosyphilis can be attributed to more frequent CSF examination and changes in diagnostic criteria in the later time period. However, despite the limitations of this and other studies, the bulk of evidence suggests that late neurosyphilis does occur less frequently than early neurosyphilis in the antibiotic era. This observation is most striking in patients also infected with HIV, and will be discussed later in this chapter. Several authors have speculated that this shift in clinical presentation is due to inadvertent treatment with antibiotics prescribed for unrelated conditions. This contention is supported by observations collected in the pre-antibiotic era (see section on symptomatic meningeal syphilis) that partial or incomplete therapy predisposes individuals infected with *T. pallidum* to develop syphilitic meningitis, meningovasculitis and ocular disease (Wile and Stokes, 1914; Moore, 1922, 1929; Moore and Gieske, 1931).

Laboratory diagnosis of neurosyphilis

Cells, protein and CSF-VDRL

The diagnosis of symptomatic neurosyphilis is based upon clinical evidence and is supported by CSF abnormalities such as pleocytosis, elevated protein and

Table 12.4 CSF abnormalities in neurosyphilis.

	White blood cells per microlitre (μl)	Protein (mg/dl)	Reactive CSF Wassermann test
Asymptomatic	0–100	< 45–100	84%
Meningeal	200–400	100–200	91%
Meningovascular	11–100	100–200	81%
Paresis	25–75	50–100	100%
Tabes	10–50	45–75	72%

Compiled from Merritt *et al.*, 1946.
The frequency of CSF abnormalities in neurosyphilis varies with the definition of each syndrome. The currently used CSF-Venereal Disease Research Laboratory (VDRL) test is likely less sensitive than its predecessor, the CSF Wassermann test (Hahn, 1961; Nitrini, 1989). In addition, reactive CSF non-treponemal serological tests are more common and CSF pleocytosis less common with increasing duration of infection.

IgG content and reactive CSF-VDRL. The diagnosis of asymptomatic neuro-syphilis is based upon the presence of CSF abnormalities alone. Mild CSF mononuclear pleocytosis, usually in the range of 10–400 WBC/μl, is character-istic of neurosyphilis; higher cell counts are seen in the early forms (meningitis and meningovasculitis) compared to the late forms (general paresis and tabes dorsalis). Mild elevations in CSF protein, ranging between 45 and 200 mg/dl are also common, again with higher values in the early compared to the late forms of neurosyphilis. The CSF-VDRL is considered to be the 'gold standard' test. However, depending upon the diagnostic criteria chosen, the CSF-VDRL may be reactive in 0–100% of individuals with neurosyphilis; the generally accepted sensitivity is 30–70% (Hart, 1986). The CSF-VDRL test is very specific. False-positive results may be obtained when the CSF is visibly blood-tinged (Izzat *et al.*, 1971; Davis and Sperry, 1979), and rarely in the absence of blood contamination (Madiedo *et al.*, 1980). Thus, a reactive CSF-VDRL establishes the diagnosis of neurosyphilis, but a non-reactive test does not exclude it. This quandary is especially difficult in evaluating patients with suspected asymptomatic neurosyphilis where diagnosis depends upon such non-specific findings as mild CSF pleocytosis or protein elevation. The frequency of CSF abnormalities in the various forms of neurosyphilis described by Merritt and coworkers (1946) is outlined in Table 12.4.

CSF treponemal tests

The application of treponemal tests to CSF remains somewhat controversial. Jaffe and coworkers (1978) examined the use of the CSF FTA-ABS test for diagnosis of neurosyphilis. These workers found that the test was never reactive in 177 patients without syphilis, but was reactive or borderline in all of 12 patients with symptomatic and asymptomatic neurosyphilis and in four (23.5%) of 17 patients with latent syphilis but not neurosyphilis. Reactive

CSF FTA-ABS was more commonly seen in those with higher serum FTA-ABS titres, and microscopic blood contamination of CSF could produce a false-positive result. A subsequent study of 94 patients from the University of Kansas Medical Center showed that the CSF FTA-ABS had a sensitivity of 100% and a specificity of 89% compared to a clinical diagnosis of neurosyphilis (McGeeney et al., 1979). A more recent study demonstrates an even lower specificity of this test: only 39% of 38 individuals with reactive CSF FTA-ABS tests were likely to have neurosyphilis based upon clinical and CSF criteria (Davis and Schmitt, 1989). The authors concluded, however, that a non-reactive CSF FTA-ABS test makes a diagnosis of active neurosyphilis unlikely. A study of CSF findings in 39 individuals with primary and secondary syphilis confirms this finding (Marra et al., 1995) and demonstrated that CSF treponemal tests may be particularly useful in excluding the diagnosis of neurosyphilis in individuals infected with HIV (see section on HIV and syphilis below).

Some authors advocate using measures of CSF intrathecal treponemal antibody production such as CSF:serum treponemal antibody ratios or indices that correct for CSF and serum albumin or IgG concentrations (Luger et al., 1981; Prange et al., 1981; Muller and Moskophidis, 1983; van Eijk et al., 1987; Wolters et al., 1988) to establish the diagnosis of neurosyphilis. However, several studies suggest that measures of intrathecal antibody production may lack sufficient specificity for clinical use. In a study of patients with primary and secondary syphilis, the CSF ITPA index was normal in two (28%) of seven patients with reactive CSF-VDRL (Marra et al., 1995) and in a study of 10 HIV-infected patients with suspected neurosyphilis, the TPHA index was normal in two (40%) of five with reactive CSF-VDRL (Tomberlin et al., 1994).

Identification of *T. pallidum* in CSF

T. pallidum may be identified in CSF by inoculation of CSF into rabbits. Although rabbit inoculation is 100% specific and quite sensitive (Turner et al., 1969), it is too cumbersome and expensive to be clinically useful. Polymerase chain reaction (PCR) can be used to detect *T. pallidum* in CSF. The limit of detection is similar to that of rabbit inoculation (Marra et al., 1998). A study of individuals with primary, secondary and early latent syphilis showed that *T. pallidum* could be detected in CSF by rabbit inoculation or by PCR in 25% of patients (Rolfs, 1997). Nonetheless, identification of the organism in CSF did not influence the efficacy of therapies that did and did not achieve treponemicidal drug levels in CSF. Thus the diagnostic importance of identification of *T. pallidum* in CSF remains to be clarified. Some experts have suggested that such identification warrants treatment in patients who have been infected for more than a year or in those who are also infected with HIV (Ronald et al., 1992).

Therapy for neurosyphilis

Penicillin therapy for neurosyphilis

Studies of penicillin treatment for neurosyphilis suffer from several inadequacies, including lack of uniformity in diagnostic criteria, in forms and dosages of penicillin administered, in outcome criteria (clinical and CSF), and in duration of follow up. Early studies emphasized total dose of penicillin administered, and often did not state the duration of therapy. Nevertheless, penicillin has become the accepted therapy for neurosyphilis.

Several studies examined the efficacy of intramuscularly administered penicillin for asymptomatic neurosyphilis. As indicated by lack of resolution or worsening of CSF abnormalities, about 9% of individuals treated with 2.4 to 9.0 million units (MU) of aqueous penicillin, amorphous penicillin, crystalline penicillin or penicillin in oil and wax failed therapy. Treatment with higher doses was usually effective (Dattner, 1949; Nichols *et al.*, 1949; Ford *et al.*, 1951; Hahn *et al.*, 1956a, b). In contrast, 21% of patients with asymptomatic neurosyphilis treated with 2.4 or 2.5 MU of benzathine penicillin failed therapy (Smith *et al.*, 1956).

The largest series of penicillin treatment of symptomatic neurosyphilis was a multicentre study of 1086 patients with general paresis undertaken by the Cooperative Clinical Group (Hahn *et al.*, 1959). Diagnosis was based upon clinical impression, and many patients had been previously treated. Patients were treated with 0.6 to more than 10 MU of aqueous or procaine penicillin; the majority received at least 2.4 MU. Forty per cent also underwent fever therapy, and 60% were followed for at least 5 years. The resolution of CSF abnormalities after treatment was similar to that seen in asymptomatic neurosyphilis; at one year following therapy, 16% of spinal fluids showed WBC counts of 5–10/μl, and WBC counts > 11/μl had 'practically' disappeared (Hahn *et al.*, 1959). Clinical improvement was seen in 30–80% of patients; those with less severe and shorter duration of symptoms had the most favourable response. Retreatment with higher doses of penicillin was of benefit only in the small number of individuals who had initially improved after therapy but subsequently worsened.

A smaller series of penicillin treatment of symptomatic neurosyphilis was published by Dattner (1949). Patients were treated with 2.0–9.0 MU of an unspecified form of penicillin. Ten per cent of 61 patients with dementia paralytica failed to resolve CSF abnormalities over a 6–56 month period. Similarly, 16% of 82 patients with meningovasculitis and 9% of 79 patients with tabes failed therapy. The majority of non-responders improved after a second course of higher dose penicillin.

Based upon the experience of the Cooperative Clinical Group, Hahn concluded in a 1961 editorial that 6–10 MU of procaine penicillin or 4.8 MU of benzathine penicillin was sufficient for all forms of neurosyphilis. No further large scale studies of therapy for neurosyphilis were conducted after that time.

In 1966, Short and coworkers demonstrated failure of 4.8 MU of benzathine penicillin to resolve CSF abnormalities in two of 26 cases of active neurosyphilis; two additional cases may have also failed therapy. More recently, Greene and coworkers (1980) described clinical progression of meningeal neurosyphilis after treatment with 7.2 MU of intramuscular benzathine penicillin, given over 3 weeks.

Case reports and small series in the mid-1970s to mid-1980s have led workers in the field to recommend progressively higher doses and different forms of penicillin as appropriate therapy for neurosyphilis. Many of these recommendations are based upon two suppositions that have not been tested: the level of penicillin in the CSF should be above 0.018 µg/ml (0.031 units/ml) for 10–14 days because this is the accepted serum treponemicidal concentration and duration of therapy required to cure early, non-neurological syphilis (Idsoe *et al.*, 1972), and recovery of *T. pallidum* from the CSF after therapy indicates treatment failure.

Neither procaine penicillin G 600 000 to 1.2 MU/day, alone or with probenecid (Lowhagen *et al.*, 1983; Yoder, 1975; Dunlop *et al.*, 1979), 2.4 MU of procaine penicillin G alone (Polnikorn *et al.*, 1980), nor as much as 14.4 MU of benzathine penicillin G (Mohr *et al.*, 1976) reliably achieves treponemicidal penicillin levels within the CSF. Virulent *T. pallidum* have been demonstrated in CSF after treatment with 2.4, 4.8 and 10.8 MU of benzathine penicillin G (Fildes *et al.*, 1918; Tramont, 1976).

In contrast, intravenous crystalline penicillin G in doses from 5 to 24 MU per day have been shown to consistently achieve treponemicidal CSF levels (Mohr *et al.*, 1976; Polnikorn *et al.*, 1980; Schoth and Wolters, 1987). Although some authors have documented CSF treponemicidal penicillin levels after intramuscular procaine penicillin G, 2.4 MU per day with oral probenecid (Dunlop *et al.*, 1979, 1981), this is not a universal experience (van der Valk, 1988). Despite the lack of clinical trials, these data, as well as experimental evidence that probenecid competes with penicillin for entry into brain (Fishman, 1966), argue that the best therapy for neurosyphilis is probably high-dose intravenous penicillin. However, well-documented instances of failure of intramuscular procaine penicillin with oral probenecid have not been reported, and the Centers for Disease Control and Prevention (CDC) (1998) recommend either regimen as shown in Table 12.5. These limitations of benzathine penicillin G have also led some experts to recommend against its use in early syphilis. Because this regimen will not eradicate organisms that have invaded the CNS in

Table 12.5   Treatment of neurosyphilis.

Aqueous crystalline penicillin G, 2–4 million units i.v. q 4 hours, for 10–14 days
or
Procaine penicillin, 2.4 million units intramuscularly once daily, plus probenecid 500 mg orally 4 times a day, both for 10–14 days

Many experts recommend the following therapy for neurosyphilis with intramuscular benzathine penicillin G, 2.4 million units weekly for 3 weeks.
Adapted from Centers for Disease Control and Prevention (1998).

early syphilis, some individuals may develop symptomatic neurosyphilis despite 'adequate' therapy for early syphilis (neurorelapse). This issue is especially pertinent to individuals infected with both syphilis and HIV and will be discussed below.

Non-penicillin therapy for neurosyphilis

Ceftriaxone is the most widely studied alternative to penicillin for treatment of neurosyphilis. Individual cases of successful treatment of asymptomatic and symptomatic neurosyphilis with ceftriaxone 1.0 gm intramuscularly (i.m.) daily for 14 days have been reported (Hook *et al.*, 1986; Cnossen *et al.*, 1995; Gentile *et al.*, 1998). In contrast, a retrospective study of ceftriaxone given i.m. for treatment of HIV-infected patients with neurosyphilis, latent syphilis and presumed latent syphilis (many of whom were eventually found to have neurosyphilis), showed a 23% failure rate using serological criteria (Dowell *et al.*, 1992). A small prospective study compared ceftriaxone 2 g intravenously (i.v.) daily for 10 days and penicillin G 4 MU i.v. every 4 hours for 10 days for treatment of neurosyphilis in HIV-infected individuals (Marra *et al.*, 1999). There was no difference in improvement in CSF measures after therapy between the two groups, but more ceftriaxone-treated subjects had improved serum Rapid Plasma Reagin (RPR) test titres after therapy. Unfortunately, there were significant differences between the two groups: more ceftriaxone-treated subjects had early syphilis and more penicillin-treated subjects had a prior episode of neurosyphilis. Because of the limitations of this study, ceftriaxone cannot be routinely recommended as an alternative to penicillin for treatment of neurosyphilis. However, ceftriaxone may be an acceptable alternative for patients with neurosyphilis and concomitant secondary syphilis.

HIV and neurosyphilis

Since the beginning of the HIV epidemic, cases of symptomatic and asymptomatic neurosyphilis and syphilitic ocular disease have been reported in HIV-infected individuals (McLeish *et al.*, 1990; Berger, 1991; Musher, 1991; Katz *et al.*, 1993; Schofer *et al.*, 1998; Shalaby *et al.*, 1997; Flood *et al.*, 1998; Inungu *et al.*, 1998; Kuo *et al.*, 1998). Many of these patients had been previously treated for early syphilis with appropriate doses of intramuscular benzathine penicillin, suggesting that they experienced neurorelapse. In addition, several reports suggest that HIV-infected individuals are more likely to fail therapy for neurosyphilis (see below). Although observations based on case reports do not provide denominator data, these reports suggest that HIV infection alters the natural course and response to therapy of syphilis and neurosyphilis.

Evidence from animal models demonstrates the importance of cell-mediated immunity in clearing *T. pallidum* from sites of infection. Immunosuppression of infected rabbits with cortisone decreases local cellular infiltration and significantly delays bacterial elimination (Lukehart *et al.*, 1981). HIV-infected rabbits (Tseng *et al.*, 1991) and simian immunodeficiency virus

(SIV)-infected macaques (Marra *et al.*, 1992) show delayed healing of syphilitic chancres. Similarly, HIV infection, and its attendant alterations in cell-mediated immunity, might decrease the ability of the host to control CNS or ocular infection.

Impaired ability of HIV-infected patients to clear organisms from the eye or CNS is particularly important to therapy of early syphilis. In the pre-antibiotic era, meningeal and meningovascular syphilis and syphilitic uveitis were most commonly seen in patients inadequately treated for early syphilis. Merritt and Moore (Moore, 1929; Merritt and Moore, 1935) argued that small amounts of therapy were able to eradicate all organisms except those that had invaded the CNS or the eye in early syphilis and led to an appropriate attenuation of the immune response. The organisms remaining in the CNS or eye were then free to multiply and produce disease. A parallel can be made to the HIV-infected patient treated with benzathine penicillin for early syphilis. This treatment does not clear *T. pallidum* from the CNS or the eye. Because of impaired cell-mediated immunity, the patient has no mechanism to eradicate persisting organisms, and remains at risk for development of symptomatic neurosyphilis or ocular disease. The results of a prospective study done at the University of Washington support this contention (Lukehart *et al.*, 1988). Seven patients with *T. pallidum* isolated from CSF before therapy for secondary syphilis had repeat CSF examinations after completion of therapy. Four of the seven patients received a single dose of 2.4 MU of benzathine penicillin. Three of the four required retreatment for neurosyphilis because of persistence of *T. pallidum* in CSF of two, and worsening of CSF parameters in the third. Two of these patients were HIV-infected, and a third became HIV-seropositive during follow up. The one patient cured by a single dose of benzathine penicillin was not infected with HIV.

The diagnosis of asymptomatic neurosyphilis in HIV-infected patients can be particularly difficult because non-specific CSF abnormalities, such as mono-nuclear pleocytosis and elevated protein (Marshall *et al.*, 1991), are often seen in HIV infection alone. This is the setting in which non-reactive CSF treponemal tests may be able to exclude the diagnosis of asymptomatic neurosyphilis. However, if CSF treponemal tests are reactive, and particularly if patients have symptoms consistent with neurosyphilis, the diagnosis of neurosyphilis remains a possibility and often merits therapy. HIV-infected patients with reactive serum serologies and ocular disease consistent with syphilis should be treated with a regimen recommended for neurosyphilis.

Response to therapy

Response in immunocompetent patients

Although clinical response to treatment of neurosyphilis has been reported in cases without CSF pleocytosis (Hooshmand *et al.*, 1972), most authors agree that evidence of CSF inflammation indicates activity of the neurosyphilitic process and therefore the likelihood of a favourable response to therapy

(Simon, 1985). CSF WBC count normally declines by 6 months after treatment and failure to normalize by one year is an indication for retreatment (Centers for Disease Control and Prevention, 1998). In a retrospective study that included nine HIV-uninfected patients with neurosyphilis, all of whom had reactive CSF-VDRL tests, CSF cell count and protein declined to normal levels by approximately 6 months after treatment (Marra *et al.*, 1996). CSF-VDRL may fall much more slowly than cells and protein.

Response in HIV-infected patients

Compared to immunocompetent patients, failure of therapy for neurosyphilis appears to be more common in patients infected with HIV. In a study of HIV-infected patients with symptomatic neurosyphilis treated with high dose i.v. penicillin, three (43%) of seven patients failed treatment at 6 months after therapy (Gordon *et al.*, 1994). Two patients showed increases in serum RPR titres, and worsening CSF parameters, including CSF-VDRL. Another patient failed clinically, with development of meningovascular neurosyphilis; serum RPR and CSF-VDRL titres had increased twofold at the time of relapse. Similarly, a recent study found that three (60%) of five HIV-infected patients with asymptomatic neurosyphilis (reactive CSF-VDRL) treated with high-dose i.v. penicillin relapsed at 5, 14, and 24 months based on fourfold increases in serum VDRL titres (Malone *et al.*, 1995). In the retrospective series discussed above (Marra *et al.*, 1996), none of the nine HIV-uninfected, but three (23%) of the 13 HIV-infected patients failed neurosyphilis therapy. All three patients failed to achieve a fourfold decline in CSF-VDRL titre at more than 1 year after therapy. In addition, normalization of CSF WBC, CSF-VDRL and serum VDRL was significantly slower in the HIV-infected subjects compared to those who were not HIV-infected.

Follow up after therapy

Careful follow up after neurosyphilis therapy is mandatory for all patients, but is particularly important for HIV-infected patients. Cerebrospinal fluid should be re-examined 3 months after therapy. For HIV-infected individuals, if CSF WBC is normal and the CSF-VDRL is non-reactive at this time, no further lumbar punctures are required. For HIV-uninfected individuals, if all CSF measures, including protein concentration, are normal, no further lumbar punctures are required. For those with persistent CSF abnormalities at 3 months after therapy (excluding protein concentration in HIV-infected individuals), CSF should be re-examined at 6 months after therapy and every 6 months thereafter until these parameters normalize. Failure of the CSF WBC count to decrease 6 months after therapy or failure of CSF-VDRL to decline fourfold (or to non-reactive if the initial titre is < 1 : 2) 1 year after therapy are indications for re-treatment. In addition, failure of CSF protein concentration to normalize at 1 year after therapy in an HIV-uninfected individual is an indication for re-treatment. Serum RPR or VDRL tests should be obtained at 3, 6, and 12 months after therapy and every 3–6 months thereafter until they are non-reactive. Failure of the serum RPR or VDRL to decline fourfold (or to non-reactive if the initial titer is < 1 : 2) at 1 year after therapy is an indication for re-treatment. These recommendations differ from those of the Centres for Disease Control and Prevention (1998) in several respects. An initial CSF examination at 3 months rather than 6 months is suggested because it decreases patient loss to follow up; CSF protein concentration is considered in HIV-uninfected individuals in determining response to therapy but is not considered in HIV-infected individuals because this measure is so frequently abnormal in HIV-infected patients; and serum non-treponemal test titre parameters are provided that are based on published data (Marra *et al.*, 1996).

References

Adams, R. D. and Merritt, H. H. (1944). Meningeal and vascular syphilis of the spinal cord. *Medicine (Balti.)*, **23**, 181–214.

Agdal, N., Hagdrup, H. K. and Wantzin, G. L. (1980). Pachymeningitis cervicalis hypertrophica syphilitica. *Acta Derm. Venereol.*, **60**, 184–186.

Arruga, J., Valentines, J., Mauri, F., Roca, G., Salom, R. and Rufi, G. (1985). Neuroretinitis in acquired syphilis. *Ophthalmology*, **92**, 262–270.

Becker, G. D. (1979). Late syphilitic hearing loss: a diagnostic and therapeutic dilemma. *Laryngoscope*, **89**, 1273–1288.

Berger, J. R. (1991). Neurosyphilis in human immunodeficiency virus type 1-seroposi-tive individuals. A prospective study. *Arch. Neurol.*, **48**, 700–702.

Berger, J. R. (1992). Spinal cord syphilis associated with human immunodeficiency virus infection: a treatable myelopathy. *Am. J. Med.*, **92**, 101–103.

Berger, J. R., Waskin, H., Pall, L., Hensley, G., Ihmedian, I. and Post, M. J. (1992). Syphilitic cerebral gumma with HIV infection. *Neurology*, **42**, 1282–1287.

Brightbill, T. C., Ihmeidan, I. H., Post, M. J., Berger, J. R. and Katz, D. A. (1995). Neurosyphilis in HIV-positive and HIV-negative patients: neuroimaging find-ings. *Am. J. Neuroradiol.*, **16**, 703–711.

Bell, F., Heath, P., Shackley, F. *et al.* (1998). Effect of combination with an acellular pertussis, diphtheria, tetanus vaccine on antibody response to Hib vaccine (PRP-T). *Vaccine*, **16**, 637–642.

Burke, J. M. and Schaberg, D. R. (1985). Neurosyphilis in the antibiotic era. *Neurology*, **35**, 1368–1371.

Byrne, T. N., Bose, A., Sze, G. and Waxman, S. G. (1991). Syphilitic meningitis causing paraparesis in an HIV-negative woman. *J. Neurol. Sci.*, **103**, 48–50.

Case records of the Massachusetts General Hospital. (1991). Weekly clinicopathological exercises. Case 32-1991. A 35-year-old man with changed mental status and multiple intracerebral lesions. *N. Engl. J. Med.*, **325**, 414–422.

Centers for Disease Control and Prevention. (1998). 1998 guidelines for treatment of sexually transmitted diseases. *MMWR*, **47**, 1–111.

Ch'ien, L., Hathaway, B. M. and Israel, C. W. (1970). Seronegative dementia paralytica: report of a case. *J. Neurol. Neurosurg. Psych.*, **33**, 376–380.

Cnossen, W. M., Niekus, H., Nielsen, O., Vegt, M. and Blansjaar, B. A. (1995). Ceftriaxone treatment of penicillin resistant neurosyphilis in alcoholic patients (letter). *J. Neurol. Neurosurg. Psych.*, **59**, 194–195.

Dattner, B. (1949). Penicillin failures in neurosyphilis. *Am. J. Syph. Gonorrhea Vener. Dis.*, **33**, 571–575.

Davis, L. E., Schmitt, J. W. (1989). Clinical significance of cerebrospinal fluid tests for neurosyphilis. *Ann. Neurol.*, **25**, 50–55.

Davis, L. E. and Sperry, S. (1979). The CSF-FTA test and the significance of blood contamination. *Ann. Neurol.*, **6**, 68–69.

Dewhurst, K. (1969). The neurosyphilitic psychoses today. A survey of 91 cases. *Br. J. Psych.*, **115**, 31–38.

Dowell, M. E., Ross, P. G., Musher, D. M., Cate, T. R. and Baughn, R. E. (1992). Response of latent syphilis or neurosyphilis to ceftriaxone therapy in persons infected with human immunodeficiency virus. *Am. J. Med.*, **93**, 481–488.

Dunlop, E. M., Al-Egaily, S. S. and Houang, E. T. (1979). Penicillin levels in blood and CSF achieved by treatment of syphilis. *J. Am. Med. Assoc.*, **241**, 2538–2540.

Dunlop, E. M., Al-Egaily, S. S. and Houang, E. T. (1981). Production of treponemicidal concentration of penicillin in cerebrospinal fluid. *Br. Med. J.*, **283**, 646.

Fildes, P., Parnell, R. J. G. and Maitland, H. B. (1918). The occurrence of unsuspected involvement of the central nervous system in unselected cases of syphilis. *Brain*, **41**, 255–301.

Fisher, M. and Poser, C. M. (1977). Syphilitic meningomyelitis. A case report. *Arch. Neurol.*, **34**, 785.

Fishman, R. A. (1966). Blood-brain and CSF barriers to penicillin and related organic acids. *Arch. Neurol.*, **15**, 113–124.

Fleet, W. S., Watson, R. T. and Ballinger, W. E. (1986). Resolution of gumma with steroid therapy. *Neurology*, **36**, 1104–1107.

Flood, J. M., Weinstock, H. S., Guroy, M. E., Bayne, L., Simon, R. P. and Bolan, G. (1998). Neurosyphilis during the AIDS epidemic, San Francisco, 1985–1992. *J. Infect. Dis.*, **177**, 931–940.

Folk, J. C., Weingeist, T. A., Corbett, J. J., Lobes, L. A. and Watzke, R. C. (1983). Syphilitic neuroretinitis. *Am. J. Ophthalmol.*, **95**, 480–486.

Ford, W. T., Wiggall, R. H. and Stokes, J. H. (1951). Penicillin therapy of asymptomatic neurosyphilis. The spinal fluid cell count as a guide to therapeutic response and re-treatment. *Arch. Intern. Med.*, **88**, 235–242.

Fordyce, J. A. and Rosen, I. (1921). Laboratory findings in early and late syphilis. Review of one thousand and sixty-four cases. *J. Am. Med. Assoc.*, 77, 1696–1700.

Gabay, E. L., Hallinan, J. and Lovett, M. A. (1983). Computerized tomographic findings in meningovascular syphilis: a case report. *Sex. Transm. Dis.*, 10, 39–40.

Gentile, J. H., Viviani, C., Sparo, M. D., Arduino, R. C. (1998). Syphilitic meningomyelitis treated with ceftriaxone: case report. *Clin. Infect. Dis.*, 26, 528.

Gordon, S. M., Eaton, M. E., George, R. et al. (1994). The response of symptomatic neurosyphilis to high-dose intravenous penicillin G in patients with human immunodeficiency virus infection. *N. Engl. J. Med.*, 331, 1469–1473.

Greene, B. M., Miller, N. R. and Bynum, T. E. (1980). Failure of penicillin G benzathine in the treatment of neurosyphilis. *Arch. Intern. Med.*, 140, 1117–1118.

Hahn, R. D. (1957). Tabes dorsalis with special reference to primary optic atrophy. *Br. J. Vener. Dis.*, 33, 139–148.

Hahn, R. (1961). Some remarks on the management of neurosyphilis. *J. Chronic Dis.*, 13, 1–5.

Hahn, R. D., Cutler, J. C., Curtis, A. C. et al. (1956a). Penicillin treatment of asymptomatic central nervous system syphilis. I. Probability of progression to symptomatic neurosyphilis. *Arch. Dermatol.*, 74, 355–366.

Hahn, R. D., Cutler, J. C., Curtis, A. C. et al. (1956b). Penicillin treatment of asymptomatic central nervous system syphilis. II. Results of therapy as measured by laboratory findings. *Arch. Dermatol.*, 74, 367–377.

Hahn, R. D., Webster, B., Weickhardt, G. et al. (1959). Penicillin treatment of general paresis (dementia paralytica). *Arch. Neurol. Psych.*, 81, 557–590.

Finne, J., Leinonen, M. and Makela, P. H. (1983). Antigenic similarities between brain components and bacteria causing meningitis. Implications for vaccine development and pathogenesis. *Lancet*, 2, 355–357.

Hart, G. (1986). Syphilis tests in diagnostic and therapeutic decision making. *Ann. Intern. Med.*, 104, 368–376.

Harrigan, E. P., McLaughlin, T. J. and Feldman, R. G. (1984). Transverse myelitis due to meningovascular syphilis. *Arch. Neurol.*, 41, 337–338.

Heathfield, K. W. (1976). The decline of neurolues. *Practitioner*, 217, 753–762.

Holland, B. A., Perrett, L. V. and Mills, C. M. (1986). Meningovascular syphilis: CT and MR findings. *Radiology*, 158, 439–442.

Holmes, M. D., Brant-Zawadzki, M. M. and Simon, R. P. (1984). Clinical features of meningovascular syphilis. *Neurology*, 34, 553–556.

Hook, E. W. III, Baker-Zander, S. A., Moskovitz, B. L., Lukehart, S. A. and Handsfield, H. H. (1986). Ceftriaxone therapy for asymptomatic neurosyphilis. Case report and Western blot analysis of serum and cerebrospinal fluid IgG response to therapy. *Sex. Transm. Dis.*, 13, 185–188.

Hooshmand, H., Escobar, M. R. and Kopf, S. W. (1972). Neurosyphilis. A study of 241 patients. *J. Am. Med. Assoc.*, **219**, 726–729.

Hotson, J. R. (1981). Modern neurosyphilis: a partially treated chronic meningitis. *West. J. Med.*, **135**, 191–200.

Hughes, G. B. and Rutherford, I. (1986). Predictive value of serologic tests for syphilis in otology. *Ann. Otol. Rhinol. Laryngol.*, **95**, 250–259.

Idsoe, O., Guthe, T. and Willcox, R. R. (1972). Penicillin in the treatment of syphilis. The experience of three decades. *Bull. World. Hlth Org.*, **47**, 1–68.

Inungu, J., Morse, A. and Gordon, C. (1998). Neurosyphilis during the AIDS epidemic, New Orleans, 1990–1997 (letter). *J. Infect. Dis.*, **178**, 1229.

Izzat, N. N., Bartruff, J. K., Glicksman, J. M., Holder, W. R. and Knox, J. M. (1971). Validity of the VDRL test on cerebrospinal fluid contaminated by blood. *Br. J. Vener. Dis.*, **47**, 162–164.

Jaffe, H. W., Larsen, S. A., Peters, M., Jove, D. F., Lopez, B. and Schroeter, A. L. (1978). Tests for treponemal antibody in CSF. *Arch. Intern. Med.*, **138**, 252–255.

Joffe, R., Black, M. M. and Floyd, M. (1968). Changing clinical picture of neurosyphilis: report of seven unusual cases. *Br. Med. J.*, **1**, 211–212.

Joyce-Clarke, N. and Molteno, A. C. (1978). Modified neurosyphilis in the Cape Peninsula. *S. Afr. Med. J.*, **53**, 10–14.

Kaplan, J. G., Sterman, A. B., Horoupian, D., Leeds, N. E., Zimmerman, R. D. and Gade, R. (1981). Luetic meningitis with gumma: clinical, radiographic, and neuropathologic features. *Neurology*, **31**, 464–467.

Katz, D. A., Berger, J. R. and Duncan, R. C. (1993). Neurosyphilis. A comparative study of the effects of infection with human immunodeficiency virus (published erratum appears in *Arch. Neurol.*, 1993, 50, 614). *Arch. Neurol.*, **50**, 243–249.

Kingery, L. (1921). A study of the spinal fluid in fifty-two cases of congenital syphilis. *J. Am. Med. Assoc.*, **76**, 12–13.

Kofman, O. (1956). The changing pattern of neurosyphilis. *Can. Med. Assoc. J.*, **74**, 807–812.

Kuo, I. C., Kapusta, M. A. and Rao, N. A. (1998). Vitritis as the primary manifestation of ocular syphilis in patients with HIV infection. *Am. J. Ophthalmol.*, **125**, 306–311.

Landi, G., Villani, F. and Anzalone, N. (1990). Variable angiographic findings in patients with stroke and neurosyphilis. *Stroke*, **21**, 333–338.

Lanska, M. J., Lanska, D. J. and Schmidley, J. W. (1988). Syphilitic polyradiculopathy in an HIV-positive man. *Neurology*, **38**, 1297–1301.

Lorentzen, S. E. (1967). Syphilitic optic neuritis. A case report. *Acta. Ophthalmol.*, **45**, 769–772.

Lowenstein, D. H., Mills, C. and Simon, R. P. (1987). Acute syphilitic transverse myelitis: unusual presentation of meningovascular syphilis. *Genitourin. Med.*, **63**, 333–338.

Lowhagen, G. B., Brorson, J. E. and Kaijser, B. (1983). Penicillin concentrations in cerebrospinal fluid and serum after intramuscular, intravenous, and oral administration to syphilitic patients. *Acta Derm. Venereol.*, **63**, 53–57.

Luger, A., Schmidt, B. L., Steyrer, K. and Schonwald, E. (1981). Diagnosis of neurosyphilis by examination of the cerebrospinal fluid. *Br. J. Vener. Dis.*, **57**, 232–237.

Lukehart, S. A., Baker-Zander, S. A., Lloyd, R. M. and Sell, S. (1981). Effect of cortisone administration on host-parasite relationships in early experimental syphilis. *J. Immunol.*, **127**, 1361–1368.

Lukehart, S. A., Hook, E. W. III, Baker-Zander, S. A., Collier, A. C., Critchlow, C. W. and Handsfield, H. H. (1988). Invasion of the central nervous system by *Treponema pallidum*: implications for diagnosis and treatment. *Ann. Intern. Med.*, **109**, 855–862.

Madiedo, G., Ho, K. C. and Walsh, P. (1980). False-positive VDRL and FTA in cerebrospinal fluid. *J. Am. Med. Assoc.*, **244**, 688–689.

Malone, J. L., Wallace, M. R., Hendrick, B. B. *et al.* (1995). Syphilis and neurosyphilis in a human immunodeficiency virus type-1 seropositive population: evidence for frequent serologic relapse after therapy. *Am. J. Med.*, **99**, 55–63.

Marra, C. M., Handsfield, H. H., Kuller, L., Morton, W. R. and Lukehart, S. A. (1992). Alterations in the course of experimental syphilis associated with concurrent simian immunodeficiency virus infection. *J. Infect. Dis.*, **165**, 1020–1025.

Marra, C. M., Critchlow, C. W., Hook, E. W. III, Collier, A. C. and Lukehart, S. A. (1995). Cerebrospinal fluid treponemal antibodies in untreated early syphilis. *Arch. Neurol.*, **52**, 68–72.

Marra, C. M., Longstreth, W. T., JR, Maxwell, C. L. and Lukehart, S. A. (1996). Resolution of serum and cerebrospinal fluid abnormalities after treatment of neurosyphilis. Influence of concomitant human immunodeficiency virus infection. *Sex. Transm. Dis.*, **23**, 184–189.

Marra, C. M., Castro, C. D., Kuller, L. *et al.* (1998). Mechanisms of clearance of *Treponema pallidum* from the CSF in a nonhuman primate model. *Neurology*, **51**, 957–961.

Marra, C. M., Boutin, P., McArthur, J. C. *et al.* (1999). A pilot randomized trial evaluating ceftriaxone and penicillin G as therapies for neurosyphilis in HIV–ACTG 145. *51st Annual Meeting, American Academy of Neurology, Toronto, Canada*, April 17–24, 1999.

Marshall, D. W., Brey, R. L., Butzin, C. A., Lucey, D. R., Abbadessa, S. M. and Boswell, R. N. (1991). CSF changes in a longitudinal study of 124 neurologically normal HIV-1-infected US Air Force personnel. *J. Acquir. Immune Defic. Syndr.*, **4**, 777–781.

McGeeney, T., Yount, F., Hinthorn, D. R. and Liu, C. (1979). Utility of the FTA-Abs test of cerebrospinal fluid in the diagnosis of neurosyphilis. *Sex. Transm. Dis.*, **6**, 195–198.

McLeish, W. M., Pulido, J. S., Holland, S., Culbertson, W. W. and Winward, K. (1990). The ocular manifestations of syphilis in the human immunodeficiency virus type 1-infected host. *Ophthalmology*, **97**, 196–203.

McNulty, J. S. and Fassett, R. L. (1981). Syphilis: an otolaryngologic perspective. *Laryngoscope*, **91**, 889–905.

Mendelsohn, A. D. and Jampol, L. M. (1984). Syphilitic retinitis. A cause of necrotizing retinitis. *Retina*, **4**, 221–224.

Merritt, H. H. (1940). The early clinical and laboratory manifestations of syphilis of the central nervous system. *N. Engl. J. Med.*, **223**, 446–450.

Merritt, H. H. and Moore, M. (1935). Acute syphilitic meningitis. *Medicine (Balt.)*, **14**, 119–183.

Merritt, H. H., Adams, R. D. and Solomon, H. C. (1946). *Neurosyphilis*. New York: Oxford.

Mills, C. H. (1927). Routine examination of the cerebrospinal fluid in syphilis: its value in regard to more accurate knowledge, prognosis and treatment. *Br. Med. J.*, **2**, 527–532.

Mohr, J. A., Griffiths, W., Jackson, R., Saadah, H., Bird, P. and Riddle J. (1976). Neurosyphilis and penicillin levels in cerebrospinal fluid. *J. Am. Med. Assoc.*, **236**, 2208–2209.

Moore, J. (1922). Studies in asymptomatic neurosyphilis II. The classification, treatment, and prognosis of early asymptomatic neurosyphilis. *Bull. Johns Hopkins Hosp.*, **33**, 231–246.

Moore, J. E. (1929). The relation of neurorecurrences to late syphilis. A clinical study of eighty-one cases. *Arch. Neurol. Psych.*, **21**, 117–136.

Moore, J. E. and Gieske, M. (1931). Syphilitic iritis. A study of 249 patients. *Am. J. Ophthalmol.*, **14**, 110–126.

Muller, F. and Moskophidis, M. (1983). Estimation of the local production of antibodies to *Treponema pallidum* in the central nervous system of patients with neurosyphilis. *Br. J. Vener. Dis.*, **59**, 80–84.

Musher, D. M. (1991). Syphilis, neurosyphilis, penicillin, and AIDS. *J. Infect. Dis.*, **163**, 1201–1206.

Nichols, F. T., Heyman, A. and Pettay, J. (1949). Penicillin therapy in asymptomatic neurosyphilis. A comparison of the effects of amorphous penicillin, penicillin in oil and wax, and crystalline penicillin G. *Am. J. Syph. Gonorrhea Vener. Dis.*, **33**, 561–570.

Nitrini, R. (1989). Treating neurosyphilis (letter). *West. J. Med.*, **150**, 213.

Noguchi, H. and Moore, J. W. (1913). A demonstration of *Treponema pallidum* in the brain in cases of general paralysis. *J. Exp. Med.*, **17**, 232–238.

O'Leary, P. A., Cole, H. N., Moore, J. E. *et al.* (1937). Cooperative clinical studies in the treatment of syphilis: asymptomatic neurosyphilis. *Vener. Dis. Inf.*, **18**, 45–65.

Polnikorn, N., Witoonpanich, R., Vorachit, M., Vejjajiva, S. and Vejjajiva, A. (1980). Penicillin concentrations in cerebrospinal fluid after different treatment regimens for syphilis. *Br. J. Vener. Dis.*, **56**, 363–367.

Prange, H. W., Moskophidis, M., Schipper, H. I. and Muller, F. (1983). Relationship between neurological features and intrathecal synthesis of IgG antibodies to *Treponema pallidum* in untreated and treated human neurosyphilis. *J. Neurol.*, **230**, 241–252.

Pulec, J. L. (1997). Meniere's disease of syphilitic etiology. *Ear Nose Throat J.*, **76**, 508–510, 512 514.

Ravaut, P. (1903). Le liquide céphalo-rachidien des syphiliques en période secondaire. *Ann. Dermatol. Syphiligr.*, **4**, 537–554.

Roeske, L. C. and Kennedy, P. R. (1996). Images in clinical medicine. Syphilitic gummas in a patient with human immunodeficiency virus infection. *N. Engl. J. Med.*, **335**, 1123.

Rolfs, R. T., Joesoef, M. R., Hendershot, E. F. *et al.* (1997). A randomized trial of enhanced therapy for early syphilis in patients with and without human immunodeficiency virus infection. The Syphilis and HIV Study Group. *N. Engl. J. Med.*, **337**, 307–314.

Ronald, A. R., Silverman, M., McCutchan, J. A., Corey, L. and Handsfield, H. H. (1992). Evaluation of new anti-infective drugs for the treatment of syphilis. Infectious Diseases Society of America and the Food and Drug Administration. *Clin. Infect. Dis.*, **15** (suppl 1), S140–147.

Rush, J. A. and Ryan, E. J. (1981). Syphilitic optic perineuritis. *Am. J. Ophthalmol.*, **91**, 404–406.

Schofer, H., Imhof, M., Thoma-Greber, E. *et al.* (1996). Active syphilis in HIV infection: a multicentre retrospective survey. The German AIDS Study Group (GASG). *Genitourin. Med.*, **72**, 176–181.

Schoth, P. E. and Wolters, E. C. (1987). Penicillin concentrations in serum and CSF during high-dose intravenous treatment for neurosyphilis. *Neurology*, **37**, 1214–1216.

Shalaby, I. A, Dunn, J. P., Semba, R. D. and Jabs, D. A. (1997). Syphilitic uveitis in human immunodeficiency virus-infected patients. *Arch. Ophthalmol.*, **115**, 469–473.

Short, D. H., Knox, J. M. and Glicksman J. (1966). Neurosyphilis, the search for adequate treatment. A review and report of a study using benzathine penicillin G. *Arch. Dermatol.*, **93**, 87–91.

Silber, M. H. (1989). Syphilitic myelopathy. *Genitourin. Med.*, **65**, 338–341.

Simon, R. P. (1985). Neurosyphilis. *Arch. Neurol.*, **42**, 606–613.

Smith, C., Kamp, M., Olansky, S. and Price, E. V. (1956). Benzathine penicillin G in the treatment of syphilis. *Bull. World Hlth Org.*, **15**, 1087–1096.

Smith, M. E. and Canalis, R. F. (1989). Otologic manifestations of AIDS: the otosyphilis connection. *Laryngoscope*, **99**, 365–372.

Solomon, H. C. and Klauder, J. V. (1921). Neurosyphilis with negative spinal fluid. *J. Am. Med. Assoc.*, **77**, 1701–1706.

Standaert, D. G., Galetta, S. L. and Atlas, S. W. (1991). Meningovascular syphilis with a gumma of the midbrain. *J. Clin. Neuroophthalmol.*, **11**, 139–143.

Stepper, F., Schroth, G. and Sturzenegger, M. (1998). Neurosyphilis mimicking Miller-Fisher syndrome: a case report and MRI findings. *Neurology*, **51**, 269–271.

Strom, T. and Schneck, S. A. (1991). Syphilitic meningomyelitis. *Neurology*, **41**, 325–326.

Suarez, J. I., Mlakar, D. and Snodgrass, S. M. (1996). Cerebral syphilitic gumma in an HIV-negative patient presenting as prolonged focal motor status epilepticus (letter). *N. Engl. J. Med.*, **335**, 1159–1160.

Terry, P. M., Glancy, G. R. and Graham, A. (1989). Meningovascular syphilis of the spinal cord presenting with incomplete Brown-Sequard syndrome: case report. *Genitourin. Med.*, **65**, 189–191.

Tomberlin, M. G., Holtom, P. D., Owens, J. L. and Larsen, R. A. (1994). Evaluation of neurosyphilis in human immunodeficiency virus-infected individuals. *Clin. Infect. Dis.*, **18**, 288–294.

Toshniwal, P. (1987). Optic perineuritis with secondary syphilis. *J. Clin. Neuro. Ophthalmol.*, **7**, 6–10.

Tramont, E. C. (1976). Persistence of *Treponema pallidum* following penicillin G therapy. Report of two cases. *J. Am. Med. Assoc.*, **236**, 2206–2207.

Tseng, C. K., Hughes, M. A., Hsu, P. L., Mahoney, S., Duvic, M. and Sell, S. (1991). Syphilis superinfection activates expression of human immunodeficiency virus I in latently infected rabbits. *Am. J. Pathol.*, **138**, 1149–1164.

Turner, T. B., Hardy, P. H. and Newman, B. (1969). Infectivity tests in syphilis. *Br. J. Vener. Dis.*, **45**, 183–196.

van der Valk, P. G., Kraai, E. J., van Voorst Vader, P. C., Haaxma-Reiche, H. and Snijder, J. A. (1988). Penicillin concentrations in cerebrospinal fluid (CSF) during repository treatment regimen for syphilis. *Genitourin. Med.*, **64**, 223–225.

van Eijk, R. V., Wolters, E. C., Tutuarima, J. A. *et al.* (1987). Effect of early and late syphilis on central nervous system: cerebrospinal fluid changes and neurological deficit. *Genitourin. Med.*, **63**, 77–82.

Vatz, K. A., Scheibel, R. L., Keiffer, S. A. and Ansari, K. A. (1974). Neurosyphilis and diffuse cerebral angiopathy: a case report. *Neurology*, **24**, 472–476.

Weismann, K. (1995). Neurosyphilis, or chronic heavy metal poisoning: Karen Blixen's lifelong disease. *Sex. Transm. Dis.*, **22**, 137–144.

Wile, U. J. and Stokes, J. H. (1914). A study of the spinal fluid with reference to involvement of the nervous system in secondary syphilis. *J. Cutan. Dis.*, **32**, 607–623.

Wolters, E. C. (1987). Neurosyphilis: a changing diagnostic problem? *Eur. Neurol.*, **26**, 23–28.

Wolters, E. C., Hische, E. A., Tutuarima, J. A. *et al.* (1988). Central nervous system involvement in early and late syphilis: the problem of asymptomatic neuro-syphilis. *J. Neurol. Sci.*, **88**, 229–239.

Yoder, F. W. (1975). Penicillin treatment of neurosyphilis. Are recommended dosages sufficient? *J. Am. Med. Assoc.*, **232**, 270–271.

Zwink, F. B. and Dunlop, E. M. (1976). Clinically silent anterior uveitis in secondary syphilis. *Trans. Ophthalmol. Soc. UK*, **96**, 148–150.

13
Rabies

Thiravat Hemachudha and Erawady Mitrabhakdi

Introduction

Rabies is one of the most feared illnesses and is widely known to man. This is readily explained by its horrifying and characteristic pictures of aero- and hydrophobia and wild agitation with an almost universally fatal outcome. However, clinical symptomatology, once believed to be unique, may be variable, particularly in those cases following exposure to virus of the insectivorous or frugivorous bat rabies variants (Hemachudha and Phuapradit 1997) and, recently, in Thai cases associated with canine rabies variants. Difference in cellular tropism either at the inoculation site or in the central nervous system (CNS) or differences in the route of spread, or both, may account for these discrepancies. These may affect different sets of neurotransmitters which in turn modulate variable neurobehavioural patterns and neuroendocrine-immune cascades. In recent years, the number of cases of rabies may also have risen because of an increasing number of travellers to rabies-endemic areas and economic migrants. Physicians should be able to give proper advice in cases of both pre- and postexposure rabies prophylaxis and be able to diagnose and to differentiate rabies from other encephalitides.

History

The association of the disease with the supernatural and the dog has been known since antiquity. The earliest record perhaps appeared in the pre-Mosaic Eshnunna Code of Mesopotamia in about 2300 BC (Rosner 1974; Baer *et al.*, 1990a; Baer, 1991; Koprowski, 1996). The name *rabies* has its root from Sanskrit, *rabhas*, in the Vedic period of India (30th century BC) that refers to the god of death and his dog as a constant companion and the emissary of death. In ancient Egyptian time, the god Sirius was imagined in the form of a furious dog. The term, *rabhas* and the Greek word *Lyssa* or *Lytta* (from the root *Lud*) and *rage* (in French) mean 'to do violence or madness'. Furthermore, in this Twentieth century rabies has also been connected to the vampire legend and the death of Edgar Allan Poe (Gomej-Alonso 1998). The term 'hydrophobia' was coined by Cornelius Celsus, a Roman in the first century AD and remains a classic description to the present. The infectivity of saliva and urine of rabid dogs was suspected since the Roman times, and thus the disease was described as poisonous (*virus* in Latin). It was not until 1804 that transmission of infection by saliva was demonstrated. Burning and cupping of the wounds of those bitten by rabid dogs had been practised since the first century and continued into the nineteenth century.

Girolamo Fracastoro (born in 1478), an Italian scientist, accurately determined the incubation period of rabies in humans. Virus spreading to the CNS by a neural route was postulated in 1769 by Morgagni, based on the symptoms of paraesthesias at the bite site. Artificial infection in rabbits by direct inoculation of the virus into the nerve also suggested a neural pathway (Di Vesta and Zagari in 1889, quoted in Baer, 1991). However, it was Pasteur's ingenious experiment that for the first time in medical history demonstrated the CNS as a prime target and proved that the disease mainly affected the brainstem ('the bulb that joined the spinal cord to the brain') (Baer, 1991). He also showed that the saliva was not the only source of the virus, but that nervous tissue was also infectious, especially when inoculated beneath the dura mater. He discovered that the virulence of rabies increased with a fixed incubation period (7 days instead of several weeks) by serial subdural passage of the virus into rabbits (referred to as a 'fixed virus'). Pasteur accidentally discovered attenuated vaccine in 1880 by injecting chickens with cholera that was left in the laboratory over the long hot summer (Haas, 1998). Attenuation of rabies virus could be obtained by passing the virus from dog to monkey and then from monkey to monkey.

Pasteur launched the science of immunology and protective vaccination on 6 July 1885 when he used his recently developed rabbit spinal cord rabies vaccine in a 9 year-old Alsatian boy, Joseph Meister and a few months later in a shepherd named Jupille (Hoenig, 1986; Baer, 1991; Haas, 1998). The development of this vaccine involved over 90 serial intracerebral passages of rabies virus in rabbits, allowing fixation of the spinal cord 6–7 days after infection. With air drying, infectivity was lost. Although Pasteur's antirabies treatment saved the lives of countless victims, it carried some serious neuroparalytic adverse effects. These were documented in 1888 by Remlinger (Baer, 1991). Rivers and Schwentker started inoculating monkeys repeatedly with homogenates of normal rabbit brain, which resulted in the first induction of experimental allergic encephalomyelitis, a useful model in studying immune-mediated encephalitis and neuritis (Rivers and Schwentker, 1935). The discovery of the 'endocellular Negri bodies' was made by an Italian physician and pathologist, Adelchi Negri in 1903. Its diagnostic value was arrived at in 1913 by Negri's wife, Lina Negri-Luzzani (Kristensson et al., 1996).

Modern cell culture rabies vaccine has proved itself to be close to an ideal immunogen based on its efficacy, few doses required and a relative lack of side-effects. Human diploid cell rabies vaccine and antirabies serum produced in mules protected all but one of 45 persons who were bitten by rabid dogs and wolves in northern Iran in 1975 (Bahmanyar et al., 1976). Since then there have been safe and potent vaccines prepared in different cell cultures such as chick embryo and Vero cells and the new purified duck embryo vaccine. Due to the serious complications of brain tissue vaccine that develop in approximately one in 400 vaccinated people (Hemachudha *et al.*, 1987a, b), in 1992 the World Health Organization (WHO) recommended limiting or abandoning the production and use of encephalitogenic and neuritogenic brain tissue vaccines (WHO, 1992).

For postexposure prophylaxis in severely bitten cases, it became obvious that antirabies serum (a more potent and relatively safe purified equine and human rabies immune globulin nowadays) plus vaccine and appropriate wound care was more effective than vaccine alone. In 1954, a rabid wolf attacked 29 people in an Iranian village. Among the 17 persons treated with heterologous immune serum-inactivated brain tissue vaccine, only one died (versus three out of 12 who had vaccine alone) (Habel and Koprowski, 1955; Baer, 1991).

Epidemiology

The number of human rabies deaths world-wide is estimated by the World Health Organization survey in 1996 to be between 35 000 and 50 000 annually (WHO, 1998). The highest incidence continued to be observed in Asia with 32 772 reported deaths (estimated to be 30 000 in India). Although rabies in Africa is relatively insignificant in terms of human mortality (238 in 1996), it is becoming a growing problem (Cleaveland, 1998). The domestic dog is the principal reservoir host in these two continents and also in South America. In specific areas, other species such as the mongooses and meerkats of South Africa, the pariah dogs and jackals of South-east Asia, and the cattle and vampire bats of South America also play a significant role in epizootic transmission (Cleaveland, 1998; Johnson, 1998).

In the USA, there has been a rabies epizootic in racoons in the mid-Atlantic and north-eastern states. Wild animals, racoon (3595), skunk (1656), fox (412) and bats (741), and domestic animals, cat (266), ruminant and equine (194), dog (111) were animals frequently reported rabid in 1996 (WHO, 1998). However, transmission from bats to humans is most common. In the USA, during 1980 and 1997, bat rabies variants (brv) have been identified in 21 of 36 cases (Noah *et al.*, 1998; MMWR, 1997b, 1998). Sixteen of these 21 cases had evidence of infection with a variant found primarily in the silver-haired bat (*Lasionycteris noctivagans*) or eastern pipistrelle (*Pipistrellus subflavus*). Only one had a definite history of a bat bite. Australia, a previously rabies-free continent, became a lyssavirus-endemic area in 1996 (Fraser *et al.*, 1996; Speare *et al.*, 1997). This new variant pteropid lyssavirus or Ballina virus (for the place where the first human infection was contracted), identified in fruit bats (flying foxes – genus *Pteropus*), is closely related to the European bat lyssavirus (EBL) – 1 and classical street rabies strains. In November 1996, the first human case with lyssavirus-like illness presenting with ophthalmoplegia and progressive limb weakness was reported in Australia (Allworth *et al.*, 1996). The second case had rabies-like encephalitis after an incubation period of 2 years (Niesche, 1998).

Of major concern in rabies is not only the human mortality but also the supply and cost of postexposure prophylaxis and the cost of disease control in animal populations. These impose a severe burden to the limited health budget, especially in developing countries. Contrary to the public's perception of the disease, almost all fatal cases of rabies in Asia did not receive postexposure treatment. In Thailand, with an average annual mortality of 70 cases, there have been over 600 000 postexposure rabies treatments administered since 1992 (Wilde, 1997). Ten per cent had vaccine and rabies immune globulin (RIG). There were 13 patients who had treatment failures between 1992 and 1997 (two in 1992, five in 1993, three in 1994, three in 1997). All but two had treatment flaws or deviation from the standard WHO recommendation. The remaining two had state of the art treatment with immediate wound cleansing and no suturing and proper administration of tissue culture rabies vaccine and equine RIG (Hemachudha et al., 1999). In the Americas, approximately 50 000 individuals (versus 183 947 in Asia in 1994) received postexposure treatment (WHO, 1996a). The public response to a single rabid kitten in New Hampshire in 1994 led to a mass immunization of 665 persons and cost about $1.5 million (Noah et al., 1996) (postexposure treatment, five doses of intramuscular tissue culture vaccine and equine RIG, for an adult in Thailand costs $70). About 10 000 individuals receive rabies postexposure prophylaxis every year in the USA (Immunization practices advisory committee, 1991). The costs of rabies control in the USA alone exceeds $300 million per year. In certain areas such as Africa, there are threats of rabies spread to wildlife leading to an emergence of new maintenance hosts and risk of endangered wildlife species extinction.

The mass application of a potent single inoculation of rabies vaccine for dogs in the 1940s was an outstanding success in the control of rabies (Johnson, 1998). Legally enforced canine rabies immunization, a practice of strict quarantine, and rigid control of stray dogs have brought canine rabies under control in North America and Europe and the disease has been eliminated from some island populations such as those of New Zealand, Japan, Hawaii, and Great Britain. However, the ecological balance of rabies infection has shifted to wild or sylvian carnivorous animals in these developed areas. Recent progress has led to the development of oral and parenteral poxvirus- and adenovirus-vectored recombinant and parenteral plasmid rabies vaccines that were successful in experimental studies in animals (Rupprecht and Kieney, 1988; Lodmell et al., 1991; Campbell, 1994; Xiang et al., 1994) and in humans (Cadoz et al., 1992). Oral immunization with modified live virus or recombinant vaccinia virus expressing the glycoprotein (G) gene of rabies virus has proved to be safe and effective in field trials in foxes (Brochier et al., 1991; WHO, 1992; Pastoret et al., 1993). This is potentially applicable for use in dogs especially in canine rabies endemic areas (almost all of Asia, Latin America, and Africa) (Haddad et al., 1994). Purified virus protein from tobacco plants infected with recombinant alfalfa mosaic virus displaying rabies glyco- and nucleoproteins successfully elicited specific virus neutralizing antibodies in mice (Yusibov et al., 1997).

Pathophysiology of infection

Rabies virus is in the Lyssavirus genus (Rhabdoviridae family). Classical rabies virus, isolated from terrestrial mammals including dogs, haematophagous and insectivorous bats, belongs to the sero- and genotype 1 and is the most prevalent world-wide (Bourhy et al., 1993; Tordo, 1996; Smith and King, 1996). Genotype classification is based on differences in the viral nucleic acid and serotype classification is based on differences in viral antigens and the antibodies they produce in the host. Rabies-related viruses are classified as sero- and genotypes 2 (Lagos bat), 3 (Mokola), 4 (Duvenhage), European bat lyssavirus or EBL 1 (genotype 5) and 2 (genotype 6), isolated from *Eptesicus serotinus* and *Myotis* bats, constitute serotype 5. A pteropid lyssavirus or Ballina virus, isolated in Australia, was recently proposed to be a new genotype 7 (Fraser et al., 1996; Ban 1997) . The bullet-shaped rabies virus contains a single, non-segmented RNA molecule of 11 932 nucleotides of negative polarity (Tordo and Poch, 1988). Transcription of the genomic RNA template into complementary messenger RNA (mRNA) by RNA-dependent RNA polymerase is required before replication. Excessive accumulation of ribonucleoprotein in the cytoplasm results in the formation of Negri bodies (Gosztonyi, 1994).

Rabies is a strict neurotropic virus infection. Different species have different levels of susceptibility, latency, and infectivity. Efficient transmission depends on the degree of aggression and efficiency of bites, as well as the amount of virus in salivary excretion. Human rabies is almost always attributable to a bite exposure. A bite to the areas with abundant nerve supply alone is not the sole determinant for rabies risk. It is also the severity of the wound (transdermal bite with bleeding), particularly if deep enough to reach the muscles, at areas where muscle surfaces contain high density of nicotinic acetylcholine receptor (AchR) that determines the likelihood of developing rabies (Baer et al., 1990b; WHO, 1992). The risk of rabies after a bite (5–80%) is about 50 times the risk after scratches (0.1–1%) (Hattwick, 1974). Binding of virus glycoprotein to nicotinic AchR leads to multiplication in the muscle cells (Murphy et al., 1973; Charlton and Casey, 1979a, 1981; Charlton, 1994). The nAchR appears to be the rabies virus receptor (Lentz et al., 1982, 1984, 1985, 1986, 1987). Rabies virus binding to nAchR is inhibited by alpha-bungarotoxin and *d*-tubocurarine. Sequence homology of amino acids between rabies viral glycoprotein and snake venom curaremimetic neurotoxins has also been demonstrated.

Monoclonal antibodies to the alpha subunit of the nAchR and monoclonal antibodies against rabies virus (anti-idiotype antibodies) specifically block viral binding *in vitro* (Burrage et al., 1985; Hanham et al., 1993). Localization of virus to the muscles may lead to variable periods of delay which, in turn, provides an opportunity for host immune clearance and for postexposure treatment (Smith et al., 1991; Hemachudha et al., 1991; McColl et al., 1993). Studies in striped skunks using polymerase chain reaction (PCR) and immmunohistochemistry demonstrated the presence of rabies antigen and genome as long as 2 months post-inoculation (Charlton et al., 1997). It remains unknown which factors – virus strain and concentration, inoculation route, genetic susceptibility or a prompt but still insufficient host immune response – control the length of this period of delay (Rupprecht and Dietzschold, 1987; Hemachudha, 1989; Charlton, 1994). The role of rabies virus persistence in bone marrow cells to explain this eclipse period is still intriguing (Ray et al., 1995).

After budding from plasma membranes of the muscle cells, virus or its genome is taken up into the unmyelinated nerve ending at the neuromuscular junctions or at the muscle spindles. Rabies virus reaches the CNS by retrograde axoplasmic flow, which can be prevented experimentally in mice by neur-ectomy and colchicine and vinblastine, and then infects and replicates again in the dorsal root ganglion and anterior horn cells (Dean et al., 1963; Baer et al., 1968; Tsiang, 1979; Bijlenga and Heaney, 1980; Lycke and Tsiang, 1987; Tsiang et al., 1989, 1991). At the dorsal root ganglion, where blood–nerve barrier is relatively scant, viral replication can be recognized and attacked by immune effectors thus producing an early clinical prodrome at the site of the bite or at the bitten extremity (Yamamoto and Ohtani, 1978; Hemachudha, 1989). Motor pathway may be preferentially involved in cases following exposure to canine rabies variant (crv). Local sensory prodromes (paraesthe-sias, itching, burning), reflecting ganglioneuronitis, can be found in as many as 30% of the cases (Hemachudha and Phuapradit, 1997). Furthermore, motor nerve is in close contact to neuromuscular junction, where virus antigen accumulation has been primarily observed.

Serial electrophysiological studies of the peripheral nerve in a patient with furious rabies, who had been bitten by a rabid dog at the left wrist and had severe aching of the left arm and hand without clinical sensory or motor deficits, revealed a denervation pattern along the left C5 to C8 region and left cervical paraspinous muscle (Mitrabhakdi et al., submitted). There was a delay of 5 days until diminished sensory action potentials were evident at the same time that the pain reached its peak. By 6 day post-onset, when there was no longer any pain, there was marked suppression of sensory action potentials with loss of pinprick sensation to the elbow and loss of joint position sense of the left hand and weakness of the hand and wrist muscles. Progression of denervation to involve contralateral C5 to C8 region and cervical muscles as well as thoracic paraspinous muscles to T8 was detected at the same time. A similar discrepancy between the appearance of local sensory prodromes and abnormal electrophysiological signs of dorsal root ganglia involvement was seen in another patient with paralytic rabies who had incurred a right leg wound and presented with severe itching on the right leg (Mitrabhakdi et al., submitted). Unexpectedly, there was no denervation sign of anterior horn cell involvement but a prolonged proximal latency of lumbosacral roots. This latter patient progressed to develop paralytic rabies within the following 2 days at which time there was still no denervation pattern. All these factors indicated a difference in neural involvement and, may be, in the pathway of spread in encephalitic and paralytic rabies.

In cases of cryptic bat rabies, where definite exposure history has rarely been obtained, the epidermis and dermis rather than the muscle, may be portals of entry (Morimoto et al., 1996; Debbie and Trimarchi, 1997). Local prodromes were reported in approximately 70% of the cases, thus may be reflecting a bias towards the sensory route (Brass, 1994; Allworth *et al.*, 1996; Hemachudha and Phuapradit, 1997; Debbie and Trimarchi, 1997; Noah *et al.*, 1998; MMWR, 1997a, b, 1998). Compared to street crv, silverhaired bat rabies variant (brv) possesses a marked difference in the structure of G protein, particularly at the attachment site for the AchR. Higher infectivity and fusogenic activity in fibroblasts and epithelial cells at lower temperature are unique characteristics of this brv (Morimoto *et al.*, 1996).

Travel time from the peripheral nerve to CNS is relatively constant (at a rate of 8–20 mm/day) and depends on the proximity of the lesion to the CNS (Tsiang, 1993). A shorter incubation period of less than 7 days can be explained by direct entry of the virus into the nerve without prior replication in the muscles as demonstrated in a patient with brachial plexus injury who had been bitten by a rabid dog (Hemachudha, 1997; Hemachudha and Phuapradit, 1997). This direct entry into the nerve has been confirmed by inoculating rabies virus into the anterior chamber of the eye of the rat (Kucera *et al.*, 1985) and also in a mouse model by inoculation of the masseter or the forelimb muscles (Coulon *et al.*, 1989; Shankar *et al.*, 1991).

Although rabies usually follows bite exposure, it can be acquired via aerosol exposure from aerosolized rabies virus in caves inhabited by rabid bats (Constantine, 1967) and in laboratory accidents with infected aerosolized tissue (MMWR, 1977). Transmission of rabies is also associated with handling and skinning of infected carcasses (Tariq *et al.*, 1991; Kureishi *et al.*, 1992), exposure of the conjunctiva, oral mucous membranes, genitalia, and skin abrasions to the saliva of rabid animals (Babes, 1912; Hattwick and Gregg, 1975). A lick by a rabid animal is dangerous only if the skin is damaged (Vibulbandhitkij, 1980). Human-to-human transmission other than corneal transplantation (Hemachudha, 1989; Fishbein and Robinson, 1993) has not been well documented (Fekadu *et al.*, 1996), although there is still a potential risk to the contact of patients with rabies since secretions are frequently virus-positive (Helmick *et al.*, 1987; Noah *et al.*, 1998; Crepin *et al.*, 1998). The transplacental route has been rarely reported in humans (Sipahioglu and Alpaut, 1985), but is well recognized in cattle (Martell *et al.*, 1973). Babies born to mothers with rabies encephalitis were found to be healthy (Lumbiganon and Wasi, 1990; Thongcharoen, 1980). Rabies can also be transmitted in experimental animals through oral-nasal routes and tracheal instillation of virus (Bell and Moore, 1971; Charlton and Casey, 1979b).

Once rabies virus reaches the CNS, rapid amplification occurs in neuronal perikarya and virus disseminates via plasma membrane budding and direct cell-to-cell transmission or by trans-synaptic propagation (Iwasaki and Clark, 1975; Iwasaki *et al.*, 1975; Perl, 1975; Charlton and Casey, 1979a; Tsiang, 1993). Following stereotaxic inoculation into the striatum, rabies virus has been shown to travel by retrograde fast axonal transport (200–400 mm/day) (Gillet *et al.*, 1986). It is not known exactly which tract is preferentially involved (Charlton *et al.*, 1996). Neurons are the CNS cells selectively involved, although infection of astrocytes and glial cells in animals and humans has been reported (Tangchai *et al.*, 1970; Iwasaki and Clark, 1975;

Iwasaki *et al.*, 1975; Matsumoto, 1975; Sung *et al.*, 1976; Tirawatnpong *et al.*, 1989). Rabies virus may use carbohydrates, phospholipids, gangliosides and neural cell adhesion molecule (NCAM or CD 56) in addition to nicotinic AchR to gain entry into the cells both *in vitro* and *in vivo* (Tsiang 1988, 1993; Castellanos *et al.*, 1997; Thoulouze *et al.*, 1998). Glial cells are significantly less susceptible than neurons to rabies virus infection *in vitro* (Tsiang *et al.*, 1983; Ray *et al.*, 1997).

Early studies in rabies-infected mice demonstrated a selective vulnerability of the neuronal cells of the limbic system, especially the hippocampus, suggesting that virus localization to this area of the brain may account for the behavioural abnormalities of the disease (Johnson, 1965b). Subsequent studies in mice, however, had discrepant results, in that hippocampus contained a minimal amount or none of the rabies virus antigen in the early stage, as determined by immunohistochemical techniques (Jackson and Reimer, 1989). Studies in skunks infected with skunk street rabies virus showed that areas that contained heavy accumulations were the motor nucleus of the vagus nerve, midbrain raphe, hypoglossal, and red nuclei (Smart and Charlton, 1992). These street rabies rabies virus-infected skunks manifested as furious rabies. All of this suggests that virus localization may not solely explain limbic sympto-matology or the diversity of the clinical manifestations.

In human rabies, clinical and laboratory evidence suggests that functional changes and clinical manifestations (including mood and behaviour, motor weakness, etc.) are due to a differential response of the various CNS regions (Hemachudha 1994). Cerebral symptoms dominate the clinical picture in furious rabies and spinal cord and/or peripheral nerve symptoms in dumb rabies. Similar regional CNS rabies antigen distribution can be found in both forms (Tirawatnpong *et al.*, 1989). There is also no correlation between the site of bite and virus localization. Brainstem, thalamus, basal ganglia, and spinal cord are preferential sites of rabies viral infection in both forms of rabies. Patients who had a survival time of 7 days or less had a greater amount of antigen-positive neurons in such structures (Tirawatnpong *et al.*, 1989). Moreover, minimal or no rabies viral antigen was found in the hippocampus and neocortex. Neuromagnetic resonance imaging studies in our two recent paralytic rabies patients as well as those previously reported cases with encephalitic rabies confirmed such brainstem predilection (Roine *et al.*, 1988; Hantson *et al.*, 1993; Laothamathas *et al.*, 1997). Inflammatory reactions are usually scant, and when they exist, do not correlate with clinical manifestations and a relative preponderance of CD4 + CD45RO + was found (Iwasaki *et al.*, 1993). During the early phase of clinical rabies (within 72 h), serum cortisol levels were significantly elevated as compared to those with viral encephalitis other than rabies and others with immune-mediated encephalitis (Hema-chudha, 1994). This indicates early stimulation of limbic structures, including the hypothalamus, which may relate to the behavioural changes. None of these patients were comatose or in a state of circulatory collapse. No rabies viral antigen could be demonstrated in the hypothalamus of some of these patients studied. Involvement of the hypothalamo-pituitary-adrenal axis with adrenal hormone toxicity also resulted in wasting syndrome and lymphoid depletion in thymus, spleen, and lymph nodes in mice (Torres-Anjel and Volz, 1988; Perry *et al.*, 1990) .

The presence and amount of virus in the CNS does not appear to determine the clinical and functional severity of the disease. Access of the virus to the CNS does not necessarily lead to rapid development of symptoms and death. High titres of virus in the brain and spinal cord can be found in animals long before clinical signs appear (Baer *et al.*, 1968). Abortive rabies and recovery from clinical rabies with or without residua have been repeatedly reported in many species (Hemachudha, 1989). As many as 20% of dogs recovered from rabies after developing clinical signs (Fekadu and Baer, 1980; Fekadu, 1988). The degree of muscarinic AchR function modifications in hippocampus of rabid dogs was not dependent on the amount of virus (Dumrongphol *et al.*, 1996). Rabies virus antigen was easily demonstrated by the immunofluorescent test in the frontal area of one paralytic patient who had quadriplegia and respiratory failure requiring ventilatory support and who was euphoric but conscious and rational at the time of biopsy, which was performed 19 days after the onset of the clinical illness (Hemachudha *et al.*, 1988c). The mechanisms mediating this susceptibility/resistance are certainly complex and involve genetic, immunological, and virological factors.

Animal host and strain may not be the major determinant for clinical manifestations, although rabies after a vampire bat bite is almost always the paralytic form (Hurst and Pawan, 1931, 1932; Nehaul, 1955; Verline *et al.*, 1975). A recent outbreak of human rabies in the Peruvian jungle transmitted by vampire bats, however, presented as the furious form (Augusto *et al.*, 1992). Furthermore, the same dog that transmitted paralytic rabies to one patient also caused classical encepalitic rabies in another (Hemachudha *et al.*, 1988c). Characterization of rabies virus isolates that caused furious and dumb rabies in Thai dogs using panels of nucleoprotein (N) and glycoprotein (G)-specific monoclonal antibodies, and genetic analysis revealed an identical pattern (Smith *et al.*, 1991). However, this is still inconclusive, rabies associated with brv differs in many respects from the classic form of crv-furious and dumb rabies. Furthermore, since 1997 we are experiencing more unusual clinical presentations and unexpected sudden death in Thai crv-rabies patients. Analysis with a panel of monoclonal antibody against N protein showed that an isolate from one such patient who died suddenly while consciousness was preserved was categorized as group 4 (found in only three of 400 canine rabies isolates, Lumlertdaecha, Queen Saovabha Memorial Institute, unpublished data). Unsuccessful immunization attempts, a widely quoted predisposing factor for paralytic rabies, were found in only seven cases (personal experience of over 100 patients, approximately one third with paralysis). This has also been the case in another report (Chopra *et al.*, 1980).

Genetically resistant strains of mice demonstrated a restriction of viral replication within the CNS, which is in turn correlated with the early appearance of CNS-neutralizing antibody (Lodmell and Ewalt, 1985; Templeton *et al.*, 1986). CD8 + T cells appear to have no role in this murine resistance (Perry and Lodmell, 1991). Lymphoid depletion due to cortisol toxicity does not explain disease susceptibility since this was observed in both infected susceptible and resistant strains of mice (Perry *et al.*, 1990). Adrenalectomy to decrease the cortisol level does not alter the development of neutralizing antibody or lethality. Virulence can also be determined by strain of virus. Fixed rabies virus injures neurons more extensively than street strains (Miyamoto and Matsumoto, 1965). Apathogenic rabies virus resulted from only one amino acid substitution at position 333 of the glycoprotein during an *in vitro* selection with antiglycoprotein monoclonal antibodies (Dietzschold *et al.*, 1983; Seif *et al.*, 1985). Rate of cell-to-cell spread, number of infected neurons, and degree of cellular necrosis were much lower in the case of this apathogenic virus (Dietzschold *et al.*, 1985). An avirulent double mutant with two amino acid substitutions, lysine to asparagine in position 330 and arginine to methionine in position 333, in the ectodomain of the glycoprotein could not penetrate the nervous system, either by the motor or by sensory route and was unable to infect motoneurons *in vitro* (Coulon *et al.*, 1998).

Successful clearance of rabies virus requires cooperation of both cellular and humoral immunity. Depletion of both T and B cells potentiates infection much more seriously than either one alone (Miller *et al.*, 1978). Similarly, adoptive transfer in immunosuppressed animals with combined T and B cells soon after infection reduced mortality in more than either cell type alone (Mifune *et al.*, 1981). Nevertheless, non-complement dependent rabies virus neutralizing antibody of any isotype is an absolute requirement for clearance of an established rabies virus infection in the CNS, as demonstrated by a successful treatment of rabies virus infected rats with a virus-neutralizing monoclonal antibody and by using a knockout mice model lacking each the individual arm of immune response (Dietzschold *et al.*, 1992; Xiang *et al.*, 1995; Hooper *et al.*, 1998). However, in order to have a rapid elimination of virus from the CNS, a strong local CNS inflammatory response is required from the early stage (Hooper *et al.*, 1998).

In view of the predilective pattern of rabies virus distribution, all rabies patients (not only one-third) should manifest as dumb rabies. Rabies virus modulates the expression of the immediate-early (*egr*-1, *jun* B, c-*fos*) and late response (encoding enkephalin) genes at particular regions of the brain (Fu *et al.*, 1993; Dietzschold *et al.*, 1996). These gene products may render neurons more susceptible to viral replication. Moreover, rabies nucleocapsid inhibits the actin-bundling effect induced by dephosphosynapsin 1, a neuron-specific protein known to exert a control on the actin-based cytoskeleton (Ceccaldi *et al.*, 1997). *In vitro* and *in vivo* experiments using cultured rat prostatic adenocarcinoma (AT3) and mouse neuroblastoma cells and suckling and adult ICR mice infected with challenge virus standard strain of fixed rabies virus showed characteristic morphological features of apoptosis, evidence of oligonucleosomal DNA fragmentation, and expression of Bax protein (Jackson and Rossiter 1997, Jackson and Park, 1998; Theerasurakarn and Ubol, 1998; Ubol *et al.*, 1998). The apoptosis is a caspase dependent programme and *Bcl*-2-transfected AT3 cells were resistant to apoptosis (Jackson and Rossiter 1997; Ubol *et al.*, 1998). Apoptosis was first observed and most marked in pyramidal neurons of the hippocampus, where there was a little infection, and in neurons scattered in the neocortex in CVS-infected adult mice. More apoptosis was evident in the brains of suckling mice than in those of adult mice. Further, the presence of rabies antigen does not correlate with the appearance of apoptosis (Jackson and Rossiter, 1997; Jackson and Park, 1998). Purkinje cells expressed viral antigen, but did not show apoptosis, whereas neurons in the external granular layer of the cerebellum did not express viral antigen, but demonstrated greater apoptotic changes. These imply that rabies virus induces apoptosis *in vivo* by both direct and indirect mechanisms. Apoptosis in human rabies, who also had dual infection with human immunodeficiency virus, was first reported by Adle-Biassette *et al.* (1996) on the basis of positive terminal deoxynucleotidyl transferase-mediated dUTP-digoxigenin nick end labeling (TUNEL) method.

Apoptosis can also be induced by the cytokine-nitric oxide process via initiation of a breakdown of sphingomyelin and ceramide production, and glutamate excitotoxicity etc. (Obeid *et al.*, 1993; Hooper *et al.*, 1995; Van Dam *et al.*, 1995; Fontana *et al.*, 1996; Merrill and Murphy, 1996). Activation of brain macrophages or microglial cells enhances the expression of the transport system X_c which is essential for glutamate release. Macrophages are also a source of quinolinic acid, a molecule acting at the N-methyl-D-aspartate receptor (Schwarcz *et al.*, 1996). Increased production of interleukin (IL)-1 alpha and diminished binding sites have been found in rabies infected mouse brain particularly in the hippocampus (Haour *et al.*, 1995; Marquette *et al.*, 1996a). Study of immunoreactive IL-1 beta and tumour necrosis factor-alpha in rabies-infected rat brains showed that these proinflammatory cytokines are produced by local microglial and infiltrating macrophages (Marquette *et al.*, 1996b). These alterations did not correlate with the presence of virus particles. The levels of NO, elaborated in rabies-infected rat brains both by resident and invading cells, correlated with the disease symptoms (Hooper *et al.*, 1995).

IL-1 can modify several hippocampal functions including electrical and hypothalamo-pituitary-adrenal (HPA) axis activities, and neurotransmitter metabolism (Ceccaldi *et al.*, 1993; Bouzamondo *et al.*, 1993; Linthorst *et al.*, 1994). Clinical as well as subclinical seizures (as evidenced by abnormal paroxysmal high-amplitude sharp wave activity in electroencephalographic recordings) have been observed as early as 1 or 2 days after the onset of clinical symptoms (Hemachudha *et al.*, 1989b; Hemachudha, 1994). It is unlikely that these cortical discharges can be explained by the presence of virus in brain cortical cells at such an early period. Regional imbalance of neurotransmitters leading to neurophysiological abnormalities or remote effects from the actual site of viral replication, particularly in the brainstem, has been postulated (Tsiang, 1982, 1985; Rupprecht and Dietzschold, 1987).

Altered neurotransmitter metabolism in terms of a decrease in potassium-evoked 5-HT release in rabies virus-infected cortical synaptosomes and an increase in gamma-amino-*n*-butyric acid transport in infected primary cortical cultures has been reported (Bouzamondo *et al.*, 1993; Ladogana *et al.*, 1994). It has been shown that there are modifications in opiate and muscarinic acetylcholine and 5-HT1D receptor affinity in mouse neuroblastoma–rat glioma hybrid cells and in rabies-infected rat brains (Munzel and Koschel, 1981;

Koschel and Munzel, 1984; Ceccaldi *et al.*, 1993). Recent studies in rabies virus-infected dog brains during its early stage showed that muscarinic AchR binding was impaired only in the hippocampus and brainstem regions (Dumrongphol *et al.*, 1996). There was no correlation between the virus distribution or amount and the degree of functional change. It is not clear whether alterations of certain neurotransmitter metabolism and receptor function are responsible for clinical diversity and whether amygdala, another region engaging in processing emotional salience of faces with specific response to fearful expressions, is also involved (Morris *et al.*, 1996). Altered electrical activities and sleep pattern changes have been demonstrated in chronically implanted mice and cats infected with street and fixed rabies virus (Gourmelon *et al.*, 1986, 1991; Tsiang, 1988). Brain IL-1 may alter serotonin metabolism which, in turn, affects the Ach system and desensitize mAchR. Clinical pictures of the patients with serotonin syndrome were remarkably similar to those in patients with furious rabies (Bodner *et al.*, 1995).

Accumulating data suggest that cellular immune responses play an important role in modifying the clinical manifestations and survival period (Hemachudha *et al.*, 1988c, 1993; Sugamata *et al.*, 1992; Weiland *et al.*, 1992; Hemachudha, 1994; Ceccaldi *et al.*, 1996). Patients with intact T-cell immunity to rabies virus with elevated levels of serum IL-2 receptor and IL-6 die faster and manifest as furious rabies, whereas those lacking such responses survive longer and clinically appear as dumb rabies (Hemachudha *et al.*, 1988c, 1993; Hemachudha, 1994). It should be noted that rabies-infected humans and mice with intact T-cell response have a similar rapid clinical course but differ in clinical expression (encephalitis in man and paralysis in mice). Nucleocapsid of rabies virus is a V beta 8-specific exogenous superantigen that also has adjuvant properties in humans (Lafon *et al.*, 1992, 1994; Astoul *et al.*, 1996). Nucleocapsid superantigen stimulates T helper 2 rather than T helper 1 lymphocytes and promotes cognate T–B-cell interaction, mediated by the superantigen bridge (Martinez-Arends *et al.*, 1995). Although nucleocapsid superantigen has been proposed to be the factor responsible for the immune accelerated death in furious rabies, immune profiles in furious rabies including levels of IL-2 receptor and IL-6 were similar to those of non-rabies and immune encephalitis (Hemachudha *et al.*, 1993; Hemachudha 1994). However, the antibody to rabies virus in furious rabies occurs earlier. Nevertheless, only 25% of rabies patients of both types develop the antibody (Hemachudha *et al.*, 1988c; Kasempimolporn *et al.*, 1991; Hemachudha, 1994). Defective N protein recognition has also been found in rabies patients (Kasempimolporn *et al.*, 1991). Moreover, natural killer (NK) cells in rabies patients were found to be defective (Panpanich *et al.*, 1992). NK cells eliminate cells that have lost major histocompatibility complex (MHC) class I surface expression. It is not known whether this defect of the NK cell response is caused by an up-regulation of MHC class I antigens or whether the virus can alter a peptide-specific NK recognition site of MHC molecules, causing cross-linking of NK inhibitory receptors 1 and 2 of p58 or 3 of p 70-NKB 1 family (Brutkiewicz and Welsh, 1995; Pazmany *et al.*, 1996). Additionally, cytotoxic T-cell response and antigen-specific cell-mediated response are also suppressed in rabies virus infected animals (Perrin *et al.*, 1996), arguing against an up-regulation of MHC class I molecules for NK defects.

Although *in vitro* experiments showed that attenuated rabies virus strains can infect lymphocytes and causes apoptosis (Thoulouze *et al.*, 1997), there is no viraemia in rabies and no circulating mononuclear cells are infected. Systemic immune dysfunctions may be affected by manipulation of the neuroendocrine control at the level of the HPA axis during the course of rabies infection (Reichlin, 1993; Ader *et al.*, 1995; McCann, 1998). IL-1 in the brain has been shown to suppress T and NK cell responses by stimulating cortisol production and by its corticotropin-releasing factor (Superstein *et al.*, 1992). Serum cortisol levels are elevated during the early stage in rabies patients, reflecting that HPA axis is intensely stimulated at the beginning (Hemachudha, 1994). However, cortisols are not responsible for peripheral immunosuppression in dumb rabies because levels were comparable among patients with dumb and furious types (Hemachudha 1997). Several neuropeptides and hormones may also be released from the neural axis during infection and can exert either inhibitory or stimulatory effects on activation, proliferation, migration, and secretions of various cell types including T, B and NK cells and macrophages (Berczi and Szentivanyi, 1996; Dunn, 1996; Weigent and Blalock, 1996). Neural regulation of immune function is also possible through the sympathetic nervous system. Thymus, spleen, and lymph nodes are richly supplied by autonomic nerve fibres. The secretions of some of them can be regulated by catecholamines released at the autonomic nerve endings and from the adrenal medulla and by pituitary hormones.

Taking these data together, paralysis in dumb rabies and in the late stage of furious rabies may result from the direct interaction between rabies virus and infected neuron in the brainstem and spinal cord by involvement of the cellular gene products and the process of apoptosis. The latter is triggered by either the direct process of virus replication or by cytokine-nitric oxide generated by local as well as migrating or invading macrophages. Rabies virus in dumb rabies may remain dormant in the CNS for a certain period. An unknown triggering event in the infected neuron, which may or may not parallel the amount of the virus, initiates the process of neuronal dysfunction. The HPA axis, sympathetic nervous system and neuropeptides are affected both in furious and in dumb forms of rabies, but to varying degrees. Diminished NK cell activity and inefficient rabies antibody production are demonstrated in both forms. However, cellular immunity is significantly suppressed in dumb rabies, attenuating the cytokine-NO damaging process. In furious rabies with accelerated death, brain dysfunctions dominate the picture. These patients would escape HPA-axis induced immune paralysis, the result of intact cellular immunity then exaggerates the cytokine-NO process and apoptosis and, simultaneously, dysregulating hippocampal functions and neurotransmitters, particularly serotonin and acetylcholine. During the preterminal phase, paralysis may then be evident.

The nature of weakness in paralytic rabies has still not been resolved. Although spinal cord motoneurons are likely to be responsible, it is not known whether motoneurons or peripheral nerve play a role from the beginning. Detailed studies of peripheral and cranial nerves showed axonal degeneration and intense demyelination (Tangchai and Vejjajjiva, 1971; Chopra et al., 1980; Minguetti et al., 1997). Deposition of IgG and complement on rabies virus positive axons in a Chinese paralytic rabies patient has been demonstrated (Sheikh et al., 1998a). Viral protein and Wallerian-like degeneration were more abundant in the ventral than the dorsal nerve roots. Periaxonal and intra-axonal macrophages were present in the roots. These suggest antibody-mediated complement dependent attack against viral particles in the axons. Our recent electrophysiological studies in three dumb rabies patients confirmed that peripheral nerve roots were the prime target but signs of anterior horn cell and peripheral nerve abnormalities were both found at the pre-terminal stage (Mitrabhakdi et al., submitted). The examination was performed serially from the early stage in one and only once during the pre-terminal stage in the other two cases. Since cerebrospinal fluid rabies antibody was absent in these three cases, as in the others previously reported (Hemachudha, 1994), or may appear only at the very late stage (Noah et al., 1998), it is unclear whether this is the result of a bystander effect from an immune attack against the virus in the axon or a pure autoimmune phenomenon. Two encephalitic and two paralytic rabies patients had a proliferation response to myelin basic protein and had a more rapidly fatal disease than the non-reactive patients (Hemachudha et al., 1988c). Molecular mimicry between Campylobacter jejuni polysaccharides and gangliosides, GM1 and GD1a, has been found in GBS patients (Sheikh et al., 1998b).

Centrifugal spread from the CNS along the neural pathways to heart and skin and to other peripheral organs, especially salivary glands and serous glands of the tongue (Li et al., 1995), is an important component of a complete rabies cycle. Salivary excretion of virus can be detected up to 14 days before the development of clinical disease in dogs (Fekadu, 1988). Intermittent secretion of rabies virus also occurs in asymptomatic dogs and dogs that have recovered from clinical rabies (Aghomo and Rupprecht, 1990) and also in rabies patients (Crepin et al., 1998). Peripheral tissues, such as the nape of the neck and cornea, can serve as diagnostic materials (Bryceson et al., 1975; Warrell et al., 1988). Since all neural and non-neural organs, except blood, are involved in the terminal phase, the organs of patients with an unexplained neurological disease should not be used for transplantation (WHO, 1992). Six cases of rabies have been reported from transplantation of cornea from donors who died of undiagnosed rabies (Hemachudha, 1989; Fishbein and Robinson, 1993).

Clinical features

Not every rabid animal bite necessarily results in clinical rabies. Rabies mortality varies from 35 to 57% in unvaccinated bite victims (Sitthi-Amorn et al., 1987; Hemachudha, 1989). The risk of developing rabies depends on both the severity of the wound, regardless of the number, and site of the exposure, and the virus content of the saliva. Transdermal bites (especially with bleeding) at the head, face, neck and hand carry the highest risk and are usually associated with a shorter incubation period; nevertheless, a bite on the leg or foot must be treated with the same urgency as bites elsewhere. In the case of rabid bats, the risk can be high even from a scratch because of the unique property of this rabies variant that can replicate effectively in non-neural cells, such as fibroblast and epithelial cells (Morimoto *et al.*, 1996). Other non-bite exposures include the inhalation of aerosolized rabies virus, corneal transplant, handling and skinning of infected carcasses, and contamination of an open wound, scratch, abrasion or mucous membrane by infected saliva or neural tissue.

Clinical features of rabies can be classified as classical and non-classical forms. The classical encephalitic (furious) and paralytic (dumb) rabies is almost always associated with canine rabies variant (crv) of genotype 1. The non-classical rabies can be found in rabies patients after exposure to virus of insectivorous or frugivorous-bat origin (genotypes 1, 5, 6 or 7) and, recently, in Thai crv-rabies patients. These atypical clinical presentations were also seen in rabies survivors.

In classical forms, once infection occurs, the clinical features can be divided into five stages, the incubation period, the prodrome, the acute neurological phase, coma, and death or recovery.

Incubation period

The incubation period for rabies is the most variable of all acute CNS infections. It is usually 1–2 months but may range from less than 7 days to 6 years (Hemachudha, 1989; Hemachudha *et al.*, 1988c,1991; Kasempimolporn *et al.*, 1991; Smith *et al.*, 1991; Panpanich *et al.*, 1992; McColl *et al.*, 1993). The cases with unusually long incubation periods (11 months, 4 and 6 years) were migrants who came to the USA from Laos, the Philippines, and Mexico (Smith *et al.*, 1991). Isolates obtained from these cases were antigenically and genetically identical to those from the countries of origin. However, most cases with reported incubations periods exceeding one year may have been due to unrecognized or trivial exposure to bats or other animals. This is particularly true in rabies endemic areas where frequent exposures are common. On the other hand, there may be no history of a bite (6% of 707 cases in Thailand between 1979 and 1985). There may have been an insignificant exposure, or exposure may have occurred so long before the onset of symptoms that it was not recognized by the patient.

Prodrome

The initial symptoms of rabies indicate the presence of virus in the CNS and dorsal root ganglion or autonomic nervous system. Except for the local symptoms at the site of the bite or a bitten extremity, these are usually vague and non-diagnostic in the form of fever, generalized muscular aching, and gastrointestinal symptoms. However, this 'local prodrome', which may present as itching, paraesthesias, tingling, burning sensations, piloerection, has to be interpreted with caution. Only an intense and progressive local reaction that starts at the wound and then gradually spreads to involve the whole limb in a non-radicular pattern or the ipsilateral side of the face is a reliable indicator of rabies (Hemachudha, 1989, 1994). Sensory function is usually intact. There is no demonstrable weakness of the bitten extremity. Rarely, these symptoms may occur distant to the site of the bite, for instance, two patients had a bite on the toes but developed severe itching in their ears as a prodrome. One of them tore his eardrum with a pencil trying to relieve these symptoms (Hemachudha, 1994). Local symptoms are equally common in patients with encephalitic and paralytic rabies and may be seen in as many as 16–80% of the cases (30% in author s experience) (Johnson, 1965a; Tangchai *et al.*, 1970; Wilson *et al.*, 1975; Kaplan *et al.*, 1986).

Acute neurological phase

Within hours or a few days after the prodrome, rabies patients enter an acute neurological phase. Two-thirds of patients suffer from an encephalitic or furious form, and the remaining present with paralysis or a condition resembling Guillain-Barré syndrome (GBS) (Hemachudha, 1989, 1994). Furious rabies patients generally die within 7 days (average 5 days) after the clinical onset, although survival may be as long as 2–3 weeks. The average length of survival is 13 days in paralytic cases. The terms encephalitic and paralysis are used to emphasize that the symptoms and signs are indicative of cerebral involvement in the former and of spinal cord and/or peripheral nerve involvement in the latter. However, deranged mental state, as seen in the case of furious rabies, may be evident in paralytic rabies, but to a much lesser degree.

Encephalitic (furious) rabies

The earliest neurological feature is hyperactivity, which may resemble an intense anxiety reaction or nervousness that can be aggravated by internal (thirst or fear, etc.) or external (bright light, loud noise, etc.) stimuli. Fever is a rather constant finding which may appear during the prodromal phase. Initially, mentation is preserved but attention span is shortened. This is followed within hours by the typical furious rabies features. There are three major cardinal signs of furious rabies.

Fluctuating consciousness. The mental status alternates between periods of progressively more severe agitation and periods of relative normality and depression. The patient abruptly becomes confused and disorientated without any warning. This bizarre behaviour usully lasts only for minutes and then abates. The patient then becomes lucid and may not recall events. As the disease progresses, confusion becomes severe and may evolve to wild agitation and aggressiveness. Between these episodes of agitation, the patient is drowsy but arousable. The period of irritability is gradually succeeded by impaired consciousness and coma.

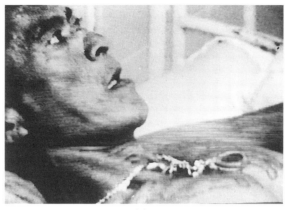

(a)

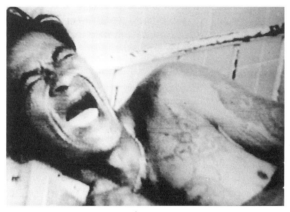

(b)

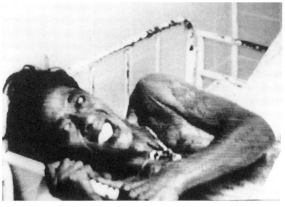

(c)

Figure 13.2 Phobic spasms in a furious rabies patient. The reactions consist of con-traction of accessory respiratory muscles and diaphragm along with a sudden increased arousal state (a). In some cases, these may be accompanied by a fearful facial expression (b) and subsequently followed by feeling of dyspnoea (c).

Phobic spasms and inspiratory spasms. Aero- and hydrophobia occur in all patients with furious rabies; however, phobic spasms may not present throughout all stages of the disease, especially once drowsiness and coma supervene. Aero- and hydrophobia can be demonstrated by blowing or fanning air on the face or chest wall of the patient and by encouraging the patient to swallow or merely offering a cup of water. This startle reaction results from spasms of the accessory respiratory muscles of the neck and diaphragm, followed by neck flexion or extension and ended with a feeling of dyspnoea. Opisthotonos is extremely rare. During these induced spasms, the patients are extremely aroused and may exhibit fearful facial expressions. Pharyngeal spasms may not necessarily be present, however, when they do exist, they may force these patients to spit their saliva, which may also be overproduced. This creates another characteristic horrible image of rabies. The first attack of hydrophobia may appear suddenly without prior experience of swallowing difficulties or pain during swallowing, arguing against a postulated conditioned reflex. One patient had his first experience of hydrophobia while taking a bath. Sensation of the soft palate and posterior pharyngeal wall remains intact but a hyperactive gag reflex is a constant finding. Intermittent inspiratory spasms, which occur spontaneously every few minutes without inducing stimuli, replace the phobic spasms once the patients lapse into coma. These inspiratory spasms actually may appear in the early stage but escape notice due to their non-intense character in the beginning and a relatively infrequent occurrence.

Signs of autonomic dysfunction. Hypersalivation is a unique feature, which persists to the pre-terminal phase. Production of 1–1.5 l of saliva in 24 h is not due to swallowing difficulties. During the confusional-agitation state, pupillary abnormalities such as fixed, dilated or constricted pupils, anisocoria, localized (at the bitten limb) or generalized piloerection, neurogenic pulmonary edema, excessive sweating, priapism as well as repeated and spontaneous ejaculations are occasionally observed.

In classic forms of furious rabies, there are usually no detectable cranial nerve deficits. Hemitract signs, such as hemiparesis or hemisensory loss, are not usually evident. Seizures are rare in furious or dumb rabies, but may occasionally be seen in fully developed rabies or during the pre-terminal phase. However, an abnormal EEG with a paroxysmal pattern of spike and wave activity with no clinical signs of seizures may be seen as early as 1–2 days after the clinical onset of disease.

Paralytic (dumb) rabies

This form of rabies is less readily diagnosed than the encephalitic form because of its lack or a lesser degree of aggression and relative sparing of consciousness. The major cardinal signs in furious rabies, described above, appear late and may be only mild in paralytic rabies. Phobic spasms occur in only one-half of the patients; however, inspiratory spasms occur in all cases during the pre-terminal phase. Weakness usually starts in the bitten extremity and then progressively involves all limbs and pharyngeal and respiratory muscles.

Bifacial paresis is as common as in sporadic GBS. In case of facial bites, weakness may initially involve facial and oculomotor muscles of the same side; however, no correlation has been found between the development of paralytic rabies and the site of the bite (Tirawatnpong *et al.*, 1989). On rare occasions, presentation as an ascending myelitis with fasciculations and loss of joint position sense, as well as pinprick sensation to the thoracic level, had been observed (Phuapradit *et al.*, 1985).

The following may be useful in differentiating paralytic rabies from sporadic cases of GBS (Hemachudha, 1989, 1994):

1   Fever is usually seen in most cases and can be found in both forms of rabies. Fever tends to be more severe as the disease progresses. Fever is absent in GBS patients once weakness develops, unless there are complications such as aspiration pneumonia.
2   Sensory function is intact in all modalities (pinprick, vibration, and joint position) in paralytic rabies patients. Except for paraesthesias at the site of the bite or in the bitten extremity, none of our rabies patients have had tingling sensations or numbness along distal extremities, as occurs in GBS cases.
3   Quadriparesis with predominant involvement of proximal muscles, loss of deep tendon reflexes, and urinary incontinence are almost always found in the early course of paralytic rabies. Urinary incontinence is unusual in GBS, especially during the early phase. Furthermore, proximal or distal muscles can be predominantly involved in equal proportion in GBS.
4   Percussion myoedema is seen from the prodrome to the pre-terminal stage in paralytic rabies. This is best elicited by percussion of the chest, deltoid, and thigh regions with a tendon hammer, and consists of mounding of a part of the muscle at the percussion site, which then flattens and disappears over a few seconds (Hemachudha, *et al.*, 1987c). It is not seen in patients with sporadic GBS, encephalitic rabies, or in those who have neurological complications from rabies vaccination of nervous tissue origin. The myoedema sign can be seen in an extreme cachectic condition, hyponatraemia, hypothyroidism, and renal failure. Myoedema during the late stage in rabies patients may be partly explained by severe hyponatraemia from the syndrome of inappropriate secretion of antidiuretic hormone.

Clinical manifestations in rabies patients after exposure to virus of insectivorous or frugivorous-bat origin (genotypes 1, 5, 6, or 7) differ in many respects from the classic forms of crv-furious and dumb rabies. Local prodromes were reported in 25 out of 40 brv-rabies patients documented between 1951 and 1997 (Brass, 1994; Allworth *et al.*, 1996; MMWR, 1996a, b, 1997a, b, 1998; Noah *et al.*, 1998). One patient had radicular pain along C8 to T2 accompanied by an inability to perform fine movements and by chorea. Two patients had objective sensory loss in one arm and the face on the same side. Ataxia was demonstrated in at least five patients and vertigo or dizziness in two patients.

During the acute neurological phase, unexpected focal neurological signs are found, weakness of the bitten extremity was recorded in eight brv-patients.

None progressed to develop dumb rabies. One had nerve conduction abnormalities of the weak limb. Myoclonus was found in six patients: generalized in two, confined to both arms in one, left arm in one, left leg and trunk in one and to both legs in the other. Segmental myoclonus progressed to a generalized pattern in two of them. Hemiparesis was demonstrated in two patients. Of these, hemisensory loss with Horner's syndrome was observed in one and asymmetry of deep tendon reflexes was observed in the other. Nine patients might have had involvement of the brainstem or cranial nerves. They presented with one or more of the following: anisocoria, bilateral ptosis, diplopia, nystagmus, pinpoint pupils, intermittent facial nerve palsy and tremor, paralysis of extraocular muscles, unilateral vocal cord paralysis. On postmortem study, one of them was found to have extensive demyelination.

Convulsive and non-convulsive seizures were found in eight patients who remained alert and coherent. One presented with status epilepticus. In Australia, the 1996 brv-patient had pain and numbness in her left arm and later developed dizziness, diplopia, complete ophthalmoplegia and progressive weakness of all limbs (Allworth et al., 1996). The most recent case (1998) had paresthaesia and rabies like encephalitis (Niesche, 1998). In the USA, where half of the cases (17 of 32 between 1980 and 1996) were associated with variants found in insectivorous bats (12 of 17 associated with silver-haired bat-Lasionycteric noctivagans or eastern pipistrelle-Pipistrellus subflavus), hydro- and aerophobia were found only in 50% of the cases (Noah et al., 1998). Phobic spasms were not described in four brv-rabies patients during 1997 (MMWR, 1997b, 1998).

In crv-rabies, weakness of the bitten extremity was observed only in patients who subsequently developed dumb rabies. Myoclonus, tremor, oculomotor abnormalities and cerebellar deficit signs were not observed. Neither hemisensory loss nor hemiparesis was observed in crv-patients. Horner's syndrome and loss of sweat on the right side of the face and trunk was seen in one crv-patient. Seizures of the non-convulsive type during early neurological phase were seen in one patient (Hemachudha et al., 1989b). Hallucinations were commonly reported in brv-patients. These were seen in only one crv-patient.

Since 1997 (April 1997 to November 1998), unusual manifestations have been increasingly seen in Thai crv-patients. Of 13 patients, five had atypical clinical features. One patient manifested with ocular myoclonus and hemichorea. The other patient had spontaneous repeated ejaculations with pleasure and did not exhibit cardinal signs of rabies until the pre-terminal phase. One paralytic rabies boy still had preserved deep tendon reflexes of all limbs until coma. The other patient with a 2-month history of dog bite to the left wrist, presenting with severe pain in his left arm and later exhibiting loss of pinprick and joint position sense and weakness of left hand, had only nocturnal agitation. He remained calm and rational during the day. There were no phobic spasms, autonomic stimulation signs nor difficulty swallowing. Monoclonal antibody analysis implicated a variant not commonly found in Thai rabid dogs (three of 400). Another patient with a severe itching at his right leg as a prodrome subsequently developed paralysis of both legs, facial and bulbar musculatures with sparing of both upper extremities. Loss of deep tendon reflexes were confined to the legs. Three of these 13 patients who remained fully awake or still arousable had sudden unexpected death.

Coma

It is extremely difficult to diagnose rabies at this stage. The two forms of rabies are indistinguishable once the patients become comatose. Inspiratory spasms are the only helpful sign in diagnosis. Special attention is required to observe the spasms in comatose paralytic rabies patients due to the generalized paralysis. In dumb rabies, alveolar hypoventilation and ventilatory failure develop before the patient becomes obtunded. In encephalitic rabies, abnormal breathing patterns and depression of consciousness appear simultaneously. Regular breathing, interspersed with inspiratory spasms, is replaced by tachypnoea and then by apneustic respiration and terminally by ataxic breathing. In paralytic rabies, these patterns are not observed. At the beginning, sinus tachycardia, disproportionate to the fever, are evident in most cases although hydration is adequate. Holter monitoring revealed evidence of a depressed R-R variability (Sunsaneevitayakul, unpublished data).These are soon followed by increasingly severe sinus bradycardia or a nodal rhythm before death. Frequently, during the pre-terminal phase, there are arrhythmias of supraventricular origin, in the form of paroxysmal atrial tachycardia and a wandering atrial pacemaker and premature ventricular ectopic beats. Prior to or at the time of hypotension, reduced ejection fraction is almost always observed by echocardiographic evaluation. Both viral involvement at the sinus or atrioventricular node and myocarditis are likely to be underlying mechanisms based on post-mortem findings and the presence of viral antigen in heart muscles (Warrell, 1976; Metze and Feiden, 1991), as well as failure to restore blood pressure with various inotropic drugs and a pacing device (Hemachudha, 1994). Coma almost always precedes circulatory insufficiency which is the prime cause of death. Aggressive attempts to save rabies patients must begin before hypotension develops. Arrhythmias may explain sudden death in our three fully alert rabies patients. Haematemesis is seen in 30–60% of patients 6–12 h before death (Kureishi et al., 1992).

Recovery

In the world literature, four patients with rabies have been reported to survive. None of them had phobic spasms or other cardinal features of rabies and all demonstrated 'usual' features of viral encephalitis. They were all regarded as atypical rabies cases. The first patient, with a bat bite (1972), had unsteady gait, dysarthria and hemiparesis (Hattwick et al., 1972). The second case (1976), following a dog bite with severe exposure, had quadriparesis, generalized myoclonus at the early stage and later developed signs of cerebellar (ataxia, dysmetria and dysdiadokokinesia) and frontal lobe dysfunctions, and bibrachial weakness (Porras et al., 1976). The third case (MMWR, 1977) had an unusual exposure to highly concentrated attenuated virus. Diagnosis of the first three patients was based on very high rabies antibody concentrations in the blood and CSF in serial observations, without definite evidence of intrathecal antibody synthesis or demonstration of viral antigen. Antibody concentrations were considered to be too high to be due to vaccine but may also occur in cases with allergic encephalitis from nervous tissue vaccine (Hemachudha et al., 1989a). The fourth case (1994) was bitten by a rabid dog with severe exposure (Lucia Alvarez et al., 1994). This case had high rabies antibody titres in both serum and CSF and a positive oligoclonal band. A recent case (case five, 1995) in Mexico, a 9-year-old boy, had severe exposure from dog bite (Baer GM, personal communication). He survived but sustained sequelae of spastic quadriparesis and dysphagia 14 weeks after the onset. All survivors were exposed to a heavy dose of the rabies virus. The first patient was bitten by a bat on the left thumb with two bleeding puncture wounds and received post-exposure prophylaxis with duck embryo rabies vaccine 4 days after the incident. The second patient had 10 days delay in postexposure treatment with suckling mouse brain vaccine. The third patient was preimmunized. The fourth and fifth patients had immediate treatment with Vero-cell vaccine, but with no rabies immune globulin. Also, in 1995, a 22-year-old Mexican crv-rabies patient was reported to survive up to 6 weeks (Guinto et al., 1995). These examples imply that once the classical path of rabies pathogenesis has been deviated, either by certain type of variant, inoculation dosage or rapidity and type of treatment, the clinical outcome can, in some cases to a certain extent, be manipulated.

Laboratory findings

Routine laboratory examination is non-diagnostic. Complete blood count is usually normal or shows mild leukocytosis with neutrophilia. Hyponatraemia is present in approximately one-third of the patients regardless of the clinical type or stage of the disease (Hemachudha, 1989). This can be explained by an inadequate intake from dysphagia and hydrophobia or inappropriate anti-diuretic hormone secretion. Hypernatraemia with polyuria has also been described but rarely occurred (Bhatt et al., 1974; Cohen et al., 1976). CSF examination reveals a normal finding in most of the cases. However, a CSF profile of mild pleocytosis (less than 30 cells/dl) with lymphocytic predomi-nance and slightly elevated protein level (less than 100 mg/dl) has been occasionally found. A pleocytosis of over 100 cells/dl (110–950) is rare.

An 8 h video-electroencephalographic (EEG) recording on a 24-year-old furious rabies patient (October, 1998) showed a well developed, low to medium amplitude, posteriorly dominant, 8–10 Hz irregular background alpha activity. Intermittent occurrence of low to medium amplitude, 2–5 Hz mixed delta activity, over the left and right temporal areas was noted as the patient became more confused. One and a half hours prior to death when the patient was obtunded, the background exhibited increasing runs of medium to high amplitude, diffusely distributed, 2–5 Hz mixed delta-theta activity.

Approximately 6 minutes prior to death, a burst suppression pattern appeared which was then followed by an electrocerebral silence (Viranuvatti, unpublished). At this stage with an EEG pattern mimicking brain death, it has been found that latencies of visual and brainstem auditory evoked potentials were within normal limit (Hantson *et al.*, 1993).

The electromyographic (EMG) pattern correlated with stages and forms of the disease (Mitrabhakdi *et al.*, submitted). Diminished sensory action potentials were found in the affected limb regardless of the clinical types at the time when the patients had a local prodrome. In furious rabies, acute denervation potentials indicative of anterior horn cell damage of the affected limb segments were found earlier and progressed diffusely to contralateral limb and rostral and caudally along the spinal cord. This was found very late in dumb rabies. F and H reflexes were markedly prolonged or absent early in the course in dumb rabies. These were subsequently followed by other demyelinating features as can be found in GBS. During the pre-terminal stage, EMG patterns were indistinguishable between nerve and anterior horn cell damage.

Computerized tomographic (CT) studies of the brain are usually unrevealing in both plain and contrast enhancement techniques (Houff *et al.*, 1979; personal experience). Rarely, multiple bilateral areas of decreased density involving both grey and white matter can be found (Newton *et al.*, 1977). Magnetic resonance imaging (MRI) in our two recent paralytic rabies patients showed gadolinium-enhancing lesions mainly in the brainstem, thalamus, hypothalamus, and grey matter of cervical spinal cord and roots (Laothamatas *et al.*, 1997) (Figure 13.1). Such brainstem and thalamus and basal ganglia abnormalities in MRI have been described in arboviral encephalitides, such as eastern equine and japanese encephalitis (Dereswicz *et al.*, 1997; Kumar *et al.*, 1997). Absence of oedema, haemorrhages, negative CT findings, and preferential involvement of brainstem can reliably differentiate rabies from other arboviral encephalitis. It has also been previously shown that the brainstem was abnormal by non-contrast MRI in two encephalitic and paralytic cases associated with brv- and crv (Roine *et al.*, 1988; Hantson *et al.*, 1993).

Differential diagnosis of furious rabies

Acute hepatic porphyria with neuropsychiatric disturbances, such as psychosis, seizures, signs of autonomic dysfunction, and involvement of the peripheral nervous system, can be confused with rabies. Fluctuating consciousness is observed in both conditions, but phobic and inspiratory spasms are seen only in rabies. A family history of the disease, ingestion of porphyrinogenic agents, abdominal pain, and dark urine colour with elevated delta-aminolevulinic acid and porphobilinogen, aid the diagnosis.

Other disease conditions mimicking rabies during the acute neurological phase include intoxication by a variety of substances, such as atropine-like

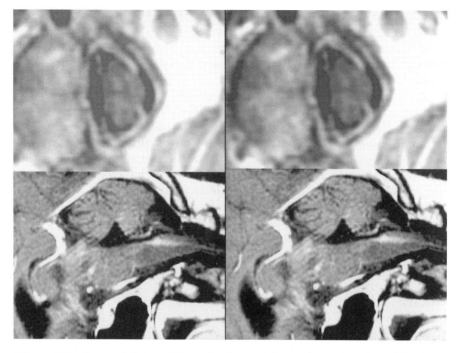

Figure 13.1   Post-gadolinium T1-weighted magnetic resonance imaging of the brain and cervical cord in paralytic rabies patients (Laothamatas *et al.*, 1997) (Reproduced with permission).

compounds, cannabis, alcohol withdrawal (delirium tremens) and tetanus. Acute serotonin syndrome in the form of encephalopathy or seizures recently described in individuals who had side effects from taking serotonin reuptake inhibitors (Bodner *et al.*, 1995) can be misdiagnosed as rabies, but may be reliably excluded by the absence of other cardinal signs of rabies. Tetanus resembles rabies only in the form of reflex spasms (Srikiatkachorn and Hemachudha, 1998). All tetanus patients have a clear sensorium. Rabies patients do not have persistent rigidity or sustained contraction of axial musculature such as the jaw, neck, back, and abdomen, as seen in tetanus. Spasms in rabies predominantly involve accessory respiratory muscles and diaphragm, whereas in tetanus, spasms occur in muscles of axial structures. Opisthotonos is far more frequent in tetanus than in rabies.

In some parts of the world where nervous tissue (sheep, monkey, and mouse brain) rabies vaccine is still widely used, allergic encephalomyelitis must be considered in the differential diagnosis. These 'accidental' complications develop in approximately one in 400 vaccinees and appear between 6 and 14 days after the first injection in over 75% of affected individuals (Hemachudha *et al.*, 1987a, b). Delayed onset and a picture of chronic progressive encephalitis have also been observed (Hemachudha *et al.*, 1988b). Neither phobic spasms, paraesthesias at bite sites, nor fluctuating consciousness are present in these post-vaccination reactions.

Differential diagnosis of paralytic rabies

Acute motor axonal neuropathy (AMAN), an axonal form of GBS, shares many similar clinical features to paralytic rabies (McKhann *et al.*, 1993; Hafer-Macko *et al.*, 1996). AMAN following *Campylobacter jejuni* infection may have preceding diarrhoea which may be mistakenly diagnosed as prodromal symptom in rabies. Quadriparesis, bilateral facial weakness and areflexia without sensory deficits are observed in both conditions. Urinary incontinence is common from the beginning in paralytic rabies. Inspiratory spasms with abnormal behaviour may appear late in the disease course and may be masked by generalized paralysis that may be severe and superimposed electrolyte and metabolic disturbances that may occur in both conditions. An acute inflammatory demyelinating form of GBS or acute motor sensory axonal neuropathy (AMSAN) and GBS-like syndrome following nervous tissue rabies vaccine has some degree of sensory deficit signs which are usually absent in paralytic rabies (Cabrera *et al.*, 1987; Hemachudha *et al.*, 1988a; Griffin and Ho 1993; Griffin *et al.*, 1996). Further, local symptoms at any one limb or one side of the face even without history of bite exposure, autonomic dysfunctions from the beginning, especially hypersalivation, abnormal pupils, and piloerection, suggest paralytic rabies.

Electrophysiological studies of the peripheral nerve cannot distinguish paralytic rabies from GBS. Demyelinating features may be found early followed by findings suggestive of both axonal and myelin damage.

Asymmetrical weakness in an unimmunized patient in an epidemic setting suggests paralytic poliomyelitis (Hurst and Pawan, 1931) or atypical forms of Japanese encephalitis (Solomon *et al.*, 1998). The Trinidad outbreak of paralytic rabies was initially thought to be poliomyelitis.

Establishing the diagnosis

Ante-mortem diagnosis of human rabies is extremely important. Delays in diagnosis result in a potential spread of contamination and an unnecessary need for post-exposure prophylaxis. Although there is no established evidence of human-to-human transmission, saliva and tracheal secretions are frequently virus positive (Helmick *et al.*, 1987; Crepin *et al.*, 1998; Noah *et al.*, 1998).

Based on clinical grounds alone, the diagnosis of furious rabies can be made with confidence when three classic or major cardinal signs are present together – fluctuating consciousness, phobic spasms and autonomic dysfunctions. However, in non-canine rabies endemic areas, such as in North America, where bats become the principal vector of rabies to humans, these clinical expressions may be variable (Noah *et al.*, 1998). Phobic spasms were found in only half (10 of 20) of the cases. However, either phobic spasms alone or presence of three or more of the following – agitation, confusion, seizures (16 of 20) or dysphagia (7 of 20), hypersalivation (10 of 20), limb pain, paraesthesias (9 of 20), limb weakness, paralysis or ataxia (three of 20) – were significantly associated with ante-mortem diagnosis (Noah *et al.*, 1998).

Local prodromal symptoms alone, although seeming severe as described by the patients, have to be interpreted with great caution since this may be modified by the patient's anxiety and fear of rabies and wound infection. A definite history of a bite, although commonly found in crv-cases, is not helpful in cases associated with brv. Of the 21 brv cases reported since 1980 in the USA, only one had a definite history of a bat bite.

Serological testing in the serum and CSF, although it should be the easiest and the most practical method, is of limited value. Rabies antibody titres of low concentrations as determined by the rapid fluorescent focus inhibition test (RFFIT) in serum could be detected in six of 31 of the non-vaccinated rabies patients tested within 1–26 days after the onset of the disease (Hemachudha, 1994, unpublished data). None of the 27 Thai non-vaccinated crv-rabies patients were CSF antibody positive to rabies virus (Hemachudha, 1994, unpublished data). All antibody positive serum samples (six of 31) were obtained within 9 days postonset (three of six within the first 3 days). This differs from cases in the Western hemisphere. Results obtained from the analysis of 102 samples from 39 cases in the USA and 16 cases in France since 1960 showed that antibody usually developed if the patients survived more than 8 days (positive serum antibody, six of 43 (14%) between days 1 and 8 versus 34 of 59 (58%) from day 9). Antibody in the CSF appeared later (positive CSF antibody, 0 of 19 between days 1 and 8 versus 10 of 28 (36%) from day 9) (Crepin et al., 1998; Noah et al., 1998).

Rabies virus may be isolated in mouse neuroblastoma cells from saliva specimens (WHO, 1992; Noah et al., 1998). This cell culture isolation is sensitive and specific, and results are known within 4–5 days; however, all samples tested must be maintained frozen after collection with no preservatives. Success rate also depends on the status of rabies antibody (87% (13 of 15) positive in antibody-negative compared to none (0 of 17) in antibody-positive patients) and the intermittence of rabies virus shedding in the saliva. False-negative results may be obtained in decomposed brain in case of biopsy or in post-mortem examination (Rudd and Trimarchi, 1989).

Results of nested PCR of RNA extracted from saliva, although sensitive, may be limited due to the intermittent nature of virus shedding and the primers used. However, the result is not affected by the status of the antibody. A 100% (10/10) sensitivity of this test in one series was achieved after the virus variants responsible for the infections were known and appropriate primers could be identified (Noah et al., 1998). Using one specific set of primers in the N gene, RT-PCR identified the presence of rabies virus in the saliva and CSF of five and two out of nine rabies patients respectively (Crepin et al., 1998). CSF contains a much lower virus concentration. These saliva and CSF specimens need a high quality collection and storage condition (−70°C) and proper handling (Hemachudha et al., 1992).

Rabies viral antigen may be detected by fluorescent antibody technique performed on frozen sections of the nuchal skin biopsy samples (Bryceson et al., 1975; Warrell et al., 1988). An examination of at least 20 sections is required to detect the rabies nucleocapsid inclusions around the base of the hair follicles (Crepin et al., 1998). The result is unrelated to the antibody status

(Noah *et al.*, 1998). Earlier studies showed that the proportion of positive results tends to increase as the disease progresses (Blenden *et al.*, 1986; Hemachudha, 1994). However, in another 26 rabies patients studied, antigen could be detected in as many as five of six (82%) patients within 4 days after onset. This number dropped to six of 10 (60%) between days 5 and 8 and to seven of 10 (70%) from day 9 (Crepin *et al.*, 1998). Detection of rabies viral antigen in corneal and salivary impression smears is unreliable.

Brain biopsy with antigen detection yielded highest sensitivity result in two series (five of six) (Hemachudha *et al.*, 1988c; Noah *et al.*, 1998). False negative results may occur when brain biopsy is performed during the first few days of the clinical illness. This may be due to a relative lack of viral antigen in the frontotemporal region and can be overcome by RT-PCR. Our experience with the nested PCR in 500 dog and five human brain samples showed 100% sensitivity without false-negative or positive results (Kamolvarin *et al.*, 1993; Hemachudha, 1994).

Data on using MRI with gadolinium contrast enhancement technique are still limited but may suggest the diagnosis of rabies once characteristic patterns appear (Laothamatas *et al.*, 1997).

In the case of post-mortem diagnosis where a full examination is not possible, brain tissue can be obtained by Silverman needle aspiration through a transorbital approach (WHO, 1992). It should be noted that only a minimal amount of brain tissue can be obtained by this technique and antigen detection by fluorescent antibody test may give a false negative result (personal experience).

Management

At present there is no specific treatment for rabies virus infection of humans once clinical signs develop. All treatment is purely symptomatic aiming to lessen the degree of aggression and to comfort the patient as much as possible. Interferon or antiviral drugs such as ribavirin, adenine arabinoside, acyclovir, inosine pronobex have been tried without success (Hemachudha, 1994; Noah *et al.*, 1998). Intrathecal or systemic administration of rabies polyclonal antibody or F (ab)2 as well as immunosuppressive therapy such as high dose steroids or antithymocyte globulin did not alter course of the disease in humans (Hemachudha, 1994). Intrathecal vaccination with a live attenuated rabies virus after the onset of clinical encephalitis has been effective in dogs (Baer *et al.*, 1975) but not in monkeys (Warrell *et al.*, 1987).

Prevention

Any bite by dogs, cats, bats, or wild animals in any part of the world, where there is wildlife or canine endemic or epizootic rabies, is a potential exposure (Hemachudha and Wilde, 1993) (Table 13.1). However, in cases encountered with bats, postexposure prophylaxis (PEP) is also appropriate even in the absence of a demonstrable bite or scratch, in situations where there is

Table 13.1   Guide for post-exposure treatment (WHO, 1996b).

Category	Type of contact with a suspect or confirmed domestic or wild [a] animal, or animal unavailable for observation	Recommended treatment
I	Touching or feeding of animals Licks on intact skin	None, if reliable case history available
II	Nibbling of uncovered skin Minor scratches or abrasions without bleeding Licks on broken skin	Administer vaccine immediately [b] Stop treatment if animal remains healthy throughout an observation period [c] of 10 days or if animal is euthanised and found to be negative for rabies by appropriate laboratory techniques
III	Single or multiple transdermal bites or scratches Contamination of mucous membrane with saliva (i.e. licks)	Administer rabies immunoglobulin and vaccine immediately [b] Stop treatment if animal remains healthy throughout an observation period [c] of 10 days or if animal is killed humanely and found to be negative for rabies by appropriate laboratory techniques

[a] Exposure to rodents, rabbits and hares seldom, if ever, requires specific anti-rabies treatment.
[b] If an apparently healthy dog or cat in or from a low-risk area is placed under observation, it may be justified to delay specific treatment (see also text).
[c] This observation period applies only to dogs and cats. Except in the case of threatened or endangered species, other domestic and wild animals suspected as rabid should be euthanised and their tissues examined using appropriate laboratory techniques.

reasonable probability that such contact occurred (e.g. sleeping person awakes to find a bat in the room or an adult witnesses a bat in the room with a previously unattended child, mentally disabled persons, or intoxicated person) (Debbie and Trimarchi, 1997). Of the 21 cases of brv-rabies patients reported since 1980 in the USA, only one had a definite history of bat bite.

A successful PEP must rely on prompt treatment whenever killing of the biting animal and immediate brain examination by fluorescence microscopy cannot be done (WHO, 1992, 1996b). Further, neutralizing antibody with levels higher than 0.5 IU/ml must be demonstrated by day 14 after initiation of PEP and be maintained throughout a year. This necessitates the need for the fifth vaccine dose on day 30. The 'provoked' or 'unprovoked' behaviour of the dog or cat is not applicable to the consideration of treatment initiation (Siwasontiwat et al., 1992; WHO, 1992, 1996b). Treatment may be discontinued, if the responsible dog or cat, but not other species, remains healthy throughout an observation period of 10 days. Observation of the biting dog or cat, but not other species, and postponement of treatment in a rabies-endemic area can be allowed in only three circumstances (WHO, 1993): (1) if there is a reliable history of dog vaccinations during the past 2 consecutive years (Tepsumethanon et al., 1991); (2) if the dog has received good care from its owner with minimal risk of exposure; (3) if there is a reasonable cause for being bitten such as feeding an unknown dog or stepping on its tail. Treatment must be initiated if the dog or cat develops abnormal signs during this observation period.

PEP consists of local wound care (thorough cleansing with soap and water, followed by a 70% ethanol or a solution of iodine), vaccine, and purified rabies immune globulin (RIG) (in case of category III-single or multiple transdermal bites or scratches or licks over mucosa) (Table 13.1) (WHO, 1996b). The wound should not be sutured. As much as possible, and all if necessary, of the RIG (human 20 IU/kg; equine source 40 IU/KG) should be injected in or around the wounds. We discourage the practice of multiple punctures to infiltrate wound with RIG which may cause additional injuries to the nerves similar to wound suturing (Hemachudha *et al.*, 1999). Each wound is pierced from one end and the needle is advanced, under the base of the wound, until the tip reaches the far edge. The needle is gradually withdrawn along with continuing delivery of the RIG. In case of multiple severe wounds where RIG is insufficient for infiltration, dilution with saline to an adequate volume has been suggested (WHO, 1996b). RIG can be administered with a delay of up to 7 days after the start of vaccine treatment. Purified equine RIG may have a small, though definite, risk of anaphylaxis, thus requiring a prior skin test.

All tissue culture rabies vaccines, human diploid cell (HDCV), purified Vero cell (PVRV), purified chick embryo cell (PCEC), and purified duck embryo (PDEV) rabies vaccine are equally safe and effective. These vaccines can be given by intramuscular (i.m.) route (at deltoid or anterolateral thigh muscle in children) on days 0, 3, 7, 14, and 30. The intradermal (i.d.) multisite regimen of '2-2-2-0-1-1', two sites on days 0, 3, and 7 and one site on days 30 and 90, is for use with PVRV, PCEC, and PDEV. The volume of the i.d. dose is one fifth of the i.m. dose per site. The i.d. multisite regimen of '8-0-4-0-1-1' is for use with HDCV and PCEC where the i.m. dose is 1 ml after reconstitution; 0.1 ml of reconstituted vaccine is given at each of eight sites, both sides of deltoid, lateral thigh, suprascapular region and lower quadrant of the abdomen on day 0, 0.1 ml at each of four sites over deltoids and thighs on day 7, and 0.1 ml at one site over deltoid on days 28 and 90. The minimal potencies of tissue culture vaccine, by an *in vivo* NIH test, proven to be efficacious in the PEP situation by i.m. and i.d. injections are at least 2.5 IU/dose and 0.7 IU/0.1 ml respectively (Chutivongse *et al.*, 1990).

Treatment should be given to an exposed person regardless of the time interval since exposure, but usually is not required after a time interval of longer than a year. Pregnancy is not a contraindication for PEP (Chutivongse *et al.*, 1995). Persons who have been previously vaccinated (either pre- or post-exposure regimen) with tissue culture or PDEV should receive two boosters on days 0 and 3 after re-exposure with no RIG treatment.

Pre-exposure vaccination is recommended for anyone at increased risk of exposure to rabies virus, including laboratory staff working with rabies, veterinarians, animal handlers, zoologists, wildlife officers and other people living in or travelling to rabies endemic areas where dogs are the dominant rabies vector species. Pre-exposure immunization schedule consists of three i.m. (one full dose) or i.d. (0.1 ml) injections on days 0, 7, and 28 at the deltoid area. This i.d. regimen has not been tested with PDEV. If antimalarial chemoprophylaxis (eg. chloroquine) is being used concurrently, i.m. injections are preferable. Laboratory staff and others at high/continuing risk of exposure should have their neutralizing antibody titre checked every 6 months. If it is less than 0.5 IU/ml a booster dose of vaccine should be given.

Acknowledgements

We are indebted to the medical residents and nurses and technicians of the Chulalongkorn University Hospital and Prommitr Hospital and Neuroimaging Center, Ramathibodi Hospital for taking care of the patients and to Professors Athasit Vejjajiva, Prida Phuapradit, Phrao Nivatvongs, Piyarat Ratanavanich, and Jiraporn Laothamatas for helpful advice. Clinical and research work was supported in part by grants from General Prayudh Charumani, Prommitr Hospital, Chulalongkorn University Hospital and Queen Saovabha Memorial Institute, The Thai Red Cross Society.

References

Ader, R., Cohen, N., Felten, D. (1995). Psychoneuroimmunology: interactions between the nervous system and the immune system. *Lancet*, **345**, 99–103.

Adle-Biassette, H., Bourhy, H., Gisselbrecht, M. *et al.* (1996). Rabies encephalitis in a patient with AIDS: a clinicopathological study. *Acta Neuropathol.*, **92**, 415–420.

Aghomo, H. O. and Rupprecht, C.E. (1990). Further studies on rabies virus isolated from healthy dogs in Nigeria. *Vet. Microbiol.*, **22**, 17–22.

Allworth, A., Murray, K. and Morgan, J. (1996). A human case of encephalitis due to a lyssavirus recently identified in fruit bats. *Commun. Dis. Intel.*, **20**, 504.

Astoul, E., Lafage, M. and Lafon, M. (1996). Rabies superantigen as a V B T-dependent adjuvant. *J. Exp. Med.*, **183**, 1623–1631.

Augusto, L. R., Percy, M. P., Edgar, T. V. *et al.* (1992). Outbreak of human rabies in the Peruvian jungle. *Lancet*, **339**, 408–411.

Baer, G. M. (1991). *The Natural History of Rabies*, 2nd edn. Boca Raton, FL: CRC Press.

Baer, G. M., Shanthaveerppa, T.R. and Bourne, G. H. (1968). The pathogenesis of street rabies virus in rats. *Bull. WHO.*, **38**, 119–125.

Baer, G. M., Shaddock, J. H., Williams, L. W. (1975). Prolonging morbidity in rabid dogs by intrathecal injection of attenuated rabies vaccine. *Infect. Immun.*, **12**, 98–103.

Baer, G. M., Bellini, W. J. and Fishbein, D. B. (1990a). Rhabdoviruses. In: *Virology* (B. N. Fields and D. M. Knipe, eds). New York: Academic Press, pp. 883–930.

Baer, G. M., Shaddock, J. H., Quirion, R. *et al.* (1990b). Rabies susceptibility and acetylcholine receptor. *Lancet*, **335**, 664–665.

Bahmanyar, M., Fayaz, A., Nour-Saleski, S. *et al.* (1976). Successful protection of humans exposed to rabies infection. *J. Am. Med. Assoc.*, **236**, 2751–2754.

Ban, E. (1997). New virus leaves questions hanging. *Nature Med.*, **3**, 5.

Bell, J. F. and Moore, G. J. (1971). Susceptibility of carnivora to rabies virus administered orally. *Am. J. Epidemiol.*, **93**, 176–182.

Berczi, I. and Szentivanyi, A. (1996). The pituitary gland, psychoneuroimmunology and infection. In: *Psychoneuroimmunology*, (H. Friedman, T. W. Klein and A. L. Friedman, eds). Boca Raton, FL: CRC Press. pp. 79–109.

Bhatt, D. R., Hattwick, M. A. W., Gerdsen, R. *et al.* (1974). Human rabies. Diagnosis, complications, and management. *Am. J. Dis. Child.*, **127**, 862–869.

Bijlenga, G. and Heaney, T. (1980). Postexposure local treatment of mice infected with rabies with two axonal inhibitors, colchicine and vinblastine. *J. Gen. Virol.*, **50**, 433–435.

Blenden, D. C., Creech, W. and Torres-Anjel, M. J. (1986). Use of immunofluorescence examination to detect rabies virus antigen in the skin of human with clinical encephalitis. *J. Infect. Dis.*, **154**, 698–701.

Bodner, R. A., Lynch, T., Lewis, L. *et al.* (1995). Serotonin syndrome. *Neurology*, **45**, 219–233.

Bourhy, H., Kissi, B. and Tordo, N. (1993). Molecular diversity of the Lyssavirus Genus. *Virology*, **194**, 70–81.

Bouzamondo, E., Ladogana and Tsiang, H. (1993). Alteration of potassium-evoked 5-HT release from virus-infected rat cortical synaptosomes. *Neuroreport*, **4**, 555–558.

Brass, D. A. (1994). *Rabies in Bats: Natural History and Public Health Implications*. Livia Press.

Brochier, B., Kieny, M. P., Costy, F. *et al.* (1991). Large-scale eradication of rabies using recombinant vaccinia-rabies vaccine. *Nature*, **354**, 520–522.

Brutkiewicz, R. R. and Welsh, R. M. (1995). Major histocompatibility complex class I antigens and the control of viral infections by natural killer cells. *J. Virol.*, **69**, 3967–3971.

Bryceson, A. D. M., Greenwood, B. M., Warrell, D.A. *et al.* (1975). Demonstration during life of rabies antigen in humans. *J. Infect. Dis.*, **131**, 71–74.

Burrage, T. C., Tignor, G. H. and Smith, A. L. (1985). Rabies virus binding at neuromuscular junctions. *Virus. Res.*, **2**, 273–279.

Cabrera, J., Griffin, D. E. and Johnson, R.T. (1987). Unusual features of the Guillain-Barre syndrome after rabies vaccine prepared in suckling mouse brain. *J. Neurol. Sci.*, **81**, 239–245.

Cadoz, M., Strady, A., Meignier, B. *et al.* (1992). Immunisation with canarypox virus expressing rabies glycoprotein. *Lancet*, **339**, 1429–1432.

Campbell, J. B. (1994). Oral rabies immunization of wild life and dogs: challenges to the Americas. In: *Lyssavirus* (C. E. Rupprecht, B. Dietzschold and H. Koprowski, eds). New York: Springer-Verlag, pp. 245–266.

Castellanos, J. E., Castaneda, D. R., Velandia, A. E. and Hurtado, H. (1997). Partial inhibition of the in vitro infection of adult mouse dorsal root ganglion neurons by rabies virus using nicotinic antagonists. *Neurosci. Lett.*, **229**, 198–200.

Ceccaldi, P. E., Marquette, C., Weber, P. *et al.* (1996). Ionizing radiation modulates the spread of an apathogenic rabies virus in mouse brain. *Intern. J. Radiation Biol.*, 70, 69–75.

Ceccaldi, P. E., Fillion, M. P., Ermine, A. *et al.* (1993). Rabies virus selectively alters 5-HT 1 receptor subtypes in rat brain. *Eur. J. Pharmacol.*, 245, 129–138.

Ceccaldi, P. E., Valtorta, F., Braud, S. *et al.* (1997). Alteration of the actin-based cytoskeleton by rabies virus. *J. Gen. Virol.*, 78, 2831–2835.

Charlton, K. M., Casey, G. A., Wandeler, A. I. *et al.* (1996). Early events in rabies virus infection of the central nervous system in skunks (Mephitis). *Acta Neuropathol.*, 91, 89–98.

Charlton, K. M., Nadin-Davis, S., Casey, G. A. *et al.* (1997). The long incubation period in rabies: delayed progression of infection in muscle at the site of exposure. *Acta Neuropathol.*, 94, 73–77.

Charlton, K. M. and Casey, G. A. (1979a). Experimental rabies in skunks: immuno-fluorescent, light and electron microscopic studies. *Lab. Invest.*, 41, 36–44.

Charlton, K. M. and Casey, G. A. (1979b). Experimental rabies in skunks: oral, nasal, tracheal and intestinal exposure. *Can. J. Comp. Med.*, 43, 168–172.

Charlton, K. M. and Casey, G. A. (1981). Experimental rabies in skunks: persistence of virus in denervated muscle at the inoculation site. *Can. J. Comp. Med.*, 45, 357–362.

Charlton, K. M. (1994). The pathogenesis of rabies and other lyssaviral infections: recent studies. In: *Lyssaviruses* (C. E. Rupprecht, B. Dietzschold and H. Koprowski, eds). New York: Springer-Verlag, pp. 95–119.

Chopra, J. S., Banerjee, A. K., Murthy, J. M. K. and Pal, S. R. (1980). Paralytic rabies. A clinicopathological study. *Brain*, 103, 789–802.

Chutivongse, S., Wilde, H., Benjavongkulchai, M. *et al.* (1995). Postexposure rabies vaccination during pregnancy: effect on 202 woman and their infants. *Clin. Infect. Dis.*, 20, 818–820.

Chutivongse, S., Wilde, H., Supich, C. *et al.* (1990). Postexposure prophylaxis for rabies with antiserum and intradermal vaccination. *Lancet*, 335, 896–898.

Cleaveland, S. (1998). Epidemiology and control of rabies. The growing problem of rabies in Africa. *Trans. R. Soc. Trop. Med. Hyg.*, 92, 131-134.

Cohen, S. L., Gardner, S., Lanyi, C. *et al.* (1976). A case of rabies in man: some problems in diagnosis and management. *Br. Med. J.*, 1, 1041–1042.

Constantine, D. G. (1967). Rabies transmission by air in bat caves. *United States Public Health Service Publication*.

Coulon, P., Derbin, C., Kucera, P. *et al.* (1989). Invasion of the peripheral nervous system of adult mice by the CVS strain of rabies virus and its avirulent derivative Av01. *J. Virol.*, 63, 3550–3554.

Coulon, P., Ternaux, J. P., Flamand, A. and Tuffereau, C. (1998). An avirulent mutant of rabies virus is unable to infect motoneurons in vivo and in vitro. *J. Virol.*, 72, 273–278.

Crepin, P., Audry, L., Rotivel, Y. *et al.* (1998). Intravitam diagnosis of human rabies by PCR using saliva and cerebrospinal fluid. *J. Clin. Microbiol.*, **36**, 1117–1121.

Dean, D. J., Evans, W. M. and McClure, R. C. (1963). Pathogenesis of rabies. *Bull. WHO.*, **29**, 803–811.

Debbie, J. G. and Trimarchi, C. V. (1997). Prophylaxis for suspected exposure to bat rabies. *Lancet*, **350**, 1790–1791.

Dereswicz, R. I., Thaler, S. J., Hsu, I. *et al.* (1997). Clinical and neuroradiographic manifestations of eastern equine encephalitis. *N. Engl. J. Med.*, **336**, 1867–1874.

Dietzschold, B., Kao, M., Zheng, Y. M. *et al.* (1992). Delineation of putative mechanisms involved in antibody-mediated clearance of rabies virus from the central nervous system. *Proc. Natl Acad. Sci.*, **89**, 7252–7256.

Dietzschold, B., Rupprect, C. E., Fu, Z. F. *et al.* (1996). Rhabdoviruses. In: *Virology* (B. N. Fields, D. M. Knipe, P. M. Howley *et al.*, eds). Philadelphia: PA: Lippincott-Raven Publishers, pp. 1137–1159.

Dietzschold, B., Wiktor, T. L., Trojanowski, J. Q. *et al.* (1985). Differences in cell-to cell spread of pathogenic and apathogenic rabies virus in vivo and in vitro. *J. Virol.*, **56**, 12–18.

Dietzschold, B., Wunner, W. H., Wiktor, T. J. *et al.* (1983). Characterization of an antigenic determination of the glycoprotein which correlates with pathogenicity of rabies virus. *Proc. Natl Acad. Sci. USA*, **80**, 70–74.

Dumrongphol, H., Srikiatkhachorn, A., Hemachudha, T. *et al.* (1996). Alteration of muscarinic acetylcholine receptors in rabies viral-infected dog brains. *J. Neurol. Sci.*, **137**, 1–6.

Dunn, A. J. (1996). Psychoneuroimmunology, stress and infection. In: *Psychoneuroimmunology* (H. Friedman, T. W. Klein and A. L. Friedman, eds). Boca Raton, FL: CRC Press, pp. 25–46.

Fekadu, M. (1988). Pathogenesis of rabies virus infection in dogs. *Rev. Infect. Dis.*, **10**, 678–683.

Fekadu, M. and Baer, G. M. (1980). Recovery from clinical rabies of 2 dogs inoculated with a rabies virus strain from Ethiopia. *Am. J. Vet. Res.*, **41**, 1632–1634.

Fekadu, M., Endeshaw, T., Alemu, W. *et al.* (1996). Possible human-to-human transmission of rabies in Ethiopia. *Ethiop. Med. J.*, **34**, 123–127.

Fishbein, D. B. and Robinson, L. E. (1993). Rabies. *N. Engl. J. Med.*, **25**, 1632–1638.

Fontana, A., Constam, D., Frei, K. *et al.* (1996). Cytokines and defense against CNS infection. In: *Cytokines and the CNS* (R. M. Ransohoff and E. N. Benveniste, eds). Boca Raton, FL: CRC Press, pp. 187–219.

Fraser, G. C., Hooper, P. T., Lunt, R. A. *et al.* (1996). Encephalitis caused by a Lyssavirus in fruit bats in Australia. *Emerg. Infect. Dis.*, **2**, 327–331.

Fu, Z. F., Weihe, E., Zheng, Y. M. *et al.* (1993). Differential effects of rabies and borna disease viruses on immediate-early and late-response gene expression in brain tissues. *J. Virol.*, **67**, 6674–6681.

Gillet, J. P., Derer, P. and Tsiang, H. (1986). Axonal transport of rabies virus in the central nervous system of the rat. *J. Neuropathol. Exp. Neurol.*, **45**, 619–634.

Gomej-Alonso, J. (1998). Rabies: a possible explanation for the vampire legend. *Neurology*, **51**, 856–869.

Gosztonyi, G. (1994). Reproduction of Lyssaviruses: ultrastructural composition of lyssaviruses and functional aspects of pathogenesis. In: *Lyssaviruses* (C. E. Rupprecht, B. Dietzschold and H. Koprowski, eds). New York: Springer-Verlag, pp. 43–68.

Gourmelon, P., Briet, D. and Court, L. (1986). Electrophysiological and sleep alterations in experimental mouse rabies. *Brain Res.*, **398**, 128–140.

Gourmelon, P., Briet, D., Clarenco, D. *et al.* (1991). Sleep alterations in experimental street rabies virus infection occur in the absence of major EEG abnormalities. *Brain Res.*, **554**, 159–165.

Griffin, J. W. and Ho, T. W. (1993). The Guillain-Barre syndrome at 75: the Campylobacter connection. *Ann. Neurol.*, **34**, 125–127.

Griffin, J. W., Li, C. Y., Ho, T. W. *et al.* (1996). Pathology of the motor-sensory axonal Guillain-Barre syndrome. *Ann. Neurol.*, **39**, 17–28.

Guinto, G., Felix, I. and Rivas, A. (1995). A case of rabies encephalitis with long survival. *Gac. Med. Mexico*, **131**, 223–228.

Haas, L. F. (1998). Louis Pasteur (1822–95). Neurological Stamp. *J. Neurol. Neurosurg. Psych.*, **64**, 330.

Habel, K. and Koprowski, H. (1955). Laboratory data supporting the clinical trial of antirabies serum in persons bitten by a rabid wolf. Bull. *WHO*, **13**, 773–779.

Haddad, N., Ben Khelifa, R., Matter, H. *et al.* (1994). Assay of oral vaccination of dogs against rabies in Tunisia with the vaccinal strain SAD Bern. *Vaccine*, **12**, 307–308.

Hafer-Macko, C., Hsieh, S. T., Li, C. Y. *et al.* (1996). Acute motor axonal neuropathy: an antibody-mediated attack on axolemma. *Ann. Neurol.*, **40**, 635–644.

Hanham, C. A., Zhao, F. and Tignor, G. H. (1993). Evidence from the anti-idiotypic network that the aectylcholine receptor is a rabies virus receptor. *J. Virol.*, **67**, 530–542.

Hantson, P., Guerit, J. M., Tourtchaninoff, D. M. *et al.* (1993). Rabies encephalitis mimicking the electrophysiological pattern of brain death. *Eur. Neurol.*, **33**, 212–217.

Haour, F., Marquette, C., Ban, E. *et al.* (1995). Receptors for interleukin-1 in the central nervous and neuroendocrine systems. *Ann. Endocrinol.*, **56**, 173–179.

Hattwick, M. A. W. (1974). Human rabies. *Publ. Hlth Rev.*, **3**, 229–274.

Hattwick, M. A. W. and Gregg, M. B. (1975). The natural history of rabies. In: *The Disease in Man* (G. M. Baer, ed.). New York: Academic Press, pp. 281–303.

Hattwick, M. A. W., Weis, T. T., Stechschulte, J. *et al.* (1972). Recovery from rabies. *Ann. Intern. Med.*, **76**, 931–942.

Helmick, C. G., Tauxe, R. V. and Vernon, A. A. (1987). Is there a risk to contacts of patients with rabies? *Rev. Infect. Dis.*, **9**, 511–518.

Hemachudha, T. (1989). Rabies. In: *Handbook of Clinical Neurology* (P. J.Vinken, G. W. Bruyn and H. L. Klawans, eds). Revised series, Amsterdam: Elsevier Science Publishers, pp. 383–404.

Hemachudha, T. (1994). Human rabies: clinical aspects, pathogenesis and potential therapy. In: *Lyssaviruses* (C. E. Rupprecht, B. Dietzschold and H. Koprowski, eds). New York: Springer-Verlag, pp. 121–143.

Hemachudha, T. (1997). Rabies. In: *CNS Infectious Diseases and Therapy* (K. L. Roos, ed.). New York: Marcel Dekker Inc., pp. 573–600.

Hemachudha, T. and Phuapradit, P. (1997). Rabies. *Curr. Opin. Neurol.*, **10**, 260–267.

Hemachudha, T. and Wilde, H. (1993). Rabies. In: *Current Therapy in Neurological Disease* (R. T. Johnson and J. W. Griffin, eds). St Louis, MO: Mosby Year Book, pp. 143–146.

Hemachudha, T., Griffin, D. E., Giffels, J. J. *et al.* (1987a). Myelin basic protein as an encephalitogen in encephalomyelitis and polyneuritis following rabies vaccination. *N. Engl. J. Med.*, **316**, 369–374.

Hemachudha, T., Phanuphak, P., Johnson, R. T. *et al.* (1987b). Neurologic complications of Semple-type rabies vaccine: clinical and immunologic studies. *Neurology*, **37**, 550–556.

Hemachudha, T., Phanthumchinda, K., Phanuphak, P. and Manutsathit, S. (1987c). Myoedema as a clinical sign in paralytic rabies. *Lancet*, **1**, 1210.

Hemachudha, T., Griffin, D.E., Chen, W. *et al.* (1988a). Immunologic studies of rabies vaccination induced Guillain-Barre syndrome. *Neurology*, **38**, 375–378.

Hemachudha, T., Griffin, D. E., Johnson, R. T. *et al.* (1988b). Immunologic studies of patients with chronic encephalitis induced by postexposure Semple rabies vaccine. *Neurology*, **39**, 42–44.

Hemachudha, T., Phanuphak, P., Sriwanthana, B. *et al.* (1988c). Immunologic study of human encephalitic and paralytic rabies. A preliminary study of 16 patients. *Am. J. Med.*, **84**, 673–677.

Hemachudha, T., Khawplod, P., Phanuphak, P. and Griffin, D. E. (1989a). Enhanced antibody response to rabies virus in patients with neurologic complications following brain tissue-derived rabies vaccination. *Asian Pac. J. Allergy Immunol.*, **7**, 49–50.

Hemachudha, T., Tirawatnpong, S. and Phanthumchida, K., (1989b). Seizures as the initial manifestation of paralytic rabies. *J. Neurol. Neurosurg. Psych.*, **52**, 808–810.

Hemachudha, T., Chutivongse, S., Wilde, H. *et al.* (1991). Latent rabies. *N. Engl. J. Med.*, **324**, 1890–1891.

Hemachudha, T., Kamolvarin, N., Tirawatnpong, S. *et al.* (1992). Ante-and post-mortem diagnosis of rabies in man and animal by PCR using nested primers. *Neurology*, **42** (suppl. 3), 370.

Hemachudha, T., Panpanich, P., Manutsathit, S. and Phanuphak, P. (1993). Immune activation in human rabies. *Trans. R. Soc. Trop. Med. Hyg.*, **87**, 106–108.

Hemachudha, T., Mitrabhakdi, E., Wilde, H. *et al.* (1999). Additional reports of failure to respond to treatment after rabies exposure in Thailand. *Clin. Infect. Dis.*, (In Press).

Hoenig, L. J. (1986). Triumph and controversy. Pasteur's preventive treatment of rabies as reported in JAMA. *Arch. Neurol.*, **43**, 397–399.

Hooper, D. C., Morimoto, K., Bette, M. *et al.* (1998). Collaboration of antibody and inflammation in clearance of rabies virus from the central nervous system. *J. Virol.*, **72**, 3711–3719.

Hooper, D. C., Ohnishi, T., Kean, R. *et al.* (1995). Local nitric oxide production in viral and autoimmune diseases of the central nervous system. *Proc. Natl Acad. Sci. USA*, **92**, 5312–5316.

Houff, S. A., Burton, R. C., Wilson, R. W. *et al.* (1979). Human-to-human transmission of rabies virus by corneal transplant. *N. Engl. J. Med.*, **300**, 603–604.

Hurst, E. W. and Pawan, J. L. (1931). An outbreak of rabies in Trinidad without history of bites and with the symptoms of acute ascending paralysis. *Lancet*, **2**, 622–625.

Hurst, E. W. and Pawan, J. L. (1932). A further account of the Trinidad outbreak of acute rabies myelitis. *J. Pathol. Bacteriol.*, **35**, 301–321.

Immunization practices advisory committee (1991). Rabies prevention – United States, 1991: recommendations of the immunization practices advisory committee (ACIP). *MMWR*, **40**, 1–19.

Iwasaki, Y. and Clark, H. F. (1975). Cell to cell transmission of virus in the central nervous system II. Experimental rabies in the mouse. *Lab. Invest.*, **33**, 391–399.

Iwasaki, Y., Ohtani, S. and Clark, H. F. (1975). Maturation of rabies virus by budding from neuronal cell membrane in suckling mouse brain. *J. Virol.*, **15**, 1020–1023.

Iwaski, Y., Sako, K., Tsunoda, I. *et al.* (1993). Phenotypes of mononuclear cell infiltrates in human central nervous system. *Acta Neuropathol.*, **85**, 653–657.

Jackson, A. C. and Park, H. (1998). Apoptotic cell death in experimental rabies in suckling mice. *Acta Neuropathol.*, **95**, 159–164.

Jackson, A. C. and Reimer, D. L. (1989). Pathogenesis of experimental rabies in mice: an immunohistochemical study. *Acta Neuropathol.*, **78**, 159–165.

Jackson, A. C. and Rossiter, J. P. (1997). Apoptosis plays an important role in experimental rabies virus infection. *J. Virol.*, **71**, 5603–5607.

Johnson, H. N. (1965a). Rabies virus. In: *Viral and Rickettsial Infections of Man* (F. I. Horsfell and I. Tamm, eds). Lippincott. pp. 814–840.

Johnson, R. T. (1965b). Experimental rabies: studies of cellular vulnerability and pathogenesis using fluorescent antibody staining. *J. Neuropathol. Exp. Neurol.*, **24**, 662–674.

Johnson, R. T. (1998). *Viral Infection of the Nervous System*. Philadelphia, Pa: Lippincott-Raven.

Kamolvarin, N., Tirawatnpong, T., Rattanasiwamoke, R. *et al.* (1993). Diagnosis of rabies by polymerase chain reaction with nested primers. *J. Infect. Dis.*, **167**, 207–210.

Kaplan, C., Turner, G. S. and Warrell, D. A. (1986). *Rabies: The Facts*, 2nd edn. Oxford: Oxford University Press.

Kasempimolporn, S., Hemachudha, T., Khawplod, P. *et al.* (1991). Human immune response to rabies nucleocapsid and glycoprotein antigens. *Clin. Exp. Immunol.*, **84**, 195–199.

Koprowski, H. (1996). Lecture on rabies on the occasion of 'The Year of Louis Pasteur'. *Res. Virol.*, **147**, 381–387.

Koschel, K. and Munzel, P. (1984). Inhibition of opiate receptor mediated signal transmission by rabies virus in persistently infected NG-108-15 mouse neuroblastoma-rat glioma hybrid cells. *Proc. Natl Acad. Sci. USA*, **81**, 950–954.

Kristensson, K., Dastur, D.K., Manghani, D.K. *et al.* (1996). Rabies: interactions between neurons and viruses. A review of the history of Negri inclusion bodies. *Neuropathol. App. Neurobiol.*, **22**, 179–187.

Kucera, P., Dolivo, M., Coulon, P. *et al.* (1985). Pathways of the early propagation of virulent and avirulent rabies strains from the eye to the brain. *J. Virol.*, **55**, 158–162.

Kumar, S., Misra, U. K., Kalita, J. *et al.* (1997). MRI in Japanese encephalitis. *Neuroradiology*, **39**, 180–184.

Kureishi, A., Xu, L. Z., Wu, H. and Stiver, H. G. (1992). Rabies in China: recommendations for control. *Bull. WHO.*, **70**, 443–450.

Ladogana, A., Bouzamondo, E., Pocchiari, M. and Tsiang, H. (1994). Modification of tritiated γ-amino-n-butyric acid transport in rabies virus-infected primary cortical cultures. *J. Gen. Virol.*, **75**, 623–627.

Lafon, M., Lafage, M., Martinez-Arends, A. *et al.* (1992). Evidence for a viral superantigen in humans. *Nature*, **358**, 507–510.

Lafon, M., Scott-Algara, D., Marche, P. N. *et al.* (1994). Neonatal deletion and selective expansion of mouse T cells by exposure to rabies virus nucleocapsid superantigen. *J. Exp. Med.*, **180**, 1207–1215.

Laothamatas, J., Hemachudha, T., Tulyadechanont, S. and Mitrabhakdi, E. (1997). Neuroimaging in paralytic rabies. *Ramathibodi Med. J.*, **20**, 149–156.

Lentz, T. L., Benson, R. J. J., Klimowicz, D. *et al.* (1986). Binding of rabies virus to purified torpedo acetylcholine receptor. *Mol. Brain Res.*, **1**, 211–219.

Lentz, T. L., Burrage, T. G., Smith, A. L. *et al.* (1982). Is the accetylcholine receptor a rabies virus receptor? *Science*, **215**, 182–184.

Lentz, T. L., Chester, J., Benson, R. J. J. *et al.* (1985). Rabies virus binding to cellular membranes measured by enzyme immunoassay. *Muscle Nerve*, **8**, 336–345.

Lentz, T. L., Hawrot, E. and Wilson, P. T. (1987). Synthetic peptides corresponding to sequences of snake venom neurotoxins and rabies virus glycoprotein bind to the nicotinic acetylcholine receptor. Proteins:structure, function. *Genet.*, **2**, 298–307.

Lentz, T. L., Wilson, P. T., Hawrot, E. and Speicher, D. W. (1984). Amino acid sequence similarity between rabies virus glycoprotein and snake venom curaremimetic neurotoxins. *Science*, **226**, 847–848.

Linthorst, A. C. E., Flachskamm, C., Holsboer, F. and Reul, J. M. H. (1994). Local administration of recombinant human interleukin-1 beta in the rat hippocampus increases serotonergic neurotransmission, hypothalamic-pituitary-adrenocortical axis activity, and body temperature. *Endocrinology*, **135**, 520–532.

Li, Z., Feng, Z. and Ye, H. (1995). Rabies viral antigen in human tongues and salivary glands. *J. Trop. Med. Hyg.*, **98**, 330–332.

Lodmell, D. L. and Ewalt, L. C. (1985). Pathogenesis of street rabies virus infections in resistant and susceptible strains of mice. *J. Virol.*, **55**, 788–795.

Lodmell, D. L., Sumner, J. W., Esposito, J. J. *et al.* (1991). Raccoon poxvirus recombinants expressing the rabies virus nucleoprotein protect mice against lethal rabies virus infection. *J. Virol.*, **65**, 3400–3405.

Lucia Alvarez, H., Ramon Fajardo, V., Elvia Lopez, M. *et al.* (1994). Partial recovery from rabies in a nine-year-old boy. *Ped. Infect. Dis.*, **13**, 1154–1155.

Lumbiganon, P. and Wasi, C. (1990). Survival after rabies immunization in newborn infant of affected mother. *Lancet*, **336**, 319.

Lycke, E. and Tsiang, H. (1987). Rabies virus infection of cultured rat sensory neuron. *J. Virol.*, **61**, 2733–2741.

Marquette, C., Ceccaldi, P. E., Ban, E. *et al.* (1996a). Alteration of interleukin-1 alpha production and interleukin-1 alpha binding sites in mouse brain during rabies infection. *Arch. Virol.*, **141**, 573–585.

Marquette, C., Van Dam, A. M., Ceccaldi, P. M. *et al.* (1996b). Induction of immunoreactive interleukin-1 beta and tumor necrosis factor-alpha in the brains of rabies virus infected rats. *J. Neuroimmunol.*, **68**, 45–51.

Martell, M.A., Ceronmontes, F. and Raulalcocer, B. (1973). Transplacental transmission of bovine rabies after natural infection. *J. Infect. Dis.*, **127**, 291–293.

Martinez-Arends, A., Astoul, E., Lafage, M. and Lafon, M. (1995). Activation of human tonsils lymphocytes by rabies virus nucleocapsid superantigen. *J. Immunol. Immunopathol.*, **77**, 177–184.

Matsumoto, S. (1975). Electron microscopy of central nervous system infections. In: *The Natural History of Rabies* (G. M.Baer, ed.). New York: Academic Press, pp. 217–233.

McCann, S. M. (1998). Introduction. In: Neuroimmunomodulation: Molecular aspects, integrative systems, and clinical advances. (S. M. McCann, J. M. Lipton, E. M. Sternberg *et al.* eds). *Ann. NY Acad. Sci.*, **840**. XIII–XIV.

McColl, K. A., Gould, A. R., Selleck, P. W. *et al.* (1993). Polymerase chain reaction and other laboratory techniques in the diagnosis of long incubation rabies in Australia. *Aust. Vet. J.*, **70**, 84–89.

McKhann, G. M., Cornblath, D. R., Griffin, J. W. *et al.* (1993). Acute motor axonal neuropathy: a frequent cause of acute flaccid paralysis in China. *Ann. Neurol.*, **33**, 333–342.

Merrill, J. and Murphy, S. (1996). Nitric oxide. In: *The Role of Glia in Neurotoxicity* (M. Aschner and H. K. Kimelberg, eds). Boca Raton, FL: CRC Press, pp. 263–281.

Metze, K. and Feiden, W. (1991). Rabies virus ribonucleoprotein in the heart. *N. Engl. J. Med.*, **324**, 1814–1815.

Mifune, K., Takeuchi, E., Napiorkowski, P. A. *et al.* (1981). Essential role of T cells in the postexposure prophylaxis of rabies in mice. *Microbiol. Immunol.*, **25**, 895–902.

Miller, A., Morse, H. C., Winkelstein, J. and Nathanson, N. (1978). The role of antibody in recovery from experimental rabies. Effect of depletion of B and T cells. *J. Immunol.*, **121**, 321–326.

Minguetti, G., Hofmeister, R.M., Hayashi, Y. and Montano, J.A. (1997). Ultrastructure of cranial nerves of rats inoculated with rabies virus. *Arq. Neuropsiquiatr.*, **55**, 680–686.

Miyamoto, K. and Matsumoto S. (1965). The nature of the Negri body. *J. Cell Biol.*, **27**, 677–682.

MMWR (1977). Rabies in a laboratory worker-New York. **26**, 183–184.

MMWR (1996a). Human rabies-California, 1995. **45**, 353–356.

MMWR (1996b). Human rabies-Connecticut, 1995. **45**, 207–209.

MMWR (1997a). Human rabies-Kentucky and Montana, 1996. **46**, 397–400.

MMWR (1997b). Human rabies-Montana and Washington, 1997. **46**, 770–773.

MMWR (1998). Human rabies-Texas and New Jersey, 1997. **47**, 1–5.

Morimoto, K., Patel, M., Corisdeo, S. *et al.* (1996). Characterization of a unique variant of bat rabies virus responsible for newly emerging human cases in North America. *Proc. Natl Acad. Sci. USA*, **93**, 5653–5658.

Morris, J. S., Frith, C. D., Perrett, D. I. *et al.* (1996). A differential neural response in the human amygdala to fearful and happy facial expressions. *Science*, **383**, 812–815.

Munzel, P. and Koschel, K. (1981). Rabies virus decreases agonist binding to opiate receptors of mouse neuroblastoma-rat glioma hybrid cells 108-cc-15. *Biochem. Biophys. Res. Commun.*, **10**, 1241–1250.

Murphy, F. A., Bauer, S. P., Harrison, A. K. and Winn, W. C. (1973). Comparative pathogenesis of rabies and rabies-like viruses. Viral infection and transit from inoculation site to the central nervous system. *Lab. Invest.*, **28**, 361–376.

Nehaul, B.B.G. (1955). Rabies transmitted by bats in British Guiana. *Am. J. Trop. Med. Hyg.*, **43**, 507–528.

Newton, T.H., Norman, D., Alvord, E.C. *et al.* (1977). The CT scan in infectious diseases of the CNS. In: *Computed Tomography* (D. Norman, ed). Berkeley, CA: University of California Press. pp. 719–740.

Niesche, C. (1998). Woman struck down by bat virus 2 years after bite. *The Australian*, 9 December.

Noah, D. L., Drenzek, C. L., Smith, J. S. *et al.* (1998). Epidemiology of human rabies in the United States, 1980 to 1996. *Ann. Intern. Med.*, **128**, 922–930.

Noah, D. L., Smith, M. G., Gotthardt, J.C. *et al.* (1996). Mass human exposure to rabies in New Hampshire:exposure, treatment, and cost. *Am. J. Public Hlth*, **86**, 1149–1151.

Obeid, L. M., Linardic, C. M., Karolak, L. A. and Hannun, Y. A. (1993). Programmed cell death induced by ceramide. *Science*, **259**, 1769–1771.

Panpanich, T., Hemachudha, T., Piyasirisilp, S. *et al.* (1992). Cells with natural killer activity in human rabies. *Clin. Exp. Immunol.*, **89**, 414–418.

Pastoret, P.P., Brochier, B. and Copens, P. (1993). Deliberate release of a recombinant vaccinia-rabies virus for vaccination of wild animals against rabies. *Microb. Rel.*, **1**, 191–195.

Pazmany, L., Mandelboim, O., Vales-Gomez, M. *et al.* (1996). Protection from natural killer cell-mediated lysis by HLA-G expression on target cells. *Science*, **274**, 792–795.

Perl, D. P. (1975). The pathology of rabies in the central nervous system. In: *The Natural History of Rabies* (G. M. Baer, ed.). New York: Academic Press, pp. 236–272.

Perrin, P., De Franco, M. T., Jallet, C. *et al.* (1996). The antigen-specific cell-mediated immune response in mice is suppressed by infection with pathogenic lyssa-viruses. *Res. Virol.*, **147**, 289–299.

Perry, L. L., Hotchkiss, J. D. and Lodmell, D. L. (1990). Murine susceptibility to street rabies virus is unrelated to induction of host lymphoid depletion. *J. Immunol.*, **144**, 3552–3557.

Perry, L. L. and Lodmell, D. L. (1991). Role of CD4+ and CD8+ T cells in murine resistance to street rabies virus. *J. Virol.*, **65**, 3429–3434.

Phuapradit, P., Manutsathit, S., Warrell, M.J., et al. (1985). Paralytic rabies: some unusual clinical presentations. *J. Med. Assoc. Thailand*, **68**, 105–110.

Porras, C., Barboza, J. J., Fuenzalida, E. *et al.* (1976). Recovery from rabies in man. *Ann. Intern. Med.*, **85**, 44–48.

Ray, N. B., Ewalt, L. C. and Lodmell, D. L. (1995). Rabies virus replication in primary murine bone marrow macrophages and in human and murine macrophages-like cell lines: implications for viral persistence. *J. Virol.*, **69**, 764–772.

Ray, N. B., Power, C., Lynch, W. P. *et al.* (1997). Rabies viruses infect primary cultures of murine, feline, and human microglia and astrocytes. *Arch. Virol.*, **142**, 1011–1019.

Reichlin, S. (1993). Mechanisms of disease: neuroendocrine-immune interactions. *N. Engl. J. Med.*, **329**, 1246–1253.

Rivers, T. M. and Schwentker, F. F. (1935). Encephalomyelitis accompanied by myelin destruction experimentally produced in monkeys. *J. Exp. Med.*, **61**, 689–702.

Roine, R. O., Hillbom, M., Valle, M. *et al.* (1988). Fatal encephalitis caused by a bat-borne rabies-related virus. *Brain*, **111**, 1505–1516.

Rosner, F. (1974). Rabies in the Talmud. *Med. Hist.*, **18**, 198–200.

Rudd, R. J. and Trimarchi, C. V. (1989). Development and evaluation of an in vitro virus isolation procedure as a replacement for the mouse inoculation test in rabies diagnosis. *J. Clin. Microbiol.*, **27**, 2522–2528.

Rupprecht, C. E. and Dietzschold, B. (1987). Editorial: perspective on rabies virus pathogenesis. *Lab. Invest.*, **57**, 603–606.

Rupprecht, C. E. and Kieney, M. P. (1988). Development of a vaccinia-rabies glycoprotein recombinant virus vaccine. In: *Rabies* (J. B. Campbell and K. M. Charlton, eds). Boston, MA: Kluwer Academic Publishers, pp. 335–364.

Schwarcz, R., Guidetti, P. and Roberts, R. C. (1996). Quinolinic acid and Kynurenic acid:glia-derived modulators of excitotoxic brain injury. In: *The role of Glia in Neurotoxicity* (M. Aschner and H. K. Kimelberg, eds). pp. 245–363. Boca Raton, FL: CRC Press.

Seif, I., Coulon, P., Rollin, P. E. *et al.* (1985). Rabies virulence:effect on pathogenicity and sequence characterization of rabies virus mutations affecting antigenic site III of the glycoprotein. *J. Virol.*, **53**, 926–934.

Shankar, V., Dietzschold, B. and Koprowski, H.A. (1991). Direct entry of rabies virus into the central nervous system without prior local replication. *J. Virol.*, **65**, 2736–2738.

Sheikh, K. A., Jackson, A. C., Ramos-Alvarez, M. *et al.* (1998a). Paralytic rabies: immune attack on nerve fibers containing axonally transported viral proteins. *Neurology*, **50** (suppl. 4), A183–184.

Sheikh, K. A., Nachamkin, I., Ho, T. W. *et al.* (1998b). Campylobacter jejuni lipopolysaccharides in Guillain-Barre syndrome: molecular mimicry and host susceptibility. *Neurology*, **51**, 371–378.

Sipahioglu, U. and Alpaut, S. (1985). Transplacental rabies in man. *Mikrobiol. Blt.*, **19**, 95–99.

Sitthi-Amorn, C., Jiratanavattana, V., Keoyoo, J. and Sonpunys, N. (1987). The diagnostic properties of laboratory tests for rabies. *Int. J. Epidemiol.*, **16**, 602–605.

Siwasontiwat, D., Lumlertdaecha, B., Polsuwan, C. *et al.* (1992). Rabies: Is provocation of the biting dog relevant for risk assessment? *Trans. R. Soc. Trop. Med. Hyg.*, **86**, 443.

Smart, N. L. and Charlton, K. M. (1992). The distribution of challenge virus standard rabies virus versus skunk street rabies virus in the brains of experimentally infected rabid skunks. *Acta Neuropathol.*, **84**, 501–508.

Smith, J. S., Fishbein, D. B., Rupprecht, C.E. *et al.* (1991). Unexplained rabies in three immigrants in the United States: a virologic investigation. *N. Engl. J. Med.*, **324**, 205–211.

Smith, J. S. and King, A. A. (1996). Monoclonal antibodies for the identification of rabies and non-rabies lyssaviruses. In: *Laboratory Technique in Rabies*, 4th edn (F. X. Meslin, M. M. Kaplan and H. Koprowski, eds). Geneva: World Health Organization. pp. 145–156,

Solomon, T., Kneen, R., Dung, N. M. *et al.* (1998). Poliomyelitis-like illness due to Japanese encephalitis virus. *Lancet*, **351**, 1094–1097.

Speare, R., Skerratt, L., Foster, R. *et al.* (1997). Australian bat lyssavirus infection in three fruit bats from north Queensland. *Commun. Dis. Intell.*, **21**, 117–120.

Srikiatkachorn, A. and Hemachudha, T. (1998). Tetanus. In: *Neurobase-Program for Personal Computers* (S. Gilman, ed.). San Diego, CA: Arbor Publishing Corp.

Sugamata, M., Miyazawa, M., Mori, S. *et al.* (1992). Paralysis of street rabies virus-infected mice is dependent on T lymphocytes. *J. Virol.*, **66**, 1252–1260.

Sung, J. H., Hayano, M. and Mastri, A. R. (1976). A case of human rabies and ultrastructure of the Negri body. *J. Neuropathol. Exp. Neurol.*, **35**, 541–559.

Superstein, A., Brand, H., Audhya, T. *et al.* (1992). Interleukin 1 beta mediates stress-induced immunosuppression via cortictropin-releasing factor. *Endocrinology*, **130**, 152–158.

Tangchai, P. and Vejjajjiva, A. (1971). Pathology of the peripheral nervous system in human rabies: a study of nine autopsy cases. *Brain*, **132**, 1497–1504.

Tangchai, P., Yenbutr, D. and Vejjajiva, A. (1970). Central nervous system lesions in human rabies. A study of 24 autopsy cases. *J. Med. Assoc. Thailand*, **53**, 471–488.

Tariq, W. U., Shafi, M. S., Jamal, S. and Ahmad, M. (1991). Rabies in man handling infected calf. *Lancet*, **337**, 1224.

Tepsumethanon, W., Polsuwan, C., Lumlertdaecha, B. *et al.* (1991). Immune response to rabies vaccine in Thai dogs: a preliminary report. *Vaccine*, **9**, 627–630.

Templeton, J. W., Holmberg, C. and Garber, T. (1986). Genetic control of serum neutralizing antibody response to rabies vaccination and survival after a rabies challenge infection in mice. *J. Virol.*, **59**, 98–102.

Thongcharoen, P. (1980). Prodrome and incubation period in human rabies. In: *Rabies* (P. Thongcharoen, ed). Bangkok: Aksarasamai. pp. 35–47.

Thoulouze, M. I., Lafage, M., Montano-Hirose, J. A. and Lafon, M. (1997). Rabies virus infects mouse and human lymphocytes and induces apoptosis. *J. Virol.*, **71**, 7372–7380.

Thoulouze, M.I., Lafage, M., Schachner, M. *et al.* (1998). The neural cell adhesion molecule is a receptor for rabies virus. *J. Virol.*, **72**, 7181–7190.

Threerasurakarn, S. and Ubol, S. (1998). Apoptosis induction in brain during the fixed strain of rabies virus infection correlates with onset and severity of illness. *J. Neurovirol.*, **4**, 407–414.

Tirawatnpong, S., Hemachudha, T., Manutsathit, S. *et al.* (1989). Regional distribution of rabies viral antigen in the central nervous system of human encephalitic and paralytic rabies. *J. Neurol. Sci.*, **92**, 91–99.

Tordo, N. (1996). Characteristics and molecular biology of the rabies virus. In: *Laboratory Technique in Rabies*, 4th edn (F. N. Meslin, M. M. Kaplan and H. Koprowski, eds). Geneva: World Health Organization. pp. 28–51.

Tordo, N. and Poch, O. (1988). Structure of rabies virus. In: *Rabies* (J. B. Campbell, K. M. Charlton, eds). Boston, MA: Kluwer Academic Publishers, pp. 25–45.

Torres-Anjel, M. J. and Volz, D. (1988). Failure to thrive, wasting syndrome, and immunodeficiency in rabies: a hypophyseal/hypothalamic-thymic axis effect of rabies. *Rev. Infect. Dis.*, **10**, 710–725.

Tsiang, H. (1979). Evidence for an intraxonal transport of fixed and street rabies virus. *J. Neuropathol. Exp. Neurol.*, **38**, 286–297.

Tsiang, H. (1982). Neuronal function impairment in rabies infected rat brain. *J. Gen. Virol.*, **61**, 277–281.

Tsiang, H. (1985). An in vitro study of rabies pathogenesis. *Bull. Inst. Pasteur.*, **83**, 41–56.

Tsiang, H. (1988). Interactions of rabies virus and host cells. In: *Rabies* (J. B. Campbell and K. M. Charlton, eds). Boston, MA: Kluwer Academic Publishers. pp. 67–100.

Tsiang, H. (1993). Pathophysiology of rabies virus infection of the nervous system. *Adv. Virus Res.*, **42**, 375–412.

Tsiang, H., Ceccaldi, P. E. and Lycke, E. (1991). Rabies virus infection and transport in human sensory dorsal root ganglia neurons. *J. Gen. Virol.*, **72**, 1191–1194.

Tsiang, H., Koulakoff, A. and Bizzini, B. (1983). Neurotropism of rabies virus. *J. Neuropathol. Exp. Neurol.*, **42**, 439–452.

Tsiang, H., Lycke, E., Ceccaldi, P. E. *et al.* (1989). The anterograde transport of rabies virus in rat sensory dorsal root ganglia neurons. *J. Gen. Virol.*, **70**, 2075–2085.

Ubol, S., Sukwattanapan, C. and Utaisincharoen, P. (1998). Rabies virus replication induces Bax-related, caspase dependent apoptosis in mouse neuroblastoma cells. *Virus Res.*, **56**, 207–215.

Van Dam, A. M., Bauer, J., Marquette, C. *et al.* (1995). Appearance of inducible nitric oxide synthase in the rat central nervous system after rabies virus infection and during experimental allergic encephalomyelitis but not after peripheral administration of endotoxin. *J. Neurosci. Res.*, **40**, 251–260.

Verline, J. D., Li-Fo-Sjoe, E., Veersteeg, J. and Decker, S. M. (1975). A local outbreak of paralytic rabies in Surinam chidren. *Trop. Geogr. Med.*, **27**, 137–142.

Vibulbandhitkij, S. (1980). Data from the rabies patients from Bumrasanaradura hospital between 1971–1977. In: *Rabies* (P. Thongcharoen, ed). Bangkok: Aksarasamai. pp. 235–251.

Warrell, D.A. (1976). The clinical picture of rabies in man. *Trans. R. Soc. Trop. Med. Hyg.*, **701**, 188–195.

Warrell, M. J., Looareesuwan, S., Manutsathit, S. *et al.* (1988). Rapid diagnosis of rabies and post-vaccinal encephalitis. *Clin. Exp. Immunol.*, **71**, 229–234.

Warrell, M. J., Ward, G. S., Elwell, M. R. and Tingpalapong, M. (1987). An attempt to treat rabies encephalitis in monkeys with intrathecal live rabies virus RV 675. *Arch. Virol.*, **96**, 271–173.

Weigent, D. A. and Blalock, J. E. (1996). Neuroendocrine peptide hormones and receptors in the immune response and infectious diseases. In: *Psychoneuroimmunology, Stress, and Infection* (H. Friedman, T. W. Klein and A.L. Freedman, eds). Boca Raton, FL: CRC Press, pp. 47–78.

Weiland, F., Cox, J. H., Meyer, S. *et al.* (1992). Rabies virus neuritic paralysis: immunopathogenesis of nonfatal paralytic rabies. *J. Virol.*, **66**, 5096–5099.

WHO (1992). 8th report of the WHO expert committee on rabies. *Technical report series*, no. 824. Geneva: WHO.

WHO (1993). Report of the symposium on rabies control in Asian countries. World Heath Organization unpublished document. WHO/Rab. Res/93.44.

WHO (1996a). World survey of rabies no. 30 (for the year 1994). World Health Organization unpublished document. WHO/EMC/ZOO/96.3.

WHO (1996b). WHO recommendation on rabies post-exposure treatment and the correct technique of intradermal immunization against rabies. WHO/EMC.ZOO 96.6.

WHO (1998). World survey of rabies no. 32 (for the year 1996). World Health Organization unpublished document. WHO/EMC/ZDI/98.4.

Wilde, H. (1997). Rabies 1996. *Intern. J. Infect. Dis.*, **1**, 135–142.

Wilson, J. M., Hettiarachchi, J. and Wijesuriya, I. M. (1975). Presenting features and diagnosis of rabies. *Lancet*, **2**, 1139–1140.

Winkler, W. G., Fashinell, T. R., Leffingwell, L. *et al.* (1973). Airborne rabies transmission in a laboratory worker. *J. Am. Med. Assoc.*, **226**, 1219–1221.

Xiang, Z. Q., Knowles, B. B., McCarrick, J. W. and Ertl, H. C. (1995). Immune effector mechanisms required for protection to rabies virus. *Virology*, **214**, 398–404.

Xiang, Z. Q., Spitalnik, S., Tran, M. *et al.* (1994). Vaccination with a plasmid vector carrying the rabies virus glycoprotein gene induces protective immunity against rabies virus. *Virology*, **199**, 132–140.

Yamamoto, T. and Ohtani, S. (1978). Ultrastructural localization of rabies virus antigens in infected trigeminal ganglion of hamsters. *Acta Neuropathol.*, **43**, 229–233.

Yusibov, V., Modelska, A., Steplewski, K. *et al.* (1997). Antigens produced in plants by infection with chimeric plant viruses immunize against rabies virus and HIV-1. *Proc. Natl Acad. Sci. USA*, **94**, 5784–5788.

14

Recurrent aseptic meningitis

Roberta L. DeBiasi and Kenneth L. Tyler

Definition of recurrent meningitis

Recurrent meningitis can be defined as two or more episodes of meningitis with an intervening disease-free interval, in which the patient is asymptomatic and cerebrospinal fluid studies are normal. Depending on the aetiology, there may be great variation in the duration of each episode (days to weeks), the disease-free interval (days to years), and the number of episodes. It is important to distinguish recurrent meningitis from chronic meningitis. In patients with chronic meningitis, CSF abnormalities are persistent, although in some patients clinical signs and symptoms may wax and wane giving the false impression of a recurrent rather than chronic process (Tucker and Ellner, 1993).

Recurrent meningitis may be bacterial or 'aseptic' in aetiology. In aseptic meningitis, no infectious organism is seen by Gram stain or isolated following bacterial culture of CSF. It is important to recognize that 'aseptic meningitis' is frequently a misnomer, as many infectious organisms, notably viruses and fungi, are important causes of 'aseptic' meningitis. Cases of aseptic meningitis are generally, but not invariably, associated with a CSF lymphocytic pleocytosis, normal glucose, and normal or mildly elevated protein. In contradistinction, almost all cases of recurrent bacterial meningitis show CSF findings typical of purulent meningitis including polymorphonuclear pleocytosis and hypoglycorrhachia. Identifying the agent(s) responsible for episodes of recurrent bacterial meningitis rarely poses a diagnostic dilemma, as almost all cases are associated with positive CSF cultures. The major issue is typically trying to identify the nature of host factors that predispose to recurrent bacterial CSF infection. Recurrent bacterial meningitis is almost always the result of an underlying immunodeficiency state (e.g. complement or immunoglobulin deficiency) or anatomical defect (e.g. Mondini malformation, traumatic basilar skull fracture) which allows direct communication between the subarachnoid space and a non-sterile site (reviewed in Kline, 1989; Adey and Wald, 1992; Schick *et al.* 1997). The subsequent discussion will focus exclusively on causes of recurrent aseptic meningitis which are summarized in Table 14.1 and 14.2.

Table 14.1   Causes of recurrent aseptic meningitis.

Idiopathic	Mollaret meningitis	
Infectious meningitis	Viral	Herpes simplex virus 1 and 2
		Enteroviruses
		Epstein-Barr virus
		HTLV-1 and Kikuchi's disease
	Other	*Cryptococcus neoformans*
		Borrelia burgdorferi
		Whipple's disease
Intracranial and intraspinal	Epidermoid and	
Tumours and cysts	Dermoid cysts	
	Other tumours	Craniopharyngioma
		Pituitary abscess
		Pituitary adenoma
		Glioblastoma
		Ependymoma
		Neurenteric cyst
		Neuroepithelial cyst
	Arteriovenous	Vein of Galen aneurysm
	Malformations	Cavernous haemangioma
Drug and chemical-induced	NSAIDS	Ibuprofen
		Sulindac
		Naproxen
		Tolmetin
	Antimicrobials	Trimethoprim-Sulfa
		Penicillin
		Cephalosporins
		Isoniazid
		Ciprofloxacin
	Miscellaneous	OKT3
		IVIG
		Carbamazepine
Recurrent inflammatory disease	Familial Mediterranean fever	
	Infantile inflammatory multisystem disease	
Connective tissue disorders	Systemic lupus erythematosus (SLE)	
	Sarcoidosis	
	Relapsing polychondritis	
	Mixed connective tissue disease (MCTD)	
Uveomeningitic syndromes	Vogt-Koyanagi-Harada	
	Behçet's syndrome	
Complement and immunoglobulin deficiency	Complement regulatory protein factor I deficiency	
	IgG subclass 3 deficiency	
Miscellaneous	Ferreol-Besnier disease	
	Headache with neurological deficits and CSF Lymphocytosis (HaNDL)	

General approach to patient with recurrent meningitis

Patients with a history of recurrent meningitis should undergo a complete general medical and neurological examination. Evaluation of cerebrospinal fluid and performance of appropriate imaging studies are essential features of the laboratory evaluation. Blood studies may also be helpful in certain

Table 14.2 Relative frequency of selected identifiable causes of recurrent aseptic meningitis*

Most Common	Herpes simplex virus
	Drug and chemical induced (especially NSAIOS and Trimethorprim-sulphamethoxazole)
Less common	Intracranial tumours and cysts
	Systemic lupus erythematosus
	Sarcoid
	Behçet's syndrome
Rare	Familial Mediterranean fever
	Uveomeningitic syndrome (Vogt-Koyanagi-Harada)
	Complement and immunoglobulin deficiency

* Epidemiological studies firmly establishing exact incidences have not been performed. Categorizaton is based on overall disease incidence, frequency of neurological involvement, and clinical experience.

conditions (Hermans *et al.* 1972; Baringer and Bell, 1993; Tucker and Ellner, 1993). Important aspects of this evaluation are summarized in Table 14.3.

Idiopathic: Mollaret meningitis

In a series of papers written in the 1940s, Pierre Mollaret described a syndrome of benign recurrent aseptic meningitis (Mollaret, 1944; Mollaret, 1945; Mollaret, 1952). Since his original description a variety of additional cases have been reported in the literature (reviewed in Hermans *et al.*, 1972; Mascia and Smith, 1984; Kwong *et al.*, 1988). There have been variations in the subsequent use of the term 'Mollaret meningitis'. Some authors have used the term to encompass essentially all idiopathic cases of recurrent aseptic meningitis, whereas others have limited its use to cases with specific clinical and CSF findings. Unfortunately, many cases were described before the advent of modern neuroimaging techniques and the availability of molecular biological tools such as CSF polymerase chain reaction (PCR) (Read *et al.*, 1997). It is likely that many cases of Mollaret meningitis described in the older literature would have been attributed to specific aetiologies if investigated using modern diagnostic tools. We suggest that the term Mollaret meningitis should be reserved for those cases of recurrent aseptic meningitis which remain of unknown aetiology after an appropriate diagnostic evaluation.

Although it is likely that cases included in the literature as Mollaret's meningitis represent a heterogeneous group of disorders, it is useful to review the clinical and laboratory features of this group, as it provides a basic overview of the syndrome of recurrent aseptic meningitis. In his 1993 review, Evans found fewer than 50 cases of Mollaret meningitis in the existing literature (Evans, 1993). Most patients present with the sudden onset of fever, nausea and vomiting, myalgia, headache, and meningismus. Kernig and Brudzinski signs occur with variable frequency. Focal neurological signs and symptoms are rarely present. There are isolated reports of patients with

Table 14.3   Evaluation of patient with recurrent aseptic meningitis.

Diagnostic category	Key findings	Disease implicated
Historical points		
● Drug Exposures	NSAIDS, trimethoprim/ sulpha, penicillin, cephalosporine isoniazid, OKT3, IVIG, carbamazepine	Drug induced aseptic meningitis
● Ethnicity	Israeli, Middle Eastern, Armenian, Greek	Familial Mediterranean fever (FMF)
	Japanese, Far Eastern, Mediterranean, Latin American	Uveomeningitic syndrome
	African American	Saroid
● Trauma	Chronic clear otorrhoea or rhinorrhoea	Anatomical CSF leak/bacterial
● Recurrent ulcers	Oral or genital – aphthous	Behçet's syndrome
	Oral or genital – blistering	Herpes simplex
● Disease-free interval	Important to distinguish chronic from recurrent episodes	
Physical exam		
● Skin	Depigmentation of hair, eyelashes (canities) and eyebrow (poliosis), skin (vitiligo), alopecia	Uveomeningitic syndrome
	Malar rash	Systemic lupus erythematosus (SLE)
	Dermal sinus tract/ectopic hair tuft ● Often at base of spine, midline spinal column, or posterior midline of skull	Intracranial epidermoid/dermoid
	Erythema migrans	*Borrelia burgdorferi* (Lyme disease)
	Palmar erythema and desquamation	Ferreol-Besnier disease
	Erythema nodosum	Sarcoid
	Thrombophlebitis	Behçet's syndrome
	Petechiae	Meningococal meningitis
	Oral/genital ulcers (see above)	Herpes simplex, Behçet's
● Ophthalmological	Uveitis	Sarcoid, Behçet's, uveomeningitic
	Choroidal tubercles	Sarcoid or tuberculosis (chronic)
	Papilloedema	Intracranial tumour
● Vital organs	Polyserositis:	FMF
	Pericardial or pleural rub, pleural effusion, heart murmur	SLE
	Organomegaly	
● Joints	Arthritis	Relapsing polychondritis, Behçet's, infantile inflammatory multi-system disease, FMF
● Neurological	Mental status	Generally unclouded in aseptic meningitis
	Nuchal rigidity/Kernig/Brudzinski signs	Non-specific
	Cranial nerve deficits	● Unusual with most recurrent aseptic meningitis and suggests chronic meningitis: e.g. syphilitic, tuberculous, fungal ● Exception: facial nerve: Lyme, sarcoid
	Focal deficits, visual field defects	Varies (see text)

Laboratory analysis

• Cerebrospinal fluid	Cell count/differential, glucose, protein		Varies with condition (see text)
	Xanthochromia		Recurrent subarachnoid bleed mimicking meningitis (e.g. AVM)
	Cytology	Large Mononuclear	Mollaret meningitis, non-specific
		Malignant	Malignancy
	Special stains	Gram, AFB	Bacterial/tuberculous meningitis
		India ink, Cryptococcal Ag	Cryptococcal menigitis
	Polymerase chain reaction		HSV, EBV, Enterovirus, *Borrelia burgdorferi* (Note: many others available for acute meningitis)
	CSF antibody studies		HSV, EBV, *Borrelia burgdorferi*, VDRL
	Culture: bacterial, viral, AFB, fungal		Viral culture insensitive
	CSF angiotensin converting enzyme		Sarcoid
• Blood	General: CBC/diff, ESR		Non-specific (see text)
	Haemoglobin electrophoresis		Sickle cell: recurrent bacterial
	Quantitative immunoglobulins		IgG3 deficiency: recurrent aseptic Other: recurrent bacterial
	Complement assays		C3b/C4b inactivator deficiency SLE Terminal complement deficiency (bacterial meningitis)
	ANA, rheumatoid factor		SLE
	Angiotensin converting enzyme		Sarcoid
	Antibody studies		*Borrelia burgdorferi*, Syphilis (VDRL/FTA-Ab), HSV, EBV, HIV
• Skin testing	Intradermal PPD		Tuberculous meningitis
	Anergy panel		If anergic: sarcoid

Radiological evaluation

• MRI	Special attention to skull base, posterior fossa and spinal canal	Intracranial and intraspinal tumours and cysts
• Computed tomography	Thin section bone windows through skull base	Occult basilar skull fracture
• Radioisotope cisternography		Cerebrospinal fluid fistula
• Chest AP/Lateral	Hilar adenopathy	Sarcoid, tuberculosis
	Pleural effusion	FMF, SLE
• Gallium scan	Diffuse uptake in lungs, parotids	Sarcoid

transient neurological disturbances including seizures, hallucinations, delirium, coma, diplopia, anisocoria, cranial nerve palsies and pathologic reflexes (Hermans *et al.*, 1972; Evans, 1993), but these abnormalities are distinctly unusual and their presence should strongly suggest consideration of other diagnoses. With the exception of fever, nausea, vomiting, and myalgia, systemic signs and symptoms are absent. Symptoms typically reach their peak within a few hours. Attacks last from a few days to a week with complete resolution of all signs, symptoms, and CSF abnormalities. The length of the asymptomatic interval between attacks is extremely variable, ranging from days or weeks to months and years. The symptom-free intervals may be longer at the beginning and in the later stages of the illness (Evans, 1993). The periodicity between attacks varies considerably both between patients and for an individual patient. Some patients with long-standing disease have noted a tendency for the attacks to become less frequent as time passes, but this is not invariable. Patients have been described with recurrent attacks occurring over nearly three decades (Tyler and Adler, 1983).

CSF findings typically consist of a pleocytosis of up to several thousand cells/μl with the remainder of CSF findings unremarkable. A mild elevation in CSF protein may occur. The presence of hypoglycorrhachia is distinctly unusual and should always raise the possibility of infectious or neoplastic meningitis. In some, but not all, cases there is a sequential progression over time in the predominant CSF cell type. Within the first 24 h pleocytosis may consist of a mixture of polymorphonuclear leucocytes (PMNs) and lympho-cytes. In some cases more than 50% of the cells are large, monocytoid cells, termed Mollaret cells. The percentage of Mollaret cells declines sharply after the first 24 h of illness. These cells are typically large (18 ± 3 μm in diameter) and irregularly round, with faint cytoplasm and fine vacuolation (Evans, 1993). They are fragile and stain only faintly, making them difficult to recognize and classify using automated cytological systems for counting and identifying CSF cells. Because of their fragility, the cells often fragment leaving behind ghost-like remnants (Hermans et al., 1972). The presence of these cells may be missed entirely if CSF is not obtained early during an attack and examined promptly. Although Mollaret speculated that these cells were endothelial in origin, subsequent electron microscopy and immunocytochem-ical studies (de Chadarevian and Becker, 1980b; Stoppe et al., 1987; Teot and Sexton, 1996) have indicated that the Mollaret cell is actually of monocyte/macrophage lineage, with characteristics of an activated monocyte (Evans, 1993). It is important to recognize that Mollaret cells are not invariably present in cases classified as Mollaret meningitis, nor are they pathognomonic for this disorder (de Chadarevian and Becker, 1980a; Crossley and Dismukes, 1990). Indistinguishable cells have been described in patients with CSF tumours and other conditions (Hermans et al., 1972). With the exception of CSF findings, laboratory studies are generally unremarkable and rarely help in the diagnosis. Some patients have a mild peripheral leukocytosis and elevated sedimentation rate.

Studies of the immunological status of patients with Mollaret's meningitis have yielded conflicting and inconsistent results. The vast majority of patients are apparently immunocompetent and lack immunological abnormalities that would explain their recurrent attacks of meningitis. There is one report of a patient with increased numbers of circulating natural killer cells during an acute attack , with normal cell numbers found 3 months later (Goldstein et al., 1986). Some patients have been reported to have elevated CSF levels of immunoglobulins (IgG), cytokines (IL-6, TNF-alpha) or other mediators (prostaglandin E2) during attacks, but data are insufficient to determine the frequency or significance of these findings.

Since the initial description by Mollaret, the pathophysiological basis of Mollaret meningitis remains obscure. Mollaret speculated about the possible role of infectious agents. As more sensitive diagnostic tests (e.g. CSF PCR) became available, subsets of cases thought to fit generally accepted diagnostic criteria for Mollaret meningitis were found to be due to herpes simplex virus (described below). Improved neuroimaging techniques including use of sequential MRI, have also led to the identification of epidermoid and other tumours in some patients (described below). Despite these advances, some cases of recurrent meningitis remain of undetermined aetiology despite exhaustive investigation. The lack of understanding about the aetiology and pathogenesis of idiopathic cases of recurring aseptic meningitis has limited investigation of treatment. A variety of treatments including antibiotics, steroids, oestrogen, and antihistamines (Tyler and Adler, 1983) have been tried in individual patients with Mollaret (idiopathic) recurrent aseptic meningitis without obvious benefit. However, specific treatments may be of benefit to patients with identifiable causes of their recurrent episodes of aseptic meningitis (see subsequent sections).

Infectious recurrent aseptic meningitis

Perhaps the single most important contribution to the understanding of recurrent meningitis has been the recognition, using newer diagnostic techniques (such as PCR), that viruses are the most frequent cause of benign recurrent 'aseptic' meningitis. As diagnostic techniques become even more sensitive, it is likely that additional infectious agents may be implicated in previously 'idiopathic' syndromes. Rare cases of recurrent aseptic meningitis caused by infectious agents may be due to fungi or bacteria rather than viruses. Among the non-viral agents most frequently implicated are *Cryptococcus neoformans* and *Borrelia burgdorferi*. It is important to emphasize that non-viral agents such as these more typically cause either acute or chronic symptoms, rather than recurrent meningitis.

Recurrent viral meningitis may be subdivided into two major categories: the first type is characterized by recurrent meningitis with each episode caused by a different virus; the second type is due to repeated episodes of meningitis caused by the same virus.

Recurrent aseptic meningitis with each episode due to a different virus is distinctly unusual. In large series of viral meningitis cases, less than 4% of patients were found to have had two or more episodes (Anderson, 1969; Klemola and Lapinleimu, 1964; Nakao and Miura, 1971). The overwhelming majority of these patients were children who experienced two episodes of viral meningitis with intervals of 1 month to 4 years between attacks. There have been rare instances of apparently immunocompetent patients who have a history of three or even four attacks of viral meningitis. In patients with recurrent viral meningitis, like their counterparts with single episodes of viral meningitis, *enteroviruses* are the most commonly implicated group of viruses. The enteroviral strains most commonly isolated are coxsackie A9, B2, B3, B5, echovirus 4, 5, 6, 7, 14, 25, 30 and poliovirus type 3, as well as mumps virus. In no case did the same virus produce more than one episode of meningitis. (Herpes simplex viruses and Epstein-Barr virus are the only viruses known to cause multiple episodes of meningitis in the same patient – described below.)

Clinical and laboratory features of these cases were unremarkable, with no increased frequency of underlying immunodeficiency, although immunological investigations were often rudimentary. This is an important point, since chronic enteroviral meningoencephalitis can occur in patients with agammaglobulinaemia (McKinney et al., 1987). In a more recent report of two normal infants with recurrent episodes of enteroviral meningitis with an interval of 1 month, sequence analysis of PCR products clearly demonstrated that the enteroviral strains causing each attack of meningitis were distinct (O'Neil et al., 1988; Aintablian et al., 1995).

Herpes simplex viruses (HSV) are the most common aetiological agents implicated when recurrent episodes of aseptic meningitis are caused by the same organism, and are almost certainly the single most common cause of benign recurrent aseptic meningitis. Following primary infection, herpes simplex viruses become latent in neural tissue, and have the capacity to reactivate periodically to produce recurrent acute episodes of disease. In adults, HSV type 2 is classically associated with aseptic meningitis, although it also accounts for about 10% of cases of HSV-related encephalitis. Conversely, HSV type 1 is more commonly associated with encephalitis and less frequently with aseptic meningitis (Craig and Nahmias, 1973; Schlesinger et al., 1995). However, this distinction is not invariant. In fact, the first virus to be isolated from a patient with recurrent aseptic meningitis was HSV-1 (Steel et al., 1982). This patient had experienced four episodes of meningitis during an 8-year period. During each episode, there was a CSF lymphocytic pleocytosis (300–900 cells/µl), a slightly elevated protein (<100 mg/dl) and a normal glucose. At the time of the last reported attack, increased CSF IgG concentration and IgG/albumin ratio were also noted. Monolayers of human embryonic lung (HEL) cells inoculated with this CSF developed cytopathic effect. The presence of HSV-specific antigens was confirmed by indirect fluorescent antibody tests and by analysis of ^{14}C-labelled polypeptides synthesized in infected cells. The role of HSV in benign recurrent aseptic meningitis has been substantially advanced by studies of patients with genital HSV infections and the application of CSF PCR for HSV DNA for diagnosis (described below).

At the time of their first episode of genital herpes, approximately 36% of women and 11% of men have symptoms of meningitis including fever, headache and nuchal rigidity (Corey et al., 1983). Approximately 20% of these patients subsequently develop recurrent episodes of meningitis. Bergstrom has reviewed the clinical and laboratory features of primary and recurrent HSV-2 meningitis (Bergstrom et al., 1990). During their first attack of meningitis, patients had a mean cell count of 431 ± 316 cells/µl (mean 85% lymphocytes) and protein of 160 ± 100 mg/dl. In subsequent attacks, the magnitude of the CSF pleocytosis and protein elevation diminished, with mean values of 280 ± 170 cells/µl (mean 94% lymphocytes) and protein of 100 ± 30 mg/dl. A critical diagnostic point was that although HSV-2 was frequently isolated (78%) and HSV-2 antigen was frequently detectable (71%) in CSF during the first episode of meningitis, cultures were never positive, nor was antigen detectable, in recurrent attacks. Conversely, evidence of CSF antibody to the HSV-2 type-specific G-2 antigen was found in only 11% of patients at the time of initial episode, but in 100% at the time of recurrences. Additional neurological complications were found concomitantly with meningitis in 37% of patients, including urinary retention, dysaesthesia, paraesthesia, neuralgia, motor weakness, and paraparesis, but subsided by 6 months in all patients. There was no correlation between the presence of these symptoms during the initial episode and their occurrence with later episodes of meningitis. This study clearly established that HSV-2 is a frequent cause of recurrent episodes of lymphocytic meningitis in patients with genital herpes, but also highlighted the inadequacy of CSF culture and antigen detection in making the diagnosis during recurrences.

With the development of sensitive PCR techniques, there have subsequently been many reports describing detection of HSV-2 specific (Picard *et al.*, 1993; Chambers *et al.*, 1994; Cohen *et al.*, 1994; Tedder *et al.*, 1994; Schlesinger *et al.*, 1995; Monteyne *et al.*, 1996) and, less commonly, HSV-1 specific DNA (Yamamoto *et al.*, 1991) in the CSF of patients with benign recurrent meningitis. We recently reported on the use of PCR to detect HSV-specific DNA in a group of 13 patients with benign recurrent lymphocytic meningitis, the largest such series described to date (Tedder *et al.*, 1994). Only 23% had a history of genital herpes, and none had lesions concurrent with their most recent episode of meningitis. Patients ranged in age from 26 to 73 (mean 39) years, were predominantly female (69%) and had experienced 3–9 (mean 4.6) attacks of meningitis over a period of 2–23 years (mean 8.4). Their CSF profiles were quite similar to that reported by Bergstrom (Bergstrom *et al.*, 1990): mean cell counts were 443 cells/μl (range 48–1600) with 58–98% lymphocytes. Protein was elevated in 85% (maximum 240 mg/dl) with normal glucose in all cases. Of the patients, 85% had HSV-specific DNA detectable in CSF by PCR, of which 91% were of the HSV-2 type. All patients with HSV-2 DNA by PCR also had HSV G-2 type specific antibodies detected in CSF. Two patients were G-2 antibody positive, but had negative PCRs.

In summary, these studies establish a number of important points: (1) among patients meeting specified diagnostic criteria who are experiencing recurrent episodes of benign lymphocytic meningitis, HSV appears to be the most important aetiological agent; (2) although HSV-1 may account for a small fraction of these cases, most are due to HSV-2; (3) episodes of recurrent HSV-2 meningitis can occur in patients without a history of genital herpes and without concurrent genital lesions, (4) viral culture is invariably negative during all but the first episode of HSV-2 induced meningitis; and (5) PCR amplification of HSV-specific DNA from CSF is a rapid and sensitive method for establishing the diagnosis. Detection of HSV-2 G-2 type-specific antibody intrathecally appears to be equally sensitive for diagnosis.

Treatment of acute episodes of herpes meningitis with intravenous acyclovir has been utilized and may decrease the duration and severity of symptoms. In patients with recurrent episodes, intermittent or continuous prophylaxis with oral acyclovir has been employed with possibly beneficial effects (Bergstrom and Alestig, 1990). Newer agents with improved oral absorption such as valacyclovir and famciclovir will likely play a greater role in the future. Duration of therapy may soon be determined by sequential measurements of CSF HSV DNA using PCR. The implications of PCR surveillance are being studied, especially with regard to neurological outcomes in recurrent HSV disease of neonates (Kimberlin *et al.*, 1996).

Epstein-Barr virus (EBV), the common causal agent of acute infectious mononucleosis, only rarely involves the central nervous system (<1% of infections). One of the most frequent neurological complications of EBV infection is aseptic meningitis. The vast majority of these cases are single episodes of acute aseptic meningitis. However, there are two reports of recurrent aseptic meningitis associated with EBV infection. One report describes a 19 year-old man who had an initial episode of aseptic meningitis coincident with primary EBV infection (Graman, 1987). He then went on to suffer seven subsequent episodes, each lasting 3–5 days, over a 1-year period. During attacks, he had a CSF pleocytosis (115–1045 cells/μl), with initial PMN predominance and subsequent transition to lymphocytes, an elevated CSF protein (62–284 mg/dl) and a normal glucose. Serum EBV titres were consistent with acute infection and included elevated IgM antibodies specific for the viral capsid antigen (VCA). Low titres of EBV-specific antibody were also found in his CSF. The patient's symptoms and CSF abnormalities resolved between episodes. The authors considered this a case of Mollaret meningitis, with EBV serving as inciting agent. They suggested that recurrent meningeal inflammation might result from reactivation of latent virus, perhaps localized in the CNS, although they provided no data to substantiate this theory. In the other reported case, a 17-year-old male with primary EBV infection and associated aseptic meningitis went on to have two subsequent episodes separated by asymptomatic intervals of 1 month and 2 years (Takeuchi *et al.*, 1989).

It would appear from these studies that EBV can cause recurrent episodes of aseptic meningitis. Establishment of the diagnosis may be difficult. Virus is almost never cultured from CSF in patients with EBV-associated aseptic meningitis. Serological studies may substantiate the presence of acute EBV infection (fourfold rise in VCA IgG or positive VCA IgM). Comparison of CSF and serum antibody titres may establish the presence of intrathecal synthesis of EBV-specific antibodies. CSF PCR to detect EBV DNA has greatly facilitated diagnosis of EBV-related CNS disease including acute meningitis (Landgren *et al.*, 1994), but positive CSF EBV PCR results have not yet been reported in patients with recurrent meningitis.

There is one described case of recurrent *histiocytic necrotizing lymphadenitis* (HNL or Kikuchi disease) associated with recurrent aseptic meningitis (Atarashi *et al.*, 1996). The patient was a 46-year-old male carrier of HTLV-I virus with a past history of at least three relapses of HNL. His sister, who was also an HTLV-I carrier, also had recurrent clinical episodes consistent with those of HNL. Kikuchi disease is a benign disorder of lymph nodes. Nodes show focal reticulum cell hyperplasia combined with patchy areas of coagulative necrosis (Unger *et al.*, 1987; Dorfman, 1987). Clinical features consist of localized, sometimes tender cervical lymphadenopathy, often associated with an upper respiratory prodrome and in some patients, with fever. The authors suggested the possibility that HTLV-I infection is relevant to the pathogenesis of HNL, although serological and ultrastructural studies have failed to confirm a specific agent in this syndrome.

There is one case report of a patient who suffered recurrent episodes of aseptic lymphocytic meningitis over many years and subsequently developed amyotrophic lateral sclerosis (ALS) (Norris *et al.*, 1975). At post-mortem there was evidence of both lymphocytic meningitis and ALS. Study of the motor neurons with electron microscopy revealed large masses of interwoven serpentine 10–15 nm tubules in some neurons that were suggested to represent viral structures. No other evidence of viral infection was found. No subsequent cases of this type have been described. Despite this single report, it is important to emphasize that the vast majority of patients with recurrent lymphocytic meningitis have a benign prognosis and do not subsequently develop either neurological sequelae or other illnesses (Tyler and Adler, 1983).

Cryptococcus neoformans is an important fungal pathogen, which commonly causes either acute or chronic meningitis. Rare cases of cryptococcal meningitis have been described in which the clinical course and laboratory features were consistent with recurrent episodes of meningitis rather than chronic infection. Examples of recurrent infection resulting from both infection with different strains of *Cryptococcus neoformans* and from re-infection with the same strain of *Cryptococcus neoformans* have been reported. Recurrences over long periods of time, even up to 6 years, have been reported (Woo and Wong, 1987). Sullivan and colleagues recently studied genomic DNA finger-printing analysis of cryptococcal DNA isolated from two HIV-positive patients who had experienced recurrent episodes of cryptococcal meningitis (Sullivan *et al.*, 1996). In one patient, the same strain persisted and caused both episodes, whereas in the other patient, a different strain was responsible for each episode. The prevalence of polymorphisms in multiple single-colony isolates from both patients also suggested that *Cryptococcus neoformans* populations may undergo microevolution. Cherniak also addressed this issue by evaluating the capsular polysaccharide glucoronoxylomannans (GXM) of isolates from patients with recurrent cryptococcal meningitis by NMR spectroscopy (Cherniak *et al.*, 1995). He found that cryptococcal isolates from later episodes had undergone a change in GSM structure compared to isolates from earlier episodes, and that this altered GSM structure affected serological properties. In distinction to these results, Magee reported a case of recurrent cryptococcal disease (2-year interval) in which isolates from each episode were characterized by pyrolysis mass spectrometry and were found to be indistinguishable from each other (Magee *et al.*, 1994). Spitzer found similar results in 11 isolates from four patients with recurrent meningitis evaluated by pulsed-field electrophoresis (Spitzer *et al.*, 1993). This suggests that cases of recurrent cryptococcal meningitis may also result from reactivation of sequestered foci of infection.

Almost all cases of recurrent cryptococcal meningitis have occurred in immunocompromised individuals, including those with HIV infection. It is predominantly in this population that cryptococcal infection should be considered as a diagnostic possibility in cases of recurrent meningitis. CSF analysis in cases of recurrent meningitis does not differ from that in acute or chronic disease. Most patients have an elevated opening pressure, lymphocytic leucocytosis ($\geq$ 20 cells/µl), elevated protein and decreased glucose. Diagnosis is rarely difficult. The presence of hypoglycorrhachia helps distinguish recurrent cryptococcal meningitis from cases of recurrent viral meningitis. Almost all patients will have a positive CSF cryptococcal antigen and CSF cultures are frequently positive. The yield of CSF cultures is enhanced by inoculating large volumes of CSF; ventricular or cisternal CSF may be culture positive when lumbar CSF is sterile.

Treatment of recurrent cryptococcal infection in immunocompromised patients is evolving. Bozzette studied AIDS patients who had completed standard therapy for primary cryptococcal meningitis and were subsequently assigned randomly to maintenance therapy with either fluconazole or placebo (Bozzette *et al.*, 1991). Of the patients receiving placebo, 37% had recurrence of cryptococcal infection at any site, including 15% with recurrent meningitis. Only 3% of patients receiving maintenance fluconazole (100–200 mg qd) had recurrence of infection in the CNS or at any body site. This suggests that maintenance therapy with fluconazole is highly effective in preventing recurrences of cryptococcal meningitis.

Aseptic meningitis is one of the common CNS manifestations of infection with *Borrelia burgdorferi* (Lyme neuroborreliosis). The possibility of Lyme disease should be strongly considered in patients with a history of tick exposure, erythema migrans or arthritis. However, it is important to recognize that neuroborreliosis can occur in the absence of any of these features. Meningitis associated with Lyme disease is typically either acute or chronic rather than recurrent. Although many patients with chronic Lyme meningitis have fluctuations in clinical signs and symptoms, documented recurrent episodes of meningitis appear to be extremely rare. There is a brief report of a 55-year-old man who had three episodes of aseptic meningitis within a 2-year period, with symptom-free periods of 7 and 16 months (Pal *et al.*, 1987). His symptoms were attributed to Lyme disease based on a positive indirect immunofluorescence antibody test and a compatible exposure history. CSF findings included lymphocytic pleocytosis of < 500 cells/µl, normal or mildly elevated protein (< 100 mg/dl), and normal glucose.

The diagnosis of recurrent Lyme meningitis may be exceedingly difficult. Infection with *Borrelia burgdorferi* is documented by positive serology. ELISAs are commonly used in screening serological tests, but positive results should always be confirmed by Western blotting (American College of Physicians, 1997; Tugwell *et al.*, 1997). The presence of Western blot confirmed seropositivity is indicative of exposure to *Borrelia burgdorferi*, but is not sufficient definitively to diagnose neuroborreliosis. Unequivocal diagnosis of neuroborreliosis requires demonstration of intrathecal synthesis of *Borrelia burgdorferi* specific antibody, demonstration of *Borrelia burgdorferi* nucleic acid in CSF by PCR, or positive CSF cultures, in a compatible clinical setting (Garcia-Monco and Benach, 1995). CSF PCR, although likely to be extremely specific for the diagnosis of neuroborreliosis, is of uncertain sensitivity. CSF cultures may require special techniques and are not routinely available in many clinical laboratories.

Because of these issues, controversy continues about appropriate criteria for diagnosis of neuroborreliosis in patients who lack evidence of CSF antibody production, nucleic acid or positive cultures. Once diagnosis has been established, intravenous administration of a third generation cephalosporin, such as ceftriaxone (2 g i.v. given in 2 divided doses), is generally considered the treatment of choice. Alternative regimens include intravenous penicillin G (5–6 million units Q6h) and oral doxycycline (200 mg/day) (Karlsson et al., 1994). Appropriate and optimal duration of therapy has not been conclusively established, but most regimens involve a minimum of 14 days up to 28 days of antimicrobials.

Whipple's disease is a rare disorder characterized by gastrointestinal symptoms, arthralgia, lymphadenopathy, skin hyperpigmentation and, in some cases, signs of CNS involvement (Knox et al., 1976; Pollock et al., 1981; Halperin et al., 1982; Relman, 1997). Gastrointestinal symptoms include abdominal pain, diarrhoea and progressive weight loss, as well as hypoalbuminaemia and steatorrhoea. Neurological complications include encephalopathy, dementia, limbic encephalitis, cranial nerve palsies, supranuclear ophthalmoplegia, ataxia, myoclonus, and oculomasticatory myorhythmia. Cases presenting as isolated aseptic meningitis are unusual. Rare cases in which manifestations appear limited to the CNS have been reported, but are unusual. Recurrent episodes of meningitis can apparently occur, although documentation of such cases is sketchy (Knox et al., 1976). Typical CSF findings in patients with Whipple's disease and aseptic meningitis include mild lymphocytic pleocytosis (< 50 cells/µl) and elevated protein. Some patients with neurological involvement have had normal CSF findings or only a mildly increased CSF protein concentration. Diagnosis has until recently depended on the demonstration of macrophages containing periodic acid Schiff (PAS) positive material in intestinal biopsy or other tissue specimens (reviewed in Louis et al., 1996). Electron microscopy of tissue may demonstrate the presence of rod-shaped (bacilliform) bodies within macrophages. Recent studies have identified the bacteria responsible for Whipple's disease as *Tropherema whippelii*. PCR tests to amplify *T. whippelii* nucleic acid have been designed, and applied to a variety of tissues and body fluids including CSF. Although these tests appear promising, the sensitivity and specificity of CSF PCR for the diagnosis of CNS Whipple's disease remains to be established (Lynch et al., 1997). As noted, cases of isolated CNS Whipple's disease have been described, but definitive diagnosis is difficult and generally requires CNS tissue specimens obtained by biopsy or at necropsy. Treatment of CNS Whipple's disease has included trimethoprim-sulphamethoxazole (one DS tablet p.o. b.i.d.), chloramphenicol (250 mg p.o. q.i.d.), and more recently ceftriaxone (2 grams i.v. b.i.d.). Reports of progressive neurological disease following penicillin and tetracycline therapy suggest that these drugs may be less suitable. Therapy must be continued for prolonged periods, perhaps up to a year, to prevent relapse.

Intracranial and intraspinal tumours and cysts

Although CNS *epidermoid and dermoid tumours* constitute only 1% of all intracranial tumours, and fewer than 1% of intraspinal tumours, they form the most important subgroup of intracranial lesions associated with recurrent episodes of aseptic meningitis (Achard *et al.*, 1990; Kriss *et al.*, 1995). Recurrent aseptic meningitis has also been reported due to an intraspinal *cystic teratoma* (Larbrisseau *et al.*, 1980). Epidermoids usually occur intracranially in the cerebellar-pontine angle or parasellar region, whereas dermoids are more commonly seen in the lumbar spine or posterior fossa (Kriss *et al.*, 1995). These tumours are not true neoplasms, but are developmental tumours caused by the inclusion of epidermal or dermal elements within the neuroaxis during embryogenesis when the ectoderm folds into a neural tube. A dermal sinus tract is created if there is incomplete fusion of the dorsal folds of the neuroectoderm, whereas complete closure yields an occult epidermoid or dermoid. Although most epidermoids are developmental, they can also be caused by antecedent lumbar puncture, specifically those performed using spinal needles with poorly fitted stylets. A similar entity located within the middle ear, known as *perichiasmatic granuloma* can occur as a complication of radical mastoidectomy (Djouhri *et al.*, 1998).

These tumours gradually enlarge and shed keratinized cells, which are subsequently degraded into cholesterol and fat. In addition to epidermal cells and epidermal debris, dermoid tumours may also contain hair, sebaceous glands, or connective tissue elements. Periodic rupture of the tumour or cyst allows entry of its contents into the subarachnoid space, triggering a chemical meningitis. Symptoms are usually of acute onset, and include fever, headache and meningismus. In most cases these symptoms resolve within 48–72 h of onset. Although these are space occupying masses, they rarely produce focal neurological deficits due to their thin capsule and malleability which allows the tumours to conform to the confines of the space in which they occur. In addition to being associated with aseptic meningitis, patients can develop recurrent bouts of bacterial meningitis. In these cases, the presence of a dermal sinus tract can serve as a neurocutaneous fistula, allowing access of bacteria (commonly *Staphylococcus aureus*) from the skin to the CSF. All patients with recurrent aseptic meningitis should be carefully examined for the presence of occult midline sinus tracts. These may be very difficult to identify, as they frequently appear as tiny dimples often associated with a tuft of hair.

CT and MRI have greatly facilitated diagnosis of epidermoid and dermoid tumours, and should be performed in all patients with recurrent episodes of aseptic meningitis. Some patients in whom a lesion is ultimately identified will initally have a series of negative studies. Some case reports describe as many as 20–30 attacks over a period of years before the lesions were successfully located (Becker *et al.*, 1984; Crossley and Dismukes, 1990; Kitai *et al.*, 1992). Several authors suggest that MRI is preferably performed at a time when patients are asymptomatic, to maximize yield. It has been suggested that at the time of an episode of meningitis, the cyst presumably may have discharged its contents and deflated, making it less visible on MRI (Aristegui *et al.*, 1998).

MRI can occasionally confirm cyst rupture by demonstrating fat droplets dispersed throughout the subarachnoid space (appearing as hypodense lesions) (Achard *et al.*, 1990).

Special CSF cytological studies may also facilitate diagnosis of dermoids tumours and epidermoid cysts. Although they are difficult to identify unless specifically searched for, the presence of fat droplets, cholesterol crystals, keratin debris, or epithelial cells on cytological examination of CSF, is virtually pathognomonic of dermoid tumour or epidermal cyst. The use of polarized light may assist visualization of keratin and cholesterol crystals in CSF. The CSF generally shows several thousand cells/μl, usually with PMN predominance shifting to lymphocytic predominance. Additional CSF findings frequently include elevated protein and mildly decreased glucose (Becker *et al.*, 1984; Achard *et al.*, 1990). Large activated macrophages have also been described, which appear indistinguishable from Mollaret cells (Carrazana *et al.*, 1989; Crossley and Dismukes, 1990). Definitive therapy of attacks of recurrent aseptic meningitis requires identification and surgical removal of the offending cyst or tumour, and correction of associated sinus tract (if present). Since the attacks of meningitis represent a reaction to chemical irritation, steroids may be useful in treatment of acute attacks or perioperatively to help reduce the severity of this inflammatory response (Becker *et al.*, 1984).

Other tumours. Pituitary and parapituitary lesions can all produce isolated episodes of aseptic meningitis, and less commonly recurrent episodes. *Craniopharyngiomas* may cause recurrent aseptic meningitis by mechanisms similar to those described for epidermoid tumours. CSF cell counts during attacks of meningitis can be in excess of 20 000 cells/μl with PMNs predominating early, shifting to lymphocytes. In one case of a ruptured craniopharyngioma, the CSF was described as 'brownish, turbid and containing small and large fat droplets' and the protein concentration was 7500 mg/dl! (Patrick *et al.*, 1974). Spontaneous haemorrhage into or infarction of a *pituitary adenoma* (pituitary apoplexy) may also lead to aseptic meningitis, presumably by allowing entry of necrotic tumour debris or blood products into the CSF. *Pituitary abscess* may also be associated with recurrent episodes of aseptic lymphocytic meningitis (Ford *et al.*, 1986; Guillaume *et al.*, 1990). The presence of visual field abnormalities, abnormalities in extraocular movements, or symptoms of pituitary hypofunction in conjunction with aseptic meningitis should suggest the possibility of pituitary apoplexy or abscess. Endocrine abnormalities may include decreased thyroid hormone and TSH, elevated prolactin, decreased follicle stimulating (FSH) and luteinizing hormone (LH), and low cortisol and ACTH. MRI and CT are clearly superior to plain radiographs in identifying pituitary lesions. In most cases, CT will detect the presence of a pituitary lesion, but MRI appears to allow for better identification of haemorrhagic changes within the lesion and better delineation of the exact anatomic extent of the mass. Treatment of pituitary apoplexy typically involves the urgent administration of stress doses of corticosteroids and trans-sphenoidal decompression of the pituitary mass. In patients with visual impairment, surgical decompression should be performed emergently. Many patients will require chronic replacement of pituitary hormones including steroids, thyroid hormone, and gonadotropins. Management of pituitary abscess includes the use of intravenous antibiotics in conjunction with surgical drainage.

Glioblastoma multiforme may be associated with a CSF pleocytosis and occasionally with symptoms of meningeal irritation, but cases of recurrent episodes of meningitis are exceedingly rare (Bernat, 1976). These tumours, by nature of their high grade malignancy accumulate abundant necrotic material or cystic components, which may rupture into the lateral or third ventricles, gaining access to the CSF. *Ependymomas* and *astrocytomas* appear to produce meningitis only rarely, and only isolated cases of each are available in the literature (Lunardi *et al.*, 1989). In all cases the tumours have been located in the posterior fossa.

Neuroepithelial cysts have been reported to occur in association with recurrent aseptic meningitis. These lesions are thought to be of developmental origin, arising from the choroid plexus or ependyma (Kuroda *et al.*, 1991). *Neurenteric cysts* have also been identified as a cause of recurrent aseptic meningitis. Weiss reported a case diagnosed by MRI, which was located posterior to the cervicomedullary junction (Weiss *et al.*, 1996).

There is one reported case of an *arteriovenous malformation* (AVM) feeding into a *vein of Galen aneurysm*, presenting with recurrent episodes of aseptic meningitis (Collins and Fisher, 1990). The mechanism responsible for these episodes remains unclear, although it was suggested that transient episodes of partial venous thrombosis involving the fistula with resultant inflammatory reaction may have played a role. The episodes of meningitis were accompanied by fever and abated spontaneously over several days. CSF analysis revealed a lymphocytic pleocytosis, mildly elevated protein and normal or mildly decreased glucose. CT scan disclosed the mass with confirmation by angiography. MRI showed the AVM feeding into a markedly dilated vein of Galen. A patient with nine episodes of lymphocytic meningitis over a 24-year period caused by a *cavernous haemangioma* has also been reported. The haemangioma was located in the lateral ventricle and was identified by MRI (Frieden *et al.*, 1990).

Drug and chemical induced meningitis

There are two mechanisms by which drugs can cause aseptic meningitis: through immune-mediated hypersensitivity reactions; or by direct chemical irritation of the meninges following cisternal, ventricular or intrathecal administration (Marinac, 1992). Unlike hypersensitivity reactions, which tend to occur immediately following drug exposure, direct meningeal irritation may be delayed up to several weeks following administration of the drug. Detergents, preservatives, radiographic contrast dyes, chemotherapeutic agents and talc have all been described to cause aseptic meningitis in this manner, generally after direct instillation into CSF. A variety of factors mediate the meningeal toxicity of drugs, including their CSF concentration, lipid solubility, particle size, ionization state, and duration of contact with the CSF (Marinac, 1992).

The drugs most commonly implicated in drug-induced hypersensitivity meningitis include the non-steroidal anti-inflammatory agents (NSAIDS), antimicrobial agents, murine monoclonal antibodies (e.g. anti-CD3), and intravenous immunoglobulins (see below). There are also two reports of carbamazepine-associated aseptic meningitis (Marinac, 1992). Drug-induced hypersensitivity meningitis typically produces a fulminant and extremely rapid (minutes to hours) onset of symptoms on re-exposure to the offending agent. Resolution of signs and symptoms of meningitis generally occurs over a period of a few days to a week following discontinuation of the agent. The exact mechanism of drug-induced hypersensitivity type aseptic meningitis is unknown (see below). Most cases do not appear to result from IgE-mediated type-1 hypersensitivity reactions, as associated systemic symptoms of hypersensitivity including urticaria, pruritus, and bronchospasm are extremely rare. Many types of drug-induced hypersensitivity meningitis, including those associated with antibiotics and non-steroidal anti-inflammatory agents are associated with intrathecal IgG synthesis and the formation of CSF immune complexes (Creel and Hurtt, 1995). In some cases antigen–antibody complexes composed of drug and drug-specific antibody have been detected in CSF, in other cases an immunological response triggered by the offending drug results in the generation of cross-reacting antibody reactive with CNS antigens. Stimulation of pre-existing anti-tissue antibody within the CNS has also been suggested as a possible mechanism (Chez et al. 1989).

NSAIDs are the most frequently implicated class of drugs causing hypersensitivity meningitis (Bouland *et al.*, 1986; Greenberg, 1988; Mifsud, 1988). In a recent review tabulating numbers of reported cases by drug, the most common inciting agents were ibuprofen (31 reports), sulindac (four), naproxen (two), and tolmetin (one) (Marinac, 1992). Ibuprofen-induced aseptic meningitis, the most common and best studied of the NSAID-associated hypersensitivity meningitides, typically occurs within weeks of beginning therapy. Common symptoms include fever, headache, stiff neck and vomiting. Patients can also develop arthralgias and myalgias, diffuse maculopapular rash, periorbital oedema, conjunctivitis, hypotension, parotitis, pericarditis, pancreatitis, pruritus, and liver function abnormalities. In rare cases, neurological symptoms such as dizziness, confusion, lethargy, obtundation, and even coma have been reported. CSF findings include leucocytosis (31–2500 cells/µl), typically with PMN predominance, elevated protein and normal to slightly depressed glucose.

The majority of patients who develop aseptic meningitis following exposure to one NSAID do not experience similar episodes with other NSAIDS, but exceptions do occur (Ruppert and Barth, 1981). The absence of cross-reactivity suggests that the mechanism of meningitis induction is not related to direct pharmacological actions of NSAIDS (e.g. prostaglandin inhibition). In one patient with ibuprofen-induced aseptic meningitis a specific cell-mediated immune response to ibuprofen was demonstrated by a macrophage migration inhibition test (Shoenfeld *et al.*, 1980). Several patients have been reported to have elevated intrathecal IgG synthesis and immune complex formation (Chez *et al.*, 1989) which normalize during the post-meningitis asymptomatic period. However, not all patients have demonstrable CSF immune complexes, suggesting that other mechanisms may be operative in inducing this syndrome (Widener and Littman, 1978). Interestingly, an increased susceptibility to NSAID-induced aseptic meningitis has been noted in patents with underlying collagen vascular or rheumatological diseases, most commonly systemic lupus erythematosus (SLE) (Ruppert and Barth, 1981). SLE or other collagen or rheumatological disease was found in 75% of reported cases in a recent series of drug-induced hypersensitivity meningitis (Marinac, 1992). Interestingly, mice prone to spontaneous development of a SLE-like syndrome develop meningitis when exposed to ibuprofen (Sands *et al.*, 1988).

Antimicrobial agents which have been identified as aetiological agents in drug-induced aseptic meningitis include, most commonly, sulphonamides and trimethoprim, but also ciprofloxacin, cephalosporins, penicillin and isoniazid. The CSF findings in trimethoprim/sulphamethoxazole-related aseptic meningitis are similar to that seen with ibuprofen-induced disease (see above), however symptoms generally occur within hours of taking the medication and abate over a period of days following cessation of therapy (Haas, 1984; Carlson and Wilholm, 1987; Joffe *et al.*, 1989; Hedlund *et al.*, 1990). Symptoms include headache, nausea, myalgia, chills, fever and confusion, as well as facial oedema (River *et al.*, 1994). Of the reported cases of trimethoprim/sulphamethoxazole-related aseptic meningitis, nearly 30% had underlying collagen vascular diseases. A striking case was reported by River in which a 15 year old developed acute paraparesis, urinary retention and paraplegia hours after receiving co-trimoxazole. This patient went on to develop typical manifestations of SLE 2 years later (River *et al.* 1994).

Ciprofloxacin-associated aseptic meningitis appears to be extremely rare. In one reported case, symptoms occurred within 2 days of starting therapy and resolved within 24 h of stopping therapy (Asperilla and Smego, 1989). The CSF showed 147 WBC/μl, with 76% mononuclear cells and 24% eosinophils, with mildly elevated protein and normal glucose. The high percentage of eosinophils has not been reported in other types of antimicrobial-induced hypersensitivity meningitis.

There are at least two reports of *penicillin*-induced aseptic meningitis (Farmer *et al.*, 1960; River *et al.*, 1994). In one of these cases, seven stereotypical episodes of meningitis occurred, associated with confusion and EEG abnormalities. Symptoms developed abruptly within a few days of exposure to penicillin. The CSF findings were typical of hypersensitivity meningitis with the exception of the development of hypoglycorrhachia during four of the seven episodes. The authors hypothesized that potential mechanisms might include deposition of immune complexes in the meninges, an intrathecal cell-mediated or humoral response to proteins bound to penicillin, or a chemical arachnoiditis. In Farmer's case, the patient had a serum sickness-like reaction 3 days after penicillin injection, followed 11 months later by biopsy-proven pachymeningitis (Farmer *et al.*, 1960).

Creel and colleagues described a case of *cephalosporin*-related aseptic meningitis in a woman who developed fever, chills, and severe back pain 5 days after receiving parenteral cefazolin (Creel and Hurtt, 1995). Her CSF showed 376 WBC/µl with lymphocytic predominance, elevated protein with initially normal glucose, followed by hypoglycorrhachia with continuation of ceftazidime therapy. Immune complexes were demonstrated in both serum and CSF. The patient improved after discontinuation of cephalosporins. However, 2 days following skin testing for cephalosporin sensitivity she had recurrence of the aseptic meningitis and became encephalopathic. She rapidly improved with intravenous methylprednisolone. Assay of her CSF drawn prior to skin testing revealed specific IgG binding to ceftazidime, but not to cefazolin or cephalexin, making a strong case for an antigen-specific humoral immune response. It is unclear if this represented soluble immune complex formation in the CSF with subsequent serum sickness (type II) or a cytotoxic reaction involving IgG directed to drug deposition in the meninges (type III).

One case of *isoniazid*-induced recurrent aseptic meningitis was reported by Garagusi (Garagusi *et al.*, 1976), in a previously healthy man receiving prophylaxis for tuberculosis. This patient experienced fever, nausea, vomiting, myalgia and mild papilloedema which recurred upon rechallenge with the drug.

Other agents. Numerous cases of *Muromonab CD-3* (OKT3)-associated aseptic meningitis have been reported. Symptoms may occur as early as following three doses of the drug or as late as 2–3 weeks following completion of therapy, but usually resolve within 24 h if therapy is discontinued. Interestingly, even when therapy is maintained, symptoms typically resolve without sequelae over 3–5 days (Roden *et al.*, 1987). CSF usually reveals lymphocytic pleocytosis (8–300 cells/µl) with elevated protein and normal glucose. The frequency with which this reaction occurs is not known definitely, but it has been reported in 2–14% of recipients (Martin *et al.*, 1988).

Although headache is a common complaint in patients receiving *intravenous immunoglobulin* (IVIG), it is usually dose-related, not associated with signs of meningeal irritation, and occurs during the infusion. In contrast, in the reported cases of IVIG-related aseptic meningitis, symptoms of meningitis usually developed on the third to fifth day of starting therapy, and as late as the seventh day after stopping therapy (Scribner *et al.*, 1994; Sekul *et al.*, 1994). The CSF leucocytosis in most cases is predominantly neutrophilic, with normal to elevated protein and normal to decreased glucose (Vera-Ramirez *et al.*, 1992). Resolution of symptoms and CSF abnormalities occur within 2 days. The prevalence of this complication is estimated at approximately 10% of recipients (Kriss *et al.*, 1995) and appears to be more common in patients receiving higher doses of IVIG (> 1 g/kg) or those with underlying neurological disorders.

Treatment for all forms of hypersensitivity meningitis includes discontinuation of the offending agent. In cases where the responsible agent is unknown, all but essential medications should be discontinued. Patients may develop severe symptoms upon re-exposure to the offending agent, so every effort should be made to avoid this possibility. Patients should discuss all new drugs, including over-the-counter medications with their physicians prior to use.

Steroids may reduce symptoms in some patients, although the symptoms generally resolve promptly when the inciting drug is stopped (Chez *et al.*, 1989).

Recurrent inflammatory disease

Familial Mediterranean fever (FMF) is a systemic inflammatory condition transmitted in an autosomal recessive manner. Many patients are of Israeli, Middle Eastern or Armenian descent. FMF is usually manifested as periodic attacks of fever, skin lesions, and serositis affecting the peritoneum, pleura and joints (Vilaseca *et al.*, 1982) associated with leucocytosis and increased acute phase reactants (ESR, C-reactive protein, fibrinogen). Periodic aseptic meningitis can also occur. George and Westfal described a 49-year-old woman with a 35-year history of multiple episodes of meningitis, fever, pleuritic chest pain, skin rash, myalgias and arthralgias (George and Westfall, 1965). CSF studies revealed WBC ranging from 121 to 520 cells/µl (10–100 % mononuclear) with elevated protein 84–127, but normal glucose. Vilaseca reported a 33-year-old man with a 13-year history of recurrent attacks of fever, lower limb rash, and aseptic lymphocytic meningitis (Vilaseca *et al.*, 1982). His symptoms recurred every 2–4 weeks, lasting 2–3 days at a time. CSF WBC ranged between 54 and 1514 cells/µl with variable predominance of either PMN (up to 80%) or lymphocytes (up to 100%). Glucose and protein were normal. Proteinuria prompted a renal biopsy, which revealed amyloidosis and led ultimately to the diagnosis of FMF. Schwabe described a 32-year-old man with FMF, who had at least five episodes of aseptic meningitis beginning at 26 years of age (Schwabe and Monroe, 1988). In each of these reported cases of FMF meningitis, neurological abnormalities were limited to meningeal signs, and all episodes terminated in 1–3 days. The possibility of FMF as a cause of recurrent episodes of meningitis should be suspected in patients with symptoms suggestive of paroxysmal polyserositis, especially if they are of the appropriate ethnic background. No specific test for diagnosis of FMF is available, although a mutation in the short arm of chromosome 16 has been reported in some families. Colchicine therapy may be useful in preventing episodes of meningitis, as well as the other manifestations of the disease.

Infantile inflammatory multisystem disease is an obscure rare illness affecting children. Its relapsing course is characterized by fever, rash, articular swelling, splenomegaly and lymphadenopathy. A recurrent aseptic meningitis may also be present, and some children develop severe psychomotor retardation (Horoupian *et al.*, 1990). Systemic manifestations are often severe and debilitating, including growth retardation and/or failure to thrive. Horoupian described a fatal case in an infant girl with symptoms beginning at 3 days of age. CSF analysis disclosed 15 WBC/µl, with depressed glucose and normal protein. She thrived the first month, and then developed irritability, low-grade fever and poor feeding. Hepatosplenomegaly soon ensued with noted developmental lag. Generalized seizures began at 2 months of age with painful swelling of elbows and knees, as well as erythema-nodosum. Over the next 2 years, these symptoms progressed. At autopsy, the leptomeninges were noted to be opaque and studded with small white nodules, and firmly adherent to the surface of the brain. The infratentorial structures were atrophic and wrapped in thickened leptomeninges. These findings were interpreted as an indolent leptomeningitis punctuated by acute exacerbations. Fewer than 20 other children with this disease have been described. Neither of the two autopsied cases had detailed neuropathological examination. The aetiology of this syndrome remains unknown; both infectious (congenital Borrelial infection) and vascular disease (Ansell, 1983), have been suggested.

Connective tissue disorders

Systemic lupus erythematosus (SLE) is associated with a spectrum of CNS complications including cerebritis, seizures, psychiatric disturbances, movement disorders, cranial nerve palsies, hemiplegia, and peripheral neuropathy (Feinglass *et al.*, 1976; Adelman *et al.*, 1986). Neurological manifestations occur in 37–82% of patients during the course of the disease, and are second only to renal complications as a cause of death (Welsby and Smith, 1977). Isolated aseptic meningitis occurs in only 2–5% of patients with previously diagnosed SLE (Welsby and Smith, 1977; Sands *et al.*, 1988). When meningitis occurs, it is often accompanied by diffuse neurological involvement including encephalopathy and myelitis. Recurrent aseptic meningitis has also been reported as a manifestation of mixed connective tissue disorder (Harris *et al.*, 1987).

Only 3% of adult SLE patients present with neurological abnormalities as the initial manifestation of SLE. Of this subgroup, recurrent aseptic meningitis as the sole initial manifestation of SLE is exceedingly rare (Canoso and Cohen, 1975; Finelli *et al.*, 1976; Welsby and Smith, 1977). Patients with SLE-associated aseptic meningitis present with fever, malaise, and meningeal signs. The CSF shows polymorphonuclear or lymphocytic pleocytosis, usually with less than 200 cells/µl, although up to several thousand cells may occur. The CSF protein is elevated and the glucose is normal or slightly decreased. In some patients with aseptic meningitis, the clinical course may progress to include intellectual deterioration, a variety of neurobehavioural abnormalities and seizures, suggestive of frank encephalitis (Adelman *et al.*, 1986). The reported patients with aseptic meningitis as their initial presentation all subsequently developed other neurological events, including transverse myelitis and optic neuritis leading to their diagnosis (Feinglass *et al.*, 1976; Welsby and Smith, 1977).

The mechanism of neurological involvement in SLE may include cerebral small vessel vasculitis as well as immune complex deposition. Reduced CSF complement levels have been described, suggesting that intrathecal immune complex formation and deposition occurs (Petz *et al.*, 1971; Hadler *et al.*, 1973). Consistent with this model, some patients with meningitis have been documented to have DNA:anti-DNA antibody complexes in the CSF (Keefe *et al.*, 1974). Antibodies against neuronal antigens may also play a role in CNS lupus, but have not yet been demonstrated in patients with aseptic meningitis (Bluestein *et al.*, 1981). Antiphospholipid antibodies may also be involved in the pathogenesis of CNS complications.

It is important to keep in mind that in addition to primary SLE meningitis, patients with SLE, especially those receiving steroids and other immunosuppressive drugs, are also more susceptible to bacterial, and fungal meningitis. They also have an increased incidence of drug-induced hypersensitivity meningitis (described above), particularly in association with ibuprofen and sulpha antibiotics.

Relapsing polychondritis is a connective tissue disorder which presents as an 'episodic yet progressive inflammation of cartilaginous structures throughout the body and recurrent inflammation of the special sense organs including the eye and the ear' (McAdam *et al.*, 1976). The disease is usually manifested by auricular chondritis, arthritis, nasal chondritis, ocular inflammation, respiratory involvement and audiovestibular damage, with any three features adequate to make the clinical diagnosis (Brod and Booss, 1988). Cartilage biopsy is confirmatory, showing intense chronic inflammatory cell response with increased plasma cell numbers, loss of chondrocytes, vacuolation of cytoplasm and nuclear pyknosis with loss of basophilia. Four patients with this disease have been described with associated aseptic meningitis, two of which had recurrent episodes occurring 2 and 3 years after their initial diagnosis of relapsing polychondritis (Brod and Booss, 1988; Ragnaud *et al.*, 1996). All patients presented with persistent headache. Additional neurological signs and symptoms including personality change, nystagmus, hyperreflexia and primitive reflexes were noted in one patient. CSF studies in all cases revealed a lymphocytic pleocytosis of 6–90 WBC/μl with normal glucose and normal or elevated protein. One patient underwent meningeal and brain biopsy which revealed lymphocytic infiltration in the meninges. Another patient had a contrast enhanced CT of the head which demonstrated thickening of the meninges, particularly in the posterior fossa. Prednisone may have produced improvement in at least one of these reported patients.

Sarcoidosis has been defined as a multisystem granulomatous disorder of unknown aetiology, most commonly affecting young adults and presenting most frequently with bilateral hilar lymphadenopathy, pulmonary infiltration, skin or eye lesions. The diagnosis is established when clinicoradiographic findings are supported by histological evidence of widespread non-caseating epithelioid-cell granulomas in more than one organ (James *et al.*, 1976). Neurological involvement has been described in 5% of patients with sarcoidosis and include cranial and peripheral neuropathies, myelopathy, hydrocephalus, intracranial or intraspinal mass or focal lesions, encephalopathy/vasculopathy, seizures and aseptic meningitis (Stern *et al.*, 1985). In Stern's review of 649 patients 5% had neurosarcoidosis, and of this subgroup 18% had aseptic meningitis. Two patients had recurrent episodes of aseptic meningitis. In another series, 26% of patients with neurosarcoidosis had aseptic meningitis (Delaney, 1977). The syndrome is characterized by headache, meningismus and sterile CSF with lymphocytic pleocytosis, increased protein and normal to low glucose. Only one patient had aseptic meningitis as the sole manifestation of neurosarcoidosis and none had it as the presenting feature of neurosarcoidosis.

Specific CSF markers for sarcoidosis potentially include elevated CSF-ACE levels (60% of neurosarcoid patients) (Scott, 1993), (β2microglobulin and CSF lysozyme (Oksanen et al., 1985). Gallium scan may show diffuse uptake in the lungs, as well as in the parotid, salivary and lacrimal glands. This, in combination with elevated serum and/or CSF ACE levels, yields a 83–99% specificity for the diagnosis of sarcoidosis (Scott, 1993). Contrast enhanced CT and MRI can be utilized to detect meningeal disease (Scott, 1993). It is assumed that granulomatous inflammation is responsible for these imaging abnormalities. Other findings that support the diagnosis of sarcoid include the presence of skin anergy, lymphocytopenia, hypergammaglobulinaemia and elevated ESR. Treatment includes initial use of steroid, often combined with other immunosuppressive agents including cyclosporine, azathioprine, and cyclophosphamide (Scott, 1993).

Uveomeningitic syndromes

Vogt-Koyanagi-Harada syndrome (uveomeningoencephalitic syndrome} is an unusual multisystem disorder whose manifestations include uveitis, alopecia, and depigmentation of the skin, hair (canities), eyebrows/eyelashes (poliosis), and iris. Neurological complications can include encephalitis and recurrent or fluctuating meningitis (Reed et al., 1958; Pattison, 1965). The disease appears to be more common in patients of Japanese, Far Eastern, Mediterranean and Latin American descent. Onset of symptoms is typically between the ages of 20 and 40 years. The usual clinical sequence consists of a meningeal phase, followed by the ophthalmic and convalescent phases. The meningeal phase of the illness may be very transient and mild enough to pass unnoticed, but can include fever, severe headache, photophobia, confusion, acute psychosis, cranial and peripheral nerve palsies, loss of sphincter control, and vestibular/cochlear dysfunction. Auditory-vestibular changes, most commonly bilateral sensorineural hearing loss (50%) are often associated with tinnitus, vertigo and nystagmus. These sequelae may also occur during the convalescent phase of the illness. The CSF may show an isolated elevation in protein, although a lymphocytic pleocytosis and increased pressure are common. The ophthalmic phase typically consists of acute, bilateral idiopathic uveitis (photophobia, eye pain, visual blurring and field defects) leading to acute glaucoma and retinal detachments. Optic neuritis is less common. Mild cases of uveitis have been described, as well as explosive cases leading to acute, permanent blindness. These two phases usually run a subacute course over several weeks, although intermittent symptoms and progression over a period of months has also been described. It is during or after these phases that the secondary manifestations appear. These may include focal areas of alopecia, vitiligo of the eyelids, periorbital areas, face, neck, trunk and back (30–70% of cases) and poliosis (40–80%), as well as persistent neurological deficits. The clinical picture usually stabilizes within a year. The aetiology of VKH remains unknown. Treatment results are inconsistent, although corticosteroids have been used with benefit in patients with acute ophthalmologic and neurologic manifestations of the disease.

Behçet syndrome is an idiopathic multisystem disorder characterized by recurrent painful oral and genital ulcers with ocular involvement (usually uveitis but also, iridocyclitis, chorioretinitis, keratitis or optic neuritis). Peak incidence is in the third and fourth decade, with males affected more commonly than females. Ulcers are usually small (< 1 cm) with a central necrotic base and can appear as single lesions, or in crops. Additional manifestations include other dermatological findings (erythema nodosum, folliculitis, and vasculitis), as well as non-destructive arthritis, colitis, venous thrombosis and pulmonary arteritis or emboli.

Neurological complications are variable in Behçet's disease, ranging from 10 to 30% of patients, and usually occur years after onset of ulcers (Wolf *et al.*, 1965; Serdaroglu *et al.*, 1989). Gille described three patients, however, in which a clinical picture of relapsing meningoencephalitis preceded the appearance of classical signs of the disease for several months or years (Gille *et al.*, 1990). Onset of neurological symptoms may be abrupt, gradual or recurrent and diagnosis may be challenging due to the variety of abnormalities on neurological examination and neuroimaging studies (Devlin *et al.*, 1995). Any part of the neuraxis may be involved, and there is no characteristic clinical pattern (Wolf *et al.*, 1965). Cranial nerve palsies, focal or generalized seizures, coma, paresis, extrapyramidal signs, neuropsychiatric disturbance, cerebellar signs, spastic paraplegia and meningoencephalitis have been reported. CSF abnormalities are consistently found (80%) when neurological symptoms are present. Pleocytosis is commonly detected, usually with 60 or less cells/μl (although as high as several thousand). There may be either a PMN or lymphocytic predominance, often with increased protein and normal glucose. The most consistent abnormalities in the CNS have been perivascular and meningeal infiltration with lymphocytes, plasma cells and macrophages, as well as small foci of softening in the grey and white matter, often in relationship to blood vessels (Wolf *et al.*, 1965). Neurological symptoms usually herald a sharp rise in mortality rate, with death occurring frequently within one year of their onset. Treatment generally involves high dose systemic corticosteroids (commonly prednisone), as well as azathioprine, and cyclosporin A.

Complement and immunoglobulin deficiency

Patients with *complement deficiency* classically are at risk for episodes of recurrent bacterial infection, including bacterial meningitis (e.g. terminal complement deficiency associated with meningococcal infection). Less commonly appreciated, however, is a predisposition toward recurrent aseptic meningitis. Bonnin *et al.* (1993) described a unique patient with complement regulatory protein factor I (C3b/C4b inactivator) deficiency whose sole clinical problem was recurrent aseptic meningitis. This 28-year-old woman of Greek origin experienced 11 episodes of acute aseptic meningitis, nine of which occurred during a 2-year period, which began abruptly with headache, fever, nausea, vomiting, neck stiffness, lethargy and fever. On each occasion there was transient CSF leucocytosis, predominantly polymorphonuclear, with elevated protein and variable glucose levels. ESR and C-reactive protein were also elevated. Each of these abnormalities resolved or were nearly normal within 5 days of onset of symptoms. Full microbiological, vasculitic, anatomic and immunological workup was normal other than a positive C1q binding assay for circulating immune complexes during two of the episodes. Throughout the 2 years, her serum complement profiles were abnormal, both during and between episodes. Total haemolytic complement activity was 50% of normal or less on all but one occasion, and there was complete absence of factor I, decreased levels of other alternative pathway proteins and normal levels of C1, C4 and C2 (characteristic of homozygous factor I deficiency). Interestingly, in the other previously reported cases of factor I deficiency, the major clinical problem was systemic pyogenic bacterial infection. This case was unique in the presentation of recurrent aseptic meningitis. The authors postulated that immune complexes that form in the CSF or cross the choroid plexus could produce an aseptic meningitis. This is of particular interest, since this mechanism has also been postulated in the pathogenesis of CNS SLE (described above).

As previously mentioned, immunoglobulin deficiencies tend to predispose patients to recurrent bacterial infections. However, *IgG subclass 3 deficiency* has been reported in association with recurrent lymphocytic meningitis in an otherwise healthy young adult woman (Snowden *et al.*, 1993). She suffered three episodes during a 5-year period and was shown to have a sustained reduction of IgG3 to below the fifth centile. Although this deficiency has previously been described in association with recurrent upper respiratory tract infection, asthma, obstructive lung disease, and enteral infections, she did not have any of these problems, nor were there any other identifiable immune defects. The authors pointed out that antibody responses involving IgG3 tend to be triggered by polymeric protein antigens such as those found in viral envelopes.

Miscellaneous

Ferreol-Besnier disease. Meyer-Lindenberg and Hotz reported an unusual case of a recurrent cutaneous syndrome associated with recurrent lymphomonocytic meningitis (Meyer-Lindenberg and Hotz, 1999). They described a 40-year-old white man with throat pain and burning sensation on the palms and soles 3 days prior to the onset of fever and severe headache. Neurological exam was unremarkable except for meningismus. Extensive reddening and early desquamation were noted in the areas of previous pain and burning. CSF examination showed 216 WBC/µl with 80% lymphocytes and monocytes (with a high proportion of large, fragile endothelial cells) and 20% PMNs, of which 50% were eosinophils. The authors point out that although the CSF cytology conforms closely to that seen in Mollaret's meningitis, an unusual feature was the high number of eosinophils. Glucose and protein were normal. Fever and headache subsided within 4 days followed by extensive desquamation of the affected skin. The patient went on to have six attacks identical to the first episode separated by disease-free intervals of 7–18 months. The cutaneous syndrome was felt to conform to the rare clinical entity of erythema scarlatiniforme desquamativum recidivans of Ferreol-Besnier, of which less than 50 cases have been reported since its first description in 1878. Although headache has been described in the prodromal phase (along with myalgias, gastrointestinal syndromes and fever), this case represented the first characterization of recurrent CSF lymphocytosis associated with this disease in the literature. The aetiology is unknown, although infectious, connective tissue disease, immunosuppression and uveomeningitic syndromes were excluded carefully in this patient.

Headache with neurologic deficits and CSF lymphocytosis (HaNDL). Berg and Williams (1995) reviewed this syndrome of episodic headache accompanied by neurological deficits and CSF lymphocytosis with symptoms occurring over a period of 1–12 weeks. In their analysis of 40 cases, 44% were noted to be male and 56% female with an age range of 7–52 years. There was no seasonal correlation, and only 24% of patients had a history of prior migraine. Neurological signs and symptoms usually consisted of hemiparesis or hemisensory changes, but also included confusional episodes or aphasia, each of which resolved within hours, or at most by 3 days. Of the patients, 73% had multiple episodes (2–20) with occurrence over 1–84 days (mean 21 days). Of these patients, 41% exhibited a deficit affecting the same region of brain, whereas in 59% different brain regions were affected with subsequent episodes. All patients were asymptomatic after recovery with follow up as long as 9 years (except one patient with headache for one year).

All patients had lymphocytic CSF pleocytosis (16–350 WBC/μl) with at least 86% mononuclear cells, predominantly lymphocytes; 91% had elevations of protein (35–247 mg/dl) and 73% had elevated opening pressure (10–40 cm H_2O). Despite the CSF inflammation, meningismus was rarely prominent. Transient focal non-epileptiform EEG changes were also found in 72%. CT scan was normal in all patients scanned; however in two of four patients who underwent MRI, several non-specific, small, high-signal areas on T2-weighted images ('unidentified bright objects' or 'UBO's) were noted without contrast enhancement.

In distinction to classic migraine, HaNDL patients did not develop chronic headaches. HaNDL also differs from hemiplegic migraine in that attacks of hemiplegic migraine occur intermittently over years rather than in the temporal clusters typical of HaNDL. In addition, the CSF is rarely abnormal in hemiplegic migraine. Status epilepticus can produce a CSF lymphocytosis, and it was postulated that some patients classified as HaNDL could actually have had unwitnessed seizures and postictal phenomena, but none had a history of subsequent epilepsy, making this less likely. The aetiology of HaNDL is unknown and has been debated in the literature. Possibilities include an inflammatory or infectious origin. One patient had echovirus 30 isolated in an attack, but this appears to be unusual (Casteels-Van Daele *et al.*, 1981). Treatment is usually symptomatic, as the attacks are brief and self-limited.

References

Achard, J.-M., Lallement, P.-Y. and Veyssier, P. (1990). Recurrent aseptic meningitis secondary to intracranial epidermoid cyst and mollaret's meningitis: two distinct entities or a single disease? A case report and a nosologic discussion. *Am. J. Med.*, **89**, 807–810.

Adelman, D. C., Saltiel, E. and Klinenberg, J. R. (1986). The neuropsychiatric manifestations of systemic lupus erythematosus: an overview. *Semin. Arthritis Rheum.*, **15**, 185–199.

Adey, G. and Wald, S. L. (1992). Chronic or recurrent meningitis. Neurosurgical perspectives. *Neurosurg. Clin. North. Am.*, **3**, 483–490.

Aintablian, N., Pratt, R. D. and Sawyer, M. H. (1995). Rapidly recurrent enteroviral meningitis in non-immunocompromised infants caused by different viral strains. *J. Med. Virol.*, **47**, 126–129.

American College of Physicians (1997). Guidelines for laboratory evaluation in the diagnosis of Lyme disease. *Ann. Intern. Med.*, **127**, 1106–1108.

Anderson, J. P. (1969). Recurrent virus meningitis. *Br. Med. J.*, **4**, 786.

Ansell, B. M. (1983). Arthritis in young children. *Br. Med. J.*, **286**, 1917–1918.

Aristegui, F. J., Delgado, R. A., Oleaga, Z. L. and Hermosa, C. C. (1998). Mollaret's recurrent aseptic meningitis and cerebral epidermoid cyst. *Pediatr. Neurol.*, **18**, 156–159.

Asperilla, M. O. and Smego, R. A. (1989). Eosinophilic meningitis associated with ciprofloxacin. *Am. J. Med.*, **87**, 589–590.

Atarashi, K., Yoshimura, N., Nodera, H., Tsukimoto, K., Beppu, H. and Kanayama, M. (1996). Recurrent histiocytic necrotizing lymphadenitis (Kikuchi's disease) in a human T lymphotrophic virus type 1 carrier. *Intern. Med.*, **35**, 821–825.

Baringer, J. R. and Bell, W. E. (1993). The evaluation of recurrent meningitis. *Hosp. Pract. (Off. Ed).*, **28**, 87–90, 96–99, 102, 105.

Becker, W. J., Watters, G. V., de Chadarevian, J. P. and Vanasse, M. (1984). Recurrent aseptic meningitis secondary to intracranial epidermoids. *Can. J. Neurol. Sci.*, **11**, 387–389.

Berg, M. J. and Williams, L. S. (1995). The transient syndrome of headache with neurologic deficits and CSF lymphocytosis. *Neurology*, **45**, 1648–1654.

Bergstrom, T. and Alestig, K. (1990). Treatment of primary and recurrent herpes simplex virus type 2 induced meningitis with acyclovir. *Scand. J. Infect. Dis.*, **22**, 239–240.

Bergstrom, T., Vahlne, A., Alestig, K., Jeansson, S., Forsgren, M. and Lycke, E. (1990). Primary and recurrent herpes simplex virus type 2-induced meningitis. *J. Infect. Dis.*, **162**, 322–330.

Bernat, J. L. (1976). Glioblastoma multiforme and the meningeal syndrome. *Neurology*, **26**, 1071–1074.

Bluestein, H. G., Williams, G. M. and Steinberg, A. D. (1981). Cerebrospinal fluid antibodies to neuronal cells: association with neuropsychiatric manifestations of systemic lupus erythematosus. *Am. J. Med.*, **70**, 240–246.

Bonnin, A. J., Zeitz, H. J. and Gewurz, A. (1993). Complement factor I deficiency with recurrent aseptic meningitis. *Arch. Intern. Med.*, **153**, 1380–1383.

Bouland, D. L., Specht, N. L. and Hegstad, D. R. (1986). Ibuprofen and aseptic meningitis (letter). *Ann. Intern. Med.*, **104**, 731.

Bozzette, S. A., Larsen, R. A., Chiu, J. *et al.* (1991). A placebo-controlled trial of maintenance therapy with fluconazole after treatment of cryptococcal meningitis in the acquired immunodeficiency syndrome. *N. Eng. J Med.*, **324**, 580–584.

Brod, S. and Booss, J. (1988). Idiopathic CSF pleocytosis in relapsing polychondritis. *Neurology*, **38**, 322–323.

Canoso, J. J. and Cohen, A. S. (1975). Aseptic meningitis in systemic lupus erythematosus. *Arth. Rheum.*, **18**, 369–374.

Carlson, J. and Wilholm, B. (1987). Trimethoprim associated aseptic meningitis. *Scand. J. Infect. Dis.*, **19** , 687–691.

Carrazana, E. J., Rossitch, E. J. JR and Samuels, M. A. (1989). Cerebral toxoplasmosis in the acquired immunodeficiency syndrome. *Clin. Neurol. Neurosurg.*, **91**, 291–301.

Casteels-Van Daele, M., Standaert, L., Boel, M., Smeets, E., Colaier, J. and Desmyter, J. (1981). Basilar migraine and viral meningitis. *Lancet*, **1**, 1366.

Chambers, S. T., Powell, K. F., Croxson, M. C., Krishnan, S. and Weir, R. P. (1994). Demonstration of herpes simplex type 2 in the cerebrospinal fluid of two patients with recurrent lymphocytic meningitis. *NZ Med. J.*, **107**, 367–369.

Cherniak, R. M., Morris, L. C., Belay, T., Spitzer, E. D. and Casadevall, A. (1995). Variation in the structure of glucuronoxylomannan in isolates from patients with recurrent cryptococcal meningitis. *Infect. Immun.*, **63**, 1899–1905.

Chez, M., Sila, C. A., Ransohoff, R. M., Longworth, D. L. and Weida, C. (1989). Ibuprofen-induced meningitis: Detection of intrathecal IgG synthesis and immune complexes. *Neurology*, **39**, 1578–1580.

Cohen, B. A., Rowley, A. H. and Long, C. M. (1994). Herpes simplex type 2 in a patient with Mollaret's meningitis: demonstration by polymerase chain reaction. *Ann. Neurol.*, **35**, 112–116.

Collins, J. J. and Fisher, W. S. (1990). Vein of Galen aneurysm presenting with recurrent aseptic meningitis and subsequent spontaneous thrombosis. *Surg. Neurol.*, **33**, 325–328.

Corey, L., Adams, H., Brown, A. *et al.* (1983). Genital herpes simplex virus infections: clinical manifestations, course, and complications. *Ann. Intern. Med.*, **98**, 958–972.

Craig, C. P. and Nahmias, A. (1973). Different patterns of neurological involvement with HSV types 1 and 2: isolation of HSV type 2 from the buffy coats of two adults with meningitis. *J. Infect. Dis.*, **127**, 365–372.

Creel, G. B. and Hurtt, M. (1995). Cephalosporin-induced recurrent aseptic meningitis. *Ann. Neurol.*, **37**, 815–817.

Crossley, G. H. and Dismukes, W. E. (1990). Central nervous system epidermoid cyst: a probable etiology of Mollaret's meningitis. *Am. J. Med.*, **89**, 805–806.

de Chadarevian, J. P. and Becker, W. J. (1980a). Mollaret's recurrent aseptic meningitis: relationship to epidermoid cysts. *J. Neuropath. Exp. Neurol.*, **39**, 661–669.

de Chadarevian, J. P. and Becker, W. J. (1980b). Mollaret's recurrent aseptic meningitis: relationship to epidermoid cysts. Light microscopic and ultrastructural cytological studies of the cerebrospinal fluid. *J. Neuropathol. Exp. Neurol.*, **39**, 661–669.

Delaney, P. (1977). Neurologic manifestations in sarcoidosis. Review of the literature, with a report of 23 cases. *Ann. Intern. Med.*, **87**, 336–345.

Devlin, T., Gray, L., Allen, N. B., Friedman, A. H., Tien, R. and Morgenlander, J. C. (1995). Neuro-Behçet's disease: factors hampering proper diagnosis. *Neurology*, **45**, 1754–1757.

Djouhri, H., Marsot-Dupuch, K., Joutel, A., Kujas, M., Brette, M. D., Artuis, F. *et al.* (1998). Perichiasmatic granuloma occuring after radical mastoidectomy: MR findings. *Eur. Radiol.*, **8**, 286–288.

Dorfman, R. F. (1987). Histiocytic necrotizing lymphadenitis of Kikuchi and Fujimoto. *Arch. Pathol. Lab. Med.*, **111**, 1026–1030.

Evans, H. (1993). Cytology of Mollaret meningitis. *Diagn. Cytopathol.*, **9**, 373–376.

Farmer, L., Echalin, F. A. and Loughlin, W. C. (1960). Pachymeningitis apparently due to penicillin hypersensitivity. *Ann. Intern. Med.*, **52**, 910–915.

Feinglass, E. J., Arnett, F. C., Dorsch, C. A. *et al.* (1976). Neuropsychiatric manifestations of systemic lupus erythematosus: diagnosis, clinical spectrum, and relationship to other features of the disease. *Medicine*, **55**, 323–339.

Finelli, P. F., Yockey, C. C. and Herbert, A. J. (1976). Recurrent aseptic meningitis in an elderly man. Unusual prodrome of systemic lupus erythematosus. *J. Am. Med. Assoc.*, **235**, 1142–1143.

Ford, J., Torres, L. F., Cox, T. and Hayward, R. (1986). Recurrent sterile meningitis caused by a pituitary abscess. *Postgrad. Med. J.*, **62**, 929–931.

Frieden, T. R., Piepmeier, J., Murdoch, G. H. and Bia, F. J. (1990). Recurrent aseptic meningitis for 24 years: diagnosis and treatment of an associated lesion (clinical conference). *Yale J. Biol. Med.*, **63**, 593–599.

Garagusi, V. F., Neefe, L. I. and Mann, O. (1976). Acute meningoencephalitis associated with isoniazid administration. *J. Am. Med. Assoc.*, **235**, 1141–1142.

Garcia-Monco, J. and Benach, J. L. (1995). Lyme neuroborreliosis. *Ann. Neurol.*, **37**, 691–702.

George, R. B. and Westfall, R. E. (1965). Periodic meningitis: an unusual manifestation of periodic diseases. *Ann. Intern. Med.*, **62**, 778–785.

Gille, M., Sindic, C. J., Laterre, P. F., De Hertogh, P., Hotermans, J. M., Selak, I. *et al.* (1990). Neurological involvement as a manifestation of Behçet's disease. *Acta Neurol. Belg.*, **90**, 233–247.

Goldstein, R., Guberman, A., Izaguirre, C. A. and Karsh, J. (1986). Mollaret's meningitis: a case with increased circulating natural killer cells. *Ann. Neurol.*, **20**, 359–361.

Graman, P. S. (1987). Mollaret's meningitis associated with acute Epstein-Barr virus mononucleosis. *Arch Neurol.*, **44**, 1204–1205.

Greenberg, G. N. (1988). Recurrent sulindac-induced aseptic meningitis in a patient tolerant to other nonsteroidal anti-inflammatory drugs. *South. Med. J.*, **81**, 1463–1464.

Guillaume, D., Stevenaert, A., Grisar, T., Doyer, P. and Reznik, M. (1990). Pituitary abscess with recurrent aseptic meningitis (letter). *J. Neurol. Neurosurg. Psych.*, **53**, 925–926.

Haas, E. J. (1984). Trimethoprim-sulfamethoxazole: another cause of recurrent meningitis. *J. Am. Med. Assoc.*, **252**, 346.

Hadler, N. M., Gerwin, R. D., Frank, M. M. *et al.* (1973). The fourth component of complement in the cerebrospinal fluid in systemic lupus erythematosus. *Arth. Rheum.*, **16**, 507–521.

Halperin, J. J., Landis, D. M. and Kleinman, G. M. (1982). Whipple disease of the nervous system. *Neurology*, **32**, 612–617.

Harris, G. J., Franson, T. R. and Ryan, L. M. (1987). Recurrent meningitis as a manifestation of mixed connective tissue disease (MCTD). *Wisconsin Med. J.*, **86**, 31–33.

Hedlund, J., Aurelius, E. and Andersson, J. (1990). Recurrent encephalitis due to trimethoprim intake. *Scand. J. Infect. Dis.*, **22**, 109–112.

Hermans, P. E., Goldstein, N. P. and Wellman, W. E. (1972). Mollaret's meningitis and the differential diagnosis of recurrent meningitis. *Am. J. Med.*, **52**, 128–140.

Horoupian, D. S., Rapin, I., Titelbaum, J. and Peison, B. (1990). Infantile inflammatory multisystem disease: clinicopathological findings and review of the literature. *Clin. Neuropathol.*, **9**, 170–176.

James, D. G., Turiaf, J., Hosoda, Y. *et al.* (1976). Description of sarcoidosis: report of the subcommittee on classification and definition. *Ann. NY Acad. Sci.*, **278**, 742.

Joffe, A. M., Farley, J. D., Linden, D. and Goldsand, G. (1989). Trimethoprim-sulfamethoxazole-associated aseptic meningitis: case reports and review of the literature. *Am. J. Med.*, **87**, 332–338.

Karlsson, M., Hammers-Berggren, S., Lindquist, L., Stiernstedt, G. and Svenungsson, B. (1994). Comparison of intravenous penicillin G and oral doxycycline for treatment of Lyme neuroborreliosis. *Neurology*, **44**, 1203–1207.

Keefe, E. B., Bardana, E. J. JR., Harbeck, R. J., Pirofsky, B. and Carr, R. I. (1974). Lupus meningitis: antibody to deoxyribonucleic acid (DNA) and DNA:anti-DNA complexes in cerebrospinal fluid. *Ann. Intern. Med.*, **80**, 58–60.

Kimberlin, D. W., Lakeman, F. D., Arvin, A. M. *et al.* (1996). Application of the polymerase chain reaction to the diagnosis and management of neonatal Herpes simplex virus disease. *J. Infect. Dis.*, **174**, 1162–1167.

Kitai, I., Navas, L., Rohlicek, C., Blaser, S., Jay, V. and Drake, J. M. (1992). Recurrent aseptic meningitis secondary to an intracranial cyst: a case report and review of clinical features and imaging modalities. *Pediatr. Infect. Dis. J.*, **11**, 671–675.

Klemola, E. and Lapinleimu, K. (1964). Multiple attacks of aseptic meningitis in the same individual. *Br. Med. J.*, **1**, 1087–1090.

Kline, M. W. (1989). Review of recurrent bacterial meningitis. *Ped. Infect. Dis. J.*, **8**, 630–634.

Knox, D. L., Bayless, T. M. and Pittman, F. E. (1976). Neurologic disease in patients with treated Whipple's disease. *Medicine*, **55**, 467–476.

Kriss, T. C., Kriss, V. M. and Warf, B. C. (1995). Recurrent meningitis: the search for the dermoid or epidermoid tumor. *Pediatr. Infect. Dis. J.*, **14**, 697–700.

Kuroda, Y., Abe, M., Nagumo, F., Neshige, R., Kakigi, R. and Tabuchi, K. (1991). Neuroepithelial cyst presenting as recurrent aseptic meningitis. *Neurology*, **41**, 1834–1835.

Kwong, Y. L., Woo, E., Fong, P. C. *et al.* (1988). Mollaret's meningitis revisited. *Clin. Neurol. Neurosurg.*, **90**, 163–167.

Landgren, M., Kyllerman, M., Bergstrom, T., Dotevall, L., Ljungstrom, L. and Ricksten, A. (1994). Diagnosis of Epstein-Barr virus-induced central nervous system infections by DNA amplification from cerebrospinal fluid. *Ann. Neurol.*, **35**, 631–635.

Larbrisseau, A., Renevey, F., Brochu, P., Decarie, M. and Mathieu, J. P. (1980). Recurrent chemical meningitis due to an intraspinal cystic teratoma: case report. *J. Neurosurg.*, **52**, 715–717.

Louis, E. D., Lynch, T., Kaufmann, P., Fahn, S. and Odel, J. (1996). Diagnostic guidelines in central nervous system Whipple's disease. *Ann. Neurol.*, **40**, 561–568.

Lunardi, P., Missori, P. and Fraiolo, B. (1989). Chemical meningitis: unusual presentation of a cerebellar astrocytoma: case report and review of the literature. *Neurosurgery*, **25**, 264–270.

Lynch, T., Odel, J., Fredericks, D. N., Louis, E. D., Forman, S., Rotterdam, H. *et al.* (1997). Polymerase chain reaction based detection of *Tropheryma whippelii* in central nervous system in Whipple's disease. *Ann. Neurol.*, **42**, 120–124.

Magee, J. T., Philpot, C., Yang, J. and Hosein, I. K. (1994). Pyrolysis typing of isolates from recurrence of systemic cryptococcus. *J. Med. Microbiol.*, **40**, 165–169.

Marinac, J. S. (1992). Drug- and chemical-induced meningitis: a review of the literature. *Ann. Pharmacother.*, **26**, 813–821.

Martin, M. A., Massanari, R. M., Nghiem, D. D., Smith, J. L. and Corry, R. J. (1988). Nosocomial aseptic meningitis associated with administration of OKT3. *J. Am. Med. Assoc.*, **259**, 2002–2005.

Mascia, R. A. and Smith, C. W. (1984). Mollaret's meningitis: an unusual disease with a characteristic presentation. *Am. J. Med. Sci.*, **287**, 52–53.

McAdam, L. P., O'Hanlon, M. A., Bluestone, R. and Pearson, C. M. (1976). Relapsing polychondritis: prospective study of 23 patients and a review of the literature. *Medicine*, **55**, 193–215.

McKinney, R. E., Katz, S. L. and Wilfert, C. M. (1987). Chronic enteroviral meningoencephalitis in agammaglobulinemic patients. *Rev. Infect. Dis.*, **9**, 334–356.

Meyer-Lindenberg, A. and Hotz, M. (1997). Ferreol-Besnier disease with associated recurrent meningitis. *J. Neurol. Neurosurg. Psych.*, **62**, 297.

Mifsud, A. J. (1988). Drug-related recurrent meningitis. *J. Infect.*, **17**, 151–153.

Mollaret, P. (1944). La meningite endothelio-leucocytaire multirecurrente benign. Syndrome nouveau ou maladie nouvelle? Documents cliniques. *Rev. Neurol. (Paris)*, **76**, 57–76.

Mollaret, P. (1945). La meningite endothelio-leucocytaire multirecurrente benigne. Syndrome nouveau ou maladie nouvelle? Documents humoraux et microbiologiques. *Ann. Inst. Past.*, **71**, 1–17.

Mollaret, P. (1952). Benign recurrent pleocytic meningitis and its presumed causative virus. *J. Nerv. Ment. Dis.*, **116**, 1072–1080.

Monteyne, P., Sindic, C. J. M. and Laterre, E. C. (1996). Recurrent meningitis and encephalitis associated with herpes simplex type 2: demonstration by polymerase chain reaction. *Eur. Neurol.*, **36**, 176–177.

Nakao, T. and Miura, R. (1971). Recurrent virus meningitis. *Pediatrics*, **47**, 773–776.

Norris, F. H., Aguilar, M. J., Colton, R. P., Oldstone, M. B. A. and Cremer, N. E. (1975). Tubular particles in a case of recurrent lymphocytic meningitis followed by amyotrophic lateral sclerosis. *J. Neuropath. Exp. Neurol.*, **34**, 133–147.

O'Neil, K. M., Pallansch, M. A., Winkelstein, J. A., Lock, T. M. and Modlin, J. F. (1988). Chronic group A coxsackievirus infection in agammaglobulinemia: demonstration of genome variation if serotypically identical isolates persistently excreted by the same patient. *J. Infect. Dis.*, **157**, 183–186.

Oksanen, V., Fyhrquist, F., Somer, H. and Gronhagen-Riska, C. (1985). Angiotensin converting enzyme in cerebrospinal fluid: a new assay. *Neurology*, **35**, 1220–1223.

Pal, G. S., Baker, J. T. and Humphrey, P. R. (1987). Lyme disease presenting as recurrent acute meningitis. *Br. Med. J.*, **295**, 367.

Patrick, B. S., Smith, R. R. and Bailey, T. O. (1974). Aseptic meningitis due to spontaneous rupture of craniopharyngioma cyst. Case report. *J. Neurosurg.*, **41**, 387–390.

Pattison, E. M. (1965). Uveo-meningoencephalitic syndrome (Vogt-Koyanagi-Harada). *Arch. Neurol.*, **12**, 197–205.

Petz, L. D., Sharp, G. C., Cooper, N. R. and Irvin, W. S. (1971). Serum and cerebral spinal fluid complement and serum autoantibodies in systemic lupus erythematosus. *Medicine*, **50**, 259–275.

Picard, F. J., Dekaban, G. A., Silva, J. and Rice, G. P. A. (1993). Mollaret's meningitis associated with herpes simplex type 2 infection. *Neurology*, **43**, 1722–1727.

Pollock, S., Lewis, P. D. and Kendall, B. (1981). Whipple's disease confined to the nervous system. *J. Neurol. Neurosurg. Psych.*, **44**, 1104–1109.

Ragnaud, J. M., Tahbaz, A., Morlat, P., Sire, S., Gin, H. and Aubertin, J. (1996). Recurrent aseptic purulent meningitis in a patient with relapsing polychondritis. *Clin. Infect. Dis.*, **22**, 374–375.

Read, S. J., Jeffery, K. J. M. and Bangham, C. R. M. (1997). Aseptic meningitis and encephalitis: the role of PCR in the diagnostic laboratory. *J. Clin. Microbiol.*, **35**, 691–696.

Reed, H. *et al.* (1958). Uveo-encephalitic syndrome of Vogt-Koyanagi-Harada disease. *Can. Med. Assoc. J.*, **79**, 451–459.

Relman, D. A. (1997). Whipple's disease. In: *Infections of the Central Nervous System*, 2nd edn (W. M. Scheld, R. J. Whitley and D. T. Durack, eds). Philadelphia: Lippincott-Raven. pp. 579–589.

River, Y., Averbuch-Heller, L., Weinberger, M. *et al.* (1994). Antibiotic induced meningitis. *J. Neurol. Neurosurg. Psych.*, **57**, 705–708.

Roden, J., Klintman, G. B. G., Husberg, B. S., Nery, J. and Olson, L. M. (1987). Cerebrospinal fluid inflammation during OKT3 therapy. *Lancet*, **2**, 272.

Ruppert, G. B. and Barth, W. F. (1981). Ibuprofen hypersensitivity in systemic lupus erythematosus. *South. Med. J.*, **74**, 241–243.

Sands, M. L., Ryczak, M. and Brown, R. B. (1988). Recurrent aseptic meningitis followed by transverse myelitis as a presentation of systemic lupus erythematosus. *J. Rheumatol.*, **15**, 862–864.

Schick, B., Draf, W., Kahle, G., Weber, R. and Wallenfang, T. (1997). Occult malformations of the skull base. *Arch. Otolaryngol.*, **123**, 77–80.

Schlesinger, Y., Tebas, P., Gaudreault-Keener, M., Buller, R. S. and Storch, G. A. (1995). Herpes simplex virus type 2 meningitis in the absence of genital lesions: improved recognition with the use of the polymerase chain reaction. *Clin. Infect. Dis.*, **20**, 842–848.

Schwabe, A. D. and Monroe, J. B. (1988). Meningitis in familial Mediterranean fever. *Am. J. Med.*, **85**, 715–717.

Scott, T. F. (1993). Neurosarcoidosis: progress and clinical aspects. *Neurology*, **43**, 8–12.

Scribner, C. L., Kapit, R. M., Phillips, E. T. and Rickles, N. M. (1994). Aseptic meningitis and intravenous immunoglobulin therapy. *Ann. Intern. Med.*, **121**, 305–306.

Sekul, E. A., Cupler, E. J. and Dalakas, M. C. (1994). Aseptic meningitis associated with high-dose intravenous immunoglobulin therapy: frequency and risk factors. *Ann. Intern. Med.*, **121**, 259–262.

Serdaroglu, P., Yazici, H., Ozdemir, C., Yurdakul, S., Bahar, S. and Aktin, E. (1989). Neurologic involvement in Behçet's syndrome: a prospective study. *Arch. Neurol.*, **46**, 265–269.

Shoenfeld, Y., Livni, E., Shaklai, M. and Pinkhas, J. (1980). Sensitization to ibuprofen in systemic lupus erythematosus. *J. Am. Med. Assoc.*, **244**, 547–548.

Snowden, J. A., Milford-Ward, A., Cookson, L. J. and McKendrick, M. W. (1993). Recurrent lymphocytic meningitis associated with hereditary isolated IgG subclass 3 deficiency. *J. Infect.*, **27**, 285–289.

Spitzer, E. D., Spitzer, S. G., Freundlich, L. F. and Casadevall, A. (1993). Persistence of initial infection in recurrent *Cryptoccus neoformans* meningitis. *Lancet*, **341**, 595–596.

Steel, J. G., Dix, R. D. and Baringer, J. R. (1982). Isolation of herpes simplex virus type 1 in recurrent (Mollaret) meningitis. *Ann. Neurol.*, **11**, 17–21.

Stern, B. J., Krumholz, A., Johns, C., Scott, P. and Nissim, J. (1985). Sarcoidosis and its neurological manifestations. *Arch. Neurol.*, **42**, 909–917.

Stoppe, G., Stark, E. and Patzold, U. (1987). Mollaret's meningitis: CSF-immunocyto-logical examinations. *J. Neurol.*, **234**, 103–106.

Sullivan, D., Haynes, K., Moran, G., Shanley, D. and Coleman, D. (1996). Persistence, replacement, and microevolution of *Cryptococcus neoformans* starins in recurrent meningitis in AIDS patients. *J. Clin. Microbiol.*, **34**, 1739–1744.

Takeuchi, M., Yamane, K., Kobayashi, I. and Maruyama, S. (1989). A case of recurrent Epstein-Barr virus meningitis. *Clin. Neurol. (Tokyo)*, **29**, 85–88.

Tedder, D. G., Ashley, R., Tyler, K. L. and Levin, M. J. (1994). Herpes simplex virus infection as a cause of benign recurrent lymphocytic meningitis. *Ann. Intern. Med.*, **121**, 334–338.

Teot, L. A. and Sexton, C. W. (1996). Mollaret's meningitis: case report with immunocytochemical and polymerase chain reaction amplification studies. *Diagn. Cytopathol.*, **15**, 345–348.

Tucker, T. and Ellner, J. J. (1993). Chronic meningitis. In: *Infectious Diseases of the Central Nervous System*, (K. L. Tyler and J. B. Martin, eds). Philadelphia: FA Davis. pp. 188–215.

Tugwell, P., Dennis, D. T., Weinstein, A. *et al.* (1997). Laboratory evaluation in the diagnosis of Lyme disease. *Ann. Intern. Med.*, **127**, 1109–1123.

Tyler, K. L. and Adler, D. (1983). Twenty-eight years of benign recurring mollaret meningitis. *Arch. Neurol.*, **40**, 42–43.

Unger, P. D., Rappaport, K. M. and Strauchen, J. A. (1987). Necrotizing lymphadenitis (Kikuchi's disease). *Arch. Pathol. Lab. Med.*, **111**, 1031.

Vera-Ramirez, M., Charlet, M. and Parry, G. J. (1992). Recurrent aseptic meningitis complicating intravenous immunoglobulin therapy for chronic inflammatory demyelinating polyradiculoneuropathy. *Neurology*, **42**, 1636–1637.

Vilaseca, J., Tor, J., Guardia, J. and Bacardi, R. (1982). Periodic meningitis and familial mediterranean fever. *Arch. Intern. Med.*, **142**, 378–379.

Weiss, M. A., Gebarski, S. S. and McKeever, P. E. (1996). Foramen magnum neurenteric cyst causing Mollaret meningitis: MR findings. *Am. J. Neuroradiol.*, **17**, 386–388.

Welsby, P. and Smith, C. (1977). Recurrent sterile meningitis as a manifestation of systemic lupus erythematosus. *Scand. J. Infect. Dis.*, **9**, 149–150.

Widener, H. L. and Littman, B. H. (1978). Ibuprofen-induced meningitis in systemic lupus erythematosus. *J. Am. Med. Assoc.*, **239**, 1062–1064.

Wolf, S., Schotland, D. and Phillips, L. L. (1965). Involvement of nervous system in Behçet's syndrome. *Arch. Neurol.*, **12**, 315–325.

Woo, E. and Wong, P. H. (1987). Recurrent meningitis of 5 years duration due to *Cryptococcus neoformans*. *Trop. Geogr. Med.*, **39**, 67–69.

Yamamoto, L. J., Tedder, D. G., Ashley, R. and Levin, M. J. (1991). Herpes simplex virus type 1 DNA in cerebrospinal fluid of a patient with Mollaret's meningitis. *N. Eng. J. Med.*, **325**, 1082–1085.

15
Tuberculous meningitis

Larry E. Davis

Introduction

Evidence of tuberculosis dates back thousands of years to the Egyptian mummies (Morse *et al.*, 1964). By the 1800s tuberculous meningitis was recognized and in 1882 Robert Koch described the tubercle bacillus.

The prevalence of tuberculosis around the world continues to increase. The current estimate of individuals infected with *Mycobacterium tuberculosis* is over 1.7 billion (Barnes and Barrows, 1993). That is over one-third of the world's population. Although there are many factors for the growth of tuberculosis, three important factors are expansion of the world's population with increased crowding of the population, increase in the number of AIDS patients throughout the world, and increasing drug resistance to *M. tuberculosis* allowing many patients with pulmonary tuberculosis to remain infective in spite of antibiotic treatment. Accompanying this expansion of patients infected with *M. tuberculosis* is an increase in patients developing tuberculous (TB) meningitis. The precise number of patients who develop TB meningitis each year is unknown. However, an estimated 8 million individuals develop active tuberculosis each year (Kochi, 1991; Barnes and Barrows, 1993). About 15% of active tuberculosis is extrapulmonary and 6% of extrapulmonary tuberculosis is meningeal. Therefore, about 70000 patients throughout the world develop TB meningitis each year and about 4000/year do so in the USA (Venna and Sabin, 1994). An increasing worry is that many of these individuals will develop TB meningitis that is drug resistant.

Currently three major problems face physicians treating TB meningitis. First, improved methods accurately to diagnose TB meningitis are needed. Second, the ability to obtain rapid, accurate antibiotic sensitivity patterns of *M. tuberculosis* isolates are becoming a necessity. Third, better antibiotic and adjunctive treatment methods of the meningitis are needed to reduce the current mortality and morbidity. This chapter will emphasize these three challenges.

Pathophysiology

M. tuberculosis is a 2–4 μm × 0.2–0.5 μm aerobic bacillus that possesses a cell wall rich in lipid (Haas and Des Prez, 1995). One of these lipids, tuberculostearic acid, is the basis of a chemical CSF test to diagnose TB meningitis. The high lipid content makes the organism hydrophobic and hence not stained by the conventional Gram stain. However, the cell wall takes up dyes such as carbolfuchsin and retains the red dye despite decolorization by acid alcohol forming the basis of acid fast stains including the Ziehl-Neelsen stain. *M. tuberculosis* replicates slowly, dividing only every 15–20 h (Haas and Des Prez, 1995).

The majority of cases of TB meningitis begin as a primary lung infection following inhalation of the bacillus with rare cases occurring after drinking infected milk (Iseman, 1996). In over 80% of individuals, the primary lung infection is asymptomatic and localized to a small area of the lower lung fields. Because mycobacteria do not secrete enzymes or toxins, they provoke little initial inflammatory reaction in the non-immune host. Over several weeks, the bacilli invade lymphatics, spread to regional lymph nodes and cause a bacteraemia. Haematogenously seeded bacilli lodge in the brain and meninges and locally slowly replicate. About 3–8 weeks into the primary infection, host immunity develops to *M. tuberculosis* and sensitized T lymphocytes and activated macrophages invade the central nervous system (CNS) travelling to the foci of infection. The bacilli are engulfed by macrophages and the foci of infection develops into a granuloma. Some macrophages fuse together forming multinucleated giant cells with their nuclei peripherally located in the cell (Langhans' giant cell). Most of the bacilli are killed by the immune process but a small number of bacilli persist as dormant, living, organisms within the cytoplasm of macrophages. The inflammatory process usually encapsulates the granuloma to form a Rich focus. Rich foci usually remain quiescent in the brain and meninges for many years, often for the life of the individual.

With ageing or immunosuppression, the dormant bacillus may reactivate in the CNS. However, in some children, the Rich foci may incompletely form or reactivate within months to a few years. When the reactivated Rich focus is located in the meninges or subgaleal brain space, *M. tuberculosis* bacilli rupture into the subarachnoid space. Dissemination of the infection occurs via the CSF and TB meningitis ensues days to weeks later.

The initial immune response in the CSF may contain both neutrophils and lymphocytes. The intensity of the inflammation rapidly increases in spite of a relatively limited number of bacilli in the CSF. Part of the intensity of the inflammation may result from a hypersensitivity reaction to antigenic material in the cell wall of the bacilli. Hypersensitivity to mycobacterial cell wall products is well recognized. Freund's adjuvant (mainly mycobacterial cell walls) is mixed with experimental antigens to boost the immune response in animals to the experimental antigen. The tuberculin skin test also relies on a hypersensitivity reaction.

Pus developing along the cerebral hemispheres settles along the base of the brain by gravity. The intense inflammation at the base of the brain often induces a vasculitis of adjacent arteries and veins (Poltera, 1977). The inflammatory reaction begins with the adventitia, then disrupts the elastic fibres, and extends to the intima. The vasculitis may cause spasm of the vessel, thrombus formation with subsequent embolization, vessel occlusion from the thrombosis, or mycotic aneurysmal dilation and rupture with focal haemorrhage. Small penetrating arteries are particularly susceptible, especially lenticulostriate arteries travelling from the middle cerebral artery to the basal ganglia (Leiguarda *et al.*, 1988). Brain infarctions develop most often in the territory of the basal ganglia, cerebral cortex, pons and cerebellum (Poltera, 1975).

Over time, the TB meningitis becomes an arachnoiditis with fibroblasts entering the exudate. The arachnoiditis or meningitis may entrap cranial nerves or may block CSF pathways. The CSF blockage commonly occurs at the opening of the tentorium (basal cisterns) with prevention of CSF from reaching the superior sagittal sinus and being absorbed. As a consequence, communicating hydrocephalus develops. Occasionally blockage occurs at the foramen of Luschka and Magendie in the cerebellum with prevention of CSF from exiting the fourth ventricle producing obstructive hydrocephalus. In some patients the arachnoiditis may extend down the spinal cord producing a pachyarachnoiditis.

The pathogenesis of tuberculomas is less well understood. The initial focus of infection occurs within the brain parenchyma and may halt becoming a small Rich focus that remains dormant for years. If bacilli become reactivated, the Rich focus may break down becoming a caseating granuloma and an expanding tuberculoma. Alternately, the initial infection may continue to grow becoming an identifiable mass before the immune process halts the growth of bacilli, walls off the granuloma, and becomes a quiescent tuberculoma. Years later bacilli in the small tuberculoma may reactivate with subsequent expansion in size. Tuberculomas cause symptoms by mass effect (increased intracranial pressure), destruction of adjacent brain, or cerebral cortex irritation with seizures.

Clinical features

Patients with TB meningitis usually present with a subacute meningitis with symptoms present for 1–3 weeks. A few patients present with an acute meningitis with prominent symptoms for only days or with a chronic meningitis with symptoms present for longer than a month. In developing countries, TB meningitis occurs commonly in children. In developed countries, the incidence of childhood tuberculosis has fallen and most of the cases occur in adults, with the highest per capita rate being in the elderly (Davis *et al.*, 1993). Individuals who are debilitated, or who have immunodeficiencies, such as AIDS, also have increased incidence (Berenguer *et al.*, 1992). Nevertheless, it is important to recognize that no ethnic group, sex, or age is spared this disease.

Initially most patients develop progressively worsening malaise, drowsiness, low grade fevers and intermittent headaches (Table 15.1). Confusion and stupor ensue. Untreated patients soon progress to semicoma. Seizures may occur before or after hospitalization and may be due to hyponatraemia, tuberculoma, hydrocephalus, brain infarction, or necrosis and cerebral

Table 15.1   Clinical presentation of tuberculous meningitis.

Common (over 50%)
   Malaise
   Headaches
   Anorexia
   Stiff neck
   Low grade fevers
   Drowsiness and lethergy

Less common (less than 50%)
   Obtundation or coma
   Papilloedema
   Hemiparesis or aphasia
   Cranial nerve palsies
   Seizures

oedema (Patwari *et al.*, 1996). If pachyarachnoiditis develops in the spinal meninges, radicular arm or leg signs and paraparesis can occur. Untreated, death virtually always occurs.

The British Medical Research Council divided the severity of TB meningitis into three stages:

stage I   = conscious, non-specific signs, and no major neurological signs;
stage II = some mental confusion with neurological signs;
stage III = stupor or coma with marked neurological signs (Medical Research
            Council, 1948).

In developing countries at least 50% of the patients are admitted to a hospital in stage 3 (Girgis *et al.*, 1998). In developed countries, patients seek medical attention sooner with only about 25% of patients being admitted in stage 3 (Davis *et al.*, 1993; Porkert *et al.*, 1997).

Co-infection with human immunodeficiency virus (HIV) does not appear to alter the clinical presentation, CSF findings, or other laboratory data (Yechoor *et al.*, 1996; Porkert *et al.*, 1997).

Laboratory findings

Systemic tests

The complete blood count may be normal, demonstrate an anaemia, or have a mildly elevated WBC. Serum tests are non-specific but hyponatraemia is seen in over half the patients (Table 15.2). Over 50% of adult patients have an abnormal chest X-ray but only 20–30% have active pulmonary tuberculosis. Intermediate strength tuberculin skin tests are positive in only about one-half of patients (Huebner *et al.*, 1993). Of those who have a negative skin test, about half of those are also anergic to other skin tests such as mumps, tetanus, and *Candida* antigens. About 10% of patients also have renal tuberculosis which is

Table 15.2   Features suggestive of TB meningitis.

Clinical and laboratory features	Liklihood of presence (%)
Progressive subacute meningitis symptoms present for 1–3 weeks	85
Hyponatraemia: Serum sodium < 135 mEq/L	75
< 125 mEq/L	45
Positive tuberculin skin test	50
CSF with pleocytosis, elevated protein and depressed glucose	85
Family members or friends with recent active TB	
Childhood TB meningitis	35
Adult TB meningitis	< 10
Neuroimaging demonstrating enhancement of basal meninges	80
Neuroimaging demonstrating a lesion consistent with tuberculoma	10–20

suggested by a sterile 'pyuria' (urinary WBCs without significant growth of bacteria on conventional media).

CSF

The CSF is always abnormal (Merritt and Fremont-Smith, 1933). The opening pressure is often elevated in the majority and occasionally is markedly elevated. The CSF contains 30 to over 1000 WBC/μl. Usually there is a mixture of lymphocytes and neutrophils with lymphocytes predominating. However, up to 15% of patients have a predominance of neutrophils (Venna and Sabin, 1994). The protein is elevated. Early in the illness the protein level usually ranges from 60 to 500 mg/dl but if obstruction to CSF pathways develops, the protein level may be 1 g/dl or higher. In over 85% of patients the glucose is depressed below 40 mg/dl but extremely low CSF glucose levels below 10 mg/dl are unusual and more typical of acute bacterial meningitis. Acid fast stains of sediment demonstrate mycobacteria in only 5–30% of cases (Davis *et al.*, 1993; Verdon *et al.*, 1996; Porkert *et al.*, 1997). Table 15.3 lists the common methods to detect *M. tuberculosis* in CSF.

Electroencephalogram

The electroencephalogram (EEG) is usually non-specifically abnormal and shows diffuse slowing which may have a focal area of marked slowing if cerebral infarctions develop (Turrell *et al.*, 1953). Occasionally focal epileptiform activity is seen, especially in patients who experience seizures. Worsening of the EEG may suggest the development of obstructive hydrocephalus.

Neuroimaging

Neuroimaging by computed tomography (CT) with contrast or magnetic resonance imaging (MRI) with gadolinium should be abnormal. MRI appears to be slightly more sensitive (Offenbacher *et al.*, 1991). The most common abnormality that is seen in over 80% of patients by CT or MRI is

Table 15.3   CSF diagnostic test for M. tuberculosis.

Test	Sensitivity (range of positive tests)
Acid-fast staining of bacteria in sediment	5–30%
Tuberculostearic acid	50–75%
M. tuberculosis isolation from routine single lumbar puncture	20–50%
M. tuberculosis isolation from 3 lumbar punctures	50–80%
Polymerase chain reaction detection of M. tuberculosis nucleic acid	50–85%
Detection of antibody to M. tuberculosis	55%
Detection of immune complexes	60%

enhancement of the meninges, especially in the basal cisterns or over the cerebral convexity (Figure 15.1) (Gupta *et al.*, 1994). The enhancement is consistent with inflammation of the meninges. Infarcts, bland or haemorrhagic, may be seen, especially in the basal ganglia internal capsules, and middle or anterior cerebral artery territories.

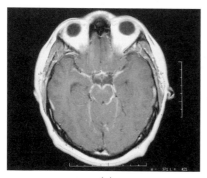

(a)

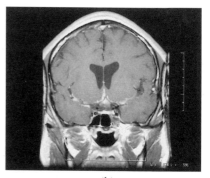

(b)

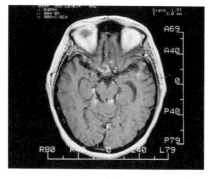

(c)

Figure 15.1   MRI (T1 with gadolinium) of a 23-year-old previously healthy male with TB meningitis. (a) Axial view demonstrating meningeal enhancement, especially in the basal cisterns. (b) Coronal view demonstrating basal meningeal enhancement. (c) MRI (T1 with gadolinium) of a 35-year-old woman in which *M. tuberculosis* was isolated from CSF. Axial view demonstrating multiple punctate granulations that enhanced in the basal cisterns.

Magnetic resonance angiography (MRA) or cerebral arteriography often demonstrates focal arterial narrowing especially in the terminal segments of the internal carotid artery and proximal segments of the middle and anterior cerebral arteries (Gupta *et al.*, 1994).

Tuberculomas are seen in about 10–20% of patients in the USA with TB meningitis, but the frequency can be above 50% in developing countries. Tuberculomas are usually located in the cerebral cortex or basal ganglia (Kioumehr *et al.*, 1994; Schoeman *et al.*, 1995). Early in the formation of a tuberculoma, there is an abundance of giant cells and the capsule lacks abundant collagen. The MRI at this stage often shows an isodense mass on T1- and T2-weighted images (Kioumehr *et al.*, 1994). As the tuberculoma matures it develops a more characteristic picture by MRI, with the mass having a low signal on T1-weighted images. Some tuberculomas demonstrate ring enhancement with gadolinium. Calcium deposits can occur in tuberculomas but are unusual. About one-third of patients with tuberculomas have more than one.

Later in the clinical course, cerebral infarctions become more common and hydrocephalus may be present. Neuroimages of the spinal cord may demonstrate pachymeningitis, spinal cord infarctions, or tuberculomas. The pachymeningitis may be diffuse or localized (Goyal *et al.*, 1997). Most focal lesions are seen as en plaque, homogeneous, uniformly enhancing, dural-based masses. The lesions appear as hyperdense on plain CT, isointense to brain parenchyma on T1-weighted MRI and isointense to hypointense on T2-weighted images.

Differential diagnosis

TB meningitis is usually a subacute meningitis and therefore must be distinguished from other causes of subacute meningitis. Table 15.4 lists the major causes of subacute meningitis that should be considered. Depending of the geographical region of the patient, fungal meningitis from *Cryptococcus neoformans*, *Coccidioides immitis*, and *Histoplasma capsulatum* should seriously be considered as their clinical and laboratory presentations are quite similar.

Making the diagnosis

Presumptive diagnosis

Table 15.2 lists the clinical and laboratory features that are suggestive of TB meningitis and the likelihood that they are found. Particularly helpful are tests suggesting the presence of a subacute meningitis, a CSF exam demonstrating inflammation (pleocytosis, elevated protein, and depressed glucose), and neuroimaging suggesting enhancement of the basal meninges or a tuberculoma. It should be noted that not every patient will have every feature and patients

Table 15.4   Differential diagnosis of subacute meningitis

Common causes
Infectious
Bacteria
  Mycobacterium tuberculosis
  Treponema pallidum
  Borrelia burgdorferi
  Listeria monocytogenes
Fungi
  Cryptococcus neoformans
  Coccidioides immitis
  Histoplasma capsulatum
Virus
  Human immunodeficiency virus
Parasite
  Taenia solium (cysticercosis)

Non-infectious
Carcinomatous meningitis
CNS sarcoidosis
Parameningeal infections (subdural empyema, epidural abscess, vertebral or cranial osteomyelitis, sinusitis, brain abscess, mastoiditis, etc.)

Less common causes
Infectious
Bacteria
  Brucella
  Mycobacterium avium intracellulare
Fungi
  Blastomycetes dermatidis
  Nocardia species
  Actinomyces species
  Aspergillus species
  Zygomycetes species
  Candida albicans
  Sporothrix schenckii
  Cladosporium
  Pseudoallescheria boydii
Virus
  Enterovirus in patient with agammaglobulinaemia
Parasite
  Toxoplasma gondii
  Angiostrongylus cantonensis
  Gnathostoma spinigerum
  Naegleria fowleri
  Entamoeba histolytica

Non-infectious
Granulomatous angiitis
Behçet's disease
Vogt-Koyangi-Harada syndrome
Chemical meningitis (foreigh bodies, sulpha drugs, etc)
Systemic lupus erythematosus
Chronic benign lymphocytic meningitis
Discharge into the meninges from epidermoid tumours or craniopharyngioma
Delirium tremens

---

may present with very atypical features. As noted in Table 15.4, a subacute meningitis does not always mean tuberculosis is the aetiology.

Tuberculin skin tests should be placed but are not always positive. A positive tuberculin skin test is suggestive but a negative skin test does not rule out the diagnosis (Huebner *et al.*, 1993). The skin test may be negative in up to 50% of patients (Haas *et al.*, 1977; Waecker and Connor, 1990; Girgis *et al.*, 1998). Most adults previously immunized with BCG vaccine as a child are tuberculin skin test negative so a positive skin test is significant (Ciesielski, 1995). A positive tuberculin skin test is less useful if the individual comes from a developing country where the prevalence of positive skin tests in adults is high. The tuberculin skin test should be placed with other skin tests for anergy. Commonly used anergy skin tests include tetanus toxoid, mumps antigen, *Candida* antigens, coccidioidin, and histoplasmin. It should be noted, however, that patients with TB meningitis may express either a selective anergy to tuberculin or generalized anergy to the entire panel of skin tests.

Definitive diagnosis

The definitive diagnosis is made from CSF by isolation of *M. tuberculosis*, identification of *M. tuberculosis* nucleic acid or proteins, and/or detection of a specific humoral immune response to *M tuberculosis*. Presently it is difficult to establish definitively the diagnosis of TB meningitis. The major reason lies in the paucity of *M. tuberculosis* bacilli in CSF. Most patients with TB meningitis have CSF that contains only 10^0 to 10^2 viable mycobacteria/ml (Davis *et al.*, 1993). For comparison, patients with pyogenic bacterial meningitis usually have from 10^5 to 10^7 bacteria/ml in their CSF and patients with cryptococcal meningitis usually have from 10^2 to 10^4 organisms/ml. Compounding this problem is the fact that mycobacteria are difficult to concentrate in CSF because the organism has a high lipid content making its buoyant density near that of CSF. Finally, the slow growth rate of mycobacterium requires weeks of incubation before a positive culture can be determined.

Culture of large volumes of CSF (10–30 ml) on three separate occasions increases the yield of a positive culture from about 30% to over 75% (Kennedy and Fallon, 1979). It has also been shown that the first few days of anti-TB therapy do not significantly affect the ability to culture *M. tuberculosis* from the CSF (Kennedy and Fallon, 1979). Thus, one does not have to withhold therapy to obtain the multiple CSF cultures. High speed centrifugation of the CSF for a prolonged period (3000 × g for 30 min) is important because the high lipid content in mycobacteria make the organism close to the buoyant density of CSF (Kent and Kubica, 1985). The standard clinical laboratory bench centrifuge used to pellet pyogenic bacteria does little to pellet mycobacteria. Table 15.5 lists the author's method of optimizing the probability of isolating *M. tuberculosis* from CSF. The concentrated CSF can be placed on solid media, such as Middlebrook 7H10, Lowenstein-Jensen, or liquid culture systems, such as the BACTEC radiometric system. Detectable mycobacteria growth on solid media often takes 4–6 weeks, but only 1–3 weeks in the BACTEC system.

Table 15.5 Optimizing successful culture of *M. Tuberculosis* from CSF.

- Remove 20–40 ml CSF from lumbar space
  Low colony count requires culture of large volume of CSF
  Highest concentration of mycobacteria are at base of brain which would be sampled by
    removal of 40 ml CSF
- Repeat lumbar puncture 3 times
  Mycobacteria can be cultured from CSF up to 1 week after onset of anti-tuberculous
    therapy
  Increases successful culture rate from ≈30% to ≈80%
- Concentrate mycobacteria in CSF
  High speed centrifugation (3000 × g for 30 min) is required to pellet mycobacteria because
    of their high lipid content
- Culture, when possible, in liquid media for *M. tuberculosis* growth
  Incubation time is shorter with liquid media, such as Bactec®, than with solid media

Since isolation of *M. tuberculosis* usually requires several weeks, there is a
need for a rapid method to diagnose TB meningitis. Ziehl-Neelsen stains of
CSF sediment are usually negative even when the culture is positive. The low
number of mycobacteria/ml present in most CSF specimens makes it very
difficult to find mycobacteria on acid-fast stains (Lipsky *et al.*, 1984; Davis *et
al.*, 1993). Several tests use CSF to detect tuberculostearic acid (cell wall
constituent of *M. tuberculosis* and a few other fungi) (French *et al.*, 1987),
antibodies to M. tuberculosis (Chandramuki *et al.*, 1989; Miorner *et al.*, 1995)
or immune complexes (Miorner et al., 1995). At present these antigen/antibody
methods appear neither highly specific nor sensitive enough to be diagnostic in
an individual patient (Patil *et al.*, 1986). The most promising diagnostic test is
the polymerase chain reaction (PCR) assay for detection of fragments of *M.
tuberculosis* DNA (Kox *et al.*, 1995). Experimental studies have found that the
test is close to the sensitivity of *M. tuberculosis* CSF cultures (Kox *et al.*, 1995;
Pfyffer *et al.*, 1996). In addition, the PCR assay may remain positive in some
patients for several weeks after anti-tuberculosis treatment (Lin and Harn,
1995). It should be noted that presently all commercial *M. tuberculosis* PCR
assays are FDA approved only for sputum and not CSF.

In this era of increasing resistance of *M. tuberculosis* to various antibiotics, it
is important not only to make the correct diagnosis but also to culture the
mycobacterium and determine its antibiotic sensitivity pattern.

In occasional patients with atypical features and localized lesions identified
on neuroimaging, it may be prudent to biopsy the involved meninges or brain.
The tissue should be cultured for tuberculosis as well as acid-fast stained and
possibly analysed by PCR for *M. tuberculosis* DNA.

Management

At present the incidence of drug resistance in CSF *M. tuberculosis* isolates is
relatively low. In a recent Egyptian study of 150 CSF isolates, resistance to
isoniazid was present in 10%, ethambutol in 7%, and rifampin in 3% (Girgis

Table 15.6 Drugs for tuberculous meningitis.

Drug	Dose (mg/kg/day) and route	Major toxicity () estimated frequency	Recommended monitoring
Isoniazid (INH)	5–10 (max 300 mg) p.o.	Hepatitis (1–2%), neuropathy (5% without pyridoxine), seizures, increased dilantin levels	Alanine aminotransferase (ALT) weekly to monthly, phenytoin levels as needed
Pyridoxine	Child: 25 mg/day p.o. Adult: 50 mg/day p.o.	To prevent INH neuropathy	
Rifampin	Child: 15 p.o. Adult: 10 max	Hepatitis (1–2%), blood hypersensitivity reactions	ALT similar to INH
Pyrazinamide	25 (max 2.5 g)	Arthralgias (5%), Hyperuriciaema, gout rash, hepatitis (1%)	Uric acid
Streptomycin	Child: 30 i.m Adult: 15 (max 1 g)	Hearing loss and vestibular imbalance (1–5%)	Audiogram baseline then monthly, tandem gait weekly
Ethambutol	15–25 p.o. (max 2.5 g)	Optic neuritis (3%), neuropathy (1–2%), rash	Monthly visual acuity and colour vision testing

et al., 1998). No CSF isolate was multidrug resistant. In a study of 30 CSF isolates from children, 17% were resistant to isoniazid (Waecker and Connor, 1990). The low incidence of drug resistance in meningeal mycobacteria in older adults likely reflects the drug sensitivity patterns present in the patients' environment decades ago when they were initially infected. Thus, the incidence of drug resistance in CSF isolates is higher in children and young adults, patients from many developing countries, and HIV-infected patients. In the near future, it is likely that additional anti-tubercular drugs will be required in the initial treatment of TB meningitis until the drug sensitivity pattern is known.

Most authorities currently recommend a three first-line drug regimen (isoniazid, rifampin and pyrazinamide) with addition of a fourth drug (streptomycin or ethambutol) (Table 15.6) (American Thoracic Society and Centers for Disease Control, 1994; Anonymous 1995; Raviglione and O'Brien, 1998). Drug resistance should be suspected if the patient has been previously treated for tuberculosis or if the individual comes from a part of the world with known high prevalence of drug resistance. In most circumstances treatment should be for 9–12 months but can be reduced to 6 months when there is an excellent clinical response or prolonged to 18–24 months if there is a poor response or known drug resistance (Moench, 1993; American Thoracic Society and Centers for Disease Control, 1994). The American Academy of Pediatrics recommends isoniazid, rifampin, pyrazinamide and streptomycin for 2 months followed by 10 months of isoniazid and rifampin (Committee on Infectious Diseases, 1992).

General principles to be followed in the treatment of tuberculous meningitis are: multiple drugs are required; drugs should adequately cross the blood–CSF barrier to achieve therapeutic concentrations in CSF; drugs should be taken on a regular basis; and drugs should be taken for a sufficient period of time to eradicate the CNS infection.

Isoniazid (INH) is a small water soluble molecule that penetrates the blood–CSF and blood–brain barriers well (Reed and Blumer, 1983). INH is bactericidal and appears to act by impairing M. tuberculosis DNA synthesis. In about 10% of individuals, INH may lead to pyridoxine deficiency and a sensorimotor distal polyneuropathy that begins 3–35 weeks into therapy. Therefore, pyridoxine 50 mg/day should be added to the regimen. Mild hepatic enzyme elevation, hepatitis, and hypersensitivity also occur. The incidence of hepatitis increases with advancing age (American Thoracic Society and Centers for Disease Control, 1994).

Rifampin is a fat soluble molecule that penetrates inflamed blood–CSF barriers well (Reed and Blumer, 1983). Rifampin is bactericidal and appears to act by impairing RNA synthesis (Holdiness, 1990; Committee on Infectious Diseases, 1992). Since rifampin induces hepatic microsomal enzymes, the drug may accelerate clearance of drugs metabolized by the liver, especially coumadin, oral hypoglycaemic agents, digitoxin, antiarrhythmic agents, and phenytoin (American Thoracic Society and Centers for Disease Control, 1994). Rifampin is excreted by the liver and hepatotoxicity has been recognized. Rifampin causes an orange discoloration to urine, saliva, and CSF.

Pyrazinamide (PZA) is a derivative of nicotinic acid, is bactericidal, easily penetrates the blood–CSF barrier, and has a unique ability to kill slowly metabolizing mycobacteria (Reed and Blumer, 1983; Moench, 1993). Streptomycin is bactericidal and penetrates inflamed blood–CSF barriers (Holdiness, 1990; Committee on Infectious Diseases, 1992). Streptomycin can lead to severe sensorineural hearing loss and hence is usually discontinued after 2 months of treatment. Streptomycin ototoxicity is increased in the elderly. Ethambutol is bacteriostatic and penetrates inflamed blood–CSF barriers somewhat poorly (American Thoracic Society and Center for Disease Control, 1994). The drug apparently interferes with RNA synthesis (Reed and Blumer, 1983; Holdiness, 1990; Committee on Infectious Diseases, 1992). This drug appears somewhat less effective than streptomycin and is usually discontinued after 2 months.

Second line antituberculous drugs include ofloxacin and ciprofloxacin, capreomycin, kanamycin, cycloserine, amikacin, clofazimine, and rifabutin (American Thoracic Society and Center for Disease Control, 1994; Anonymous, 1995).

Treatment of tuberculomas is generally similar to that of TB meningitis (Afghani and Lieberman, 1994). However, it has been recognized that occasionally tuberculomas can appear or expand in the face of appropriate tuberculosis antibiotic therapy (Afghani and Lieberman, 1994). New clinical symptoms may develop due to the tuberculomas (Teoh et al., 1987).

It is well recognized that poor compliance in taking the medications may result in clinical relapses with the development of drug resistant mycobacteria.

Therefore, when the patient is discharged and begins an outpatient treatment programme, institution of directly observed therapy should be entertained. Thrice weekly treatment programmes are available to make this easier (American Thoracic Society and Center for Disease Control, 1994; Raviglione and O'Brien, 1998).

In addition to anti-tubercular drugs, adjunctive therapy with corticosteroids has been recommended for severely ill patients. Several studies (Kumarvelu *et al.*, 1994; Schoeman *et al.*, 1997; Girgis *et al.*, 1998), but not all (Kaojaren *et al.*, 1991; Chotmongkol *et al.*, 1996), have reported fewer deaths and less neurological sequelae in patients given either prednisone (children – 4 mg/kg/day) or dexamethasone (adults – 12–16 mg/day, children 8 mg/day) for the first 1–2 months of therapy. In general, patients with more severe meningitis (stages II and III) have benefited the most. If the likelihood of the diagnosis is not high, one should consider omitting the corticosteroids as use of corticosteroids without appropriate drug therapy can worsen other infectious causes of subacute meningitis.

Since these drugs have known adverse reactions, it is advisable to obtain baseline measurements of serum hepatic enzymes, bilirubin, creatinine, uric acid, and a complete blood count including a platelet count (American Thoracic Society and Center for Disease Control, 1994). These values will help determine if there is pre-existing renal or liver disease that may require modification of drug dosages. The overall frequency of adverse reactions for a four-drug regimen is about 8% if streptomycin is given and 3% if ethambutol is given (American Thoracic Society and Center for Disease Control, 1994).

The management of increased intracranial pressure is often a challenge. While the CSF pressure may be only mildly elevated on admission, it can dramatically increase should complications such as hydrocephalus, thrombosis of draining veins and sinuses, or brain oedema develop. CT scans are helpful should papilloedema develop or the patient deteriorate. In children early in the clinical course, increased intracranial pressure may sometimes be managed with repeated lumbar punctures to remove CSF and with acetazolamide (30 mg/kg/day in three divided doses p.o.) to reduce CSF formation (Visudhiphan and Chiemchanya, 1979). However, often a ventriculo-peritoneal shunt is required for long term reduction of the intracranial pressure.

In successful treatment, the CSF slowly returns to normal. CSF cell counts lower by 50% during the first month but may not become normal for a year (Kent *et al.*, 1993). CSF glucose becomes normal in 1–2 months and protein becomes normal by 12 months or longer. CSF cultures should be sterile by the first month but PCR results may remain positive for a month (Lin and Harn, 1995).

Prevention

One major protective effect of BCG is to confine a primary tuberculosis infection to the lungs and to prevent its haematogenous spread through the activation of macrophages and subsets of T lymphocytes (Ciesielski, 1995). Thus, while there continues to be controversy as to whether childhood

Table 15.7   Prognosis of tuberculous meningitis by MRC stage on admission.

Outcome	MRC stage I (%)	MRC stage II (%)	MRC stage III (%)
Survived			
Full recovery	71	56	13
Permanent neurological sequelae	16	13	16
Died	13	31	71

Based on 1038 patients with tuberculous meningitis analysed from eight studies published over the past 12 years (Ogawa *et al.*, 1987; Davis *et al.*, 1993; Misra *et al.*, 1996; Verdon *et al.*, 1996; Yechoor *et al.*, 1996; Porkert *et al.*, 1997; Girgis *et al.*, 1998).

immunization with BCG is effective in preventing subsequent pulmonary tuberculosis, there is considerable evidence that childhood immunization with BCG vaccine reduces the risk of developing TB meningitis (Rodrigues *et al.*, 1993).

Prognosis

Based on eight different studies of tuberculous meningitis published over the past 12 years (1038 patients), the outcome of this disease is still poor. Fifty per cent die, 15% survive with permanent neurological sequelae (poor outcome) and 35% survive with a full recovery or minimal sequelae (good outcome). The stage on hospitalization is the single most important predictor of outcome (Table 15.7). Only 13% of patients admitted with stage I disease died while 71% of those admitted in stage III died.

Other poor prognostic factors include the presence of miliary tuberculosis, delay in onset of treatment, being very young or old, presence of a debilitating condition, and very abnormal CSF (very low glucose or elevated protein) (Molavi and LeFrock, 1985).

Neurological sequelae include hemiparesis, paraparesis, quadriparesis, aphasia, mental retardation, dementia, blindness, deafness, cranial nerve palsies, epilepsy, and hypothalamic and pituitary dysfunction.

Acknowledgements

Supported by Research Service, Department of Veterans Affairs. The author thanks Drs Blaine Hart and Roland Lee for helping to prepare the MRI scans of patients with TB meningitis.

References

Afghani, B. and Lieberman, J. M. (1994). Paradoxical enlargement or development of intracranial tuberculomas during therapy: case report and review. *Clin. Infect. Dis.*, 19, 1092–1099.

American Thoracic Society and Centers for Disease Control (1994). Treatment of tuberculosis and tuberculosis infection in adults and children. *Am. J. Respir. Crit. Care Med.*, **149**, 1359–1374.

Anonymous (1995). Drugs for tuberculosis. *Med. Let.*, **37**, 67–70.

Barnes, P. F and Barrows, S. A. (1993). Tuberculosis in the 1990s. *Ann. Intern. Med.*, **119**, 400–410.

Berenguer, J., Moreno, S., Laguna, F. *et al.* (1992). Tuberculous meningitis in patients infected with the human immunodeficiency virus. *N. Engl. J. Med.*, **326**, 668–672.

Chandramuki, K., Bothamley, G. H., Brennan, P. J. and Ivanyi, J. (1989). Levels of antibody to defined antigens of *Mycobacterium tuberculosis* in tuberculous meningitis. *J. Clin. Microbiol.*, **27**, 821–825.

Chotmongkol, V., Jitpimolmard, S. and Thavornpitak, Y. (1996). Corticosteroid in tuberculous meningitis. *J. Med. Assoc. Thai.*, **79**, 83–90.

Ciesielski, S. D. (1995). BCG vaccination and the PPD test: what the clinician needs to know. *J. Fam. Pract.*, **40**, 76–80.

Committee on Infectious Diseases (1992). Chemotherapy for tuberculosis in infants and children. *Pediatrics*, **89**, 161–164.

Davis, L. E., Rastogi, K. R., Lambert, L. C. and Skipper, B. J. (1993). Tuberculous meningitis in the southwest United States. *Neurology*, **43**, 1775–1778.

French, G. L., Chan, C. Y., Cheung, S. W. *et al.* (1987). Diagnosis of tuberculous meningitis by detection of tuberculostearic acid in cerebrospinal fluid. *Lancet*, **2**, 117–119.

Girgis, N. I., Farid, S. Z., Mansour, M. M. *et al.* (1998). Tuberculous meningitis, Abbassia Fever Hospital – Naval medical research unit no. 3 – Cairo, Egypt, from 1976–1996. *Am. J. Trop. Hyg.*, **58**, 28–34.

Goyal, M., Sharma, A., Mishra, N. K, Gaikwad, S. B. and Sharma, M. C. (1997). Imaging appearance of pachymeningeal tuberculosis. *Am. J. Roentgenol.*, **169**, 1421–1424.

Gupta, R. K., Gupta, S., Singh, D. *et al.* (1994). MR imaging and angiography in tuberculous meningitis. *Neuroradiology*, **36**, 87–92.

Haas, C. W. and Des Prez, R. M. (1995). Mycobacterium tuberculosis. In: *Principles and Practice of Infectious Diseases*, 4th edn. (G. L. Mandell, J. E. Bennett, R. Dolin, eds). New York: Churchill Livingstone. pp. 2210–2243.

Haas, E. J., Madhavan, T., Quinn, E. L. *et al.* (1977). Tuberculous meningitis in an urban general hospital. *Arch. Intern. Med.*, **137**, 1518–1521.

Holdiness, M. R. (1990). Management of tuberculous meningitis. *Drugs*, **39**, 224–233.

Huebner, R. E., Schein, M. F. and Bass, J. B. (1993). The tuberculin skin test. *Clin. Infect. Dis.*, **17**, 968–975.

Iseman, M. D. (1996). Tuberculosis. In: *Cecil Textbook of Medicine*, 20th edn. (J. C. Bennett and F. Plum, eds). Philadelphia: W.B. Saunders. pp. 1683–1689.

Kaojaren, S., Supmonchai, K., Phuapradit, P., Mokkhavesa, C. and Krittiyanunt, S. (1991). Effect of steroids on cerebrospinal fluid penetration of antituberculous drugs in tuberculous meningitis. *Clin. Pharmacol. Ther.*, **49**, 6–12.

Kennedy, D. H. and Fallon, R. J. (1979). Tuberculous meningitis. *J. Am. Med. Assoc.*, **241**, 264–268.

Kent, S. J., Crowe, S. M., Yung, A., Lucas, C. R. and Mijch, A. M. (1993). Tuberculous meningitis: a 30 year review. *Clin. Infect. Dis.*, **17**, 987–984.

Kent, P. T. and Kubica, G. P. (1985). *Public Health Mycobacteriology: a Guide for the Level III Laboratory*. Atlanta GA: US Department of Health and Human Services, Public Health Service, Centers for Disease Control. pp. 31–36.

Kioumehr, F., Dadsetan, M. R., Rooholamini, S. A. and Au, A. (1994). Central nervous system tuberculosis: MRI. *Neuroradiology*, **36**, 93–96.

Kochi, A. (1991). The global tuberculosis situation and the new control strategy of the World Health Organization. *Tubercle*, **72**, 1–6.

Kox, L. F. F., Kuijper, S. and Kolk, A. H. J. (1995). Early diagnosis of tuberculous meningitis by polymerase chain reaction. *Neurology*, **45**, 2228–2232.

Kumarvelu, S., Prasad, K., Khosla, A., Behari, M. and Ahuja, G. K. (1994). Randomized controlled trial of dexamethasone in tuberculous meningitis. *Tuber. Lung Dis.*, **75**, 203–207.

Leiguarda, R., Berthier, M., Starkstein, S., Nogues, M. and Lylyk, P. (1988). Ischemic infarction in 25 children with tuberculous meningitis. *Stroke*, **19**, 200–204.

Lin, J. J. and Harn, H.-J. (1995). Application of the polymerase chain reaction to monitor *Mycobacterium tuberculosis* DNA in the CSF of patients with tuberculosis meningitis after antibiotic treatment. *J. Neuro. Neurosurg. Psych.*, **59**, 175–177.

Lipsky, B. A., Gates, J., Tenover, F. C. and Plorede, J. J. (1984). Factors affecting the clinical value of microscopy for acid-fast bacilli. *Rev. Infect. Dis.*, **6**, 214–222.

Medical Research Council (1948). Streptomycin in tuberculosis trials committee. Streptomycin treatment of tuberculous meningitis. *Lancet*, **I**, 582–596.

Merritt, H. H. and Fremont-Smith, F. (1933). Cerebrospinal fluid in tuberculous meningitis. *Arch. Neurol. Psych.*, **33**, 516–536.

Miorner, H., Sjobring, U., Nayak, P. and Chandramuki, A. (1995). Diagnosis of tuberculous meningitis: a comparative analysis of 3 immunoassays, an immune complex assay and the polymerase chain reaction. *Tubercle Lung Dis.*, **76**, 381–386.

Misra, U. K., Kalita, J., Srivastava, M. and Mandal, S. K. (1996). Prognosis of tuberculous meningitis: a multivariate analysis. *J. Neurol. Sci.*, **137**, 57–61.

Moench, T. (1993). Tuberculous meningitis. In: *Current Therapy in Neurologic Disease*, 4th edn (R. T. Johnson and J. W. Griffin, eds), Philadelphia: B.C. Decker. pp. 119–122.

Molavi, A. and LeFrock, J. L. (1985). Tuberculous meningitis. *Med. Clin. N. Am.*, **69**, 315–331.

Morse, D., Brothwell, D. R. and Ucko, P. J. (1964). Tuberculosis in ancient Egypt. *Am. Rev. Tuberc.*, **90**, 524–541.

Offenbacher, H., Fazekas, F., Schmidt, R. *et al.* (1991). MRI in tuberculous meningoencephalitis: report of four cases and review of the neuroimaging literature. *J. Neurol.*, **238**, 340–344.

Ogawa, S. K., Smith, M. A., Brennessel, D. J. and Lowy, F. D. (1987). Tuberculous meningitis in an urban medical center. *Medicine*, **66**, 317–326.

Patil, S. A., Gourie-Devi, M., Anand, A. R. *et al.* (1996). Significance of mycobacterial immune complexes (IgG) in the diagnosis of tuberculosis meningitis. *Tubercle Lung Dis.*, **77**, 164–167.

Patwari, A. K., Aneja, S., Ravi, R. N., Singhal, P. K. and Arora, S. K. (1996). Convulsions in tuberculous meningitis. *J. Trop. Pediatr.*, **42**, 91–97.

Pfyffer, G. E., Kissling, P., Jahn, E. M. I. *et al.* (1996). Diagnostic performance of amplified *Mycobacterium tuberculosis*. Direct test with cerebrospinal fluid, other nonrespiratory, and respiratory specimens. *J. Clin. Microbiol.*, **34**, 834–841.

Poltera, A. A. (1975). Vascular lesions in intracranial tuberculosis. *Pathol. Microbiol.*, **43**, 192–198.

Poltera, A. A. (1977). Thrombogenic intracranial vasculitis in tuberculous meningitis: a 20 year post mortem survey. *Acta. Neurol. Belg.*, **77**, 12–19.

Porkert, M. T., Sotir, M., Parrott-Moore, P. and Blumberg, H. M. (1997). Tuberculous meningitis at a large inner city medical center. *Am. J. Med. Sci.*, **313**, 325–331.

Raviglione, M. C. and O Brien, R. J. (1998). Tuberculosis. In: *Harrison s Principles of Internal Medicine*, 14th edn (A. S. Fauci, E. Braunwald, K. J. Isselbacher *et al.*, eds). New York: McGraw-Hill. pp. 1004–1014.

Reed, M. D. and Blumer, J. L. (1983). Clinical pharmacology of antitubercular drugs. *Pediatr. Clin. N. Am.*, **30**, 177–193.

Rodrigues, L. C., Diwan, V. K. and Wheeler, J. M. (1993). Protective effect of BCG against tuberculous meningitis and miliary tuberculosis: a meta-analysis. *Intern. J. Epidem.*, **22**, 1154–1158.

Schoeman, J. F., Van Zyl, L. E., Laubscher, J. A. and Donald, P. R. (1995). Serial CT scanning in childhood tuberculous meningitis: prognostic features in 198 cases. *J. Child. Neurol.*, **10**, 320–329.

Schoeman, J. F., Van Zyl, L. E., Laubscher, J. A. and Donald, P.R. (1997). Effect of corticosteroids on intracranial pressure, computed tomographic findings, and clinical outcome in young children with tuberculous meningitis. *Pediatrics*, **99**, 226–231.

Teoh, R., Humphries, M. J. and O'Mahony, G. (1987). Symptomatic intracranial tuberculoma developing during treatment of tuberculosis: a report of 10 patients and review of the literature. *Q. J. Med.*, **63**, 449–460.

Turrell, R. C., Shaw, W., Schmidt, R. P. *et al.* (1953). Electroencephalographic studies of the encephalopathies II. Serial studies in tuberculous meningitis. *Electroencephalogr. Clin. Neurophysiol.*, **5**, 53–63.

Venna, N. and Sabin, T. D. (1994). Tuberculous of the nervous system. In: *Current Diagnosis in Neurology*, (E. Feldmann, ed.). St Louis: Mosby. pp. 117–125.

Verdon, R., Chevret, S., Laissy, J-P. and Wolf, M. (1996). Tuberculous meningitis in adults: Review of 48 cases. *Clin. Infect. Dis.*, **22**, 982–988.

Visudhiphan, P. and Chiemchanya, S. (1979). Hydrocephalus in tuberculous meningitis in children: Treatment with acetazolamide and repeated lumbar puncture. *J. Pediatr.*, **95**, 657–660.

Waecker, N. J. and Connor, J. D. (1990). Central nervous tuberculosis in children: a review of 30 cases. *Pediatr. Infect. Dis. J.*, **9**, 539–543.

Yechoor, V. K., Shandera, W. X., Rodriguez, P. and Cate, T. R. (1996). Tuberculous meningitis among adults with and without HIV infection. *Arch. Intern. Med.*, **156**, 1710–1716.

16

Ehrlichiosis and the nervous system

Larry E. Davis, Christopher D. Paddock and James E. Childs

Introduction

The first description of an ehrlichial infection came from Algeria in 1935, where research dogs developed a fatal haemorrhagic illness after becoming heavily parasitized by the brown dog tick, *Rhipicephalus sanguineus*. Examination of peripheral blood smears showed basophilic bodies in the cytoplasm of monocytes (Donatien and Lestoquard, 1937). The organism responsible for this disease was subsequently named *Ehrlichia canis*, and is now recognized to have a world-wide distribution. At least seven additional ehrlichial pathogens of animals have been identified in the subsequent 60 years. Human disease attributable to an *Ehrlichia* species was initially discovered in Japan in 1953. The disease, named sennetsu fever, is a mononucleosis-like illness caused by *E. sennetsu*. The first documented case of human ehrlichial infection in the USA occurred in 1986 (Maeda *et al.*, 1987). In this report, a 51-year-old man developed a non-specific febrile illness with marked thrombocytopenia and anaemia after sustaining multiple tick bites on a trip to Arkansas. Examination of the peripheral blood smear revealed basophilic inclusions in the cytoplasm of his circulating monocytes. The patient's serum demonstrated a high titre of antibody reactive with *E. canis*; initially, this veterinary pathogen was thought to be the causative agent. In 1991, a novel bacterium was isolated from the blood of a febrile patient from Fort Chaffee, Arkansas (Dawson *et al.*, 1991). The bacterium, subsequently named *Ehrlichia chaffeensis*, is antigenically and genetically similar to *E. canis* and is now recognized as the agent of human monocytic ehrlichiosis (HME). A second ehrlichial pathogen of humans in the USA was identified from patients in Wisconsin and Minnesota in 1994. These patients developed an illness similar to HME, but inclusions were observed almost exclusively in neutrophils rather than in monocytes (Bakken *et al.*, 1994). A novel *Ehrlichia* species has since been isolated from patients with this disease (termed human granulocytic ehrlichiosis, HGE). This species is antigenically and genetically similar to the *E. equi* and *E. phagocytophilia*, recognized veterinary pathogens of horses, dogs, sheep and cattle. This bacterium has yet to formally named and is generally referred to as the agent of HGE.

Biology

Ehrlichiae are small (0.5–1.5 µm), obligate intracellular pathogens classified among the family *Rickettsiaeceae* (Rikihisa, 1991). These Gram-negative bacteria are unable to utilize glucose, and use glutamine or glutamate to synthesize adenine triphosphate (Rikihisa, 1991). The genus *Ehrlichia* is loosely organized into three 'genogroups'. Each contains a species that causes disease in humans, as well as several veterinary pathogens. In addition to members of the genus *Ehrlichia*, genogroup I (*E. canis* genogroup) contains *Cowdria ruminantium*, genogroup II (*E. phagocytophila* genogroup) contains *Anaplasma* species, and genogroup III (*E. sennetsu* genogroup) contains *Neorickettsia* species (Walker and Dumler, 1997).

Ehrlichiae appear to infect target cells by attaching to membrane receptors on the host's leucocytes and inducing phagocytosis (Webster *et al.*, 1998). The resultant endosome, however, fails to develop into a mature phagocytic or lysosomal vacuole, and there is no fall in pH and no digestion of the endosomal components by lysosomes. Ehrlichiae reside and divide within endosomes, producing intracytoplasmic aggregates of bacteria called morulae. The morphology of morulae vary among ehrlichial species with regard to their size, number of individual ehrlichiae, and the presence of a fibrillar matrix (Popov *et al.*, 1998). Individual morulae can contain more than 50 bacteria (Popov *et al.*, 1998). Individual bacteria are released from mature morulae in the host cell cytoplasm into the extracellular space by cell lysis or by exocytosis with fusion of the vacuole membrane with the plasma membrane (Rikihisa, 1991).

Epidemiology and natural history

Human ehrlichioses caused by *E. chaffeensis* or the HGE agent have been reported throughout broad, albeit discontinuous regions of the USA (Eng *et al.*, 1990, Fishbein *et al.*, 1994; McQuiston *et al.*, 1999). Human infections with one or both of these agents, and perhaps antigenically-related ehrlichial species, have also been documented in Europe (Lotric-Furlan *et al.*,1998; Christova and Dumler, 1999), South America (Ripoll *et al.*, 1999), and Africa (Uhaa *et al.*, 1992). Forty-seven states have reported one or both types of ehrlichiosis (Figures 16.1 and 16.2), although some of the cases from individual states have resulted from travel to endemic locations rather than local acquisition of infection. The peak incidence of HME and HGE occurs from May to August (Fishbein *et al.*, 1994; Bakken *et al.*, 1996). Cases of HGE continue to occur during the fall months (Comer *et al.*, 1999b). The variation in the seasonal distribution of reported cases of HME and HGE reflects activity periods of their different tick vectors.

The majority of HME cases have occurred in the southeastern and south-central states (especially Oklahoma, Missouri, Arkansas, and Texas), while most cases of HGE have occurred in north-central and northeastern states, particularly New York, Connecticut, Minnesota, and Wisconsin (McQuiston *et al.*, 1999). The male predominance of reported cases of both HME and HGE

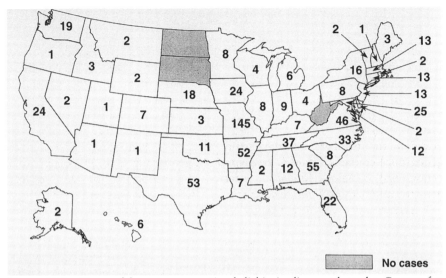

Figure 16.1 Cases of human monocytic ehrlichiosis diagnosed at the Centers for Disease Control, Atlanta GA, 1986–1997. Data from Mcquiston *et al.*, (in press).

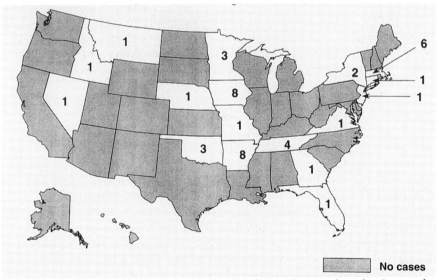

Figure 16.2 Cases of human granulocytic ehrlichiosis diagnosed at the Centers for Disease Control, Atlanta GA, 1986–1997. Data from Mcquiston *et al.*, (in press)

likely represents increased exposure to ticks through more outdoor activities. The diseases can occur in any age group, but the majority of symptomatic infections appear to occur in adults over 40 years of age (Fishbein *et al.*, 1994; Everett *et al.*, 1994; Bakken *et al.*, 1994). Perinatal transmission of HGE has been described (Horowitz *et al.*, 1998c).

The majority of cases of ehrlichiosis represent sporadic transmission. However, episodes of clustered disease involving communities (Standaert *et*

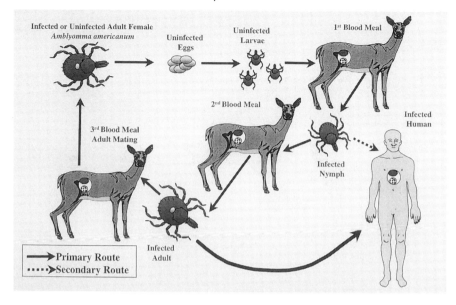

Figure 16.3 A life cycle for *Ehrlichia chaffeensis* demonstrating the primary and secondary routes of spread.

al., 1995) or occupational groups, particularly military recruits (Peterson *et al.*, 1989; Arguin *et al.*, 1999), have occurred following a common exposure to areas with high tick infestations.

E. *chaffeensis* and the agent of HGE are maintained in nature as complex zoonoses, with ticks acting as the vector (figures 16.3 and 16.4). A primary tick vector of HME is the lone star tick, *Amblyomma americanum* (Anderson *et al.*, 1993). White-tailed deer are an important source of blood meals for adult and immature stages of *A. americanum*. Experimentally infected white-tailed deer can maintain a bacteraemia for at least 24 days (Dawson *et al.*, 1994), and naturally infected deer have been found in the southeastern United States (Lockhart *et al.*, 1997). Humans become infected with E. *chaffeensis* following the bite of an infected nymph or adult tick. Based on seasonal distribution of cases of HME and infection rates observed in adult and nymphal ticks, adults appear to be the most important stage for transmitting the agent to humans (CDC, unpublished data; Burket *et al.*, 1998).

The principal vector responsible for transmission of HGE in the Northeast and upper Midwest is *Ixodes scapularis*, the black-legged or deer tick (Pancholi *et al.*, 1995; Telford *et al.*, 1996). In the western USA, *I. pacificus* may represent an important vector (Richter *et al.*, 1996). In Europe, *I. ricinus* is a vector incriminated in transmission of the HGE agent to humans (Dumler and Bakken, 1998; Petrovec *et al.*, 1999). The HGE agent may persist in the wild in a deer tick-rodent cycle, similar to the maintenance cycle of *Borrelia burgdorferi* (Telford *et al.*, 1996). Epidemiological and natural history data suggest that nymphal *Ixodes* ticks are the most important stage involved in transmitting the HGE agent to humans.

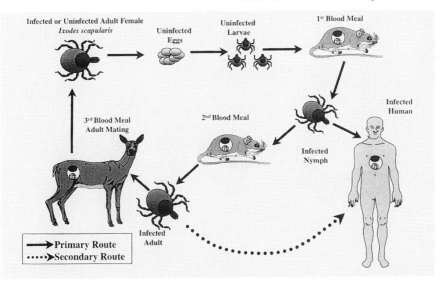

Figure 16.4   A life cycle for the agent of human granulocytic ehrlichiosis demonstrating the primary and secondary routes of spread.

Ticks are capable of transmitting a wide array of human pathogens, and dual human infections with ehrlichiae and other agents have been reported. Among the described coinfecting pathogens are *Rickettsia rickettsii*, the agent of Rocky Mountain spotted fever (Sexton *et al.*, 1998); *B. burgdorferi*, the agent of Lyme disease (Nadelman *et al.*, 1997; Trotta *et al.*, 1997); and *Babesia microti*, an agent of babesiosis (Mitchell *et al.*, 1996). In an area of New York state where HGE is endemic, up to 53% of captured ticks were infected with the HGE agent and 26% of captured ticks were infected with both the HGE agent and *B. burgdorferi* (Schwartz, *et al.*, 1997).

Pathophysiology

E. chaffeensis primarily infects mononuclear cells, especially macrophages and monocytes, and to a lesser extent lymphocytes. Occasionally *E. chaffeensis* may be seen in immature granulocytes, particularly in persons with unusually severe disease (Maeda *et al.*, 1987; Paddock *et al.*, 1993, 1997). In infected patients, *E. chaffeensis* is most readily identified in fluids and tissues with abundant mononuclear cells, including blood (figure 16.5), cerebrospinal fluid, spleen, bone marrow, lymph nodes, liver sinusoids, and lungs (Dunn *et al*, 1992; Dumler *et al.*, 1993; Paddock *et al.*, 1993; Marty *et al*; 1995). However, the ehrlichioses are systemic infections, and with careful inspection, ehrlichiae may be seen in virtually any organ (Marty *et al.*, 1995).

The target cells of the agent of HGE are granulocytic leucocytes, predominantly neutrophils (Bakken *et al.*, 1994). However, localization of the HGE agent in macrophages, endothelial cells, and fibroblasts has also been described

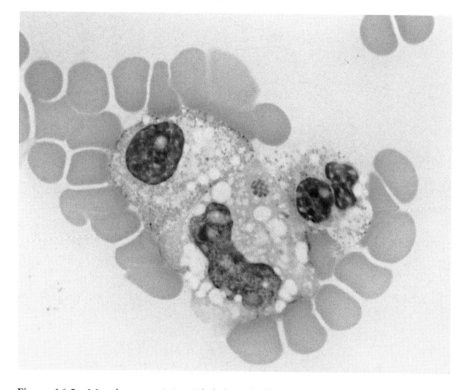

Figure 16.5 Morulae containing *Ehrlichia chaffeensis* in cytoplasm of a peripheral blood monocyte from a patient with fatal human monocytic ehrlichiosis.

(Walker and Dumler, 1997). Cells susceptible to the HGE agent express CD15s, a cell-surface molecule that is necessary for binding to and infection of the host cell by the bacterium (Goodman *et al.*, 1999).

Exactly how ehrlichiae cause disease in humans is poorly understood. Ehrlichiae do not cause vasculitis and endothelial damage like that characteristically seen in other rickettsial diseases. However, ehrlichial infections may elicit perivascular inflammatory infiltrates in many organs (Marty *et al.*, 1995; Walker and Dumler 1997; Grant *et al.*, 1997) and may directly kill infected leukocytes (Rikihisa, 1991; Popov *et al.*, 1998). Experimental mouse models of *E. chaffeensis* infection (Winslow *et al.*, 1998) and granulocytic ehrlichiosis (Hodzic *et al.*, 1998a) have been developed. Although these models do not completely reproduce all disease manifestations observed in humans, they may assist in examining pathogenic host immune responses to ehrlichiae.

Similarly, the pathogenic mechanisms responsible for central nervous system (CNS) manifestations of ehrlichial infections are incompletely characterized. Histopathological evaluation of CNS tissues from patients with fatal HME associated with severe encephalopathy may show no discrete lesions in the meninges or brain (Ratnasamy *et al.*, 1996). In other patients, perivascular infiltrates composed of lymphocytes, plasma cells and macrophages are observed in the leptomeninges (figure 16.6) and Virchow-Robin spaces

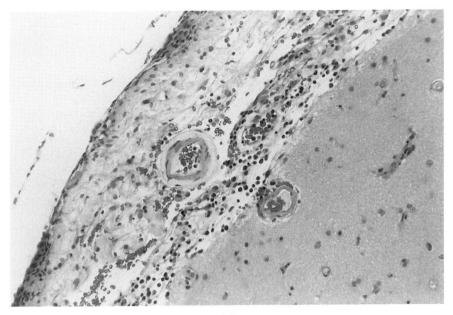

(a)

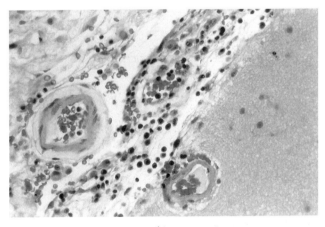

(b)

Figure 16.6 (a) Perivascular lymphoplasmacytic infiltrate in the leptomeninges of a patient with meningitis caused by *Ehrlichia chaffeensis*. (b) Higher magnification of (a). (Photography courtesy of Stephen Hunter, MD, Emory University School of Medicine).

(Marty *et al.*, 1995; Grant *et al.*, 1997). It has been suggested that ehrlichial meningitis occurs as a result of the inflammatory response to infection of perivascular macrophages by *E. chaffeensis* (Walker and Dumler, 1997). Subdural and meningeal hemorrhages, as well as subdural hygromas, have been reported from patients with severe CNS involvement (Dumler *et al.*, 1991;

Standaert et al., 1998). However, discrete lesions involving brain parenchyma have not been described.

For unknown reasons, CNS manifestations of HGE are noted with far less frequency than with HME, although meningitis may also occur in this form of ehrlichiosis (Walker and Dumler, 1997). Clinical experience with this form of the disease is relatively recent, and perhaps as yet unrecognized CNS manifestations associated with HGE may be observed as more patients are evaluated (Standaert et al., 1998).

Clinical features

In general, the clinical features of HME and HGE overlap to a substantial extent (Table 16.1). As mentioned earlier, meningitis and other CNS signs are reported more frequently with HME. The incubation period for both diseases is typically 1–2 weeks; most patients develop symptoms 5–10 days following the bite of an infecting tick. The frequency of asymptomatic ehrlichial infections is unknown and difficult to assess. Surveillance of military recruits who develop antibodies reactive with Ehrlichia spp. antigen following intense exposures to ticks in field training exercises suggests that as many as 60–70% of individuals infected with ehrlichiae do not develop disease (Yevich et al., 1995; Arguin et al., 1999). However, as these studies have not been able to differentiate between asymptomatic seroconversion to a known pathogen and infection by an antigenically related organism, these data require cautious interpretation.

The most common symptoms of HME and HGE are fever, headache, myalgia, and malaise (Eng et al., 1990; Fishbein et al., 1994; Bakken et al., 1996; Aguero-Rosenfield et al., 1996) (see Table 16.1). Patients with HME often have gastrointestinal symptoms that include nausea, vomiting, diarrhoea, and anorexia. Gastrointestinal complaints are observed in more than 50% of patients with HME, but are seen less frequently (30–40%) in patients with HGE (Bakken et al., 1996). A mild, short-lived rash that involves mainly the trunk with sparing of the hands and feet occurs in about one-quarter of adult patients with HME, although rash may occur in as many as 60% of paediatric patients infected with E. chaffeensis (Barton et al., 1992; Schutze and Jacobs, 1997). The rash has no unique characteristics and has been reported to be macular, papular, maculopapular, and occasionally petechial (Fishbein et al., 1994). A rash is rarely noted in patients with HGE (Bakken et al., 1996).

As many as 10% of patients with ehrlichial infection develop a more complicated illness, which may include involvement of the pulmonary, cardiovascular, or nervous systems. Acute respiratory distress syndrome, toxic shock syndrome, profound hypotension, cardiomyopathy, pancarditis, and pulmonary and gastrointestinal haemorrhaging have been reported (Eng et al., 1990; Fichtenbaum et al; 1993; Fishbein et al., 1994; Bakken et al., 1996; Jahangir et al., 1998). These complications typically develop in the second week of the illness. Concurrent human immunodeficiency virus (HIV) infection

Table 16.1 Clinical features of ehrlichiosis

Common (greater than 50%)	Patients* (%)
Fever	98
Malaise	79
Headache	78
Myalgias	73
Chills/rigor	66
Anorexia	56
Less common (10–49%)	
Nausea	48
Arthralgias	36
Non-specific rash	28
Cough	26
Lymphadenopathy	23
Diarrhoea/abdominal pain	21
Confusion	20
Meningismus	13
Uncommon (less than 10%)	
Hypotension	
Myocardial complications	
Acute respiratory distress syndrome	
Pneumonia	
Secondary bacterial infections	
Hepatomegaly	
Jaundice	
Seizures	
Stupor or coma	

* Data taken from 273 patients with HME or HGE reported in the following literature: (Eng *et al.*, 1990; Fishbein *et al.*, 1994; Bakken *et al.*, 1994; Everett *et al.*, 1994; Aguero-Rosenfeld *et al.*, 1996)

can complicate the clinical course, and fatalities have been reported from this patient population (Paddock., *et al.*, 1993, 1997).

Neurological features

Over three-quarters of patients with either HME or HGE develop a mild to severe headache during the course of their illness (Table 16.2). However, few develop mental status changes. Generalized weakness and myalgias are commonly present and some patients have an elevated serum creatinine phosphokinase. Unusual neurological findings include marked muscle weakness (Hammill *et al.*, 1992), dysgeusia (Everett *et al.*, 1994), and paresis (Grant *et al.*, 1997). Long-term neurological sequelae including bilateral foot drop, speech impairment, and diminished reading and fine motor ability have been described in children following severe disease (Schutze and Jacobs, 1997).

Table 16.2   Neurological features in HME and HGE*

General ehrlichiosis (> 75% patients)
Headache
Myalgias
Lethargy, rare confusion

Meningitis syndrome (10% of HME patients)
Severe headache
Meningismus
Lethargy to confusion
Photophobia
Cranial nerve palsies (CN 3, 4, 5, 7)

Encephalitis/encephalopathy syndrome (~ 10% of HME patients)
Marked confusion
Obtundation to coma
Seizures
Hyperreflexia to clonus
Ataxia

---

* Ehrlichial meningitis and encephalopathy are most frequently associated with HME and rarely with HGE; data from Ratnasamy *et al.*, 1996; Bakken *et al.*, 1996, 1998; Grant *et al.*, 1997; Standaert *et al.*, 1998). Some patients may develop a meningoencephalitis with features of both encephalitis and meningitis.

Meningitis syndrome

Features typical of a meningitis syndrome develop in about 10% of HME patients (see Table 16.2). These patients develop a severe headache, stiff neck, lethargy, photophobia, and occasional confusion. Neurological signs may develop at the onset or somewhat later in the illness. Cranial nerve palsies may develop in patients with HME or HGE. Palsies of the third and fifth nerves have been described in patients with HGE (Bakken *et al.*, 1998), and fourth and seventh nerve palsies have been reported in patients with HME (Everett *et al.*, 1994; Carter and Miller, 1997; Grant *et al.*, 1997). The duration of neurological symptoms is 1–3 weeks with treatment but can be longer if treatment is delayed. Since patients with HGE may be simultaneously infected with *Borrelia burgdorferi*, it is possible that the meningitis and nerve palsies in some patients are due to CNS Lyme disease (Ahkee and Ramirez, 1996). However, there is abundant evidence that *E. chaffeensis* directly infects the CNS. Morulae of *E. chaffeensis* have been visualized in CSF monocytes of infected patients and polymerase chain reaction (PCR) methods have been used to detect ehrlichial DNA in cerebrospinal fluid (CSF) (Dunn *et al.*, 1992; Ratnasamy *et al.*, 1996; Standaert *et al.*, 1999). *Ehrlichia chaffeensis* has been isolated from CSF of patients with HME (Standaert *et al.*, in press).

Encephalitis/encephalopathy syndrome

Up to 10% of patients with HME develop signs suggestive of an encephalopathy or encephalitis (Ratnasamy *et al.*, 1996; Standaert *et al.*, 1998), although the absence of discrete inflammatory infiltrates in brain parenchyma suggests that most patients with CNS signs develop their symptoms from an encephalo-pathy rather than an encephalitis. These patients become confused, obtunded, or comatose. When reported, coma generally occurs in untreated patients 1–2 weeks after onset of disease.

Patients with HME-induced encephalopathy may develop broad-based gait, hyperreflexia and clonus (Harkess *et al.*, 1990; Ratnasamy *et al.*, 1996). Generalized seizures have been reported for patients with HME (Ratnasamy *et al.*, 1996) and HGE (Bakken *et al.*, 1996). Some patients have features of a meningoencephalitis with CNS signs and cranial nerve palsies.

Peripheral nervous system syndrome

The peripheral nervous system appears to be involved less than the CNS. The most common picture described is limb weakness. This may involve all limbs and has been called a demyelinating neuropathy, myelitis, and peripheral neuropathy (Maeda *et al.*, 1987; Bakken *et al.*, 1998). Variants of this have included an apparent brachial plexopathy with weakness of one arm (Aguero-Rosenfeld *et al.*, 1996; Horowitz *et al.*, 1996) and an external ophthalmo-plegia, ataxia, and limb weakness similar to that seen in the Miller-Fisher variant of Guillain-Barré syndrome (Bakken *et al.*, 1998).

Laboratory findings

Abnormalities in several standard laboratory tests may provide early pre-sumptive clues to the diagnosis of the human ehrlichioses. Patients character-istically develop leucopenia, thrombocytopenia, and elevations in liver transaminase levels (Fishbein *et al.*, 1994; Aguero-Rosenfeld *et al.*, 1996; Schutze and Jacobs, 1997) (Table 16.3). Patients may not demonstrate all three abnormalities, and the abnormalities may be absent on initial presentation (Fishbein *et al.*, 1994). Cytopenias are characteristically noted in the first week of illness, and may return to normal in the second week of disease, even in some untreated patients. Approximately 50–75% of patients with HME or HGE develop leucopenia in the first week of illness, with the nadir generally between 1.5 and 4.0 cells $\times 10^9/l$ (Dumler and Bakken, 1998; Fritz and Glaser, 1998). Lymphocytopenia is frequently noted in patients with HME and HGE, and neutropenia has been reported in patients with HGE (Aguero-Rosenfeld *et al.*, 1996). Thrombocytopenia has been reported in 70% of patients with ehrlichial infection, with platelet counts generally between 50 and $150 \times 10^9/l$ (Dumler and Bakken, 1998; Fritz and Glaser, 1998). In some patients with severe disease, platelet counts may plummet to $< 20 \times 10^9/l$, and these patients may risk spontaneous haemorrhages (Dumler *et al.*, 1991; Paddock *et al.*, 1993; Bakken *et al.*, 1996). Anaemia is a less frequently observed finding, but may occur in as many as 50% of patients with HME and HGE. Bone marrows of cytopenic patients are generally normocellular, suggesting that

Table 16.3 Laboratory findings in ehrlichiosis

Common (greater than 50%)	Patients* (%)
Leukopenia	66
Lymphocytopenia	66
Elevated aspartate aminotransferase	84
Elevated alanine aminotransferase	77
Thrombocytopenia	69
Less common (10–49%)	
Anaemia	49
Elevated erythrocyte sedimentation rate	33
Elevated BUN and creatinine	26
Uncommon (less than 10%)	
Elevated creatinine phosphokinase	
Elevated bilirubin	
Depressed albumin	
Elevated fibrin split products	

* Data taken from 273 patients with HME or HGE reported in the following literature: Eng et al., 1990; Fishbein et al., 1994; Bakken et al., 1994; Everett et al., 1994; Aguero-Rosenfeld et al., 1996.

leukopenia and thrombocytopenia are due to peripheral events, resulting in sequestration or destruction of these elements (Dumler et al., 1993).

Mildly or moderately elevated levels of aspartate aminotransferase and alanine aminotransferase occur in 70–90% of patients with ehrlichial infection (Everett et al., 1994; Aguero-Rosenfield et al., 1996). Alkaline phosphatase levels are usually less affected. A variety of other abnormal laboratory test results may occur in patients with ehrlichial infection, including elevated serum creatinine phosphokinase levels (Hammill et al., 1992; Shea et al., 1995) and C-reactive protein (Lotric-Furlan et al., 1998). Electrolyte abnormalities, particularly mild to moderate hyponatraemia, are frequently noted in patients with severe disease (Everett et al., 1994; Schutze and Jacobs 1997).

CSF findings

An abnormal CSF profile (generally pleocytosis and/or an elevated CSF protein value) is most often seen in patients with mental status changes; in the largest series of patients studied, 71% of patients with HME who presented with confusion, disorientation, or delirium demonstrated one or more CSF abnormality (Table 16.4). In patients with no obvious cognitive impairment, only 11% had an abnormal CSF (Ratnasamy et al., 1996). Reported CSF leucocyte counts in patients with ehrlichial meningitis range from 1 to 1400 cells $10^6/l$; highest cell counts have been seen in children and in adults >60 years of age. Lymphocytes are the predominant cell type in approximately 75% of patients with pleocytosis, although a neutrophilic predominance may be seen in nearly

Table 16.4   CSF in HME with CNS involvement

Opening pressure	Normal
Cells	Leucocyte pleocytosis (1–1400 cells/mm^3) predominately mononuclear cells
Protein	Normal to mild elevation (30–200 mg/dl)
Glucose	Normal to borderline low ($\geq$ 35 mg/dl)
Morulae	Positive in rare instances
Culture	Positive in rare instances
PCR	Positive in rare instances

Range of values based on the following references: Harkess *et al.*, 1990; Dunn *et al.*, 1992; Fishbein *et al.*, 1994; Ratnasamy *et al.*, 1996; Standaert *et al.*, 1999.

25% of cases, particularly early in the course of the illness (Golden, 1989; Ratnasamy *et al.*, 1996; Standaert *et al.*, 1998). In contrast to other bacterial meningitides, hypoglycorrhachia is seen in relatively few patients and is generally mild when noted (Fichtenbaum *et al.*, 1993; Ratnasamy *et al.*, 1996; Standaert *et al.*, 1998). Moderately elevated CSF protein values (e.g. 0.60–2.00 g/l) are reported in approximately 75% of patients with HME meningitis (Ratnasamy *et al.*, 1996). Morulae of *E. chaffeensis* are rarely identified in CSF mononuclear cells in persons with severe HME, and *E. chaffeensis* DNA has been amplified from CSF by using PCR (Dunn *et al.*, 1992; Ratnasamy *et al.*, 1996). *E. chaffeensis* has also been isolated from the CSF of patients with HME (Standaert *et al.*, 1999).

Neuroimaging

The cranial computed tomogram (CT) is usually normal (Ratnasamy *et al.*, 1996). A non-contrasted magnetic resonance image (MRI) frequently is also normal. However, the MRI with gadolinium may show enhancement of the meninges consistent with meningitis (Ratnasamy *et al.*, 1996; Bakken *et al.*, 1998). Focal areas of cerebral oedema or haemorrhage are usually absent.

Electroencephalogram

In obtunded or comatose patients, the EEG often demonstrates non-specific slowing of background activity (Eng *et al.*, 1990; Ratnasamy *et al.*, 1996). Seizure foci or focal areas of delta waves have yet to be reported.

Establishing the diagnosis

The clinical presentations of HME and HGE may be notoriously non-specific, and the differential diagnoses for these infections may be quite broad. However, suspicion of ehrlichiosis should increase if a patient presents in the spring through fall months with a febrile illness with no other obvious cause, and: recalls a tick bite or exposure to ticks in the preceding 3 weeks; lives in or

Table 16.5   Diagnosis of ehrlichiosis

Serology against *E. chaffeensis* or HGE agent by indirect immunofluorescence assay

    4-fold antibody rise or fall in acute and convalescent phase serum titre

    Single titre of ≥ 64 with compatible history

    Most common method of making diagnosis

Polymerase chain reaction assay of blood, CSF or tissues

    Still experimental with unknown sensitivity

Morulae seen in leucocytes on blood or buffy coat smear, bone marrow aspirate, or tissue sections

    Only in acute febrile stage of illness and hard to find

Isolation of *E. chaffeensis* of HGE agent from blood, CSF, or tissues

    Difficult, lengthy, and often negative

---

has travelled through an area where the diseases are endemic; has leucopenia, thrombocytopenia, or elevated liver transaminase levels, or: develops clinical signs of meningitis or encephalitis. As many as one third of patients lack leucopenia or thrombocytopenia at clinical presentation, and a normal or elevated leucocyte or platelet count should not rule out the diagnosis. Treatment decisions should be based on a presumptive diagnosis developed from epidemiological and clinical clues, including those described above, and never delayed for results of confirmatory laboratory tests.

The differential diagnosis of ehrlichial infections includes several illnesses associated with tick bites: Lyme disease (*B. burgdorferi*), Rocky Mountain spotted fever (*R. rickettsii*), tularemia (*Francisella tularensis*), Colorado tick fever (*Coltivirus sp.*), and babesiosis (*Babesia sp.*) (Spach *et al.*, 1993; White *et al.*, 1998). Other diseases to consider include leptospirosis (*Leptospira sp.*), murine typhus (*R. typhi*), epidemic typhus (*R. prowazekii*), Q fever (*Coxiella burnetti*), typhoid fever (*Salmonella typhi*), infectious mononucleosis (*Epstein-Barr virus*), infectious endocarditis, meningococcal meningitis (*Neisseria meningitidis*), and various viral hepatitides.

The diagnosis can be established by several methods (Table 16.5). In order of their routine application, these are: serological tests to measure specific antibody titres, detection of morulae in peripheral blood or CSF leukocytes, detection of ehrlichial DNA by PCR of blood or CSF, direct detection of ehrlichiae in tissue samples by immunohistochemistry, or by isolation of the bacteria.

The majority of patients with HME or HGE are diagnosed by serological tests, and the most widely available antibody test is the indirect immunofluor-escence assay (IFA) (Fishbein *et al.*, 1994; Nicholson *et al.*, 1997). The IFA can detect immunoglobulin G (IgG) or IgM antibodies in the patient's serum or plasma that are reactive with *E. chaffeensis* or with the agent of HGE (Nicholson *et al.*, 1997). Prior to the isolation of the human ehrlichial pathogens, the veterinary pathogens *E. canis* and *E. equi* were used as surrogate antigens for screening human serum samples.

Serum samples from humans infected with one of the human ehrlichial pathogens do not usually cross-react with rickettsial antigens; however, varying degrees of cross-reactivity among antigens derived from the different *Ehrlichia* species have been noted (Dumler *et al.*, 1995, Comer *et al.*, 1999b). Because this cross-reactivity among ehrlichial species is seen in 10–30% of patient serum, samples should be tested against both antigens when possible. When antibodies are detected against both agents, differences in endpoint titre may be useful for ascribing the exact cause (Comer *et al.*, 1999a) . A probable diagnosis of ehrlichiosis can be made in a person with a compatible illness and a single titre of ≥64 (or higher in some laboratories). A confirmed diagnosis of ehrlichiosis can be made in a person with compatible illness with a fourfold change in antibody titre in acute- and convalescent-phase samples (Fishbein *et al.*, 1994; Comer *et al.*, 1999b). Results of the IgG IFA test are frequently negative in the first week of illness, when most patients initially present for care, and a negative serological result for the acute-phase sample does not exclude the diagnosis (Childs *et al.*, 1999; Horowitz *et al.*, 1998b). Documenting seroconversion to ehrlichial species is the most widely recognized method to confirm the diagnosis; however, this method requires collection of a second serum sample 3–6 weeks after the acute illness. If HGE is suspected or diagnosed, additional serological tests for *B. burgdorferi* (Lyme disease) and *Babesia* species (human babesiosis) should be considered, as patients may be coinfected with these agents (Ahkee and Ramirez, 1996; Nadelman *et al.*, 1997).

Identification of intraleucocytic morulae in blood smears, CSF sediment, or bone marrow aspirates has the advantages of being specific, rapid, and simple to perform. However, morulae are seldom identified in blood samples from patients with HME, so diagnostic sensitivity can be low (Standaert *et al.*, in press; Childs *et al.*, 1999). Morulae are more frequently seen in samples from patients with HGE, although successful visualization of infected cells depends largely on the experience and perseverance of the microscopist (Bakken *et al.*, 1996; Horowitz *et al.*, 1998b). In one series of patients with HGE, the percentage of granulocytes with detectable morulae was generally less than 1%, but could be as high as 41% (Bakken *et al.*, 1994). The peripheral blood smear should be stained with an eosin-azure type stain (Wright's, Diff-Quik, Giemsa, or the like). *Ehrlichia*-infected patients may have depressed leucocyte blood counts that make examination of the smear more difficult; experienced technicians are invaluable to properly identify the morulae.

PCR assays to identify DNA from *Ehrlichia* species in blood, CSF, and serum are used with increasing frequency. Numerous publications report on the results obtained using PCR primers specific for both *E. chaffeensis* and the HGE agent on human samples (Everett *et al.*, 1994; Aguero-Rosenfeld *et al.*, 1996; Comer *et al.*, 1999a). Comparisons of results obtained from culture-confirmed patients are encouraging, and identification of ehrlichial DNA by PCR targeting a number of genes suggests this will be a sensitive method for diagnosing both HME and HGE infections (Horowitz *et al.*, 1998b; Childs *et al.*, 1999; Standaert *et al.*, in press). Although PCR testing appears to be a sensitive method for detecting ehrlichiosis, in at least one patient PCR testing of

CSF was negative while culturing yielded an *E. chaffeensis* isolate from CSF after 50 days (Standaert *et al.*, in press). Although PCR has served a useful purpose in diagnosing HGE in several clinical series (Bakken *et al.*, 1994; Everett *et al.*, 1994), it should be noted that PCR tests are not standardized, and the analytic and diagnostic sensitivities and specificities of these assays still require assessment. The isolation of Ehrlichia species from blood, CSF, or other tissues requires a research laboratory, and primary isolation can take up to 7 weeks (Dawson *et al.*, 1991; Paddock *et al.*, 1997; Horowitz *et al.*, 1998b; Standaert *et al.*, in press). The sensitivity of isolation as compared to other laboratory procedures has been investigated in only a few circumstances, as culturing of these organisms is seldom undertaken (Horowitz *et al.*, 1998b; Childs *et al.*, 1999; Standaert *et al.*, in press).

Management

As with other rickettsial diseases, treatment decisions for the patient with a presumptive diagnosis of HME or HGE, should be based on clinical and epidemiological findings. Confirmatory tests, particularly serology, are primarily retrospective and should not be used to influence decisions regarding initiation of appropriate antibiotic therapy. Doxycycline (100 mg twice daily by mouth for 7–14 days) is the drug of choice for adults and for children infected with *Ehrlichia* spp. Tetracycline (25 mg/kg/day) may also be used in adult patients with ehrlichial infection. Rifampin has successfully been used in a limited number of patients for whom tetracyclines are contraindicated (e.g., pregnant women) (Buitrago *et al.*, 1998). *In vitro* antibiotic studies have found that doxycycline and rifampin are bactericidal against *E. chaffeensis*. Penicillin, ceftriaxone, chloramphenicol, ciprofloxacin, erythromycin, co-trimoxazole, and gentamicin were ineffective (Brouqui and Raoult, 1992). Similar *in vitro* antibiotic sensitivities have been reported for the agent of HGE (Klein *et al.*, 1997).

With appropriate therapy, patients characteristically defervesce within 24–48 hours. In fact, failure to respond to a tetracycline antibiotic within the first 3 days should suggest infection with an agent other than ehrlichiae. Patients with severe illness may require longer courses of treatment. Other symptoms subside over the next 2 weeks, although headaches, generalized weakness, and malaise may persist for several weeks after recovery from the acute febrile illness. Leucopenia and cytopenia typically correct 2–3 weeks after the onset of disease, although anaemia may appear during this time (Fishbein *et al.*, 1994). Patients with ehrlichial meningitis usually improve on treatment over 1–3 weeks. The CSF of these patients may continue to show a pleocytosis for at least a week after the acute illness. In patients with encephalopathy caused by ehrlichial infection, recovery is usually complete but it may take several months (Everett et al., 1994). Neurological sequelae have been reported in some paediatric patients with severe HME (Schutze and Jacobs, 1997).

Patients with severe ehrlichial infections may develop a variety of secondary infections, including disseminated candidiasis, invasive pulmonary aspergillosis, *Cryptococcus neoformans* pneumonia, and herpes simplex virus and cytomegalovirus infections (Fritz and Glaser, 1998). These opportunistic infections may result from alterations in neutrophil and CD4 lymphocyte function (Dumler and Bakken, 1998).

It is unknown whether prior infection confers immunity in patients, although reinfection of the same patient with the agent of HGE has been reported (Horowitz *et al.*, 1998a).

Prognosis

For most patients, the prognosis is excellent. In healthy patients with relatively uncomplicated disease, a full recovery is expected even if neurological signs developed during the course of the illness (Ratnasamy *et al.*, 1996). However, particularly severe infections and poor outcomes have been recorded in patients with pre-existing immune dysfunction, including HIV infection, malignancy or iatrogenic immunosuppression (Paddock *et al.*, 1993; Marty *et al.*, 1995, Bakken *et al.*, 1994; Dumler and Bakken, 1998).

If complications develop, such as myocarditis, acute respiratory disease, or shock, the prognosis is worse. An estimated 2–5% of patients die from complications of ehrlichial disease (Eng *et al.*, 1990; Bakken *et al.*, 1994; McQuiston *et al.*, 1999).

Prevention

The key to preventing ehrlichiosis is to avoid being bitten by an infected tick. In persons exposed to tick-infested habitats, prompt careful inspection for and removal of crawling or attached ticks remain important methods to prevent disease. Rapid discovery and removal of a newly attached tick lessens the risk of infection, as ticks appear to require 24–48 h of attachment to a host before ehrlichiae can be transmitted (Katavolos *et al.*, 1998; Hodzic *et al.*, 1998b). Prophylactic administration of doxycycline after a tick bite is not indicated since the overall risk of infection is low. No vaccine for ehrlichial infection is currently available for humans.

Acknowledgements

Supported in part by the Research Service, Department of Veterans Affairs.

References

Aguero-Rosenfeld, M. E., Horowitz, H. W., Wormser, G. P. *et al.* (1996). Human granulocytic ehrlichiosis: a case series from a medical center in New York state. *Ann. Intern. Med.*, **125**, 904–908.

Ahkee, S. and Ramirez, J. (1996). A case of concurrent Lyme meningitis with ehrlichiosis. *Scand. J. Infect. Dis.*, **28**, 527–528.

Anderson, B. E., Sims, K. G., Olson, J. G. *et al.* (1993). *Amblyomma americanum*: a potential vector of human ehrlichiosis. *Am. J. Trop. Med.*, **49**, 239–244.

Arguin, P. M., Singleton, J., JR., Rotz, L. D. *et al.* (1999). An investigation of possible transmission of tick-borne pathogens via blood transfusion. *Transfusion*, **39**, 828–833.

Bakken, J. S., Dumler, S., Chen, S-M. *et al.* (1994). Human granulocytic ehrlichiosis in the upper Midwest United States. A new species emerging? *J. Am. Med. Assoc.*, **272**, 212–218.

Bakken, J. S., Erlemeyer, S. A., Kanoff, R. J. *et al.* (1998). Demyelinating polyneuropathy associated with human granulocytic ehrlichiosis. *Clin. Infect. Dis.*, **27**, 1323–1324.

Bakken, J. S., Krueth, J., Wilson-Nordskog, C. *et al.* (1996). Clinical and laboratory characteristics of human granulocytic ehrlichiosis. *J. Am. Med. Assoc.*, **275**, 199–205.

Barton, L. L., Rathore, M. H. and Dawson, J. E. (1992). Infection with *Ehrlichia* in childhood. *J. Pediatr.*, **120**, 998–1001.

Brouqui, P. and Raoult, D. (1992). In vitro antibiotic susceptibility of the newly recognized agent of ehrlichiosis in humans, *Ehrlichia chaffeensis*. *Antimicrob. Agents Chemother.*, **36**, 2799–2803.

Buitrago, M. I., Ijdo, J. W., Rinaudo, P. *et al.* (1998). Human granulocytic ehrlichiosis during pregnancy treated successfully with rifampin. *Clin. Infect. Dis.*, **27**, 213–215.

Burket, C.T., Vann, C. N., Pinger, R. R., Chatot, C. L. and Steiner, F. E. (1998). Minimum infection rate of *Amblyomma americanum* (Acari:Ixodidae) by *Ehrlichia chaffeensis* (Rickettsiales; Ehrlichieae) in southern Indiana. *J. Med. Entomol.*, **35**, 653–659.

Carter, N. and Miller, N. R. (1997). Fourth nerve palsy caused by *Ehrlichia chaffeensis*. *J. Neuroophthalmol.*, **17**, 47–50.

Childs, J. E., Sumner, J. W., Nicholson, W. L., Massung, R. F., Standaert, S. M. and Paddock, C. D. (1999). Outcome of diagnostic tests using samples from culture-proven cases of human monocytic ehrlichiosis: implications for surveillance. *J. Clin. Microbiol.*, **37**, 2997–3000.

Christova, I. S. and Dumler, J.S. (1999). Human granulocytic ehrlichiosis in Bulgaria. *Am. J. Trop. Med. Hyg.*, **60**, 58–61.

Comer, J. A., Nicholson, W. L., Sumner, J. W. *et al.* (1999a). Diagnosis of human ehrlichiosis by PCR assay of acute-phase serum. *J. Clin. Microbiol.*, **37**, 31–34.

Comer, J. A., Nicholson, W. L., Olson, J. G. and Childs, J. E. (1999b). Serologic testing for human granulocytic ehrlichiosis at a national referral center. *J. Clin. Microbiol.*, **37**, 558–564.

Dawson, J. E., Anderson, B. E., Fishbein, D. B. *et al.* (1991). Isolation and characterization of an *Ehrlichia* sp. from a patient diagnosed with human ehrlichiosis. *J. Clin. Microbiol.*, **29**, 2741–2745.

Dawson, J. E., Stallknecht, D. E., Howerth, E. W. *et al.* (1994). Susceptibility of white-tailed deer (*Odocoileus virginianus*) to infection with *Ehrlichia chaffeensis*, the etiologic agent of human ehrlichiosis. *J. Clin. Microbiol.*, **32**, 2725–2728.

Donatien, A. and Lestoquard, F. (1937). Etat actuel des connaissances sur les rickettioses animales. *Arch. Inst. Pasteur Alger.*, **XV**, 142–187.

Dumler, J. S., Asanovich, K. M., Bakken, J. S. *et al.* (1995). Serologic cross-reactions among *Ehrlichia equi*, *Ehrlichia pagocytophilia*, and human granulocytic *Ehrlichia*. *J. Clin. Microbiol.*, **33**, 1098–1103.

Dumler, J. S. and Bakken J. S. (1998). Human ehrlichioses: Newly recognized infections transmitted by ticks. *Ann. Rev. Med.*, **49**, 201–213.

Dumler J. S., Broqui, P., Aronson, J., Taylor, J. P. and Walker, D. H. (1991). Identification of *Ehrlichia* in human tissue. *N. Engl. J. Med.*, **325**, 1109–1110.

Dumler, J. S., Dawson, J. E. and Walker, D. H. (1993). Human ehrlichiosis: hematopathology and immunohistologic detection of *Ehrlichia chaffeensis*. *Hum. Pathol.*, **24**, 391–396.

Dunn, B. E., Monson, T. P., Dumler, J. S. *et al.* (1992). Identification of *Ehrlichia chaffeensis* morulae in cerebrospinal fluid mononuclear cells. *J. Clin. Microbiol.*, **30**, 2207–2210.

Eng, T. R., Harkess, J. R., Fishbein, D. B. *et al.* (1990). Epidemiologic, clinical, and laboratory findings of human ehrlichiosis in the United States, 1988. *J. Am. Med. Assoc.*, **264**, 2251–2258.

Everett, E. D., Evans, K. A., Henry, B. and McDonald, G. (1994). Human ehrlichiosis in adults after tick exposure. Diagnosis using polymerase chain reaction. *Ann. Intern. Med.*, **120**, 730–735.

Fichtenbaum, C. J., Peterson, L. R. and Weil, G. J. (1993). Ehrlichiosis presenting as a life-threatening illness with features of the toxic shock syndrome. *Am. J. Med.*, **95**, 351–357.

Fishbein, D. B., Dawson, J. E. and Robinson, L. E. (1994). Human ehrlichiosis in the United States, 1985-1990. *Ann. Intern. Med.*, **120**, 736–743.

Fritz, C. L. and Glaser, C.A. (1998). Ehrlichiosis. *Infect. Dis. Clin. North Am.*, **12**, 123–136.

Golden, S. E. (1989). Aseptic meningitis associated with *Ehrlichia canis* infection. *Pediatr. Infect. Dis. J.*, **8**, 335–337.

Goodman, J. L., Nelson, C. M., Klein, M. B., Hayes, S. F. and Weston, B. W. (1999) Leukocyte infection by the granulocytic ehrlichiosis agent is linked to expression of a selectin ligand. *J. Clin. Invest.*, **103**, 407–412.

Grant, A. C., Hunter, S. and Partin, W. C. (1997). A case of acute monocytic ehrlichiosis with prominent neurologic signs. *Neurology*, **48**, 1619–1623.

Hammill, W. W., Wilson, M. B., Reigart, J. R. *et al.* (1992). *Ehrlichia canis* infection in a child in South Carolina. *Clin. Pediatr.*, **31**, 432–434.

Harkess, J. R., Stucky, D. and Ewing S. A. (1990). Neurologic abnormalities in a patient with human ehrlichiosis. *South. Med. J.*, **83**, 1341–1343.

Hodzic, E., Ijdo, W. I., Feng, S. *et al.* (1998a). Granulocytic ehrlichiosis in the laboratory mouse. *J. Infect. Dis.*, **177**, 737–745.

Hodzic, E., Fish, D., Maretzki C. M., De Silva, A., Feng, S. and Barthold, S. W. (1998b). Acquisition and transmission of the agent of human granulocytic ehrlichiosis by *Ixodes scapularis* ticks. *J. Clin. Microbiol.*, **36**, 3574–3578.

Horowitz, H. W., Aguero-Rosenfeld, M, Dumler, J. S. *et al.* (1998a). Reinfection with the agent of human granulocytic ehrlichiosis. *Ann. Intern. Med.*, **129**, 461–463.

Horowitz, H. W., Aguero-Rosenfeld, M. E., McKenna, D. F. *et al.*, (1998b). Clinical and laboratory spectrum of culture-proven human granulocytic ehrlichiosis: comparison with culture-negative cases. *Clin. Infect. Dis.*, **27**, 1314–1317.

Horowitz, H. W., Kilchevsky, E., Haber, S. *et al.* (1998c). Perinatal transmission of the agent of human granulocytic ehrlichiosis. *N. Engl. J. Med.*, **339**, 375–378.

Horowitz, H. W., Marks, S. J., Weintraub, M. and Dumler, J. S. (1996). Brachial plexopathy associated with human granulocytic ehrlichiosis. *Neurology*, **46**, 1026–1029.

Jahangir, A., Kolbert, C., Edwards, W. *et al.* (1998). Fatal pancarditis associated with human granulocytic ehrlichiosis in a 44-year old man. *Clin. Infect. Dis.*, **27**, 1424–1427.

Katavolos, P., Armstrong, P. M., Dawson, J. E. and Telford III, S. R. (1998). Duration of tick attachment required for transmission of granulocytic ehrlichiosis. *J. Infect. Dis.*, **177**, 1422–1425.

Klein, M. B., Nelson, C. M. and Goodman, J. L. (1997). Antibiotic susceptibility of the newly cultivated agent of human granulocytic ehrlichiosis: promising activity of quinolones and rifamycins. *Antibicrob. Agents Chemother.*, **41**, 76–79.

Lockhart, J. M., Davidson, W. R., Stallknecht, D. E., Dawson, J. E. and Howerth, E. W. (1997). Isolation of *Ehrlichia chaffeensis* from wild white-tailed deer (*Odocoileus virginianus*) confirms their role as natural reservoir hosts. *J. Clin. Microbiol.*, **35**, 1681–1686.

Lotric-Furlan, S., Petrovec, M., Zupanc, T. A. *et al.* (1998). Human granulocytic ehrlichiosis in Europe: clinical and laboratory findings for four patients from Slovenia. *Clin. Infect. Dis.*, **27**, 424–428.

Maeda, K., Markowitz, N., Hawley, R. C. *et al.* (1987) Human infection with *Ehrlichia canis*, a leukocytic *Rickettsia*. *N. Engl. J. Med.*, **316**, 853–856.

Marty, A. M., Dumler, J. S., Imes, G., Brusman, H. P., Smrkovski, L. L. and Frisman, D. M. (1995). Ehrlichiosis mimicking thrombotic thrombocytopenic purpura. Case report and pathological correlation. *Hum. Pathol.*, **26**, 920–925.

McQuiston, J. H., Paddock, C. D., Holman, R. C. and Childs, J. E. (1999). Human ehrlichioses in the United States. *Emerg. Infect. Dis.*, **5**, 635–642.

Mitchell, P. D., Reed, K. D. and Hofkes, J. M. (1996). Immunoserologic evidence of coinfection with *Borrelia burgdorferi*, *Babesia microti*, and human granulocytic *Ehrlichia* species in residents of Wisconsin and Minnesota. *J. Clin. Microbiol.*, **34**, 724–727.

Nadelman, R. B., Horowitz, H. W., Hsieh, T-C. *et al.* (1997). Simultaneous human granulocytic ehrlichiosis and Lyme borreliosis. *N. Engl. J. Med.*, **337**, 27–30.

Nicholson, W. L., Comer, J. A., Sumner, J. W. *et al.*, (1997). An indirect immuno-fluorescence assay using a cell culture-derived antigen for detection of antibodies to the agent of human granulocytic ehrlichiosis. *J. Clin. Microbiol.*, **35**, 1510–1516.

Paddock, C. D., Suchard, D. P., Grumbach, K. L. *et al.* (1993). Brief report: fatal seronegative ehrlichiosis in a patient with HIV infection. *N. Engl. J. Med.*, **329**, 1164–1167.

Paddock, C. D., Sumner, J. W., Shore, G. M. *et al.*, (1997). Isolation and characteriza-tion of *Ehrlichia chaffeensis* strains from patients with fatal ehrlichiosis. *J. Clin. Microbiol.*, **35**, 2496–2502.

Pancholi P., Kolbert C. P., Mitchell P. D. *et al.* (1995). Ixodes damini as a potential vector of human granulocytic ehrlichiosis. *J. Infect. Dis.*, **172**, 1007–1012.

Peterson, L. R., Sawyer, L. A., Fishbein, D. B. *et al.* (1989). An outbreak of ehrlichiosis in members of an army reserve unit exposed to ticks. *J. Infect. Dis.*, **159**, 562–568.

Petrovec, M., Sumner, J. W., Nicholson, W. L. *et al.* (1999). Identity of ehrlichial DNA sequences derived from *Ixodes ricinus* ticks with those obtained from patients with human granulocytic ehrlichiosis in Slovenia. *J. Clin. Microbiol.*, **37**, 209–210.

Popov, V. L., Han, V. C., Chen, S. M. *et al.* (1998). Ultrastructural differentiation of the genogroups in the genus *Ehrlichia*. *J. Med. Microbiol.*, **47**, 235–251.

Ratnasamy, N., Everett, E. D., Roland, W. E. *et al.* (1996). Central nervous system manifestations of human ehrlichiosis. *Clin. Infect. Dis.*, **23**, 314–319.

Richter, P. J., Kimsey, R. B., Madigan, J. E. *et al.* (1996) *Ixodes pacificus* (Acari:Ix-odidae as a vector of *Ehrlichia equi* (Rickettsiales: Ehrlichieae). *J. Med. Entomol.*, **33**, 1–5.

Rikihisa Y. (1991). The Tribe *Ehrlichieae* and ehrlichial diseases. *Clin. Microbiol. Rev.*, **4**, 286–308.

Ripoll, C. M., Remondegui, C. E., Ordonez, G. *et al.* (1999). Evidence of rickettsial spotted fever and ehrlichial infections in a subtropical territory of Jujuy, Argentina. *Am. J. Trop. Med. Hyg.*, **61**, 350–354.

Schutze, G. E. and Jacobs, R. F. (1997). Human monocytic ehrlichiosis in children. *Pediatrics*, **100**, E10.

Schwartz, I., Fish, D. and Daniels, T. J. (1997). Prevalence of the rickettsial agent of human granulocytic ehrlichiosis in ticks from a hyperendemic focus of Lyme disease. *N. Engl. J. Med.*, **337**, 49–50.

Sexton, D. J., Corey, G. R., Carpenter C. *et al.* (1998). Dual infection with Ehrlichia chaffeensis and a spotted fever group rickettesia: a case report. *Emerg. Infect. Dis.*, **4**, 311–316.

Shea, K. W., Calio, A. J., Klein, N. C. and Cunha, B. A. (1995). Rhabdomyolysis associated with *Ehrlichia chaffeensis* infection. *Clin. Infect. Dis.*, **21**, 1056–1057.

Spach, D. H., Liles, W. C., Campbell, G. L. *et al.* (1993). Tick-borne diseases in the United States. *N. Engl. J. Med.*, **329**, 936–947.

Standaert, S. M., Clough, L. A., Schaffner, W. *et al.* (1998). Neurologic manifestations of human monocytic ehrlichiosis. *Infect. Dis. Clin. Pract.*, **7**, 358–362.

Standaert, S. M., Dawson, J. E., Schaffner, W. *et al.* (1995). Ehrlichiosis in a golf-oriented retirement community. *N. Engl. J. Med.*, **333**, 420–425.

Standaert, S. M., Yu, W., Scott, M. A. *et al.* (in press). Primary isolation and molecular characterization of *Ehrlichia chaffeensis* from seven patients with human monocytic ehrlichiosis. *J. Infect. Dis.*

Telford, S. R., Dawson, J. E., Katavolos, P. *et al.* (1996). Persisting DH. Perpetuation of the agent of human granulocytic ehrlichiosis in a deer tick-rodent cycle. *Proc. Natl Acad. Sci. USA*, **93**, 6209–6214.

Trotta, R. F., Hospenthal, D. R., Bennett, S. P. *et al.* (1997). Human monocytic ehrlichiosis with concurrent Lyme antibody seroconversion. *Infect. Dis. Clin. Pract.*, **6**, 401–405.

Uhaa, I. J., Maclean, J. D., Greene, C. R. and Fishbein, D. B., (1992). A case of human ehrlichiosis acquired in Mali: clinical and laboratory findings. *Am. J. Trop. Med. Hyg.*, **46**, 161–164.

Walker, D. H. and Dumler, J. S. (1997). Human monocytic and granulocytic ehrlichioses. Discovery and diagnosis of emerging tick-borne infections and the critical role of the pathologist. *Arch. Pathol. Lab. Med.*, **121**, 785–791.

Webster, P., Ijdo, J. W., Chicoine, L. M. and Fikrig, E. (1998). The agent of human granulocytic ehrlichiosis resides in an endosomal compartment. *J. Clin. Invest.*, **101**, 1932–1941.

White, D. J., Talarico, J., Chang, H. G. *et al.* (1998). Human babesiosis in New York state: review of 139 hospitalized cases and analysis of prognostic factors. *Arch. Intern. Med.*, **158**, 2149–2154.

Winslow, G. M., Yager, E., Shilo, K., Collins, D. N. and Chu, F. K. (1998). Infection in the laboratory mouse with the intracellular pathogen *Ehrlichia chaffeensis*. *Infect. Immun.*, **66**, 3892–3899.

Yevich, S. J., Sanchez, J. L., Defraites, R. F. *et al.* (1995). Seroepidemiology of infections due to spotted fever group rickettsiae and *Ehrlichia* sp. in military personnel exposed in areas of United States where such infections are endemic. *J. Infect. Dis.*, **171**, 1266–1273.

Index